HANDBOOK OF ADOLESCENCE

HANDBOOK OF ADOLESCENCE

Psychopathology
• Antisocial Development •
Psychotherapy

Carl P. Malmquist, M.D.

NEW YORK • JASON ARONSON • LONDON

To all who have shared their
ideas with me and have patiently awaited
the fruition of this work

Contents

HANDBOOK OF ADOLESCENCE

Chapter One

Adolescent Psychological Development

ADOLESCENT DEVELOPMENT: FAMILY INFLUENCES

What factor exerts the most significant influence on adolescent development? Is it primarily intrinsic psychological processes in the individual? Is it intrafamilial processes? Is it the broader social environment? Or do the genes and physical development remain paramount? While the days of rigid adherence to one or another of these positions are over, an implicit commitment to one of them as the most influential is still utilized by those in routine contact with adolescents.

Three main parent-child influences operate on adolescent socialization:

1. Quantitative interactions in terms of the frequency of contact and its correlative intensity.

2. Qualitative factors such as the manner in which people relate within a given family. (A given family operates in terms of all the overt and covert feelings and values with which clinicians deal.)

3. Opportunities to test and reevaluate the social techniques within a family and the outside world. (Powerful relationships, developed earlier in the context of dependency and attachment, have been massively reinforced by early initiation, duration, and the quality of exclusivity present in families. When preadolescent experiences occurred in the context of mutual respect, a modeling experience based on admiration of adults is most likely.[1] In turn,

personal expertise, a power position in the family, and community status also enhance the development of respect.[2])

Parental Consistency. One of the most cited factors in the literature, parental consistency is something all parents should practice in their child-rearing. In a cognitive sense, consistency acquires significance from the stability it provides in assimilating the chaotic stimuli of the world. In addition, it provides a stabilizing ego component in terms of organizing the outer environment with the inner world of strivings, controls, and impulses. All learning processes require a certain baseline of consistency if learning is to take place. Lack of consistency leads to a set of experiences which may appear arbitrary, capricious, and subject to the whims of the moment. Much remains to be determined from longitudinal and naturalistic studies of families with respect to the impact of degrees of parental inconsistency. Such variations as both parents being consistent in their inconsistency, sporadic inconsistencies, parental splits with one parent relatively more consistent than the other, all contribute to undesirable variations. Sex of the child cross-examined with the sex of the parent is also important, as are the various "nuisance variables" related to social class.

Once they enter the realm of the clinical, studies and reports continue to elaborate the adverse impact of inconsistencies in one parent or both. The inconsistencies may be based on retrospective evaluation of data or clinical elucidation of ongoing behaviors. Assignments of some type of causal weightings to the antecedent parental behavior are made, but debate reigns as to whether the main emphasis should be on inconsistency in enunciation of rules, or whether emphasis should be placed on lack of enforcement of expectations and norms. Several studies point to associations of parental inconsistency with delinquency.[3] Others point to the impact on behavior disturbances in the emotional realm.[4] Other studies have compared adolescent boys exhibiting antisocial trends to a control group, matched otherwise for age and paternal occupation, and found the former group wanting.[5] Significantly more parental inconsistency was present in the parents of aggressive boys. Another group of 450 juveniles were seen in a clinic setting where they presented with primary complaints of disobedience, hostility, temper outbursts, restlessness, excitability, bullying, aggressiveness, and domineering behavior.[6] Conflict between parents and child-rearing was prominent. Such conflict is in agreement with follow-up studies of boys like the Cambridge-

Somerville Youth Study, in which erratic discipline was significantly related to criminality under certain conditions.[7] In this study there was a strong association with antisocial development when parental inconsistency was coupled with low affection in the family matrix. The explanations offered involved types of settings in which there was an absence of rewards for conformity. If certain behaviors are inconsistently valued or enforced, doubt may be raised as to their value, raising the probability of the adolescent's taking his chances with them. A poorly integrated family, in which there is a quality of unpredictable over-reactivity, is frequently seen with impulsive adolescents.[8] A variety of stresses may disrupt the brittle family stability. In such cases as the onset of puberty itself, the adolescent may be selected, due to his provocative proclivities, to serve as the family scapegoat.[9]

Disciplinary Techniques. A second major factor operating within families and socialization processes, disciplinary techniques, will be more thoroughly discussed in chapter 7, but is noted here as one of the major influences on child development. Isolation of one such variable fails to convey adequately the picture of the processes involved. This leads to models utilizing a host of dichotomous variables such as love, hostility, autonomy-restrictiveness, with intermediate subdivisions. In this context, the complexity of the variables becomes obvious when one considers sex differences, changes that can occur over the course of development in parent, child, and family, the various physical disciplines that may be used, degrees of parental affection, the addition or omission of cognitive justifications, and responses to aggression in the child.

Cognitive Explanations. The degree of cognitive explanations is another factor operating in socialization. To what degree (if any) do parents attempt to justify how they direct their own lives and that of the family by making explicit their rationale? Relevant questions here are the extent to which explanations are made, as well as the overlap with consistency factors. Levels exist as to the analysis of this factor as well. One simple approach is to take a group of adolescents and attempt certain cross-correlations, seeking significance. For example, failure of parents to set a time at which the adolescent is expected to be home at night might be found to correlate significantly with a wide variety of certain types of sexual experiences.[10] Or, the lack of a curfew might be found to correlate with a general factor of parental indifference to the activities of their adolescent offspring.

The matter of parental awareness of the current norms of adolescent behavior may induce different parental attempts at justification. This can vary from the parent who accommodates to the adolescent culture to one who holds to his own ideas on behavior—for adolescents and adults—but who continues to justify his position. Given the same hypothetical adolescent in each situation, we would be more likely to predict different responses. Consideration would have to be given to the adolescent's level of intellectual functioning as well (not primarily in terms of his intelligence quotient, although that would not be irrelevant, but in terms of his ability and desire to assimilate cognitive justifications). Motivational components have not been mentioned so far, but presumably parents with a greater need to give rational explanations for their decisions differ from those who do not, at least in this one important dimension. Whether this is due to differences in parental cognitive structures on some genetic or reinforced basis, or a part of a compulsive personality organization of the parent, need not concern us in this context. It is more significant to determine what type of parent personality is more likely to justify. In turn, variables in the personality of the child can lead to accommodation or protest. The point at which explanations are given is also important; explanations given ex post facto are qualitatively different from those made before the fact.[11]

Autonomy.   Degrees of autonomy are a fourth factor operating in the socialization of youths within families. What are the factors operating for a given adolescent to participate with a minimal degree of anxiety outside his home? While in some ways this reflects parental security to permit independence, in other cases it may reflect a push from within the adolescent to secure his autonomy from earlier anxieties. In this context, autonomy serves both defensive and developmental goals. Development of autonomous inner controls requires an exposure to diverse social experiences in a peer group. In a way, the peer group setting provides the adolescent with an opportunity to test his own internalized views of the world versus alternatives. Overprotection makes this exposure threatening and stymies self-reliance.

Internalization processes in girls appear to be slower than in boys, explainable as retarded autonomy for girls. Adolescent boys, who are more dependent on family controls, are seen as more socially incompetent and deficient in certain ego functions.[12] Maternal over-restrictiveness with boys is more prevalent in delinquent populations than in controls, and is correlated with hostility, feelings of isolation, and resentment.[13]

ADOLESCENCE AS A DEVELOPMENTAL PHENOMENON

It is not as controversial as it once was to maintain that adolescents, like others, are subject to great variation in their daily functioning. Adolescents have had time to develop various neurotic conflicts and certain definitive characterological traits. Perhaps the former may bother the adolescent less than someone who is slightly younger, or much older, possibly because there is hope that the neurotic suffering is more temporary. The adolescent also has more devices available to "act out" his conflicts. Hope of environmental solutions for individualized neurotic conflict may coalesce with a great upsurge to change many deleterious things in the adolescent's world. By the post-adolescent period, ensuing despair may be related to disillusionment. However, for a majority of adolescents, neurotic conflicts exist alongside the more intact personality functions. Only under particular types of stress or crises, when feelings of oppression are induced, are intrapsychic disequilibriums produced. At that time regressive signs and symptoms may become more overt.

For the less prominent crises and disequilibriums there is a constant shift back and forth between neurotic, or even psychotic, levels of ego functioning and less conflicted states. Such a formulation in terms of equilibriums introduces the notion of dynamics in terms of a balance between contending forces. These are not the forces of physics, but rather a manner of explanation relying on this type of hypothesis. In terms of a structural model of personality—id, ego, and superego—a disequilibrium may occur if any or all of these structures as well as, or in addition to, conflicts with the external world. While an adolescent may be handling his drives in a gratifying manner, he may not be appraising the external world in a realistic manner. Drive gratification may be occurring in a setting of adapting to the world in a self-punitive manner. Or, while ideals may be met, drives may be left in a state of suspended animation. Accompanying these possibilities may be an objectively threatening situation of conflict in the world. Changes may occur in the drive level, particularly in adolescence. This may be seen in the ego and in the demands adolescents begin to make on themselves in terms of their own ideals and aims as well as of institutional norms.

Shifts in the dynamic balance do not occur only from upsets in the external or internal circumstances of an individual. During adolescence shifts occur on the basis of changes which are a concomitant part of the developmental processes themselves. These developmental processes may be used to illustrate how disturbances occur, but one must first examine the progression of changes in the following: (1) impulses, (2) ego structure, (3) object relations, and (4) ideals and social relations.

Impulses. Impulses may change with respect to quantity as well as quality. The former is noted in the onset of preadolescencence in which an increase in drive activity is seen. This operates with respect to undifferentiated types of pregenital activities as well as sexual and aggressive components. The preadolescent is seen as someone who is hungrier, greedier, crueler, dirtier, more inquisitive, boastful, narcissistic, and inconsiderate. It is not merely a matter of more than, or less than, but also of different kinds of feelings and urges which cannot be handled with the safety of the latency age. Yet in most cases the adolescent is still involved in the predicament of living in the midst of the same family unit with his intensified feelings. The struggle with his aggressive impulses, which will be played out within the family of origin, can be contrasted with a culture in which the aggression of young people can be channelized outside the family or local community.[14] Enemies who threaten from without, whether realistically or by trumped-up propaganda, give adolescents a greater opportunity to join a common cause against an external threat. This has been observed in present-day Israel as well as in Nazi Germany.

Ego Structure. Changes in the structure of the ego include the entire range of shifts which occur in ego functioning. The adolescent counterbalances shifts in impulsivity and unpredictability by exaggerated and frequent use of defensive efforts to keep himself under better control. This puts the ego in a precarious state because of the increased demands being placed on it from many sources. There may be alternations between indulgences and strenuous efforts to ward off discharge if breakthroughs have taken place.

Object Relations. When early attachments, which are intense and exclusive, are too threatening to be maintained within the same format as earlier, object relations change. The need for autonomy may take the form of abandonment or reinforcement of earlier object ties. How is this witnessed? It is seen in a variety of behaviors—disparagements, indifference, insolence, revolt, and protest—not just directed against people to whom the adolescent was once closely attached, but to the institutions and beliefs which represent them. It is not surprising that adolescents can at one moment be the most virulent of creatures and a moment later feel themselves helpless and in need of support. As a corollary, the closer earlier ties have been, the more stormy the upheaval may be when it comes.

Ideals and Social Relations. To effect the loosening of ties, a restructuring of the strivings and inhibitions of the adolescent is required, since too many earlier aspirations are based on imitations and assimilations of parental models. The search for an eternal ideal in early adolescence may take the form of hero-worship, or the use of some parental substitute, although it appears that the degree of closeness of this type of figure or institutional representation of the parent is beginning to lose favor among many young adolescents. Increasingly, many adolescents tend to adopt the mores of their contemporary peer groups or join causes which stand in stark opposition to parental ideals. A naive belief that peer-group emulation is the result of a reasoned consideration of alternatives is common, but when the boundaries between the value systems, beliefs, and practices of youths and their parents become blurred, difficulties in revising ego-ideals and superego structures de facto become even more difficult and prolonged. What is important is to determine which type of adolescent upheaval and protest is most conducive to resolution of developmental arrests.

DEVELOPMENTAL ALTERATIONS IN
ADOLESCENTS AND THEIR FAMILIES

A perennial question, phrased half in jest among families with adolescents, is, Who will best be able to survive the struggle? It might be better to ask which family members need the most assistance, or even to consider that the family unit itself may need help as a group. This viewpoint does not mean that the adolescent and his family exist in a state of perpetual conflict, for many adolescents may have a relatively smooth transition through the rites of passage without stormy variations. But the adolescent period of development does possess a set of problems and challenges very different from preadolescence. Earlier developmental landmarks and conflicts continue to exert an influence via the epigenetic principle of things reaching an ascendancy at different points and remaining to aid or hinder a personality, but while these earlier phenomena are not to be ignored, something above and beyond this view is required. Even in the strictly biological realm, witness the difference in sexual impulses related to the increased hormonal level ensuing at puberty as compared to preadolescence. Adolescence as nothing but a recapitulation of earlier conflicts is an archaic view wherein the adolescent was seen as seeking attachments primarily for the purpose of reworking oedipal feelings.

Altered Dependency Needs. One of the main developmental tasks an adolescent must learn is different ways of dealing with dependency needs. While part of this involves a need to redirect sensuous attachments away from family members, there is also the parallel need to seek new sexual outlets. To give up the former and attain the latter in a setting outside the home is one of the basic developmental goals. In some ways this is merely another way of raising the question of man's need first to separate his sexual attachments from his family of origin and then redirect them so that sensual and tender components can be fused. Not to achieve this means the possibility of perpetuating sexuality with overtones of degradation by splitting object ties to whom are directed on the one hand the tender feelings and on the other the sensual.[15]

Family interactional patterns also undergo a realignment during adolescence. The peer group and buddy system of the latency-age child provide a temporary stability from the parental vantage point, and permit the child new yet serious attachments outside the home. In the absence of emotional conflict, the security of the child and his affectional needs are not seriously threatened by abandonment, nor are the parents. These shifts in affectional attachments accompany cognitive shifts which gradually permit the adolescent to achieve diverse human relationships.

Unlike thought processes during latency, which are tied to concrete-operational modes, the beginning of formal thought processes permits a greater degree of transcendence. These changes in cognitive abilities give the ego greater capacity for control and direction of impulses, further heightening the imagination feeding the development of the ego-ideal to permit commitment to various ideologies. While many risks are taken in terms of which ideals may appeal to the adolescent at any given moment, the need for emancipation can be attested to by those adolescent casualties who have never risked at all. One of the major revisions required for the adolescent boy is to see himself as independent and assertive toward females rather than as dependent and submissive. For the adolescent girl it is not so much a matter of loosening the attachment to the mother, per se, but revising her concept of where and whom will provide an adequate set of attachments outside the family to meet her needs and expectations as an acceptable female in terms of sex-role identity. For both the boy and the girl it is a matter of convincing themselves that they do not really need their parents to survive, and that their parents will survive without them as well.

Loosening of ties is carried on simultaneously in two realms: within the psychological world of the adolescent personality, and in the objective relationships with other people in external reality. Loosening also occurs in modifying the superego, and in attacking that for which the parents have stood. Although a classical view emphasizes the need to attack due to the awareness that the parents have concealed many intimacies, which the adolescent may view as betrayal to sensuality in place of his newly found idealistic aims, other factors are of equal importance. Objective failings in the parent, which can be more validly appraised in affective and cognitive terms, contribute to this process.

Again, rather than viewing adolescent anger toward parents as just a displacement from a resentment of parental intimacies, it is too simplistic to say that frustrating parental qualities exist which can no longer be denied. This is typically seen in the boy who condemns his father's passivity toward females and begins to detect it in other activities and innumerable facets of his father's daily life. The chronically disillusioned father is all too prone to give rise to a disillusioned son. The girl is then more likely to react not only to her sexual enlightenment about what her parents' private life may have been like, but to see that much of the mystification concerning what her adult mother did may have been a response to the conflicts and disappointments in the mother herself; that the hypochondriasis, moodiness, somatization, and anger of her mother has really been an obscuring device. The result is confusion—the substitution of false issues for what actually transpired during earlier years.

Family Conflicts Revealed. The mystification process during adolescence results in an unmasking, so that previous conflicts within a family no longer remain clouded.[16] In more severe types of adolescent and family psychopathology there is an added component of personal fault, for to detect mystification is to alert the adolescent to conflict which has been concealed. The process is subtle, for many things occur and are experienced in the course of development which remain cloaked. Most common are acknowledging factual occurrences, but not denying their meaning. A mother says to her adolescent daughter, "Whatever makes you think we didn't want you? We had you, didn't we?" Or, more subtly, the adolescent is told how he feels, which is the projected parental feeling. The father says to his adolescent daughter, "You must feel bad about what you're doing with Tom." In this case, too many overdetermined influences are operating. The father may feel bad, not about what his daughter is doing, but rather about something in his own personal life, or even about the potential loss of his daughter. If the daughter confronts him about this mystification process, she is likely to meet an angry denial and a retreat into abstractions about the loose morals of the contemporary generation.

Another example is that of a depressed, acting-out girl of fifteen who is told by her parents that they are unhappy because they cannot go out for an evening as they fear what she might do when they are away. Further, they tell her that her father has refused a promotion in rank and salary at his job because this would mean more time away from home due to travelling. The girl feels that these are fraudulent accusations, and that the reason for restrictions on her parents' life is a desire of the mother to have her father around the house more to assist her with the work and management of the children, coupled with a lack of desire on their part to go out themselves. If the adolescent confronts her parents, she is told she is an ungrateful and disrespectful person who does not realize the sacrifices her parents have been making for her. In other words, she is being told she has an obligation to see her parents' acts on the level, and with the meaning, that they are saying is present. Not to accommodate in this manner is to be ungrateful.

In many cases the issue may never get beyond the legalistic assessment of rights and duties. The substance of content is cloaked under accusatory gestures. The frequent pattern is a girl who has been transgressing in some minor way. Although staying out late, truanting, or staying away from home are considered delinquent acts in terms of juvenile court statutes, they are more significant in a psychological sense as indicative of something within the family matrix in the realm of mystification devices.

> Consider a sixteen-year-old adolescent girl who feels she should be able to make her own dates and not specify where she will be, nor when she will return home beyond some absolute limit, such as 1 A.M. on weekends. To provide this data to her parents is considered an undue interference. Her father labels this "being a

good father." The mother smugly comments that the daughter gets away with everything. When the daughter protests too vigorously, an argument results and at times progresses to cursing and physical blows. This is taken as further confirmation of unruly tendencies and lack of respect toward her parents. The girl insists this has all resulted from the confusion she experiences when at home. When she is home she wants to escape, but she is not sure from what. She realizes on reflection that it is not merely due to the arguments, nor to the debate on rights and duties over how much freedom she should have, but she has not been able to see that all of these measures conceal the mystification in the relationships between members of the family which have been safely handled prior to adolescence, but are now no longer contained in this manner.

The Need to Maintain The Status Quo.   Perhaps the most cogent applications of mystification formulations during adolescence occur from the need for maintaining the status quo in families. Vagueness and befuddlement serve a purpose in family life, in which people are perceived as different from what they actually say or do. The family members may not be aware of this perceptual aberration, but by observing the different perceptions of family members, the befuddlement becomes clear. Witness the need of the adolescent to emancipate himself, which requires an alteration in the family stability. If parental needs to maintain preconceived schema are prominent, the threat from a realignment is high. The need to avoid such confrontation can extend to ludicrous lengths in which all but the family see the avoidance.

A sixteen-year-old boy ran away from home several times. When he was younger, he stayed away for a day or two at a time, and at fourteen tried interstate "escapes." The usual approaches of warnings, family therapy, and correctional institutions for running away did not alter his behavior. When first seen for treatment, he was undergoing a thirty-day trial of living in an apartment with two other boys with similar propensities. The parents were paying the rent on the condition that he see a psychiatrist for some time during this thirty-day interval. In the initial interview, the mother reassured the boy that she was sympathetic to his desires to try being away from home since she was sure he wanted to return. He insisted he really did not wish to return home. At the peak of this confrontation, the mother retreated into what was an attack: "You don't know what you're doing. You don't really understand." Under protest that he did understand, the mother could reassure herself that he thought he did understand, but really did not. "That's why we've insisted that you see a psychiatrist." Fortunately, this boy was old enough, and possessed enough ego strength, to reject therapy under the terms which his mother offered.

Emergence of Severe Psychopathology. Similar concepts have been employed to describe the nonmutual complimentary relationships present in families where someone has been diagnosed as schizophrenic. Maintenance of rigid role structures by intense pseudomutuality have been described.[17] Although these mechanisms need not necessarily result in schizophrenia, they appear prone to induce severe conflict in individuals caught up in these processes and leave them vulnerable to psychotic episodes. In the following case, a fifteen-year-old girl developed personality changes six months before becoming overtly psychotic.[18] According to her mother, June was:

TABLE 1

Before	*After*
told me everything	does not tell me what is going on inside her
went everywhere with me	wants to be by herself
was very happy and lively	often looks unhappy; is less lively
liked swimming and cycling	does not do this so much but reads more
was "sensible"	is "full of boys"
played dominoes, drafts, and cards at night with mother, father, and grandfather	is not interested in these games anymore; prefers to sit in her room and read
obedient	disobedient and truculent
never thought of smoking	smokes one or two cigarettes a day without asking permission
believed in God	does not believe in God

In the six months between her first perception of the changes in June and the onset of what we recognized as a psychotic breakdown, June's mother had consulted two doctors about the changes which she regarded as an expression of "illness" and perhaps evil. "It's not June, you see. That's not my little girl." Neither doctor could see evidence of illness or evil in June. To the doctors, on the other hand, these changes were normal maturational, culturally syntonic expressions of growing up and achieving greater autonomy. The girl was completely mystified, because, although she was becoming more autonomous, she still trusted her mother. As her mtoher repeatedly told her that her developing autonomy and sexual maturation were expressions of either madness or badness, June began to feel ill and feel evil. One can see this as praxis on her part to attempt to resolve the contradiction between the processes of her own maturation and her mother's barrage of negative attributions about them.

From our standpoint, June appears confused. She feels she has a lovely mummy, she begs forgiveness for being such a bad daughter, she promises to get well. Although at this point she is complaining that "Hitler's soldiers are after her," not once in many interviews does her mother make any other complaints about June except to attack as bad or mad those processes of development that we regard as most normal about her.

As will be discussed in more detail in other chapters, the adolescent may try to communicate in a vague way about the bind of feeling trapped. Since it may require the soul of a poet to put it well, as well as the therapeutic ear of a poet to hear it, the mystification processes are missed. In some cases more overt efforts by the adolescent to reveal the types of family disillusionment are met with angry rebuffs and denials by parents, and by counselors and therapists as well. This may involve minor revelations (a father is discovered not to be the success portrayed, but rather a flunky who puts in meaningless hours behind a desk in a family business). Or it may involve more dramatic and devastating material, such as the discovery by a girl that her idealized father has been maintaining a mistress for ten years, which can lead to dramatic acting out on the part of the adolescent. The destruction of identification models in these cases is a significant developmental possibility which may be hard to recoup. Some of the revelations may sound so exaggerated that the therapist begins to view them as projections or psychotic distortions, which can trigger the ultimate despair in the adolescent, particularly if he senses a hesitancy in the therapist to bring it up with the parents.

VARIETIES OF ADULT RESPONSES
TO ADOLESCENT BEHAVIOR

Avoidance of closeness and denials of hostility in family interaction can be followed by acting out or psychotic episodes during adolescence. There are, however, adult and parental responses more specific to the emergence of adolescence itself. In part, these adult responses borrow from the contemporary set of

myths propagated about adolescents which are often mutually
contradictory and therefore impossible to refute. While adolescents
may be viewed by some as a repository of the projected hates and
wishes of society, therefore to be condemned, punished, or ostracized, they may also be viewed as reacting to the corruption of the
world which they have been exposed to and had little part in
creating. Implicit in this are ever-present questions about responsibility and choices for one's behavior. These types of incongruent
polarities can be examined in terms of adult-parent responses to the
adolescent. In this section, earlier developmental influences and
conflicts are acknowledged but temporarily bypassed for purposes
of explicating the more immediate responses. The more handicapping types of patterns that are present when intense family and
individual conflicts exist are similarly acknowledged, but not dwelt
on here. The following illustrations show a variety of responses
which may extend to flamboyant situational occurrences.[19]

The Adolescent as a Dangerous Being.   This transcultural theme
is often explained in terms of puberty rites and prolonged periods of
apprenticeship or subservience to protect the integrity of adults or
their property. In this sense, the dangerous adolescent is seen as a
power threat within the family unit. This explanation is very like the
Darwinian and Freudian theories on the origin of the family. Both
aggressive and sexual overtones are present in the adolescent as
threat, and only observations and dynamic formulations from
specific family units can illustrate the details. The threat may vary
from that of a more vigorous and attractive youth to the opposite-
sexed parent, extending out to other areas of socialization which
have not been easily resolved. The very use and emphasis of phrases
to describe adolescents as "explosive" or "a seething cauldron of
hates" or "like a train on the loose" betray the threat and fear. When
the threat is not comfortably dealt with directly, it may be seen in
reaction formations. Rather than overt expressions of fear from the
dangerous object, the expression is in terms of the danger of the
adolescent in a world of threatening people and situations. This is a
type of overprotective device to deal with parental hostilities, and it
may have emerged in the context of adolescence.

The Adolescent As A Tempter.   The seeming freedom of the
adolescent appeals to parents in many ways. While this may be a
rekindling of old and unresolved desires, it can also be a response to
the adolescent as a recognizably appealing person in his own right

at this time. It is no longer kid's play when heterosexual outings or meetings occur once secondary sexual characteristics have developed, followed by menstruation or seminal emissions. All of the intellectual preparation for these events, either in the home or from sex-education classes, do not seem to have remedied the variety of emotional responses present in a given family based on their predisposed attitudes and conflicts.

A few of the more prominent of these are:

1. Parents whose own security and narcissism are contingent upon the need for an immature and dependent child will be threatened by any warning sign of adolescent maturity—sexual or otherwise. When the outward sexual signs of this maturity occur, they are viewed as a threat to the parental security system which elicits countermeasures to suppress or undermine such developments.

2. Parents who have never resolved many of their own repressed conflicts about sexuality have not been able to handle this with ease even in the earlier years of their children's lives. At that time, denial and repression were more effective. Expressions of disgust or repulsiveness about sexual activity may have succeeded earlier, but the adolescent may not be turned off so readily later. Conflict is raised in terms of remaining at a more infantile, or relatively asexual, level of sexual life, versus asserting oneself as a sexual being. When the assertion becomes too conspicuous, the issue is joined with the parent who has been avoiding the acceptance of his own sexuality.

3. A parent may take an intense interest in the vicissitudes of the adolescent's sexual groping. While re-experiencing some of his own groping, there is a feeling of confirmation regarding his own maturity as he witnesses the ineptness of the adolescent in action.

4. A direct sexual attraction for the adolescent may raise the anxiety and guilt level of the parent. Responses may vary from parental avoidance of expressions of affection to enjoying the acting out of the adolescent in a vicarious manner. In some families incestuous activity may result. All of this may coexist with strict limits being set by the parents on activities outside the home in which caution is urged, or rejection conveyed if the adolescent appears to be seeking attachments outside of the family. The threat of child loss leads to parental efforts to undermine it. These operations are rarely verbalized in terms of the not-too-covert desires. This occurs in contexts of pre-existing marital conflict when a parent responds with envy to the sexual prowess or pleasures

witnessed in the adolescent. The mother may experience envy for the
potential she believes present in her daughter and for her son's
relative freedom. The need to experience, perhaps for the first time
themselves in a long time, drives such parents to prying inquisitive-
ness.

5. Not just heterosexual impulses toward the adolescent may be
aroused, but autoerotic, homosexual, and polymorphous perverse
impulses. The resultant conflict and disequilibrium may induce
philandering or engaging in perverse escapades.

6. That fictional parent who healthfully stands back at just the
right distance and views the sexuality of their adolescent offspring
as just a culmination of another stage of psychosexual development
has at least a theoretical or statistical possibility.

The "Sick" Adolescent.   In some ways the sick adolescent is a
variant of the dangerous-object theme. Parents' expectations,
reinforced by society and professionals, stress adolescence as a
period of great instability. By extension, it follows that psychopathology can be expected to emerge. The most intriguing question is,
how frequently are psychopathological responses in adolescents
socially induced? Szasz has raised some provocative questions
about the nature of hospital commitments, but even these questions
do not completely justify the mental-illness appellation for the
adolescent.[20]

Are distraught adolescents mentally ill? Or are they really
attempting to communicate their personal problems? While sick-
ness achieves some secondary gains, illness may be a high price to
pay for a problem in impaired human relationships. Predisposing
organic diatheses for some types of behavioral traits do not fully
explain why some adolescents begin to react in certain ways that are
viewed as sick or unstable. And there is the large rate of residual
deviants among adolescents, as well as in other age groups, a
problem never singled out as the cause of personal, familial, or social
pathology.[21]

The common notion that adolescent behavior is equivalent to
psychopathology on the loose too often leads to loss of self-esteem in
the adolescent. Too many of the inevitable conflicts associated with
the developmental phase of adolescence are labelled as signs of
illness rather than as developmental conflicts. The optimal job of
the therapist is to take the private language, distortions, and
anxieties of these adolescents and their families and translate their
cryptic signals into words that prevent anomalous development.

This puts one of the initial therapeutic tasks with adolescents on the level of linguistic analysis, although it is not a literal translator but a sensitive, sophisticated clinical unraveler which is needed.[22] This is not a plea to view adolescence as no different from any other phase of life, but to see it as having its own set of difficulties in which drive levels, feelings, and object relations are on a more intense and fluctuating level that need not be viewed as strictly pathological.

Parental Envy of Adolescents. Mothers whose attractiveness and vigor are waning often do not feel admiration for their adolescent daughters. Fathers, trapped in a life of routine and discipline, frequently have their envy kindled by the opportunities of their sons—a phenomenon witnessed in almost all social groups with young competitors. This is accentuated by an emphasis on youth, beauty, and slimness in females and physical fitness and muscularity in males. The phenomenon of *athlete's neurosis*, which peaks in the fifth decade of life, often occurs when adolescents are still living at home.[23] Athlete's neurosis is seen in males who have over-valued their health and fitness prior to middle age, when they find themselves developing persistent neurotic symptoms in response to minor physical injuries.

Envy may also manifest itself in competitive participation with adolescent offspring. Mothers attempt to act and dress like their adolescent daughters, or become flirtatious and competitive with their daughter's boyfriends. In some situations where the father is absent, the mother and daughter may double-date, and occasionally a boyfriend of intermediate age alternates his attentions between mother and daughter. This competition may go so far as to result in their mutual pregnancy by the same boyfriend. Alternating sadomasochistic relations between the mother and daughter may emerge under the stress of jealousy and resentment. To the one who loses and is down, a martyred role is available which can easily be switched should a victory come on the morrow.

Parental Mourning. The empty nest syndrome experienced by middle-aged women whose children have left home often precipitates an increase in drinking. A feeling of emptiness results from loss of the attachments, anticipations and excitements attendant upon having children to nurture. Mothers who attempt to delay the departure of children are inevitably unsuccessful; in situations where the parent prevents the loss of their adolescent by maintaining the childhood tie, a psychopathological variant of development exists. In some cases the anticipation of loss in the parent has begun so early that the child never really entered adolescence. To permit the final completion of the separation and individuation processes begun during infancy requires a fair degree of ego autonomy and development in parents as well as adolescents. Old and unresolved object ties and depressive tendencies may well interfere.

The Adolescent As An Object of Curiosity. This response is elicited when the adolescent is viewed as a curious specimen to be examined like a puzzling technological creation, alternately frightening and amusing. While feelings of tenderness accompany the curiosity, it may be also used defensively to avoid closeness. An element of derogation may be involved as well, similar to any strange sect or deviant group under scrutiny.

DEVELOPMENTAL STAGES OF ADOLESCENCE: PREADOLESCENCE

It is both illogical and confusing to discuss adolescents as a homogeneous group. The range in years spans five to ten, which means that we are dealing at one end of the spectrum with a junior-high-school-level individual and at the other end with a college-age or older individual. Hence the developmental phenomena of adolescence are more easily dealt with by division into three stages:

Preadolescence commences with the first psychological changes accompanying alterations in hormonal functioning, and includes the period preceding and shortly after the onset of pubertal changes. This is a transitional period between latency and midadolescence which lasts about eighteen to twenty-four months. Changes occur in behavior as a result of these psychological changes so that it is desirable to consider them separately for heuristic purposes.

Midadolescence lasts until the mid-teens, and most characteristically involves the dissolution of peer group attachments. A greater closeness on the one-to-one level is begun, but while greater personal intimacy is sought by the adolescent, adherence to norms and ideologies of a group or institution different from that of the parents flourishes.

The onset of *Late Adolescence* is difficult to place in terms of a chronological year. Mid-teen for one adolescent might be fifteen, and for another it might be seventeen or eighteen. During this period a more intense concern about the adolescent's personal future in terms of commitment to a vocation and love relationships appears to take

from some part of her body, such as her nose. In some cultures there may be a secondary gain from the attribution of religious significance to this.

There are also superego implications in terms of the girl's self-appraisal. She may avoid taking pride in her body as an object of self-love, vanity, interesting clothes, and coquettishness. This need not be interpreted as masculine, but it may be a flight into intellectual interests in which narcissistic gratifications will be met apart from her body.

In other adolescent girls, anxiety about menstruation and its meaning, and the response of others to it, takes on a compulsive quality of preoccupation with tones of hypochondriasis. Pain and discomfort associated with menstruation readily lend themselves to this. The narcissism of the girl becomes transferred into keeping her "treasure chest" intact and safe from injury. Premenstrual irritability permits a greater release of aggression, either on a primary basis or associated with other paraphernalia. Is the fact that some courts treat menstruation as an extenuating circumstance in connection with a crime representative of a response to masculine guilt toward women, or an action based on confirmable evidence that women are more prone to aggressive acts during menstruation and hence should be viewed as less liable? Such special handling is another manifestation of the narcissistic view of herself as someone who desires special consideration. By extension, the girl may over-evaluate herself so that her ideation is that the male who gets her is receiving a special prize worthy for a prince. Carried too far, this makes her so precious that no man deserves the prize and she avoids contamination with "dirty" activities.

Masochistic Aspects of Menstruation. From the educational changes in families and the culture within the past generation, menstruation does not have the traumatic implications it once had for many girls. When menstruation occurs it is viewed as something to be expected. Although details of the process are still unknown, it is seen as an inherent part of maturing as a female and necessary for pregnancy. Therefore, it appears that the educational mission has accomplished a great deal at this time for a large number of girls, and to a lesser extent boys, regarding the trials and tribulations of menstruation. What remain are some of the idiosyncratic responses in certain girls as well as the incorporation of conflicts about menstruation into existing and previously unresolved conflicts. A mixture of fantasy and personal distortion remain. Female attitudes toward the monthly flow in terms of enduring such an inconvenience and suffering with magnanimity can be viewed as part of an identification process with mothers or older women to form this type of group identity with females. Others add that these types of attitudes are part of what is a normal feminine masochistic attitude toward pain and discomfort.[25]

This raises questions concerning this component of female character structure. Feminine masochism has been viewed by some as an inherent part of female character, particularly in classical psychoanalytic theory. The usual developmental occurrences, such as menstruation, defloration, and parturition are seen as biological analogs to the female suffering in a psychological and social sense. These formulations stress the inability of the girl to accept having an opening in herself in place of a phallus. An opening which periodically bleeds is something humiliating, and not a source of pleasure. Discovery by the girl that she lacks a phallus plus the menarcheal experience are the traumata in female development. To master the traumata a denial of femininity occurs along with masculine identification. The prepubertal girl who has not yet menstruated but has some emerging secondary sexual characteristics finds herself at the peak of discontent with the opposite sex, presumably from her absorption in her own changing body and the low level of feedback to assist her in gaining awareness of what is transpiring within her own body. Commencement of menstruation itself facilitates differentiation of fantasies and anticipations from reality, and provides a greater ability to perceive and organize what has been happening. In that sense, the discomfort of menstruation is viewed as serving an integrative function in the psychosexual development of a woman.[26]

Without entering into the intricacies of the theory of masochism at this point, males react in a variety of ways to menstruation. A mixture of horror, disgust, and avoidance in the form of cultural mores has frequently been commented upon. This appears to be related to fears of the pubertal boy which are related to his awareness of the bloody state of the girl. In most boys, such adverse reactions do not persist on a conscious or an unconscious level. In some males a variety of masochism called feminine masochism evolves in which the boy unconsciously identifies with the humiliated woman, such as an oedipal mother.[27] The accompanying fantasies of these boys reveal themes of being mutilated, beaten, or giving birth. By vicariously experiencing feminine humiliation, the boy is permitted to retain his de facto male state. However, it is interesting that more boys who are conflicted in this area will later seek to become women surgically. Again, we do not know if cultural factors operate to restrict as many woman from seeking surgical alteration.[28] Even in cases of feminine masochism in boys, similar to girls who seek humiliating predicaments, the behavior is not solely a wish for punishment but a device to assert and maintain control. They arrange or provoke humiliating punishments.

If one does not accept the theory of inevitable feminine masochism as a significant variable determining the response of the girl to menstruation, antecedent developmental phenomena, and current interpersonal material become significant. Of course, this does not deny that many girls may have prominent masochistic tendencies on the basis of the developmental factors. Such factors become relevant in terms of the comfort or degree of protest a girl has about the changes occurring in her body. More broadly, how does the girl feel about what she sees as her future in a family or society as a woman? Problems of gender identity and overall identity, as they have developed from her early years, put a particular strain on the occurrence of the menses if there has been pre-existing confusion. Parental attitudes toward the girl, as well as the type of marital situation of her parents, bear significant weight as well. In this regard the attitude of the parents toward women becomes an ongoing agent of great importance. A mother who has been overtly or silently protesting her gender and role cannot help having a great impact on the responses of her daughter. This is seen in silent suffering, or badgering the pubertal girl with warning and restrictions that makes menstruation seem like an onerous burden to endure.

Witnessed societal factors, such as the greater freedom and opportunity given boys, accentuate ambivalences. Much has been written about the protest of women in this century regarding subservient roles. A crucial balance appears to reside somewhere between exaggerated protest against women's subservience and a pride and acceptance of the attributes of femininity without an implication that these are in some way inferior. If such things as attractiveness to boys, an appealing physique, and a capacity for child-bearing have little appeal, a potential for conflict during adolescence and later is present. The response of others to puberty in the girl appears crucial in this respect, for if she senses others perceiving her as attractive and desirable, it appears to be more important than meeting criteria of absolute beauty. This is seen in the therapy of adolescent girls, as well as in observations in schools and social settings. What may puzzle the girl is a withdrawal of her father from the closeness which previously existed, which may be misinterpreted as a rejection of her budding femininity rather than a protective device. Later in life they may have conflicts over attempts to secure an occupational identity while needing much reassurance from men.[29]

Sexual Anxieties in Preadolescent Boys. Changes in physique related to secondary sexual characteristics lead to accompanying psychological concerns. While masturbatory activity does not commence with puberty but exists in various forms from early childhood into latency, it has a new meaning during preadolescence. Ejaculation is contingent upon the maturation of the prostate and seminal vesicles, which occurs during puberty. Nocturnal emissions do not usually start until the midadolescent period (about age thirteen). The meaning of ejaculation and emissions varies for the boy as menstruation does for the girl.

Even with education about seminal emissions, the boy may experience anxiety when they occur. Part of this is associated with the lack of choice and control as to occurrence, and part with the vividness of the dreams which often accompany nocturnal emissions. The matter of lack of control is seen in the dream content which involves themes of a homosexual or incestuous nature involving mothers, sisters, cousins, or teachers. Whether the pressing nature of overt sexual fantasies in the boy is directly connected with the biological phenomena of hormones or stimulation from filled seminal vesicles, which has no parallel in girls, or whether it is primarily due to the psychological elaboration of fantasies, is difficult to decide.

Whatever the basis, the result is a restlessness. Erections occurring in the midst of a group setting, or an all-male setting such as an athletic event like wrestling, can be humiliating and lead to shame. Superego development, as verified by religio-cultural edicts which prohibit sexual thoughts as well as acts, leads to guilt reactions in the vulnerable adolescent. When ejaculation occurs as a willful act of choice by masturbating, the adolescent also experiences guilt. Concerns of an earlier age that physical injury, insanity, or permanent sexual impairment may result have been modified recently by educational means, but guilt from such acts still persist from their officially being condemned by most Judeo-Christian cultures. The psychological fantasies which accompany masturbation can induce an even deeper guilt. In some cases obsessive ruminations about the possible ill effects of masturbation, or self-condemnation for giving in to one's urges, is a displacement from other sources of guilt and anxiety.

Simultaneous with autoerotic activities, the beginnings of turning to heterosexual objects for gratification emerge in the form of crushes. Crushes are primarily directed toward someone of the same sex. This is the use of others similar to that seen in play-acting, which gives a hysterical or neurotic quality to many adolescent relationships. The narcissistic basis for these attachments is seen in the fawning quality of adoration present toward the idol or hero. The idol consumes thought processes and time of the young adolescent, and he may desire to be near him, know more about him, or have some relic of his such as something he has worn, touched, or signed. In part this is on a preobject choice level since the relationship is not based on mutuality. It is basically one of narcissistic identification which contributes to ego-ideal development, a part of superego alteration which occurs at this stage and utilizes other adults to lessen the internalized directives which have been so heavily influenced by parental models. This shift in expansion permits a lessening of the close dependency tie as well, but the adolescent is then left vulnerable to slights from idols who may be indifferent, if not outright rejecting. This is another source contributing to the mood lability of the young adolescent.

A different type of precariousness results when the crush is directed to an adult whose own conflicts regarding homosexual attractions to adolescents have not been resolved. A threat exists from those who seek out contacts through vocational choice. From the side of the adolescent, the transiency of the crush may prevent the prolonged involvement which results in homosexual activity. In some of these situations the occurrence of sexual activities which are pleasurable and reassuring in the dependency context may lead to fixations. Institutional alterations may provide a bulwark against too strong an attachment of this type by permitting a shift to fulfilling the ideals of some type of institutional group. By such a dilution safety is added.

In addition, sublimatory and aggressive discharge may be available. Linkage to the same sex is seen when the initial seeking of competency is to impress the peer group of the same sex. For boys this involves athletic or scholarly prowess, while for girls it involves beauty, social, or educational attainment. Only later does the shift to preferring admiration from a heterosexual object occur. All of this emphasizes the importance of the peer group for the early adolescent. The mores of this group in the form of dreams, styles, and tastes predominate over the dictates of other normative groups. Some refer to the language, customs, and approaches of the group as an independent adolescent culture.

Telephoning.   The activity of telephoning is associated with the pressures toward safe love relationships.[30] The typical adolescent, while using the telephone, employs a variety of postures accompanied by erotic gyrations and contortions. The feet may be up in the air and the head down, while conversational content is filled with double meanings, staccato-like assaults, gossip, and direct advice about personal goings-on. Throughout the intimacies, physical distance is maintained by virtue of the literal distance. Yet a voice is available, while sexual references and feelings remain safe. The phone further permits distance and safe separation from parents. Twenty-four-hour-a-day telephone exchanges for adolescents to call at any time which have developed in many of the metropolitan areas are part of this picture.

Dancing.   Another illustration of multiple needs being met in the peer group is dancing. Both sexual and aggressive impulses are expressed by the various maneuvers, directly and symbolically. However, dancing is tantalizing in that it is closer to foreplay than telephoning. This is seen in the bewildering pattern of constant change in dance styles. Observe the partial drive discharge buttressed by defenses which results in a compromise. While the rolling of the pelvis and thrusting of the hips are not too concealed, they are the ultimate permissible. The rules of the game may even require that the dancers rarely touch and never kiss. There is good reason why some religious groups fastened on dancing as lewd. It was geared to prevent the consequences of extending the evening's activities after the dance which could lead to adverse social consequences.

The Predicaments of Preadolescence.   An alteration in previous types of controls is reflected in preadolescence. In part this is based on weakened superego directives to internalized authorities which contributed to superego formation. There are reasons why adults get upset by prodromal indications of what is to come. Besides reactivating or stimulating their own impulses, parents are bothered by what may seem a general regression in the course of socialization of their child. What they are not aware of is that such behavior is not only inevitable but actually progressive in a developmental sense. Judging by external behaviors, qualities of unpredictability, fused with oral demands, surge to the fore. From the urgency of these behaviors arise petty pilfering, lying, destructive acts, and other digressions. Boys as well as girls may alternate in their cleanliness and lavatory habits. Exaggerated styles of dress emphasizing rags or worn and torn clothing permit the compromise of messiness with a mockery of adult conformity and neatness. Overt acts of cruelty or bullying may occur. In the sexual realm, polymorphous activity can vary from mutual masturbation to seducing younger children and being used by older adolescents or adults. In this setting, concentration on academic subjects may lessen temporarily.

Weakening of the primary identifications of the preadolescent with his family finds expression in the following cluster of developmental phenomena:[31]

1. Conflict of double standards—individual child still parent-loyal, peer-group code basically anti-adult (Result: new waves of guilt and shame in both directions)
2. Embarrassment about open submission to adult politeness and good-manner codes
3. Shamelessness in language and behavior, bravado through flouting of health and safety rules, special joy in risk-taking
4. Avoidance of too open acceptance of adults in official roles, even of those very much liked (teachers and parents, for example)
5. Loyalty to peers and risk-taking in their favor, even where they are personally despised or feared
6. Openly displayed freshness against authority figures.
7. Deep-seated revulsion toward any form of praise or punishment which seems to be perceived as infantilizing
8. Safety in homosexual groupings; view of the other sex as hunter's trophy rather than in terms of interpersonal relationships
9. Negative loading of any form of official acceptance of help from adults, pride in "taking it bravely" at any price
10. Low prestige of verbal communication with the trusted adult, hesitation about communicating feelings and emotions
11. Apathy toward adults as partners in play life, unless it is a group game situation
12. Increase in contagion power of behavior by peers, especially those five degrees tougher and a few years older than parents would feel comfortable with

Psychological Dangers. Several psychological dangers are possible in the preadolescent period:

1. The strong urgency of drive-based activities, poorly modulated by ego and superego, can lead to overt antisocial conduct. A sequence of labeling processes in a community may commence. This pushes the adolescent toward confirming these behaviors as part of his self-concept, which tends to be perpetuated.

2. Reinforcement for some behaviors leads to establishing these dispositions as rewarding in their own right. This is seen in the gratifications available from antisocial peer or gang activities, as well as in various kinds of sexual behavior such as homosexuality. Since the preadolescent is often a lonely and self-centered being, with weakened allegiances and ties, he is subject to the transient attachments of peer groups and heroes.

3. If the adolescent's behavior leads to chronic anxiety, increased defensive efforts by the ego will lead to symptom formation and possibly neurotic conflict. Present frustrations can cause past disappointments and rivalries to become reactivated. The need to avoid the closeness of old emotional attachments within the family operates here as well.

4. The mistake (perpetuated by organizations whose purpose is to advise and educate parents) that the parent should be the pal of the adolescent serves to complicate developmental processes. When adults, who are at the center of many of the child's conflicts, behave as peers, they become too close to the sources of anxiety which the child is defending against. The solution is for parents to accept the instability in the preadolescent even though they are not able to intervene helpfully by many of the techniques suitable when the child was younger. By preadolescence, disillusionment with parents has progressed. Since fantasies become more difficult to maintain, parents are seen realistically. It is a developmental necessity for any set of parents, no matter how adequate they have been in their overt parenting roles, to be abandoned by their offspring.

Since this is a period of ego and superego weakness as well, many of the previous parental criticisms and disappointments receive their delayed comeuppance. An unfortunate byproduct is the bitterness that may ensue from the perplexity of what is occurring, supplemented by well-meaning advice from almost everyone. The most disappointed parents are those who have tried to maintain mutual respect in their home and perhaps have practiced equality, consistently disowning a position of authority with their children. When preadolescence arrives, these parents are offended that their child needs to extend separation and independence. In a sense, even a parent who is completely anti-authoritarian cannot expect the upsurge of desires and reactivated infantile fantasies to have no impact. "To grow in strength, to mature, to become clever, is automatically translated by him into the fall and decline of the parents. When he feels grown up, father and mother appear childish to him; when he feels proud of his own knowledge, the parents seem stupid; the boy's masculinity is synonymous for him with the father's impotence, his social success with seeing the father as a failure."[32]

MIDADOLESCENCE

Characteristics. Midadolescence is often seen as synonymous with adolescence in a strict sense. While earlier childhood has directed much of its efforts at securing object ties that will not be abandoned, and middle-childhood has permitted the child to expand his relationships based on a place within his family if conflict has not been too great, adolescence must undo this to some degree while not totally abandoning it. The preadolescent begins to relate to friends on a narcissistic basis, but in midadolescence the shift to the heterosexual object becomes primary. This, reinforces old and new anxieties about relationships to people of all ages. Hence, mounting anxieties and unlimited hopes may be present simultaneously, since potentialities seem unlimited. When something appears to threaten the unlimited potential, sadness predominates. This makes evaluation of the meaning of midadolescent behaviors, as well as prediction of the final outcome in terms of psychopathology, very difficult.

What is the sine qua non psychologically for an adolescent to emerge into a heterosexual life? Heterosexual life does not imply heterosexual activity in a genital sense (for this no more is required than a biologically intact body which can perform coitus). But which developmental processes permit tenderness and attachment to flourish? If excessively close affectional ties are present within the same-sexed peer group, delay in heterosexual shifts occur. Heterosexuality cannot take place by a parental fiat, as in "Now you may go seek a relationship with a girl (boy) outside our family." Nor would going through the motions of securing heterosexual relationships truly represent heterosexuality. Instead, superego directives which have decreed the avoidance of heterosexual life must be altered to permit it. In part this can be affected by parental permission, and in part a weakening of inhibitions to accompany the increase in drive life is necessary. Ideally, gradual alteration in superego permissiveness occurs, rather than an abrupt or overwhelming alteration. Previous development of strong controls, utilizing guilt and shame, when overthrown abruptly, can usher in manic-like excitability or depression. Realizing the finality of parental loss can further contribute to depressive possibilities. Expectations, real or fancied, of exceeding parental attainments also contribute as does resentment about parental failings.

Behaviorally, most adolescents alternate between exaggerated dependence and criticism of parental ways with regression to earlier ways of being good. Reappraisal of parents permits a more balanced view. To the extent that attacks on parental integrity succeed in provoking counterattacks by the parents, the adolescent gains further internal permission to free himself and pursue his attachments elsewhere. However, this is rarely reassuring to the family which finds its stability threatened or disappearing. Earlier masochistic trends in the adolescent can push this type of provocation to extremes which go beyond what is necessary, leaving permanent wounds. Parental firmness and limit-setting elicit protest, but they also provide something to fight against. Narcissistic overevaluation of self makes it difficult to give up the powerful parent who continues to stand for and offer what the adolescent does not try out on his own.

Fantasies and Their Offshoots. At midadolescence the role of fantasy assumes preeminence. Fantasies and daydreams are used as transitory phenomena between narcissism and heterosexual object-finding.[33] Their most accommodating aspect is their evanescence, as perceptions of earlier life and attachments feed into them. Similar to dreams, in fantasies all manner of conquests can be achieved, as well as a safe return. In this connection, fantasies accompanying masturbation are of interest as normal developmental manifestations, but the manifest content is always accompanied by unconscious latent content. The latter is a result of defenses against undisguised wishes which are not permitted conscious elaboration. Fantasy provides a compromise, allowing a partial gratification of desires still denied or conceded. There is a predicament in masturbation for the adolescent even apart from the superego dictates he has assimilated against the act. While masturbation gives him a feeling of independence from requiring external objects for sexual gratification, at the same time it makes him dependent on an autoerotic activity. Boys appear to be more responsive to physiological tension, and more prone to be aroused by fantasies to masturbation without actual exposure to another person.[34] This is contrary to some beliefs that girls are more prone to fantasize. Many fantasies take place when superego control and ego functioning are not fully active, such as before going to sleep or upon awakening. Pregenital components utilizing sado-masochistic, voyeuristic, exhibitionistic, or bestial themes are used.

Accompanying tendencies to daydream are a parallel phenomenon—depersonalization. Feelings of estrangement from the body may be a response to heightened anxiety. A state of flatness, reflecting an impoverished ego, may be the most frequent manifestation of self-observation in adolescence. The adolescent speaks of himself as "dead" or "having the blahs."

While daydreams are ego syntonic, feelings of unreality in depersonalized states are not, which is closer to levels of psychotic disorganization. Many adolescents experience these phenomena in transient forms. When clinicians become aware of them, they are most likely to view them as part of a schizophrenic process or as accompaniments of anxiety or obsessional diagnoses.

One part of superego functioning concerns itself with self-observation. This is one facet of reality testing which tends to promote regressive and depersonalized states when it lacks balance. To appraise oneself in any critical or praiseworthy manner is contingent upon knowing and observing what one does. Not to know and observe interferes with this, yet this is precisely what may be desired by the adolescent. Truthfulness in the development of higher forms of cognitive operations appears to be dependent on the integrity of superego functioning.

An example of heightened self-observation in adolescence is keeping a daily record or diary.[35] Since the sex-role standard in the contemporary United States views this as feminine behavior and therefore something passive, diary-keeping is more common among girls. To the degree that the adolescent cannot, or does not, translate desires into some type of activity, the diary hears about them. The diary assumes qualities of an objective nature in which the adolescent is able to stand back and observe himself. The fuss made over the privacy of the diary is striking in view of the many ways in which adolescents leave it lying about to be found accidentally. Keeping such a record has a quality of object-orientation. yet an appraisal of others is possible in terms of feelings and wishes and the possibility for realistic reappraisal as well as desires. For some, the writing begins to assume greater reality than life itself, and may accentuate withdrawal tendencies. While avoidance of acting out may be facilitated, role-playing without participation may be encouraged.

The following extract from Anne Frank's *The Diary of a Young Girl*,[36] written while she hid in an attic with her family during World War II to escape the Nazis, illustrates these points:

Thurs.

Dear Kitty,

My longing to talk to someone became so intense that somehow or other I took it into my head to choose Peter.

Sometimes if I've been upstairs into Peter's room during the day, it always struck me as very snug, but because Peter is so retiring and would never turn anyone out who became a nuisance, I never dared stay long, because I was afraid he might think me a bore. I tried to think of an excuse to stay in his room and get him talking, without it being too noticeable, and my chance came yesterday. Peter has a mania for crossword puzzles at the moment and hardly does anything else. I helped him with them and we soon sat opposite each other at his little table, he on the chair and me on the divan.

It gave me a queer feeling each time I looked into his deep blue eyes, and he sat there with that mysterious laugh playing around his lips. I was able to read his inward thoughts. I could see on his face that look of helplessness and uncertainty as to how to behave, and, at the same time, a trace of his sense of manhood. I noticed his shy manner and it made me feel very gentle; I couldn't refrain from meeting those dark eyes again and again, and with my whole heart I almost beseeched him: oh, tell me, what is going on inside you, oh, can't you look beyond this ridiculous chatter?

But the evening passed and nothing happened, except that I told him about blushing—naturally not what I have written, but just so that he would become more sure of himself as he grew older.

When I lay in bed and thought over the whole situation, I found it far from encouraging, and the idea that I should beg for Peter's patronage was simply repellent. One can do a lot to satisfy one's longings, which certainly sticks out in my case, for I have made up my mind to go and sit with Peter more often and to get him talking somehow or other.

Whatever you do, don't think I'm in love with Peter—not a bit of it! If the Van Daans had had a daughter instead of a son, I should have tried to make friends with her too.

I woke at about five to seven this morning and knew at once, quite positively, what I had dreamed. I sat on a chair and opposite me sat Peter... Wessel. We were looking together at a book of drawings by Mary Bos. The dream was so vivid that I can still partly remember the drawings. But that was not all—the dream went on. Suddenly Peter's eyes met mine and I looked into those fine, velvet brown eyes for a long time. Then Peter said very softly, "If I had only known, I would have come to you long before!" I turned around brusquely because the emotion was too much for me. And after that I felt a soft, and oh, such a cool kind cheek against mine and it felt so good, so good. . . .

I awoke at this point, while I could still feel his cheek against mine and felt his brown eyes looking deep into my heart, so deep that there he read how much I had loved him and how much I still love him. Tears sprang into my eyes once more, and I was very sad that I had lost him again, but at the same time glad because it made me feel quite certain that Peter was still the chosen one.

It is strange that I should often see such vivid images in my dreams here. First I saw Grandma so clearly one night that I could even distinguish her thick, soft, wrinkled velvety skin. Then Granny appeared as a guardian angel; then followed Lies, who seems to be a symbol to me of the sufferings of all my girl friends and all Jews. When I pray for her, I pray for all Jews and all those in need. And now Peter, my darling Peter—never before have I had such a clear picture of him in my mind. I don't need a photo of him, I can see him before my eyes, and oh, so well!

Yours, Anne

Love. The natural history of the emergence of heterosexual involvement to the point of being in love has a double aspect. The observer sees various preparatory steps, while the adolescent sees an unpredictable phenomenon. From the same-sexed attachments of preadolescence, a shift toward large heterosexual groups occurs during midadolescence. In time, smaller sub-groups break off. Within these, first attachments occur which are known for their simultaneous intensity and fickleness in terms of the ease with which they shift. Several boys and girls in the group may go with other members in the same group and rotate. Within this framework the commencement of physical contact in the form of kissing or petting takes place. Physical gratification does not seem the primary goal, but rather a mixture of contact and exploration, as well as the excitement of the new experience. Renewal of the caressing and touching of earlier dependency experiences is another accompaniment. From these groups within the larger group, some initial outings occur in the form of couples. The demands adolescents can make on each other may arouse anxiety. Old jealousies and possessiveness are resurrected with a need to back away. Being in love on one night may be followed by a call from the partner on the next night terminating the relationship.

No set format is possible for the pursuit of heterosexual activities in an age that grants much leeway to experimentation. While some early relationships lead to sexual involvement, a great many fluctuate on the level of heavy petting and masturbation. Intercourse may be sought by the boy with someone with whom he has no close associations.

For others, sexual experimentation may lead to going all the way. An interesting by-product is the heightening of sex-role practices. *Resonance phenomena* permit tendencies of the opposite sex to be conceded safely to the opposite sex, which can then be enjoyed by virtue of loving these properties in the loved object.[37]

The adolescent has a readiness for feeling affective tenderness. When it occurs, an added dimension is given to heterosexual life. When the first physical explorations give way to the emergence of tenderness, it is as though one has given way to the other. What remains is the need to fuse them, which remains impaired in a great many adolescents and adults.

Many factors contribute to promote attraction to a partner who can absorb the feminine component for a boy and the masculine component for a girl. Absorption permits further polarization of sex identity, but blocks in accomplishing this may lead to premature attempts to establish sex role by flights into early marriage in a desperate attempt to demonstrate that the adolescent truly is a boy or girl.

Heterosexual Shifts.   Common are the varieties of choices that come to the fore for the adolescent in the realm of heterosexual object choices of a serious nature. Those adolescents for whom separation processes from parents have been indecisive have remnants of a need to hurt or avenge the parents. During adolescence these emerge via angry attacks and reproaches. The girl who has retained a strong attachment to her father is likely to resent the incompetent manner which her mother uses to manage the house and care for her father.

Persistence of feelings that her father has been wronged are seen in the appeal for these girls of boys who are failures or outcasts. The choice varies: in one case it is a boy who has been a chronic school failure and has had home difficulties with his parents; in another case it is a member of a minority group who appeals to the sensitized part of the girl; in others it may be the boy with delinquent tendencies who appeals to her feeling that she needs to help and understand him in a way no one else can.

The limitations of choices made on these bases are seen by way of the instability in these situations. The needs of delinquent boys themselves can rarely be resolved by the adolescent girl, although a flight into marriage may be tried or a pregnancy achieved. The choice of the girl is governed by her unresolved needs to compete and give more successfully than she believes took place in her own home, and thus to select a boy on the basis of his being maligned or poorly treated. Success under these circumstances has a price in terms of guilt from the ramifications which can arise.

An attractive fifteen-year-old, with hair combed over her eyes, from a middle-class background, wore an expensive fur coat over extremely casual clothes more in keeping with her peer group. A similar split was seen in her attitude, which alternated between "little girl" and "woman." Over the past year therapy became indicated through the power demands which the girl had forced. Typically, she did not come home on time, and complained of being "picked on" when her parents objected. Moody periods of staying by herself and fantasizing about when she could leave home were accompanied by feelings of wanting to hurt her parents. Her father was mortified by her shift to "total inappropriateness and contempt for what we have worked so hard for." Her revenge extended to the point of ridiculing promises she made and a pattern of chronic lying since, "They don't trust me." Her parents were baffled by the boy she idealized. While the girl was a bright but sporadic student, the boy was a school dropout. Although she stated she had known him for a year, their first meeting had been casual and for the preceding six months he had been in a correctional facility where she was unable to see him. She exchanged passionate letters with him dealing with how she would wait for him. While no one understood *him*, he was the only one who understood *her*.

Until her mother had an unexpected pregnancy (at the time the girl was entering puberty) she had felt understood at home. But "That was a stupid thing for my mother to do since she can't manage what she has and moans about how much she has to do now."

A boy needs a heterosexual relationship in which he can be secure that sexual activity with a girl he knows, and toward whom he feels tenderness, does not carry a threat of retaliation by another male. He also needs reassurance that the girl will not use sexual activity as a form of manipulation for demands he is not capable of fulfilling. For his own psychological security he must be willing to take a stand and approach a girl without being overwhelmed by anxiety, and it follows that he must not see girls as too threatening to take a personal risk. The operating anxiety pertains to fears of pregnancy, venereal disease, or getting caught.

There are other psychological conflicts, but he has objective fears as well (the fear of inflicting pain, or the derivative of being unable to separate following the act). Other fantasies pertain to fears of losing control, becoming dependent on the girl or sexual activity, or humiliation after he commits himself.

Homosexual Possibilities.   Homosexual love leading to homosexual acting out emerges during the midadolescent period. In both sexes, the obvious factor of massive reinforcement of a pleasurable type of behavior coming at a time of heightened desire and genital receptiveness combine to make this a favored type of sexual outlet for some adolescents.

More specific factors may operate with boys. A strong maternal identification can be a predisposing factor. An absent father, or a passive, withdrawn male in the home, coupled with a controlling and intimidating mother, is common. In boys who tend toward a homosexual object choice, a strong and poorly resolved oedipal tie to an older woman, or an incestuous representative, acts to restrict interest in the female. Generalization of females as sexually forbidden objects is not confined to earlier objects of attachment. In some boys the derivative form of the vagina dentata fantasy, has fears of being devoured in any close relationship with women. Derivatives of this fantasy are not simply those of the vagina literally possessing teeth; instead anxiety is raised about the vagina as a dangerous place to trust a prized part of the body.

In girls the dispositional tendencies toward a homosexual object choice may be related to an envy of boys which has taken the form of contempt or attempts to be one of the boys. These girls wish to protect or take care of other girls the way a father has taken care of a wife. Not being able to provide adequately for a girl may lead to intense jealousy or envy. In classical psychoanalytic formulations of penis envy, these feelings are tied up with the disappointment in not having a penis as something that forever bars the girl from being a boy.

In other cases the dependency of the girl on a maternal figure is so great and unresolved that risking the loss of this caring object is too great. The need not to lose the maternal figure is a correlative part of the equation, together with demands made on the girl by other family members. This leaves the girl hesitant to exchange this type of relationship for another and she remains the obedient and trusting little girl.

Even to raise the question of homosexual behavior, indicating the possibility of homosexuality as a developmental outcome, requires explanation. As with any other line of development, there are similar behaviors and distinguishing psychopathological development can be difficult. This is not a mere academic exercise, for the psychological consequences of a diagnostic appraisal which is too inclusive or exclusive are not inconsequential. Beyond the psychological, there are the adverse social consequences of such a categorization. In turn, the perception that others see them as different can further exacerbate anxiety and discomfort. This can lead to association with those described as similar and avoidance of those who might reveal the true self. Experimental evidence has shown how individuals react when they feel different from others.[38]

Therefore, the limitations of our clinical ability to predict an outcome of homosexual development must be kept constantly in mind, especially since the prevalence of homosexual activities rises during adolescence. Many of the criteria used to appraise behavior as perverse are inapplicable to childhood and adolescence. Once it is recognized that the occurrence of homosexual behavior does not establish homosexuality, the types of criteria useful with adults are seen as not helpful. The distinction between overt and latent homosexuality is not useful when appraising overt adolescent acts, such as mutual masturbation. Distinctions between sexual passivity and activity have always suffered in terms of what these mean in behaviors or fantasies. For example, the partner on top during intercourse might not be the most active at all; while intrusion can occur along with great passivity. Most important prognostically is the question of relative reversibility. Even if the acts appear well entrenched, there is a difference if they are integrated within the personality and ego-syntonic or dystonic.

While external genitalia permit the cognitive operation in the child of deciding if his anatomy meets the criteria for a boy or girl, the sense of maleness or femaleness is more complex.[39] On this groundwork many oedipal themes are enacted in both positive and negative senses, based partly on a conceptualization of anatomical differences. A preference for a parent of the opposite sex during the oedipal period will correspond to the adult model of heterosexuality, and vice versa. Whatever seems to predominate at that period cannot be taken as a guide to later psychopathology. Preferences in individual children are heavily influenced by pre-oedipal experiences and the personalities of adults in the home. It is obvious that in the ensuing years, the boy who prefers males and avoids females is not necessarily emerging as a future homosexual during latency, but establishing himself in terms of masculine identity. Similarly, we do not view the girl who, during her elementary school years, prefers associating with boys rather than girls as someone who is manifesting well-developed heterosexual ties, but perhaps as someone who is not comfortable with her sense of femaleness.

The necessary but not sufficient component for homosexuality to emerge as a preferred sexual object choice in adolescence, and to be maintained, requires at least one of the following:

1. Variations in biological endowment which perhaps tend toward greater dispositions to homosexual object choices
2. A narcissistic factor, wherein the adolescent chooses a same-sexed partner in his own self-image rather than permitting the components of his personality to be sought and displaced in a member of the opposite sex with whom he can develop a love relationship
3. Developmental experiences in the years before adolescence which promote and reinforce homosexual tendencies (these may have been from the early oral or anal period, or have taken place during the phallic phase by way of enormous emphasis on the phallus and phallic abilities
4. Fixations of excessive attachment or dependency for a certain parent
5. Exposure to traumatic experiences at a sensitive period, such as those connected with witnessing intercourse or childbirth, premature seductive behaviors from adults toward the child, or fear of genital injury connected with a horror of the female body or perception of the male genitals as ugly

However, even if all these factors are present, a homosexual outcome still cannot be predicted. Too many chance circumstances intervene to permit prediction with any degree of reliability. How the above necessary, but not sufficient, factors occur, and also at what developmental period they occur, is important. This means the balance between heterosexuality and homosexuality during the developmental period is so precarious, and so many influences can operate favorably or adversely, that only weightings with a low degree of probability can be given until adolescence is over and the final object choice established.[40]

With these strictures in mind, once adolescence has arrived there are signs and symptoms customarily used as indicators of sex-role conflict which may eventuate in an adult homosexual character:

1. Maintenance of a pattern of preferred or exclusive homosexual activity which arouses little anxiety or guilt in the adolescent
2. Lack of heterosexual interests or activities as well as masturbation involving heterosexual themes
3. Masturbation fantasies primarily with homosexual themes or sado-masochistic content
4. Earlier developmental fixations originated by family configurations which have permitted or fostered strong female identifications in the boy and male identifications in the girl possibly due to absent or inadequate parenting by the same sex, or parental conflict

These conflicts are frequently in operation at the time of adolescence; the pattern for boys is that of the weak father and domineering, harsh mother, and for girls a similar dread of the mother with a feeling of intense aggression that emerges in adolescence.

5. An enormous amount of conscious anger and rage accompanied by few heterosexual interests

Two seemingly unrelated phenomena occur: one is a fear and anxiety concerning any type of sexual activity in which, when the conscious hostility has abated for a period, the threat of sexuality arouses fear; the other is a series of heterosexual performances in which the overcompensatory demonstration of coital stamina betrays something that must be disquieting to the mental equilibrium of the adolescent. In some of these cases, reaction formations emerge against the anxiety in the form of ascetic pursuits alternating with excessive indulgence in sensual exploits. The pseudomasculinity serves to deny the latent female wishes in the boy and simultaneously permits aggression against the contemptible female who is felt to be part of themselves.

6. A persistent love relationship with an older member of the same sex, based on homosexual love, which may have been initiated by a homosexual surrender

At that time a cognitive awareness occurred. The danger is in the form of regressive features in which the sexual object is the original parental love object.[42] It is interesting to see how in some cases the adolescent permits himself to be used or abused by the adult once a relationship has commenced, although there may also be fights and make-ups. In one case a quite attractive sixteen-year-old girl had been carrying on this type of relationship with a seventy-year-old woman for three years. She initially made inquiry about therapy on her own, using a false name "so that I can see her and know I won't lose her."

7. Homosexual behavior may recur if it is abruptly curtailed (Conversely, homosexual behavior may be expressed in many neurotic or neurotic character problems, such as thefts)

THE EGO IN ADOLESCENCE

The psychology of the ego is a fitting topic for a monograph in its own right, but a synopsis will be given of the relevant developmental material pertaining to adolescence. Ego functioning in adolescence is of great interest since it encompasses a period of life in which both pathological and conflict-free functioning are evident in extreme manifestations. This is particularly striking in dealing with the experiential component of adolescence, real and sought for: the feeling of bodily and psychological relationship with time and content variables which may involve either a feeling of uninterrupted continuity with what went before, or ego fragmentation.[43]

The ego as the seat of experience assumes predominance in adolescence. But it is only the beginning of exploration. The experiential component of the adolescent is not taken as the core of adolescent psychology, but rather a means to what lies behind certain modes of experiencing and what reactions are set in motion. The biological impetus to action stirs the adolescent as no other period is capable of doing with the same intensity. How the adolescent copes with the upsurge of demands, and proceeds to the development of a more perfect type of mental structure, the hypothesized ego, is merely another viewpoint on adolescence: a functional definition arising out of interaction from both the physical aspects of the body and its drive derivatives and the impingement of the environment. A few of the distinctions in terms of ego psychology will be given in the course of this discussion.

Unconscious Contributions. While the focus of this material is on the ego utilizing a structural viewpoint, topographical formulations regarding maturational systems operate as well. This is to emphasize that though the behaviors of the adolescent appear overt and compelling, they are also complex manifestations of drive life. Conscious, preconscious, and unconscious intent permeate different thoughts, acts, and feelings. While the psychology of adolescence can longitudinally attempt to confine itself solely to aspects of consciousness, this omits so many of the determinants of behavior that the psychology of the adolescent is oversimplified to a distorted degree. While routine acts may not require complex formulations of multiple motives, as a rule multiple motivations are prominent in the interpersonal area as well as in the intrapsychic sphere.[44] The goal is to avoid the fallacy of confining motivational formulations to symptom formation or psychopathology.

Having set this as a working principle, let us modify it to a practical principle that unless there is a need to look beyond the obvious, little may be gained by doing so when dealing with large numbers of adolescents. (Clearly, when some course of deviant development appears, or symptoms are emerging, we must look beyond the apparent.)

A great deal of the psychological life of the adolescent, unless he is conflicted, involves ego functions in which conflict may be present but not controlling. Nor is it desirable to utilize knowledge and portray idealistic or altruistic strivings of the adolescent as nothing but derivatives from drives and therefore something to be criticized. This type of degenerate fallacy is all too prominent where a little knowledge is a dangerous thing. First of all, the end result of the act has to be evaluated on its own merits, and secondly this may be a very desirable technique for the adolescent to secure gratification and hence greater psychological integration. The resultant act is not a disguise but a tapered end result which has been permitted this expression by the ego. Danger occurs when filtering by the ego is absent or minimal. Only a small amount of experience can be conscious at any one time, and resort is had to the vast realm of preconscious explanations which permit integration to extend beyond the immediate, yet not involve the repressed or unavailable.[45] Many of the efforts of past perceptions, affects, acts, and cognitive processes are available in the preconscious reservoir and some of the object representations which continue to shape behavior and self-image.

A provocative issue, especially pertinent to the adolescent, concerns the relative degree of unconscious content compared to that of the past several preceding decades. There is a possibility that there is relatively less unconscious content in the psychological make-up of the contemporary adolescent. While many acts or thought processes are carried out in the absence of a self-reporting system which satisfactorily accounts for why we think and act the way we do, it may be that there is less need to repress what was previously handled in such a manner.

Lack of repression does not affect formulations about the level of primitive unconscious motivation operating by primary process criteria and involving prelogical cognitive operations characteristic of id functioning. Instead it involves unconscious motivation connected with ego and superego functions, which pertain more to the area of fantasies and daydreams, and the implications for the adolescent in society if they are kept less repressed and organized.

Many fantasies and daydreams involve elaborations of wishes and goals, but they also help delineate the adolescent from others. Failure to repress certain drive derivatives may interfere with the delineations of the body and self, and the autonomies of each, and make the adolescent more prone to periodic questions regarding who is a friend and who is an enemy. There is a tendency to experience himself as participating with and through others. While sociologists theorize about this as a shift from an inner-directed to an outer-directed man, psychologically it leaves the individual vulnerable to slights, disappointments, and seeing himself as wronged. It is a short step to see himself as being a victim of society which therefore deserves the results of his vented rage. The result is that much of what may have been repressed into the unconscious ego stays conscious. Other defense operations are utilized more readily, and the balance between the unconscious ego shifts to the conscious.

The Ego as Organizer. Another by-product of this shift is that the capability of the ego to organize experiences becomes impaired. In contrast with the pressing needs connected with id-based activities, a certain degree of time and leisure are required to organize myriad experiences. Part of this is related to the development of the reality-testing part of the ego (discussed later) without which perceptions, thinking, feelings, and decision-making stay on a preconscious level. Put another way, delays or distortions of development of secondary process thinking are more likely to occur. With fewer demands from the environment to handle feelings and impulses via fantasies or sublimations, qualities associated with secondary process thinking are affected adversely.

Inherent to the development of secondary process thinking is the interposition of delays between wishes and gratifications. With the pressing upsurge for gratification in adolescence, another developmental crisis is presented in terms of whether further elaboration of these types of thought processes will occur. What might be taking place under the impact of cultural change is a neglect of one mode of thought for another.

While the most mature mental organizations utilize much that is not realistic or logical, the distinction is between regression in the service of the ego for creative activities versus impulse-dominated types of activities which utilize few creative processes. The gradual ability to tolerate ambiguity, which has been evolving since infancy, assumes increased significance at adolescence. This is not only from the drive upsurge, but from the relevance for furthering internalization processes as well as self-representations. If cognitive and perceptual activities such as reasoning, recall, memory, decision-making, and imagining are to proceed in place of immediacy, the adolescent must have the opportunity for delay.

In one sense we have come full circle with the adolescent as well as with our culture. For a long time the emphasis was on the inhibited person while now the quantitative problem has shifted to those little given to introspection or the use of imagination. The need for the concrete and the experiential rather than the abstract and reflective has assumed pre-eminence. It is as though the weakened ability to tolerate delay heightens aggression and impulsivity but does not lead to other types of solutions for dealing with desires.

The role of modeling, identification, and internalization is vitiated either by the adolescent who does not perceive the model as necessary, or by options which bypass delay and do not permit the time to further these processes within the adolescent. In this sense conflict itself fosters delay and the type of pondering which leads to decision-making. This is not an argument to justify a line of development toward obsessional neuroses, but an indication of danger if certain types of cognitive ego functions do not develop by the time adolescence is reached.

Rather than confining their techniques to denial or repression as does the younger child, the adolescent is expected to renounce or postpone gratification. Since immediate solutions for conflict are not always available, the ability to tolerate indecision becomes an important measure of ego strength. In summary, various factors contribute to impulsive qualities in contrast to secondary process thinking. These are not exclusive, but rather overlap and involve such things as cultural opportunity not to delay, mechanisms for handling frustration, use of certain cognitive ego functions and identification models, and exposure to the need for delay and tolerance of conflict.

Continued Ego Growth. The essential antecedents required for continued ego growth during adolescence are:

1. A maturation of perceptual processes, so that a progressive differentiation and selectivity can respond to stimuli with greater refinement than when the child was younger. Reality testing must progress, so that guided and modulated demands can be made. The ego must achieve sufficient distance from both the id and the external world to maintain autonomy. Without the former the adolescent is prone to act out impulsively to an exaggerated extent; without the latter the adolescent is no better than a bundle of reinforcement schedules without personal integrity.

2. A degree of reality testing sufficient to interact without severe distortion must be present. Included in any semblance of adequate reality appraisal are such fundamentals as delineation of other people, separating objects in the world from one another and from one's self, and a delineated body- and self-image. It becomes a matter of degree, coupled with the vulnerability of a given adolescent to distorted boundaries.

The most common distortion is the use of projected identifications, in which the adolescent expects others to react according to his projected needs. There are also distorted body perception experiences accompanying an increase in narcissism. Confusion about gender identity is discussed in a separate chapter.

A sufficient degree of correspondence must be present for a given individual to ensure that his personal and social life are not bent in the direction of misinterpretations. Not all parts of reality can be given equal importance in view of the heightened importance possessed by some parts of the body, such as the mouth or body shape.[46]

How closely the self-image of the adolescent corresponds to how others see them fluctuates between two extremes. In some respects they overvalue themselves, while in others they downgrade themselves to a degree that is pathological. While these exaggerations correspond to adolescent mood swings, in other respects they reflect unique superego development. Obviously, conflict distorts this view of reality. With adolescents, distortion occurs when there are discrepancies between private myths conflicting with those of the larger world. To maintain family myths in the face of contrary experiences, or behaviors that defy them, is not only a distortion of reality but is one more factor enhancing psychopathology.

3. By adolescence a flexible use of fantasy should have been achieved. This is not the world of fleeting part-objects of infancy, nor

the childlike playing out of the latency-age child. Fantasy is required to aid in the delay of gratification when interferences from reality conflict with what is desired and can also be used for creative, academic, or vocational pursuits. Without fantasy, enjoyment of the arts is impossible beyond a purely sensory level.

4. Verbal and cognitive abilities representing true inner and outer reality serve several goals. In terms of ego development they are related to abstract thought processes, to the ability to confirm perceptions with others by verbalization, and to the substitution of thoughts for action. Language is a precise and flexible way of interacting with others, which shows subtle shades of meanings with respect to loves and hates that need not be acted on. Precision allows reformulations of how one views the world, for the inaccessible can be challenged verbally. The more precisely he can verbalize what is happening, the closer the adolescent is to an asymptote of reality testing. Yet the adolescent can escape precision by using private language: personal privacy is distinguished from delusion formation which is not subject to confirmation, verbal or otherwise.

The adolescent is also vulnerable to the overvaluation of words. This dovetails with the use of intellectual defenses in which verbalizations assume more real qualities than experiences. Magic and ritual, private and public, resort to verbal incantations. When pushed to the psychopathological this is seen in personal or public emphasis on obsession as an end in itself. Variations in linguistic styles and expressions in adolescents under stress reveal their vulnerability, most dramatically during psychotic episodes when a regression to concretism, metaphor, allusion, babbling, or mutism occur.

Although refinement of defensive processes permits further control of drive life under ego domination, it is in the realm of maturation of adaptive devices where adolescent growth is seen most vividly. Conflict-free ego developments are the well-known sequences of development studied in normal psychology (motor development, perception, and cognitive development in Piagetian modes, as well as perfection of preconscious thought processes which foster adaptation to the environment with a minimum of effort). These adaptations occur in daily activities as well as in areas where the complicated meshing of biological talents with psychological adaptations produce achievements. The need for social reinforcement is seen most clearly in artistic or athletic achievements, as an unconscious process of refinement.

Conflict-Free Ego Functioning. A difference exists between ego functions which are conflict-born and the conflict-free functions, which originate independently. A conflict-free ego sphere does not mean this part of the ego is immune from conflict, but that secondary conflicts may develop (the distinction being that in primary autonomy certain ego activities develop independent of conflict, and therefore are not drive-dependent). There is still a connection with drive discharge, and primary autonomous functions can, in time, become involved in conflict. The most common example of impairment in an originally conflict-free function is interference with motor reactions. Earlier in history this was strikingly observed in hysterical paralysis. Conversely, functions used in the course of drive gratification, or defensively against drives, or in conflict resolution, can undergo a change of function and become a means of adaptation referred to as the development of secondary autonomy.[47] While the origin of these functions has begun in conflict, they can become emancipated in a secondary way.

Adaptation involves processes connected with both conflict-born and conflict-free areas of the ego. While greater conflict is seen during adolescence, more adaptive abilities are present, both in the sense of primary and secondary autonomy. In this the ego is described adaptively. Combinations of defensive and adaptive activities are seen where sexual or aggressive drives are transformed into more neutral activities. By this process of neutralization, derivatives of the sex drive may be sublimated to achieve gratification (desexualization), while aggressive derivatives are handled in the form of tapered expressions, which emerge as competitive pursuits or channeled aggression into creative ventures. The closer to the surface the sexual or aggressive drives are, the anxiety is more threatening. In turn, the adolescent is more coerced and experiences less freedom.

Systematics of the Adolescent Ego. This background permits us to consider some of the theoretical issues concerning the ego in adolescence. The fluctuating state of the ego does not have the same implications for someone past adolescence.

Theoretically, there is an advantage in appraising the ego during adolescence from the changes in drive organization that are occurring. In addition, the ego's reactive qualities of adapting, or failing to adapt, to new and different environmental demands can be seen more easily in statu nascendi. The strength of ego development from preceding experiences undergoes a type of experimental evaluation. Without the presence of adequate devices to buffer the adolescent against new demands of increasing magnitude, acting out may occur. Certain ego activities may lag in development or take on a quality of exaggerated precocity. Neurotic symptoms or peculiarities of character may emerge.[48]

In other cases conservative tendencies to protect what functioning does exist tend toward withdrawal. One difficulty that emerges with the onset of puberty is where the ego growth that should have occurred during latency is not present. Leisure to facilitate mechanisms to handle impinging stimuli by receptive and integrative devices may have been kept at the more disorganized level characteristic of the oedipal or preoedipal child.

While some of these children have been products of family or social disorganization, others have been exposed to excessive stimulation. Overstimulation may take the form of erotic aggressive behaviors which keep the child in a state of suspended animation. In this predicament the child cannot terminate tension and is blocked from integrating these activities. The upsurge of drives at puberty tends to be overwhelming due to deficient cognitive controls. Not only may learning be interferred with by the prominence of sexual and hostile feelings and impulses, but autonomous ego functions may be impaired.

In the absence of earlier identifications and internalizations which strengthen self-control, the adolescent enters a period of greater stress with predisposed vulnerabilities. From deficient internalization, the dependency on external objects as the primary or sole regulator of self-esteem is striking. Related to this deficit is the absence of the progressive utilization of language.[49] These phenomena are not so much regressive as developmental abortions of ego functions that are required if adolescence is to be confronted on its own terms.

It is important to realize that not everything in adolescent disequilibrium is a failure of defenses to control anxiety or other painful affects. Symptoms may be a result of the strength of drive expression. There may also be an inability of the ego to direct the impulses into areas where discharge is possible. In other words, symptoms can result from the crude state of the ego not being adequate to handle the more advanced demands made on it.[50]

Defense mechanisms are used to control or stabilize ego states and behaviors; however, other devices such as adaptive techniques exist. There are also restitutive or compensatory techniques. Ego deformations result when the adolescent withdraws from activities or interests which threaten him. In some cases this leads to ego splitting and disociative phenomena.[51] These devices are not independent, since they may be used either together. Even utilization of defense mechanisms cannot be viewed as an isolated phenomenon, since these, too, may have adaptive aspects. To deny, avoid, or intellectualize will have ramifications in terms of how any individual reacts. While a certain behavior may be adaptive for a given adolescent, this does not mean that conflict should be avoided with the outside world (witness the adolescent ego which challenges the status quo).

The phenomena of adolescent mourning and mood swings are inevitable—and necessary—occurrences in the normal psychology of the adolescent. These phenomena are associated with the increased narcissistic quality in which objects outside the self are not sought out. Depersonalization experiences result from ego splitting, and the accompanying phenomenology involves intellectual or philosophical quests directed to establishing identity. The duration indicates how upsetting object shifts are, and how tenaciously they may strive to maintain the narcissistic position. When narcissistic gratification has been highly dependent on parental ties and indulgences, the need for emancipation and new object ties induces even more profound ego states of moodiness.

Adolescent homesickness has not been studied in enough detail for what it can teach us. Instead it has been handled cavalierly as a manifestation of separation anxiety. While narcissistic withdrawal at the expense of the objective world seems to produce a heightened state of ego experience, what is usually experienced, in addition to mood swings, is an impoverished ego state from the "giving up of the world." When efforts are made to rediscover the world via new object ties euphoric states may appear and be superseded by depressive states when old object ties make their claim. Seeking new experiences alternates with old patterns in which neither are totally acceptable and phase-specific cyclothymia results. Moods, in contrast to the reactive qualities of affective states, do not relate to any specific content or object but rather become attached to varying feelings, thoughts, and acts. Moods are a sensitive barometer of the adolescent's state of mind or ego state.[52]

SPECIFIC EGO FUNCTIONS

The ego functions significant in the life of the adolescent are:

1. Reality testing
2. Executive ego functions
3. Cognitive ego functions
4. Object relationships
5. Autonomous functions
6. Synthetic functions
7. Defense mechanisms

Early precursors of ego functioning are conceptualized in the literature in terms of the purified pleasure ego, in which everything good or pleasurable is part of the ego and everything bad or discomforting is not. As the ego evolves it views itself as part of the self but not in the broadest sense. As a hypothetical construct, the ego is usually defined either functionally or experientially. While early theorizing postulated that the ego differentiated from the id by modifications induced by contact with external reality, Freud came to believe that certain ego functions have an inherent biological basis in the individual and develop in their own right.[53] Hartmann viewed this as an early undifferentiated matrix from which ego functions developed.[54] Ego development is discussed in terms of the development, interaction, and operation of its separate functions.

Reality Testing. When one of the most important ego functions, reality testing, is impaired, the ramifications for all the other functions of life are profound. There are three ways this occurs in adolescence:

1. An impaired sense of reality can lead to depersonalization experiences and the perennial "Who am I?"

2. If the impairment proceeds to a degree where the adolescent is not sure of what reality is, his testing of reality has been compromised. Severe cases show blurred object boundaries. This may represent psychotic behavior or temporary fluctuation of an ego state in the adolescent.

3. Without adaptation, the best intentions and abilities lie dormant or lead to maladaptive choices. While early psychoanalytic theory formulated this in terms of the pleasure principle subsuming itself to the reality principle, cognitive psychology has emphasized

the terms of the child going from a self-centered to an objective view of the world.[55]

Recent Piagetian theory has used the concept of egocentrism as a lack of differentiation in some area of subject-object interaction.[56] Of great relevance to the reality-testing function is the characteristic of formal operational thought, which permits the adolescent to conceptualize the thoughts of others. A common difficulty is the failure to pay attention to the preoccupations of others compared to the adolescent's own concerns. This not only may predispose the adolescent to misinterpret others, but his egocentrism may cause him to believe that others are more concerned—positively or negatively—about him than they really may be. It is as though the adolescent were living in front of an audience.[57]

Pushed to an extreme, lack of differentiation manifests itself in adolescent megalomania. When it is pointed out that the original ideas have been available for some time, the adolescent continues to feel superior since he believes he went through the same processes of original thought as the individuals who made the prior discoveries.

Both family expectations and social realities contribute to adolescent reality problems. A parent who invests his need for omnipotence in a child fosters fantasies of specialness. In the contemporary world adolescents can quickly become immersed in a level far beyond their capacities or talents. A distorted view of things gives a special importance. Depressions and outbursts of rage can be expected during the transition to a world in which far less importance attaches to the individual.

Executive Functions.   Such diverse activities as basic locomotion, manipulation, and language, are executive functions of the ego. Masturbation has been discussed, but in terms of executive ego functioning, questions should be raised about it occurring to excess. This is not because of possible physical harm, but because when an adolescent masturbates routinely several times daily he may suffer from ego dyscontrol. These behaviors must be seen as developmentally different during adolescence.

Cognitive Ego Functions.   The widest variety of psychological activities studied by normal psychology are listed here as an extremely important area of ego functioning since they involve perception, reasoning, and memory. Their intact functioning goes a long way toward furthering successful mastery of the environment. Difficulties show up in the form of impairment in abstract thinking, predominance of egocentric thought patterns, reliance on magical hopes, difficulties in giving expression to feelings, and on to the cognitive correlations of schizophrenia, perhaps one of the earliest and most subtle signs of such a deviation.

Object Relationships. As the sine qua non of human development, object relations include such theoretical topics as attachments, dependency, narcissism and shifts from the self to the broader world of objects.[59] Deviations vary from psychotic courses of development, manifested in object fusions and misconstructions, to a paranoid community. Common varieties of this function in adolescence are seen in dependency expectations and reactions to disappointments. Crushes and hero-worship are encompassed in this area, as are attachments to inanimate objects or animals, such as pets or horses. Rejection and slights in human relationships with peers and adults is a major theme. The whole area of identification is only mentioned as one crucial variable in terms of adolescent object relationships.

Autonomous Ego Functions. Autonomous ego functioning is separate from ego functions based on conflict. The point requiring emphasis with all of the autonomous functions is that the ego is far more than a developmental by-product of how it responds to drives.[60] That the ego has an independent course of development which requires assessment at all stages is obvious, and so is the fact that one or more of these autonomous functions have the potential for conflict. Even when it emerges during adolescence, conflict is neither inevitable nor permanent. Accommodations and variations account for some of the uneven progression and regression of functions where there is a startling aptitude in one area with malfunction in others. It is difficult in some cases to evaluate the extent to which a disturbance of autonomous functions has progressed. Is it a temporary lag, an inhibition stemming from neurotic conflict, or a result of earlier and undetected arrests in the development of a certain function which have become apparent during adolescence? These possibilities challenge the best of clinicians.

Synthetic Ego Function. The most basic defense of the ego which sustains an individual and protects him against psychological dissolution is the synthetic ego function.[61]

Organizing function is a more descriptive phrase since it includes elements of differentiation as well as integration. A number of experiences have occurred in the ego over the course of development, some from environmental stimuli and some from internal stimuli, and they have all required some type of assimilation and integration. Synthesis serves to reconcile conflicting ideas or unite contrasts. The establishment of causal thinking by way of a sequential chain is a requirement for synthesis—a problem originally posed for psychology and philosophy in the modern age by the philosopher David Hume, who stressed the unpredictability of any future event based merely on its occurrence in the past.[62] Spatial or temporal proximity provides a causal nexus based on habitual associations.

Within cognitive psychology, Piaget went far beyond this in efforts to give a developmental nexus to the idea of causality in the child. The infant originally seemed to form causal associations between his own acts and resultant events. A subjective feeling of causality was associated with the consequences of his own acts, which led philosophers to call this free will. Hence, psychological impulse of the child is taken as the cause of occurrences. However, the infant originally did not have such a volitional sense of his own movement, so the explanation was later imposed. In fact, up to the period of adolescence there is difficulty in expressing causal relationships.[63] Until what Piaget referred to as a function of organization, or a regulatory function of the intellect, is present, a consistent explanation by logical deduction is difficult, if not impossible.

While failure to give causal explanations may be little more than a developmental problem, when causal explanations do occur they have similarities to the process of secondary elaboration in dreams. This gives greater plausibility to the primary process content which does not obey the rules of logic as known in the waking state. While awake, apparent contradictions and inconsistencies are handled by their elimination from ego scrutiny.

The most typical manifestation seen in the adolescent is rationalization for his behavior, while the more fragile adolescent is likely to summon semi-plausible explanations. The need to explain what is happening is connected with some degree of cognitive satisfaction and anxiety reduction. The limitation is that these values may be attained at the cost of achieving a synthesis. For some, the thought disorder emerges under the classification of dementia praecox, which begins in adolescence. In others, periodic states of confusion or disorganization result. If the integration is successful, it promotes not only a broader and more objective view of the world but it may foster creativity by way of synthesizing diverse sources of information or data.[64]

Defense Mechanisms in Adolescence. Defenses are so important they are given a separate section. Only the most important defenses employed by the adolescent will be reviewed under two main groupings:[65]

Defenses Against Attachments to Objects

Displacement
Reversal of Affect
Increase in Narcissism
Regression

Defenses Against Impulses

Repression and Denial
Asceticism
Intellectualization
Noncompromise
Isolation

Defenses against attachment to objects arise more prominently during adolescence due to increased striving for autonomy. The goal is to change the situation in which the adolescent has grown up or to alter the responses of people in the environment. Old object ties, with their loves and hates, are what pose the conflict that elicits defensive efforts.

Displacement mechanisms are most clearly seen when the adolescent leaves the family. This need not be a literal leavetaking, but a withdrawal to the status of a boarder in the home. Rather than gradually severing object ties within the family matrix, the adolescent leaves in an exaggerated way, seeking attachments elsewhere. Parental substitutes are sought with individuals or institutions.

The substitute may have to be quite far removed or disguised from the original parent. Unresolved longings show up in fluctuation from one type of attachment to another. For some adolescents this takes the form of ambivalent attachments to and attacks upon groups. Fleeting close attachments followed by angry rejection to churches or political institutions may serve such purposes. Individuals often serve as foils which arouse competitive jealousies in parents as well.

Other adolescents adopt parental roles and therefore disown the childlike state by ministering to those more dependent or younger.

The vulnerability of the adolescent to corrupt demagogues becomes clear when the displacement mechanism is clarified. The adolescent trying to separate from the family may replace them with what really are other family members in disguise. Unfortunately, it is common to choose a leader or hero whose ideals provoke serious difficulties. The adolescent with conflicts in the area of authority figures is quite vulnerable to turbulent periods of violent protest or pacifism. Yet by displacements the adolescent feels more comfortable internally, since he has temporarily removed his anxiety about other close attachments.

Reversal of affect in adolescents is used when they cannot achieve the degree of object separation which displacement permits. Rather than seeking displaced objects, they war within themselves and their family with overtones of strong hate and protest. Their ambivalence is such that they cannot effectively separate; they are compelled by old loves to ask for independence, but in reality do little about it. This shows up in passive-aggressive features mixed with active sarcasm about parental ways. In this way a masochistic bond is maintained to the family since compulsive disobedience is just as crippling as compulsive obedience.

To make reversal of affect work, two subsidiary mechanisms are needed. Denial of past and present attachments is coupled with reaction formations which preclude sympathy or attitudes of respect. An ominous transition is seen when the adolescent ego experiences hostility as intolerable and proceeds to project hate onto others and then to protect himself. An ego rupture leading to an outburst of violence may occur. In other cases the hostility may be directed against the self as a depression with moody withdrawal punctuated by attempts at escape.

> An attractive fifteen-year-old girl fell in love with a series of boys. They were all quite appealing to her, and she often tried to avoid returning home. This led to parental conflict. While home she either attacked her parents' boring existence or found herself feeling guilty about her attacks on them. Letters to her friends, left about her room by her to be discovered, were filled with comments about her hate for her parents. At other times sadness for her parents interfered with her ability to enjoy herself when she was out. A miscarried attempt at reversal of affect had resulted in a moody, depressive-prone adolescent.

Narcissism has been mentioned in a developmental context. As a defense it is employed when attachments outside the family are difficult to achieve. Narcissism can affect the ego and superego. Grandiose fantasies of unlimited potential or power, or fantasies of achieving great success or popularity are from the ego. Those dominated by a strong superego display suffering or self-sacrifice. Hypochondriasis can be a defense against attachment to objects.

Regression occurs on both ego and id levels, serving to maintain old object ties, and tempering separation anxieties from parents. In extreme cases regression may be to a level of primary identification with objects where characteristics of the self become fused with others and vice versa. Blurring of object boundaries leads to projection as well. Another possibility is the development of the "as if" character structure, discussed elsewhere. In this the main technique of relating to others is by taking on the attributes of someone else. This is not relating to these objects but merely trying to be like them. Genuine affect is blocked and its submergence threatens the defensive balance. Such an escape from feelings and attachments is a precarious one.

Related is a "fear of emotional surrender,"[66] or of involving oneself in any close relationship. In some cases this has overtones of sexual fears, in which passivity is the threat. Emotional closeness or love implies a type of submitting to another to be maltreated. This is either resisted or surrendered to.

When defenses against attachments fail and the adolescent is prevented from emancipating, impulses emerge and defenses are created. The first attempt is usually denial, or disowning the impulses. While temporarily successful in allowing the trappings of family life to be maintained with a younger child, this is an unwieldy defense. Repression of impulses serves to avoid confrontation, but if perpetuated leads to the avoidance of many activities and gratifications.

Asceticism implies a protest against some (and sometimes all) impulses. It may extend against basic physiological needs such as sleep and food. This is an instinctual anxiety where the ego is threatened with being overwhelmed. Gradations between degrees of impulse gratification and being inundated by impulses appear to be lost. Pleasure comes to the fore and the ego interferes with pleasurable experiences accompanying drive gratification.

Some of these defenses become obsessional when attempts are made—by way of rituals or gestures—to ward off drives. Masochistic pleasure, in which suffering becomes one of the main sources of gratification, also appears in some cases. Starvation periods to the extreme of anorexia nervosa alternating with bulimia illustrate the ever-present tendency to indulge in massive breakthroughs of impulse life, leading to orgies followed by condemnations for beastliness and purification rites.

For some, little acts of denial are accumulated only to sanction indulgence to a limited extent (witness the fads concerning diets). Physical exercises or muscle-building programs may be used with a certain degree of suffering as well. In other cases techniques of superego bribery are permitted, in which a given set of practices permits other types of indulgences.

Intellectualization is available from cognitive development which permits abstract thinking to take place with a passion. To use this capacity defensively requires, in addition, that the social setting be one where thought processes are valued. Intellectualization seeks to make a connection between drives and ideational content. In this way drives are perceived as more under ego control which can operate in the area of words and intellect as an active coping device to handle aggression. Various philosophical, political, and ethical discussions reflect this defense.

Most striking is the discrepancy between the commitment to the intellect and the heated passion typically present in discussions. Rationalizations and displacements are often required to maintain the intellectual position, perhaps because the defense is being challenged in the discussion. In fact, arguments mirror the conflicts against which the adolescent is defending himself. As adolescence progresses defensive operations participate in a definitive character structure which shape special aptitudes or choices of work or continued schooling. Of course, the danger with any defense is that it may be pushed to an extreme. When this occurs with intellectualization, the risk becomes psychopathological in the form of crippling obsessional ruminations rather than action and rational decision-making.

Noncompromise is a defense against impulses modeled on taking a rigid and nonarguable position about something parents or authorities have set careless standards about. It occurs in the behavioral or ideational areas that are most threatening to the adolescent.

An adolescent boy, whose mother was a prostitute, assiduously avoided any contact with girls. He entered a seminary and thereafter devoted his intellect to creating a world where sexual needs were subject to elimination by higher pursuits. This comprom-ise revealed the condensation of intellectualization with noncompromise. An adolescent girl, whose parents engaged in several extramarital affairs, demanded not only absolute loyalty in any potential marriage of her own, but found it intolerable as an adolescent for herself or a boy she dates to go out with others—an example of the all-or-nothing nature of noncompromise.

In a sense these positions have a connection to reaction formations by their rigid adherence to a position that may become exaggerated or caricatured. The main threat is that parents or peers are indulging in behavior an adolescent cannot comfortably entertain, even on an ideational level. Hence, an uncompromising position is taken against anything with traces of such indulgence.

Isolation refers to the separation of affect from content: a situation that could arouse anxiety becomes attached to something else. A degree of ego splitting is required, in which either affect or ideation are repressed. If this does not happen, a displacement of the affect to some other situation or object occurs. Isolation is also used to defend against the loss of objects. Blos discusses a similar defense which he calls "uniformism," in which the adolescent adopts a code of behavior permitting him to divorce feelings from action in the struggle of the ego against early object ties or drives.[67] In this solution sexuality may not be denied, but codified through the norms of a group. Experiencing emotion becomes progressively split off from the peer-sanctioned norm for behavior. While affect suffers, there is a semblance of security by way of the shared code of the group. Mutual dependency needs and recognition of sameness in one another's external behaviors permits the adolescent to avoid experiencing the affect that goes with personal involvement.

ADOLESCENT CHARACTER STRUCTURE

Questions related to adolescent character structure are a segment of the broader and more complex area of character formation in general. There are questions specifically germane to adolescence. Conversely, material pertaining to the changes of character structure in adolescence have relevance for the broader problem of character structure. To what extent are the character changes in adolescents the relatively final arbiters of the ultimate character structure of an individual? What are the developmental changes in character structure which occur during the course of adolescence? Has character structure been so decisively formed by the time adolescence is reached that what transpires is a matter of consolidating what has already been shaped?

Traits and Character Structure.   The problem of character traits, temperament, and dispositional tendencies is related to that of character structure. Some of the clinical difficulties are discussed later. In this section we will discuss the problem as a set of relatively fixed traits, attitudes, and types of responses. On the one hand there are unique differences which give individuality to a particular adolescent; on the other hand, stability is contingent upon a predictable environment in which behaviors elicit expected responses from others. This view of character gives greater recognition of the environment and culture than did earlier psychoanalytic formulations. Early formulations were drive-based, such as Abraham's emphasis on character traits being related to a certain level of drive development or fixation.[68] Problems such as the influence of oral erotism or character, determinants of the anal character, and how these early types of character formations developed to a genital level were once key questions.

Although inherited dispositional tendencies and upbringing were seen as significant influences, the stress was on elements of infantile sexuality which became excluded from adult sexual life or which continued to have the greatest influence on certain character traits. What resulted was a certain sum of instinctual reactions toward the environment. The position was maintained that the final determination of character was reached when the genital level was attained. Fused with the stage theory of character-determination was the economic model where the genital stage was parallel to narcissistic libido being transformed into object libido as a condition for object love to occur. Rather than the environment determining a certain character structure, it was the attainment of the genital stage which determined how one would participate in his milieu. The definitive event for character was the Oedipus complex, in view of the bearing this had on how the child would feel toward those with whom he interacted. Yet, having stated this, Abraham pointed out that setting up norms for normal character development was not something that psychoanalysis wished to do. They were too aware of the wide variations in individuals as well as the contributing factors of race, nationality, social class, and what could be induced by changing external circumstances.[69] Mutability of character was recognized both within the realm of psychopathology, in which shifts from oral to anal trait-dominance could occur, and also within the wide norms tolerated as nondeviant in which adaptation was the keynote.

Later developments gave more emphasis to the role of the ego. Reich introduced the defensive aspects of the ego as decisive, so that character came to be viewed as the typical mode of reaction of the ego to the id and the outer world.[70] This shift did not displace earlier formulations, but became a supplement. What has evolved today as the common theme in character development is the adaptive function served by a given character structure. Character structure is not merely the result of drive transformation, but of certain ego techniques and adaptations. Nor do these ego functions remain confined to a defensive status for a final contribution to character. Rather, what begins as a defense against certain drives can change.

Character Syntheses: Individuation. Character synthesis has been viewed as the essential therapeutic task to be mastered by the adolescent,[71] and as such, is crucially related to establishing ways for the ego to maintain equilibrium. The more these ways bind anxiety, or reduce conflict, the less conspicuous the character structure of any adolescent is. However, while the ultimate goal is a smooth, functioning integration, the changes occurring in personality organization of the adolescent rarely happen without some disruption or instability. In part this is due to the shift in drive life, although shifts within the ego itself give some flexibility. As in any other stage, developmental changes require new adaptations and solutions.

Blos has four necessary preconditions if adolescent character formation is to proceed: (1) a period of second individuation, (2) handling residual traumas, (3) maintenance of ego continuity, and (4) emergence of a sexual identity.[72] The first refers to the loosening of object attachments that have remained since earlier childhood. This is not conceptualized solely as a looseness from external objects, but as a disengagement from internalized representations of objects. Toward these internalized objects a mixture of hate and love exists which contributes to the particular type of personality structure. More specifically, not only does superego development take a particular twist contingent upon these object relations, but certain personality traits are reinforced.

Actually, the individuation, which is best accomplished in adolescence, is the culmination of one of the necessary and universal steps of development: diminishing emotional dependence on others. By biological necessity a mother-infant symbiosis takes place in which, over time, a transformation occurs into object relationships.

Mahler views the symbiosis of infancy as the necessary precursor for establishment of intrapsychic separation-individuation.[73] She has posited four subphases of separation as occurring during the infantile period:[74]

1. *Differentiation* occurs, beginning at five to six months and lasting to about one year of age, in which there is a gradual decrease of bodily dependence.

2. At approximately ten to fifteen months, a phase of *practice* takes place which overlaps with the phase of differentiation. In this period there is a great investment in motor skills and exploration of the environment.

3. *Rapprochement* lasts from age fourteen to twenty-two months. During this period the infant becomes more concerned with his mother's whereabouts when he separates from her.

4. Gradual separation is again attained during the period from twenty-five to thirty-six months, which is the product of attaining *object constancy*. This has an accompanying verbal progression and a sense of time which permits delay of gratification and more endurance of separation.

These early subphases are mentioned to indicate the developmental anlage of separation processes which continue throughout latency, and recrudesce in adolescence. As a group, these four subphases are considered in their totality as the first major separation stage.

Adolescence is viewed as the second major period of individuation.[75] The required shift in object relations in this period leads to a heightened vulnerability for psychopathology which cannot accurately be assessed by a brief glimpse of behavior. At any one time behavior can appear intact or regressed. During adolescence the main task of individuation is freedom from the degree of control that internalized objects have exerted. To the degree that this is handicapped, the adolescent is restricted to replications, substitutions, and displacements from these objects under a facade of autonomy. Failure to lay a gradual groundwork during earlier childhood for this individuation creates a set of antecedents from which character problems are likely to flourish. Overt parental support is further weakened during adolescence. Successful accomplishment of disengagement from the dependency objects—internal and external—is a hallmark of ego maturation as well as ego strength. Conversely, failure to disengage is indicative of fixation in the manner of handling drives and impairment in certain ego functions. Unless the adolescent has the freedom to handle drives in ways different from earlier ones, and to interact with different objects, he will be unable to make and maintain contacts on a mature level. Signs of failure to accomplish this appear in such ego disturbances as acting out, extreme negativism, violent protest, learning disabilities, depressive moods, and self-destructive activities.

Regressive tendencies are pervasive as part of the disengagement process. These tendencies can enhance development, or ensure that further separation and individuation will not occur. Enhancement takes place when the more advanced ego of the adolescent regresses, so that earlier types of drive expressions, object relationships, and conflicts can be reinvoked and integrated or abandoned. If this can be accomplished, a relative shift in the balance from id to ego takes place and the character structure takes on greater stability and predictability.

Regression may also be used to ensure that individuation does not take place. A frequent example is the occurrence of exaggerated efforts at separation, which are guaranteed to maintain the individual in subservient roles to others. Leaving home to live in disorganized settings, persistent truancy as a protest maneuver, or acts of exaggerated bravado are possibilities. Pushed far enough, different forms of institutionalization are the inevitable result. This is the ultimate in regressive dependency, whether the place of confinement is a hospital, a foster home, or a correctional facility. Institutionalization allows the adolescent the luxury of shifting responsibility to others to make decisions for him, thereby subverting separation and individuation as he simultaneously protests vehemently about the way he is being treated.

Handling Residual Traumas. A second condition for adolescent character development to proceed is containment of traumatic occurrences from earlier years. The concept of trauma entails several historical and theoretical issues. Trauma is not used in terms of any one single event, nor is it used in a restricted sense of a particular type, such as a sexual trauma. Yet specificity is needed for explanation, such as how traumatic occurrences contribute to adolescent character structure. Traumatic occurrences can mean everything from older notions of an overwhelming environment whose stimulation breaks through a stimulus barrier to pathogenic influences in general. Therefore, a brief digression into the meaning of the concept of trauma is necessary.[76]

From the perspective of ego development, a traumatic situation is experienced as helplessness in the face of accumulating excitation, which can be provoked by external as well as internal threats. Trauma can also occur in harmless environments which produce anxiety in a particular person on the basis of pre-existing constellations. Therefore, any event for which the defensive armamentarium is insufficient has the potential for trauma. Time permitting, and an ego adaptiveness or defense being available, a disequilibrium does not occur since characterological stabilization allows assimilation by the ego.

Yet the ego-syntonic solution is not necessarily permanent. Acknowledging individual differences and sensitivities, there is susceptibility during developmental periods in which characterological devices previously operating no longer suffice. Further, the enormous impact of a given environment is vitally important in terms of how a certain event will be reacted to. For example, a cohesive group with good leadership is far more able to tolerate adversity than is the lone individual among enemies. It is the latter situation, under the threat of trauma, which permits brainwashing. For the adolescent, the presence of identification models or peer groups can similarly contribute to the neutralization of what might otherwise be experienced as traumatic incidents.

What is an internal threat to the ego of one child may not be to another. External events to a particular child may be experienced as raising a particular type of anxiety, such as object loss or superego disapproval. Something wished for which appears close to fulfillment can also function as a trauma, such as a threatening sibling being injured, although some character structures might assimilate the event as ego syntonic. When events once traumatic no longer function in this manner, a state of potential helplessness or panic has been avoided by certain types of character developments.

Maintenance of Ego Continuity.   A third necessity for adolescent character development is a continuity of the ego. This pertains to the historical continuity of an identity essential to avoid ego fragmentation. The perpetual postponement of confrontation with the changes in demands being made on the adolescent is an ever-present danger. Adolescence may also be the time when discrepancies are perceived between what has been maintained as part of a family myth system and what the family configuration really is. This may precipitate acting out or psychotic regression. Lack of continuity between myths inculcated and internalized, and the perception of contradiction, disrupts the hoped-for continuity. Some individuals in their fourth and fifth decades are still using adolescent solutions to the awakening of family fraudulence. A sense of personal intactness and generational continuity are by-products of ego development from younger years and make a fundamental contribution to the stability of character structure in adolescence.

Emergence of a Sexual Identity. Though it will be discussed more thoroughly later, sexual identity is mentioned here as a necessary factor in the development of character structure. During adolescence less fluctuation in sexual identity is possible. Persistence of ambiguity regarding sexual identity during adolescence leads to confusion if bisexual identifications are too overt. Once adolescence has arrived, ambivalence has a drastic impact on character functioning, partly due to self-concept, but also because there is so little environmental acceptance of it after puberty.

ACHIEVEMENT

General Aspects. As with many of the other topics covered in this chapter on general aspects of adolescence, texts are written about any one topic. This is particularly so with regard to the problem of achievement. Comments could be restricted to a conventional approach dealing with academic achievement, or to subsequent vocational performance. There is also the problem of creativity, which can hardly be ignored as an achieving type of task or performance. Should creativity be restricted to artistic endeavor, or should it include the creative delinquent as well? In the same vein, athletic performance may involve aspects of achievement as well as creativity.

Perhaps the tenor of adolescent views and reactions to achievement is conveyed best by a statement about the culture which says, "The comparatively striking feature of American culture is its tendency to identify standards of personal excellence with competitive occupational achievement. In the pure type, the value attached to achievement does not comprehend the person as a whole, but only his accomplishments, emphasizing the objective results of his activity."[77] It is this cultural position which has given impetus to the backlash of a counter-culture which questions achievement as a hollow myth, or at best appraises it in terms of a skill that will sell.[78]

Three perspectives to achievement have held sway in academic writings: (1) a moralistic perspective, (2) an intellectual approach with a heavy emphasis on intelligence and cognition, and (3) a personality-social dimension.[79] Moralistic approaches to achievement place it in the context of a fusion of behaviors being rewarded in a sense of tangibility and virtue. The adolescent who applies himself, develops good study habits, is honest, dedicated, and assiduous, will not only get good marks but be promoted in the system to higher academic standing in the future. If the verbal and memory skills, which are correlated with academic achievement, are not in his repertoire, his diligent application may still be rewarded by advancement in some other field, such as a skilled trade, for which he strives to advance in a manner analogous to advancement in other fields; the emphasis is on diligence to service. So went the theory. The moralistic, if not inspirational, quality of the advocates of the hard-work school of rewards has elicited much criticism and mockery at times. Yet it would seem that the majority of achieving adolescents operate by such diligence. For those who seek the easiest rewards of advancement within the existing system, using the techniques maintained by most school systems appears to be the best guarantee.

The Role of Intelligence.   Once measurement of intelligence was introduced, another dimension of achievement emerged. Initial formulations stressed correlations, so that cross-group comparisons were put in terms of middle-class youths being greater achievers than lower-class youths based on differences in measured intelligence between the groups. Despite the continuing debate about the nature of intelligence, the basic issue pertains to whether intelligence tests measure anything independent of cultural opportunities, or whether they reflect primarily opportunities. Clearly, there remains a far-from-perfect correlation between IQ scores and academic achievement, when two students with the same measured intelligence achieve quite differently. Most relevant was Terman's follow-up study with individuals with very high IQ scores in which many failed to attain more than quasi-skilled occupational positions and showed very little of what anyone would describe as creativity.[80] This pointed out that intellectual factors alone, whatever their source, are insufficient to account for achievement.

Stress on Multiple Factors.   Terman's study led to investigation of multiple factors involved in achievement and a search for a single determining factor. Some stressed social variables, while others stressed psychological or personality factors.

A number of approaches are available within the personality-social-structure dimension, including motivational factors, variance in individual abilities, values, interpersonal and family dynamics, and peer influences. Social structure operates as a class status, modified by differences in socialization experiences within a class or ethnic group. Variations within such groups in training for independence and achievement, and the impact of the school as a social system in promoting achievement, competence, and the impact of teacher-pupil relations are all relevant. Several studies have been done on each of these factors in what seems like a never-ending quest for the roots of achievement.

Permeating discussions of achievement is the old question of how it is to be defined or measured. Most approaches take an instrumental approach based on competent task performance, or attainment of a certain status level. McClelland and his associates view the origins of achievement motivation in terms of learned motives for which training in excellence and mastery are the antecedents of achievement. The relationship of competition to self-esteem is seen as significant when there is failure to meet standards of excellence held out by the culture in the form of parental representatives inducing negative affect in the child. When competitive demands for meeting standards of excellence are met, they induce positive affect.[81] How attainment of standards of excellence by the adolescent are to be attained remains debatable. A circular quality is inherent in assessing achievement in terms of getting good grades, when getting good grades is also viewed as a mark of achievement. It is the same with other measures, such as attaining membership in certain social or academic groups, all of which have been used in different studies evaluating the adolescent achiever.

Evaluating Performance. Differentiating hierarchies of achievement in terms of performance attainments presents the same problems. Is one student achieving more by being on more committees than another? An eight-year follow-up of high school students found little relationship between occupational status or social prominence as an adult and social prominence in high school.[82] Is a higher grade point average to be taken as a valid index of greater achievement? While marks in high school are the most effective predictor of performance in college for groups of adolescents, exceptions are notable in both directions.[83] There is also the matter of relative continuity in skills, abilities, and habits. If intelligence is held constant, to what extent does the intensity of drive level toward goals become the main arbiter of achievement? This opens the entire grab bag of factors relevant to why certain ambitions have developed.

Modes of ambition are important as well. While two groups may be equally ambitious, their goals may vary widely.[84] One may seek to advance to a position of dominance or recognition within a group by virtue of a position or title; another individual seeks plaudits for his performance per se—be this in solving mathematics or running the hundred-yard dash. A further distinction is the relative degree of attainment for those who will be rewarded when their performance is something the group applauds, versus an internalized standard which persists in the absence of such external rewards. The former is achievement based on pleasing others versus the self. When achievement motivation is appraised in terms of fantasies with this theme on the Thematic Apperception Test (TAT), it appears related to the quality of the performance of certain tasks and the predominance of certain goals.[85] Yet longitudinal follow-up on groups of those rated high on achievement by this criterion during adolescence have failed to find any upward intergenerational mobility.[86] A deficit in the TAT as a measuring instrument is revealed in the discrepancy between tapping certain fantasies on the TAT pictures and how the child actually performs in the future.

Gender Differences.   Gender differences are a significant variable in achievement. Cultural norms influence the importance of social activities for girls; even though girls surpass boys in high school grades, they are less likely to enter college.[87] The self-esteem of most girls is more contingent on success in social relationships than on school grades. In a national survey of adolescents, assets for achieving popularity and social acceptance were mentioned three times as often by girls as boys as one of their worries.[88]

From a different perspective, female patients in the lower-middle-class are much more prone than their male counterparts to use their physical assets to get ahead—not only in high school by charming male teachers, but later in the business world as well.[89] In the past ambitious girls, not oriented toward a professional career, began to achieve in terms of what they anticipated the type of husband they marry will need to achieve. In time, this appears to continue via achievements through their children. At least for some women, this is now changing but raises other types of problems.

Several other variables operate with respect to achievement such as self-esteem. Success in any venture which has been assigned cultural value is likely to increase esteem, yet those who have an adequate sense of personal worth to begin with are more likely to achieve success in their undertakings. Similarly, the ambitious are more likely to achieve if other factors are constant. Certain types of cognitive traits, such as curiosity and seeking new ways of doing things, favor achievement. A belief that the environment is more under internal control, rather than subject to external whimsy, also favors a better performance academically.[90]

The Role of Anxiety. Anxiety in relationship to achievement is a timeworn yet still fascinating topic. Thirty years ago an attempt was made to study the implications of social anxiety on effective learning and mobility strivings.[91] Teachers and psychologists were observed to connect high anxiety with striving, since the latter was viewed as an anxiety-reduction maneuver. However, the gist of subsequent studies has been to show an inverse relationship between anxiety level and either school or test performance. High anxiety level is also seen as associated with low self-esteem.[92]

A different research strategy sought to evaluate the impact of anxiety about test performance and cheating.[93] Shelton and Hill studied forty-nine boys and sixty-two girls from a middle-class high school with the hypothesis of determining if the relationships between test conditions, anxiety, and cheating could be evaluated. Students were first told that they were to make up as many English words as possible from the word generation in eight minutes. After this, another test was given to measure anxiety about achievement. Third, another test was given and timed so that the students could not complete it. The next day the subjects were divided into three groups: *success* (They were told they had produced five to seven more words than a sample of good students from a different high school); *failure* (They were told they had produced five to seven words less than those in a hypothetical high school); and *controls* (No feedback information was given). The original number of words constructed was counted, but the papers were returned ostensibly uncorrected, accompanied by a master list of all possible words. *Cheating* was defined as the difference between the number of original words produced and those the subjects circled on the subsequent master list. Of the 111 subjects, 53 percent cheated. The results are impressive in that 56 percent of the success group cheated— apparently because the students had an enormous need to achieve even when it "didn't count." It might also have been possible that their insight into the fraudulent nature of their performance impelled them to try to keep up a false level.

While 61 percent of the failure group cheated, even 43 percent of the control group, who knew nothing about the relative standing, cheated. The groups were then divided into high, moderate, and low regarding achievement anxiety. A comparable percent of those in the success and the failure groups (91 and 83 percent respectively) cheated when anxiety was high, but even in those with a low level of anxiety, one-third cheated. Interpretations of these empirical findings stir many unresolved biases. Do they express a weakening of our moral fabric? In psychodynamic terms, do the findings reflect less internalization operating, or rather norms of achievement which have been so internalized that there is a need to meet them even under circumstances which mean nothing? The results do not basically change even when the comparison is made with specific, known friends instead of reference being made to an unknown reference group in another high school.[94]

The Impact of the Youth Culture.   Today, the entire question of achievement is being re-appraised by adolescents, as well as by many others, who see the concept as implying nothing more than the values of a dominant group. In recent decades, formulations of a youth culture have been used in discussions of the anti-intellectual oppositional values of the youth group.

The youth culture was originally described by Parsons in terms of two main criteria:[95] (1) an opposition to the adult world and what it stood for, and (2) the dominant influence of the sex-role standard in defining the behaviors, attitudes, and attributes of what is masculine or feminine. Such things as athletic prowess, sex-appeal, and an attractive personality are related to masculinity, while sex-appeal and popularity are related to femininity. Even at the time of Parson's study in the early 1950s, the youth culture was seen as giving little status to academic achievement. While academic achievement was tolerated if the other assets of the sex-role standard were present, it was not given much status in its own right. This work confirmed earlier formulations of academic indifference, or the acceptability of the gentleman's seat, as congruent with the sex-role standard.

The study by Coleman in 1961 supported this position.[96] Adolescents in ten high schools were ranked. Being an athletic star, or popular, was ranked ahead of being a brilliant student. Girls chose being a social leader or popular in preference to being a brilliant student as something they wanted to be remembered for. High academic achievers were less likely to be part of the leading crowd, but even more, those viewed as having high ability were not likely to be high achievers, illustrating the impact of the social setting which may be adverse to scholarship when it is possible. This was even more conspicuous among adolescent girls than boys. Of forty-nine girls in the leading crowd, not one wanted to be remembered as a brilliant student. Later, these girls will fear success.[97]

Academic achievement is viewed as particularly alien to the sex-role standard in males when it is combined with feminine characteristics and bookishness. It appears that for an athletic boy scholarship does not seem to matter—pro or con—which conveys the impact of athletics in the contemporary world of adolescents.

Personal attributes associated with academic success have long been known besides intelligence. High verbal ability, high self-esteem, a belief that actions count, and internalized controls, are usually cited. Argument has not centered on the value of these attributes, but rather on their source, nature, and ability to be developed once periods of development have been completed. Apart from individual factors, the interacting influences of the family, school personnel, teaching techniques, social class, and ethnic, religious and racial variables, all become relevant. Studies based on social class origins using grades, IQ scores, achievement motivation, and upward mobility goals show these to be class-correlated.[98]

Family Influences. Economic and political factors affect family influences on academic achievement. While a smaller number of boys from lower socio-economic families graduate from college, the likelihood of those ranked as possessing high ability to graduate was sixty-six times as high as boys who ranked with low ability coming from the same backgrounds.[99] In one sense, this begs the question as to what determines ability, but it also demonstrates that whatever such attributes are, they exert an influence. Of course, many longitudinal factors operate: low-income families receive poorer nutrition, poorer medical care for physical illnesses, a need to rely on community mental health facilities for emotional or learning problems, and living quarters which are either crowded or not conducive to fostering good learning habits. In some cases, direct economic need requires an adolescent to work for money, and although those adolescents who have a combination of achievement-promoting factors going for them can handle this, pursuits such as reading or participating in cultural events may have to be sacrificed. For others, lack of funds directly interferes with the opportunity to continue school.

Certain socialization and cultural patterns in homes are additional determiners of achievement. Elder has classified these into four influences: (1) achievement and training for independence, (2) goals, training, and ability, (3) modeling influences of parents for achievement and education, and (4) impact of the absence of a father.[100]

Families with achievers tend to have both explicit and implicit standards of excellence set by parents. Socialization practices have parental warmth, coupled with specific training for achievement and independence which the child performs autonomously, assuming responsibility for his actions. The research methodology employed in one study asked mothers what age their sons were expected to do such things as entertain themselves, make their own decisions, and work hard without assistance.[101] Of course, any survey study, based on what parents report, must be viewed with skepticism. All of these studies appear plagued by a lack of sufficiency in explanations. Perhaps the complexity of variables vitiates conclusions. The need to function in an independent and autonomous manner is probably as great in families in the lower socio-economic brackets, which are noted for their low contribution of achievers. Therefore, studies which find the mean age of achievement and independence training in preadolescents and mothers to be significantly higher in the working class than in the middle class may mean little.[102]

Subtle distinctions between a child being able to manage and being ranked as independent still leaves a large gap in achieving mastery. On the other hand, clinical work demonstrates the adverse impact, by the time adolescence is reached, of family configurations stressing the need for high achievement and independence. While the report may indicate that mothers of boys with high motivation are competent and aggressive, and demand these qualities in their sons, it is but a stone's throw to the adolescent who reacts to such demands by rebellion and negativism. The influence of mothers on achievement was seen in a Kagan and Moss study where boys who rated high on achievement from grade school to young adulthood were closely protected by their mothers in the first three years, but were thereafter placed under strong demands to achieve.[103] Maternal acceleration in elementary years was highly correlated with achievement behaviors of sons.

A cross-cultural study in Brazil found that an authoritarian father induced a feeling in a son that he has two alternatives available to him: revolt or submission.[104] This corresponds with observations of the reactions of fathers who are insecure in their own attainments and are put under further strain with a son who has the potential to compete or exceed him. However, all types of situations are possible. A son may identify with a dominant father, and if the father is a high achiever this may lead to emulation. Ambiguities and lack of agreement on what dominance implies permeate studies, which either fail to state this or attempt to compare studies using different criteria for dominance. Some use overt ratings of an observer, some employ psychometric devices, and others are aware of the covert and manipulative ways in which dominance can be exerted. While general socialization practices, such as explicit parental demands for academic achievement, disciplinary techniques for failure based on rational considerations, and the low use of physical punishments may all be relevant to the internalization of norms toward academic achievement, they would seem to provide a valid baseline in the absence of contravening influences from elsewhere.

Parental goal-setting, the second important family practice contributing to achievement, is influential if two qualifications are met: parental goals which correspond with the abilities of the adolescent to meet them, and lack of personal or social conflict to negate parental goal-setting. This clearly illustrates the lack of independence in these variables. Parental conflicts about achievement can induce neurotic conflict in a child, but even without this too much stress can result in overachievement before adolescence is reached. At adolescence, a negativistic protest intervenes. While some adolescents take the alternative of withdrawing into a fantasized world of achievement, some do not limit their protest to academic failure.

A fifteen-year-old, promoted in elementary school years to the extent of skipping one grade, began a progressive academic decline in junior high school. His mother was divorced during his infancy and put her hopes for achievement in her two sons. Much of her life revolved around intellectual pursuits, although her attainments had been minimal. While the eldest, at eighteen, went through a transient period of failure in high school, he did perform successfully in college. It was about the time of his phasing out that the younger boy began to lose interest in classes and become truant. At fifteen, the boy was dismissed from school and spent most of his days engaging in minor delinquencies. His mother alternated between telling him to leave home and taking him back when he arrived disheveled and hungry after days or weeks on the loose. While neither his measured IQ of 140, nor his mother's ambitions, sufficed to permit him to stay in school, when interviewed he was carrying a book, used in courses at a local college, which he was reading and underlining on his own. Much more is relevant here than distorted handling of parental ambition, but it is possible to surmise that a great many situations of dissonance between parental goals and academic achievement are in similar categories.

Dissonance between the adolescent and his parents is frequently seen when the former has a mediocre ability academically but the parents have set an unrealistic level of attainment for him. This may not result in the type of delinquency in the above case, but it may influence the personality by its effects on self-esteem. It may also affect the ability to take chances and induce a chronic feeling of failure.

Sociological theorists have stressed that for some adolescents the conflict may not be within the individual or family so much as within the type of social organization which does not provide adequate opportunities. Historically, this appears to have been particularly true with minority groups. Currently it is seen despite ostentatious attempts to give a few talented minority adolescents added support and permission to achieve. In fact, the number of court cases will increase from the competition over admissions to particular programs.

An important variable is parental belief in the future being controllable. While this has a low salience among South American mothers, it is strikingly present in German and Japanese mothers, whose belief in the future appears in early training for responsibility. Sons are supposed to be hard-working and conscientious with the expectation that hard work will be rewarded by these mothers.[105] The relationship between these child-rearing practices to later depressive-proneness opens up the question of the relationship between achievement and depression witnessed clinically in many age groups. Coleman found parental aspirations in black families unrealistic for their children in terms of what achievement was most feasible.[106] The problem is complicated by the maintenance of the myth, enforced in public schools, which appears largely irrelevant to the dilemmas of the lower-class child. Frustration and anger are reasonable responses.

Long-range consequences of frustrated expectations show up in the black adolescent who has been falsely led to believe in open opportunities despite his background and abilities. Again, some raise the issue that this is primarily a problem of lower-class parents absorbing the cultural impetus to achieve but lacking the means to translate *how* to their children. Whether the how is a mater of parental training techniques and/or a cultural problem is not clearly known. We do not even know why achievement becomes internalized in some and not in others. This issue raises the whole problem of internalization of aspirations and prohibitions in the course of development.

To what extent does parental modeling influence the development of achievement? Does the de facto occupation of a father—say as a skilled laborer—have more influence on the son's achievement goal than hopes that his son will be a doctor? Immediately, a complex number of variables precludes simple answers. It is less likely that the skilled laborer will practice, in his daily life, intellectual pursuits utilizing verbal skills than will the father who is at an occupational level where such pursuits are routinized. Studies have indicated that lower-class boys with college ambitions actually reject their fathers' occupations, an example of negative occupational role.[107] In a study of 194 Stanford students, one-third of the lower-class students reported their father as the most important parental influence, as compared to two-thirds of a random example, and three-fourths of the lower-class students cited their mothers as the dominant parental influence.[108]

Relevant are data pertaining to upward mobility in families and across class and occupational lines. Paternal modeling is not the sole or even the most significant influence for academic achievement in a male adolescent. The educational level and ambition of the mother for her sons may well be determiners, just as a highly intelligent father may be the model for academic achievement in a daughter. Modeling is not a sufficient explanation for these processes, and more complex motivations need consideration.

Modeling influences must not be confined to parents either, since siblings, relatives, teachers, and heroes all exert some effect. The peer influence is seen in the McDill and Coleman study which involved 600 students in their freshman and senior high school years.[109] There was a significant finding that ambitious youths seek out friends with similar interests and goals. Membership in a high-status group of this type is a better predictor of college plans among senior boys and girls than the educational levels of either parent, and is only slightly less so at the freshman level.

The absence of a father is another confused variable regarding achievement. Data must be considered separately for boys and girls, and conclusions are further handicapped because pure cultures, in which a parent does not remarry or have other attachments rarely exist. Studies based on such mixed groups must be viewed with skepticism. Conclusions are often reached wherein a greater incidence of fatherless homes among blacks is said to account for less ambition and achievement among black adolescents. When enormous numbers of other variables are involved, such as socio-economic status, maternal ambition, reaction of the mother to an absent father, the reason for the father's absence, the age at which the father left, the age of the mother, family size and ordinal position, family practices regarding ambition and independence, the abilities, opportunities, and personality variables of the adolescent, any type of conclusion must be tentative. There might even be an advantage where black, or lower-class, youths are not exposed to the failure model of a father in such circumstances. It is not solely, or perhaps even significantly, father absence that can explain academic achievement or failure.

The family size and configuration and their impact on a given child may be far more important in terms of external characteristics and personality dynamics. Many studies have directed themselves to appraising the relationship between the number of children in a family and achievement motivation as well as academic attainment. They almost all conclude that an inverse relationship exists.[110]

Bossard explains this by the influence of family size on socialization practices.[111] Increasing numbers of children are associated with greater parental leadership and dominance, in which the parent becomes the prime decision-maker. There is also a diluted contact with each child and a replacement of parents by older children in the performance of rearing functions. This frequently means less interest in the academic work of each child. What theoretical formulations can be made regarding the effect on achievement? The further question of what determines family size is also relevant. Apart from religious influences in Roman Catholic families up to the 1960s, family planning may largely reflect the upward mobility variable, the emancipation of women from procreation. Cross-correlations between economic conditions and family size operate with attendance at poorer quality schools. Recent studies emphasizing the importance of early years on cognitive and verbal abilities bear out the impact of the adverse effects of a large number of young children when the mother must manage them all by herself.

Family configurations include a wide variety of possibilities and one despairs of shorting out their influences. This is so despite the large number of studies purporting to do this. The original stimulus for investigating configurations came from two sources. Psychodynamic studies teased out the subtle implications within families and the impact on individual development. A second source was data revealing that first-borns have an exaggerated representation among achievers or notable men. Yet, is this due to the first-born status or some other dependent variable? Explanations involve the exclusivity such a child receives, higher parental expectations, or the motivation of the first-born to remain ahead. Methodology in these studies is subject to criticism, particularly in studies which compare first-borns with others. Some even lump only-children with first-borns. Others include families with one or ten children.

Thus, an interesting longitudinal study which compared forty-six pairs of first- and second-born children from fifteen months to pre-adolescence, concluded that mothers were more critical and demanding of first-borns although they stimulated them verbally more than the second-born. The study concluded that the second-born received less warmth initially but by the preschool period began to receive more. It was hypothesized that this interfered with doing things independently. Obviously, this has little relevance for larger families.[112]

Again, the displacement theory, whereby an eldest child is replaced, and held to lead to status sensitivity toward authority figures, would not operate the same, if at all, in families with different numbers of children.[113] Differences in gender composition and sequences of birth should also be specified, along with the spacing between children and parental age at birth. Many cultural and ethnic factors operate with respect to sex and ordinal position and their relationship to educational achievement. Perhaps many of these variables are mediated by differential socialization practices, or parental responses, depending on the particular position of a child in the family structure.

Finally, notice must be taken of factors operating independently of the family and personal context. These are broad aspects concerned with social setting which not only involves socio-economic studies but also the impact of institutional settings or peer influences. The methodologic problem is to control other variables, such as IQ, and then study the effect of one variable.

For example, if a group is homogeneous with respect to other variables, what is the impact on achievement if socio-economic status varies? Of course, the oversimplification is that one can isolate the effect of one such variable. Hence, a study such as that of Sewell and Armer in which a multiple regression analysis concluded that the neighborhood an adolescent occupies accounts for less than 2 percent of the variance in college aspirations.[114] However, only 25 percent of the variance in college aspirations was accounted for by all other factors—leaving a substantial margin of variability. Another problem in such group data is the failure to account for variations within groups. We would have little idea if the 2 percent (for which neighborhood appeared to be influential) were weighted in terms of race, religion, or sex. Idiosyncrasies of individual personality development are, by acknowledgment, bypassed in these approaches. Subsumed under neighborhood is a presupposition of uniformity in schools, teachers, facilities, and communication, which may not be so for neighborhoods comparable in other respects. Coleman's study concluded that it was not facilities or curriculum that accounted for the greatest variance in verbal ability scores at the ninth and twelfth grade levels with adolescents, but the quality of the student body.[115] This refers to plans of the student to attend college, perception by teachers of student quality, attendance, and families owning encyclopedias. Most of these are pre-existing qualities in the student. Teacher quality was greater in effect than either curriculum or the type of faculty.

FAILURES AND ACHIEVEMENT:
DROPOUTS AND THE DISADVANTAGED

Studies.   Adolescents who fail to achieve have personal difficulties and social liabilities far in excess of their numbers. The Coleman Report on the equality of educational opportunity suggested, in accord with the above material, that home influences were the most important predictors of who would profit from school.[116] In terms of population, about fifty million children and adolescents attend school, which represents approximately one-quarter of the country's population. The 1967 Sizer Report studied the fifteen largest cities in the United States and found that 31 percent of the children who completed ninth grade failed to graduate from high school.[117] Six percent of children who start fifth grade never enter senior high school.

For male dropouts in one of these cities the rate of unemployment was 15 percent higher than for high school graduates. In another city, 48 percent of males with high school diplomas were unemployed. A tentative conclusion reached in the Sizer Report, and felt to be true by others, is that the contemporary high school diploma has little to offer. Only one study has compared dropouts favorably to those who finish high school.[118] Contrary results are well-documented.[119]

Hathaway, Reynolds, and Monachesi have done a follow-up study on 1,000 male and 812 female high school dropouts in a state-wide study of adolescents in Minnesota.[120] [121] This study began in 1953 when the boys were in ninth grade, and between 1962 and 1966 a follow-up study was made of 1,000 boys in a control group, picked randomly from the same high school. The boys had a mean age of twenty-eight on follow-up. Results indicate a deplorable waste.

Adolescent dropouts become the future laborers of America. If they are lucky, they become skilled laborers. Even if a dropout is intelligent, he is likely to gravitate into the group of slightly skilled laborers, or the unemployed. In this study, 14 percent of the dropouts were at or above the 64th percentile in intelligence test scores, which represents the top 36 percent of the population intellectually. The dropouts were downward in social mobility compared to their fathers, they fathered more children than the controls, and had a higher proportion of criminal histories (37 percent of the dropouts had committed crimes at a misdemeanor level or higher, while only 9 percent of the controls had done so). Girls present a similar adverse picture, although a less dramatic one.

All of this should not be taken as an indication that the solution for dropouts is the continuance of a coercive system of education. There are too many questions about the value of a high school diploma to opt for this solution. To presume that a relatively uniform system of education, such as the public schools, should suffice for almost all adolescents is naive, if not destructive. However, there is no way to attend a trade or vocational high school which carries the same level of status and achievement.

To drop out may achieve more self-respect at the time than the two available options. Temporary affiliation with a dropout peer group, perhaps extended for a few years in the military, soon leads to alienation and disaffection. There are other consequences which do not show up in the statistics of the Hathaway-Reynolds-Monachesi study which must be kept in mind as well: personal conflict, acting out, and other types of self-destructive behaviors.

The Disadvantaged. In many ways the disadvantaged are also failures of the system. They make an exaggerated contribution to the dropout problems and fail to achieve in an academic sense, but—more important—in their personal lives. Schools and their representatives come to exemplify the frustrations which bar achievement and give a sense of personal competency. On the other hand, schools should not be used as foils against which disadvantaged youths flail their grievances and disappointments.

Lack of adaptation to the needs and norms of the lower and middle-classes shows up in schools' preoccupation with rules and regulations. Enforcement of the Puritan ethic on a group for which it is largely irrelevant produces contempt. The Horatio Alger story is basically a middle-class success story, not one for the millions in the ghettos to emulate. Rather than a successful experience, school is all too often something to be tolerated—or even an experience with an adverse impact on self-esteem because of repeated failures.

Studies on the impact of teacher expectancies on children have been devastating in their academic and personality consequences for the disadvantaged. Teacher expectations are that the disadvantaged will do poorly academically. Children perceive this and react to it in two ways: (1) negativistic behavior, to exaggerate in a defensive manner a contempt for school and what it stands for, and (2) an adverse effect on self-concept whereby the children do not perceive themselves as able to achieve in school. Especially do boys—black or white—get perceived by teachers as asocial, aggressive in verbal and physical ways, hyperactive, and tense.[122] Many more boys are viewed as brain damaged either within school systems in poor neighborhoods struggling with large numbers of these youths, or in public and community clinics.

Whether this reflects an accurate diagnostic assessment, free from class bias, or whether it is an oversimplified approach is not clear. It is possible that antecedents such as prenatal defects, poor obstetrical care, and nutritional factors load the dice toward the poor having a greater incidence of organicity. But many factors determine whether these children are behaving as they would from an injured brain. The self-fulfilling prophecy too often operates with respect to meeting expectations of a teacher as to performance level, and by assigning something physically wrong as etiological.

Of course, many explanations are given—genes, father absence, social disorganization—but the result is the same. The expectation that performance will be impaired is set; with the disadvantaged child the presumption is that they are deficient until proven otherwise.

An enormous significance is put on language ability and verbal expressivity for every level of academic achievement as well as later in the world of vocational success. But it is exactly in terms of competing for success that the arugment becomes circular and the task seems hopeless. Educators who foster intervention programs with the goal of having the disadvantaged catch up presume that this is what the poor, the blacks, and the disadvantaged want. While some of them do, those now running the system want it even more because they believe in it. Reasons are usually articulated poorly, as in "technocracy needs people with these abilities."

There are definite advantages to verbal abilities for attainment of certain goals, but it is a value preference in contrast to behavior patterns which do not adapt so readily to the norms of public education: impulsivity, challenges to authority, and emphasis on the kinesthetic. While some of these behaviors are reflections of personality traits, and are appraised as such by the clinician, they are often grouped in school systems as detrimental behaviors to be changed. While attempts to develop language skills, cognitive abilities, and intellectual interests should not be opposed, a caveat must be sounded in two respects: (1) To accomplish these goals as an institutional task is in itself a value judgment which must be clearly dealt with through individual children and families as well as institutions. (2) There are many questions about whether intervention succeeds even when it is tried. This judgment is based on empirical results as well as on theoretical appraisal of what is required for lasting results in terms of intervention in the life of the child, his family, and his culture. More pervasive is the difficulty in evaluating whether even the limited results seen in studies are transferable from the experimental settings in which they are carried out to society at large.

In this context, achievement is often viewed by boys as feminine, and incongruent with male sex-role identity. High-achieving boys believe teachers see them as achieving by way of feminine virtues.[123] Schools mainly staffed by women, and functioning as nurturers in many ways, are seen as feminine institutions. It is of interest that high-achieving adolescent girls believe they are perceived as masculine in view of their nonconformity in seeking achievement and independence. The main image of the school is the inculcator of rules and conformity. The teacher is not seen as someone who presents cultural or intellectual stimulation, but rather as a socializer of the child by introducing rules.[124] Couple this with the sex-role standard of the adolescent boy in which autonomy, self-initiative, and a need to emancipate are present, and it becomes

unlikely that a youth from a culturally disadvantaged area will wish
to conform and begin learning.

WORK

Achievement in adolescents is not separate from vocational
development. Too many discussions treat vocational choice as a
discreet area of development—perhaps related to academic achievement for college attendance. The close relationship between work,
personality development, and functioning is often ignored, despite
its important implications for sex-role identity and self-esteem. All
this points up the confusion over what is considered vocational
behavior.

Sociological Perspective. Occupational and industrial sociology
views work as another social institution in which man participates,
that takes on its meaning through the mores of a given culture.
Labor and manpower economics are related fields which contribute
to the occupational viewpoint. A developmental perspective requires
appraisal of such things as knowledge about vocations, why certain
vocations are given certain values, relationships between childhood
aspirations and those of adolescence, as well as eventual adult
choices. An ego focus raises questions about the role of changing ego
functions with respect to vocational aspirations. There is the
complex interaction of psychological variables within an individual
and his family which lead to vocational choices, failures, and
disappointments.

At the turn of the century, occupational psychology was
preoccupied with the psychology of individual differences. The era
of psychological testing gave rise to a vocational psychology based
on an effort to measure traits related to occupational choice. Such an
approach had value when choosing personnel for discreet tasks, but
had major limitations in making predictions about vocations, as
well as the compatibility of certain vocations. However, many
occupations tapped complex and diverse vocational goals.

Complex variables do not remain fixed indefinitely. Shifts in the
personality equilibrium occur in time as a reaction to changing
environmental conditions. What finally relegated trait measurement from a position of dominance in vocational work to that of a
more limited role was the realization that vocational problems were
more complicated than predicting whether a person had the ability
to perform isolated tasks on a job. Broader learning models had to be

utilized, in addition to developmental and motivational aspects. The developmental approach gained ground in the 1940s from publications emphasizing research problems involving vocational aspirations as basically developmental problems[125]

Borow lists four concerns in a psychological approach to vocations:[126]

1. Attention needs to be given to a theoretical framework which can generate hypotheses about vocational choice and interpret empirical findings.

2. What are the stimulus variables relevant to the development of career behavior? For example, what meaning do certain child-rearing practices have? What is the relationship, (if any) between certain courses in school with respect to vocational planning and behavior? Does counseling of any type have a significant influence? What part do other life experiences play regarding vocation?

3. Very little is known about the childhood roots of vocational motivation. While clinicians who do intensive therapy are able to detect a confluence of trends in people, they have an opportunity to work on a different level from that witnessed with the millions who plan on a more circumscribed basis. Outside of such clinical situations, there is a dearth of longitudinal studies.

4. Research approaches limited to data on aspirations in choice of vocation as outcome variables are too limited, and should be rejected in favor of a concept of occupational behavior.

Basic Approaches: Developmental. Four major approaches to vocational choice have been used: (1) a developmental approach, (2) child-rearing practices, (3) psychoanalytic formulations, and (4) socio-cultural influences. A developmental perspective stresses age-related stages of thinking about vocational choice.[127] The three relevant periods, all based on changing cognitive abilities, are: fantasy, tentativeness, and realism. The period of *fantasy* is dominant up to preadolescence, or about age eleven, when vocational thoughts are not related to personal assessment of intellectual or personal attributes. The child is dominated by stereotypes and wishful thinking. The *tentative* period lasts from age eleven to seventeen. The developmental shift occurs by age thirteen or fourteen with a realization that training and ability are prerequisites. By age fifteen or sixteen personal values gain influence, and by age seventeen a synthetic process merges interests, abilities, and values. A *realistic* period of choice comes toward the end of the seventeenth year, when a vocational life-plan is worked out. Various possibilities are thought out prior to a commitment. In viewing the 1951 work of Ginzberg, the lock-step manner in which these formulations are made is striking.[127] Choice of vocation is rarely the outcome of a series of sequentially structured changing views on jobs. For the disadvantaged, these formulations may have even less relevance.

Super's self-concept theory, one of the most detailed developmental theories of vocational choice, considers vocational behavior in terms of interactions between an individual and his environment.[128] During the course of adolescence, vocational attitudes become more complex and reality-oriented in terms of self-concept. Super hypothesizes two major stages of vocational development in adolescence: exploration and establishment. The exploratory stage includes three phases of vocational development: a tentative phase of choice, in which interests are still diffuse and unrealistic; a transitional phase; and a trial phase, with minimal commitment.

The establishment stage extends into late adolescence and has an initial trial with commitment and stable advancement. In each stage a series of developmental tasks involves crystallizing, specifying, and implementing a vocational choice. Instability of vocational plans among young adolescents occurs when preferences are inconsistent with other choices. A follow-up a year after high-school graduation indicates that only 17 and 26 percent of boys and girls respectively retain the occupational plans they made in the ninth grade.[129] Ability profiles are more valid predictors of later occupational plans than either the plans of the young adolescent or measures of vocational interest.

Child-rearing Viewpoints. Child-rearing viewpoints on vocational behavior are a specific version of person-environmental interaction theories. Roe employed a sophisticated approach based on developmental and motivational psychology to integrate the job functions of certain occupations and the personality attributes of potential employees.[130] Motives for occupational choice and satisfaction were investigated. Two dimensions were employed: groups and levels. The former corresponds to a factorization of interests into eight primary work categories: service, business, contact, organization, technology, outdoor, science, general cultural, and arts and entertainment. Levels deal with a hierarchical arrangement of occupations within groups according to training and skill requirements. In any type of classification, things become arbitrary and overlapping to some extent: as an illustration, many occupations under the science group, such as medical specialists, university and college faculty, or veterinary work, have much more to do with service in terms of function than with science. This led to an emphasis on the differential influences of family experiences which give an impetus in childhood toward occupational choices.[131]

Roe's two-way classification was coupled with dominant child-rearing approaches based on emotional concentration on the child, avoidance of the child, and acceptance of the child. Combining these testable hypotheses is feasible if, for example, a child exposed to avoidance later makes occupational choices not involving interpersonal contact (a technology or science choice). However, attempts to confirm such hypotheses have had limited results, due to the crudeness of research instruments and the simplicity of experimental design.

In most research of this type, we do not expect a straightforward relationship between parental attitudes and later personality variables. Not only do other factors in the environment intervene over the course of development—especially during adolescence—but the complexity of family psychodynamics does not result in one-to-one relationships. At present, predictions about occupational outcome are no better than going from choices to transitions.[132] This is seen in attempts to predict choices made in the educational careers of scientists.[133]

No one is attacking the importance of family relationships on emerging vocational choices during adolescence. It is just that vocational choices are related to so many variables that prediction and assortment become difficult. Work involving motives, achievement, childhood, and family antecedents are all relevant. Zytowski estimates that 80 percent of American males want to work, and continue to do so, even if they have an income sufficient for their needs. If this is so, it tells us something of great significance about the boy whose work has little meaning for him. Although this is currently confused by the social and political alienation of a great many adolescents who stress their opposition to work in the form in which they witness it, it is all the more impressive that training for something that is meaningful appears lacking. Data about the lack of meaning of investing in high schools is more impressive. At most, about 10 percent will graduate from college.[134]

It is not surprising that working class males stress the prime value of work, apart from economic necessity, is to give them something to occupy themselves. To an extent, this is a perpetuation of the ethos of their high school years. In a random study of 401 men, one-third gave a negative reason for working, such as having nothing else to do, or not knowing what they would do with their time.[135]

Most studies give short shrift to the occupational plans of girls, although this may change in the future due to increasing protestations by women's groups and a more active stance by adolescent girls. It comes as a surprise to many that the adolescent girl will spend an average of twenty-five years of her adult life working in the labor force. Having children leads only to a temporary absence for most women, who eventually return to work. The mean age of the American woman-worker is about thirty-eight years.[136]

Almost no studies have dealt with the problem of predicting career choice among adolescent girls.[137] In part, this is associated with the close connection for girls between education and age at the time of marriage. Girls who perform poorly academically, or have low academic interests, are more likely to become involved in affairs leading to early marriage. Elder noted that a 1967 U.S. census survey found that two-fifths of girls aged eighteen and nineteen who were not in school were married and living with a spouse, compared to less than 2 percent of those girls who were full-time college students.[138] Poor academic performance is not the sole variable operating here. Various types of family and personal situations are weighted toward early marriage and few vocational plans for girls.

Psychoanalytic Viewpoints. Psychoanalytic theory has relevance for occupational psychology. It is not that there is a psychoanalytic theory about work, but rather that any type of significant pattern that occurs in life involves multiple aspects of personality functioning. Apart from the overt aspects of development, subtle and idiosyncratic processes operate. This makes for difficulty in assessing such formulations in terms of empirical testing to confirm or abandon them, which is more viable when discreet variables are measured.

While early formulations attempted to unravel vocational choice in terms of derivatives from impulses which cannot be expressed, shifts in theoretical formulations have permitted material to be encompassed without becoming oriented to a "nothing but" explanation. Unfulfilled aggressive wishes, for example, may lead to an occupation gratifying wishes, such as prize-fighting. They may also take a more rarified form, such as a career as an army man or even a super-salesman. These are mentioned as some possibilities and to indicate the multitude of possibilities.

Ego functioning, may see defensive operations influencing occupational choice. Continuing the example chosen, an individual with prominent aggressive trends may handle them by way of reaction formations so he engages in an occupation emphasizing peace or non-violence. This sort of person may be violently opposed to war. The principle of overdetermination guarantees that a large number of intrapsychic, interpersonal, and environmental components get considered with their different strengths in individuals to determine how and why certain occupational choices are made.

Some studies attempt to utilize psychoanalytic theory in studying occupational choice. Nachmann tested the hypothesis that males who enter law or dentistry had strong, dominant fathers, while those who enter social work had weak, inadequate, or absent, fathers.[139] This data supported the hypothesis, noting the childhood homes of future lawyers demonstrated open acceptance of aggression, compared to repression of aggression in homes of future dentists. Segal also found personality trait differences between student occupational choices.[140]

In a general way, psychoanalytic theory has contributed to the vocational dilemmas of the adolescent population by its realization, based on clinical observations, that lack of satisfaction and pleasure in work may be the result and the cause of a conflicted personality. Freud went so far as to put work and sex on the same level by referring to normality in terms of the ability to love and work. He saw work as an essential for civilization to endure: "The communal life of human beings had, therefore, a twofold foundation: the compulsion to work, which is created by external necessity, and the power of love, which made the man unwilling to be deprived of his sexual object—the woman—and made the woman unwilling to be deprived of the part of herself which had been separated from her—her child. Eros and Ananke [love and necessity] have become the parents of human civilization, too."[141] While Freud saw work in terms of a necessity, predicated upon renunciation of the pleasure principle in the course of childhood socialization, he also noted this alone would not suffice to keep man working. It was rather the emotional relationships—libidinal attachments of people to each other—which were necessary to keep man working. Without the pleasurable quality, obtained through work taking the place of gratifying childhood impulses, a pattern of work would not continue. This formulation raises provocative questions about both schooling and subsequent work if the element of personal gratification and human attachments are deficient.

Subsequent study focusing on the ego led to a perspective of work serving many functions. If work in some manner is considered at least partly connected with aggressive drive, gratification through work can be viewed as a setting for drive reduction. Executive ego functioning would be the vehicle. Robert White presents a case against motivational theories based on drive reduction, such as a psychoanalytic theory of instinct.[142] He posits that the efforts a human puts forth to effect environmental changes are accompanied by, and lead to, feelings of efficacy and competency. Rather than viewing these as derived from basic drives—sexual or aggressive— White sees them as utilizing "independent ego energies" which motivate people to explore and be curious. Some might question the need for primary drive theory and substitute a set of secondary drives as learned phenomena in toto. Those who wish to abandon drive theory as a common source for action in humans, would substitute environmentally determined elicitors.

Much of White's thinking is similar to that of Ives Hendrick, who proposed "executant" ego functions to control or alter the environment.[143] He was impressed by the enormous effort man uses to change his environment. Governing executant functions is a work principle whose aim is mastery of the environment. Lantos contrasted two kinds of pleasure in children's play: the function itself and that in achievement outside the activity itself.[144] Work is related to the latter, which is not undertaken for its own sake but to ensure self-preservation. Pleasure in work achievement is an ego reaction, in contrast to libidinal pleasure.

Menninger estimated that 75 percent of patients coming to psychiatrists suffer from an incapacity to obtain satisfaction in their work, or the inability to work.[145] He believed that work becomes pleasurable as certain external and internal conditions are met. Externally there must be: (1) a minimum of compulsion, (2) positive group feeling among workers, (3) absence of excessive discomfort or fatigue, (4) pride in the product or service given, and (5) a conviction that the work is useful and appreciated. Internally there must be relative freedom from (1) guilt associated with pleasure, and (2) neurotic compulsion to work or not to work.

The latter types of situations take us into the psychopathology of work, which involves family conflict in the course of development. These may manifest themselves in over- or underachievement in work.[146] Erikson's psychosexual stages, parallel to latency, of industry versus inferiority, give a direct emphasis to work and achievement.[147] Attitudes toward work and adaptation are seen in the context of psychosocial development as well as in peer relationships and toward the authority of parents and teachers. In all of these psychoanalytic formulations, certain themes are regnant. An emphasis on childhood experiences and epigenesis as having a significant place in later vocational development is prominent. In some, impulses are given a primacy not seen in other theories of vocational choice, even within the ego, and psychosocial influences are stressed.[148]

In perspective, the value of psychoanalytic theory regarding work is that if sufficient data were available on the developmental and social experiences of a given child, we would be able to have a precise picture of why certain types of choices related to vocation occur. Conversely, the most cogent reconstructed picture might be possible for why an adult has made the choices he has. For some, social determinants in adolescence play a relatively greater role, while for others family experiences are crucial. This perspective allows us to see how individual adolescents, if disturbed psychiatrically, may continue to function adequately in terms of school or work while others with less severe psychopathology may become handicapped more easily in the realm of work.

Socio-cultural Influences. Economic factors cannot be ignored when appraising the vocational picture presented to an adolescent. Whatever the antecedent developmental, familial, and depth factors have been, unless the economy is in a position to fulfill individual prospects within its occupational structure, it will come to nought. Individual aspirations, as well, cannot be gratified within society's impersonal context.

One of the most important things in work satisfaction appears to be the *setting* in which it takes place. Specifically, this means that the interpersonal context, on a peer or supervisory level, emerges as extremely important. The adolescent senses conflict in any hierarchy. To what extent they develop and feel loyalty to a bureaucracy, even though their talents may make them mobile within the economy, is a crucial question. A paradoxical factor is what the adolescent realistically observes between the inverse relationship of number of working hours in some status occupations, and the declining number of hours in others. Executive or professional jobs have a work-week climbing to sixty hours a week, while the average work-week has declined from about seventy hours a week in 1850, and forty-four hours in 1940, to thirty-seven and a half hours in 1960.[149]

The obvious question is, "Is it really worth it?" Even for the most mundane occupations, it will probably be necessary to keep running in place just to maintain a horizontal occupational status. Except for the most menial task, continued training, either in off-working hours or on the job, will be promoted. Such continuing educational devices as refresher courses, in-service training, increased numbers of meetings, courses, or institutes are in the offing. If the predictions of our labor economists are accurate, job obsolescence is such that a worker may need retooling two or three times during his working life for new positions. This will be advantageous not only to the adolescent who sees himself as someone with multiple interests wanting to acquire different skills and talents, but to those whose continued curiosity permits them not to stagnate. Personality rigidities that prevent easy transitions to new demands and those whose state of super-specialization makes transition difficult will be at a disadvantage.

In addition to these economic factors, *socio-cultural influences* affect the work choices of the adolescent. Whether social class is mainly a reflection of occupational level, or vice versa, is unresolved because of their interlocking nature. Implicit throughout is the value-system of occupation as well as working. Complexities in evaluation of social class are well-known, and involve such things as family income, source of income, status of the father's job, education of family members, location and type of residence.

Occupational prestige, as eluctable as it is, is a prime factor in how adolescents think about jobs. From about age twelve, jobs are thought of in terms of a rank order which seems related to the status-conferring power of a job. Status can be a nebulous entity. Those who write on the problem of job status refer to it being determined by such things as: level of education required for a job (a surgeon whose training requires an average of fourteen years of post-high-school training), source and amount of monetary returns, special skills which are not readily learned by others, personal autonomy (a minimum of direction from others and freedom to do one's thing), influence on other people or social groups, public recognition (a political position or professional athlete), the degree of enjoyment or luxury associated with a given job, the physical versus the intellectual aspects of the work.

However this heterogeneous grouping is finally weighted, data are impressive in terms of prestige rankings of specific occupations. Rankings for ninety occupations from 1947 were repeated in 1963, and the two sets correlated at a .99 level.[150] No substantial changes occurred, illustrating societal conservatism in this respect. The six highest occupational rankings in terms of rank were: U.S. Supreme Court Justice, physician, nuclear physicist, scientist (in general), government scientist, and state governor. Actually, nuclear physicist and scientist in general were tied for third, and the last two tied for fourth. Nuclear physicist moved from eighteenth in 1947 to a tie for third-place in 1963. The six lowest occupational rankings ranked from lowest upward are: shoe-shiner, street-sweeper, garbage collector, sharecropper (one who owns no livestock or equipment), soda-fountain clerk, and laundry clothes-presser.

Another interesting trend is the shift in occupations from 1947 to 1963. The following moved upward by five or more notches: chemist, lawyer, instructor or teacher in public schools, electrician, policeman, carpenter, and labor union official. The following moved downward by five or more rankings: diplomat in the foreign service, mayor of a large city, head of a department in a state government, banker, owner of a factory employing over a hundred people, artists who exhibited in galleries, musician in a symphony orchestra, farm owner and operator, radio announcer, manager of a small store in a city, travelling wholesale salesman, playground director, and farmhand. The impact on the adolescent in terms of occupational prestige can be seen when it is noted that high school athletic coaches are rated above owners of factories employing a hundred people, artists, symphony musicians, novelists, economists, newspaper reporters, and columnists.

Social-class status permits some guarded conclusions. Socioeconomic status is one significant variable among many. No direct relationship was found to exist between social-class origins and levels of aspiration-attainment. Factors discussed earlier do operate: family, ethnic background, ordinal position, models, and value systems. Abilities, attitudes, and intelligence need consideration, as high aspirations are positively correlated with these factors.

Vocational Failure. In recent years joint problems of achievement and vocation have been looked at from the perspective of youths considered culturally disadvantaged. Studies have involved different disciplines. Controversy does not center upon the disabilities of the disadvantaged, but on remedial and preventive efforts which fail to reveal consistent gains. Factors relevant to the adverse vocational development of the disadvantaged can be listed as:

1. Limited cognitive opportunities to stimulate intellectual development
2. Discrepancies between aspirations that have developed and what is realistically sensed as practical
3. Exposure to cultural and aesthetic factors which favor kinesthetic or motor abilities, inhibitions over expressivity of affect, but which, with a few major exceptions such as in the arts or athletics, are handicaps in terms of verbal and intellectual development
4. Affective blunting or defensive withdrawal from living in overcrowded settings with minimal privacy
5. Limited social contact with those in other social classes, ethnic backgrounds, or neighborhoods
6. Higher incidence (from multiple causes) of broken homes, absent fathers, and larger families with the impact of this on modeling, identification, and matriarchal power in families.
7. Lack of opportunity to witness the rewards of conformity and dedication to the working goals of the system
8. Greater exposure to higher delinquency groups, distrust and hatred of authority figures, externalization mechanisms taking precedence over internal ones as a control mechanism over impulses
9. Inferior schools, teachers, subjects, and facilities
10. A view that fate and chance, rather than personal effort or autonomy, take precedence
11. Lack of occupational inheritance possibilities in terms of sons succeeding, or wanting to succeed, in their fathers' jobs, opposed to a family indoctrinating and expecting a son to follow in his father's footsteps (there may also be a forced acceptance of menial work similar to that which relatives have done for economic survival)

VOCATIONAL CHOICES

As indicated above, no single factor governs the attitudes and feelings about work which develop at the beginning of adolescence. Cutting across these headings, it appears that certain factors play such a major role in any discussions of work, once adolescence is achieved, that they cannot be ignored.[151]

1. *Personality development* in terms of traits, attitudes, interests, neurotic conflicts, under- or overachievement, family socialization, and psychodynamic patterns are assets or liabilities not easily circumvented.

2. *Constitutional factors* operate by way of givens that are probably least subject to modification. While few argue that the physique of a professional athlete or the musical ability of a Mozart can be developed, for some endowments, the modifiability potential becomes arguable. Intelligence is one of these, in terms of the degree to which it is basically determined by genic assortment versus environmental exposure.

3. *Social organization* and *historical trends* are difficult to alter within any short-term period. While government and institutions may attempt to shift trends through scholarships and more funds for schools and teachers, the problem is the maintenance of such ad hoc devices to affect social change. Consider the difficulties of raising the status of certain occupations, such as maintenance employees, who may be in short supply despite increasing salaries and shorter work-weeks.

4. Influences from current social standing and convictions of families, relatives, and friends above and beyond the personal assets and liabilities of an adolescent are based on all of the above. Social standing is not confined to established norms or assets. Fashions and fads come and go, giving advantages to those who luck out at a particular historical period. A black in the United States at the present time has more opportunity than at almost any time in history. With larger numbers of adolescents receiving high school diplomas and college degrees, relative opportunity from mere possession of a degree is diminishing.

5. *Social-role characteristics* elicit certain vocational pursuits. Personality characteristics dovetail with this as well, since personality traits in ego functioning go with certain occupations. Conversely, avoidance of other occupations which do not fit a certain personality configuration occurs.

6. *Values* and *norms* of an individual exert a guiding influence on vocational choice during adolescence. The ego-ideal influences a range of occupational choices. Dedication to service, pursuit or avoidance of high income, a need to help or succor, are mediated via ideals in this manner. Superego influences operate to restrict certain choices. An example would be a type of sales work viewed as exploiting, or a military career for others.

Discussion of factors impinging on the adolescent confrontation of work have used the perspective of academic or clinical insights. While many of these have relevance to their own particular framework, a criticism is that they may not have much relevance to some of the organizational dilemmas in which the adolescent finds himself and how this contributes to conflict. Most germane in this respect for large numbers of human beings is the lack of connection between schooling and subsequent life. It is not that the overworked and nebulous term "relevance" need become the final arbiter of what schools should do, but rather that the goals of a compulsory and universal system of education have not been made clear.

Now that children no longer need protection from the factories which exploited them, the efficacy of a system of compulsory education is under question. Few would care to argue that the accomplishment of such a system has been to educate the child, although the goal may have been to accomplish this. While some knowledge is absorbed, those poured through the system could hardly be described as receiving more than the basics. In fact, almost all of the claims listed throughout the history of American public education have never occurred.[152]

At various times, one or another accomplishment has been presented as justification for schooling: achieving social mobility, eliminating class distinctions, fostering economic mobility, democracy, or the production of responsible adults who contribute to their country's welfare. In its early form—besides keeping children out of factories—one of the best byproducts of education may have been to channel some children into vocational or trade schools. However, this became a two-track system, with social discrepancy for those weeded out rather than a place of sufficient status to attract many. How effective vocational schools are in their training is a valid question in its own right. There is little evidence that industrial and governmental growth were contingent upon what was happening to those in the public school system. It is even questionable how much a strictly technical education on a university level, such as engineering, has to do with the type of work that is performed once a job is secured.

This does not mean that the adolescent years in school may not have served other functions. For some, it may have been fun. For others, schooling may have enabled them to meet certain regulatory standards to later get a job, such as in teaching or a civil service position. For a few, it passed time until they could secure some other life goal, such as marriage, even though when many were ready to join the work force later on they lacked useful qualifications. For others with talent, time, money, and motivation, schooling may have served as a gateway to permit them to continue receiving higher education on a college, graduate, or professional level.

In this manner, the school system serves as a major device for limiting occupational choice. According to Caplow, "It does this in two ways: first by forcing the student, who embarks upon a long course of training, to renounce other careers which also require extensive training; second, by excluding from training, and eventually from the occupations themselves, those who lack either the intellectual qualities (such as intelligence, docility, aptitude) or the social characteristics (such as ethnic background, wealth, appropriate conduct, previous education) which happen to be required."[153] The result is a tracking system which early feeds into promoting those who perform well on taking tests, reading, IQ tests, and teacher recommendations, all heavily weighted toward those who fit into an approach with little critical appraisal or questioning.

In almost all vocational sequences—from the most menial positions to those based on many years of schooling—the overriding accomplishment of the school appears to be its role as a moralizing and socializing agent to produce conforming people. Conformity includes demands for discipline, obedience, punctuality, and self-control, which are virtues necessary for society to function efficiently and to permit industrial growth. For those youths who have had difficulty in adapting to the system, there is a channeling over a period of time into poorer schools with even less pretense of any educational mission. Although there is a bias operating against certain ethnic or racial groups, it appears to operate in the direction of maintenance of overall class rigidities. One product of this channeling process is seen when the Selective Service System has operated.[154]

If one were to challenge not only the school's mission as a socializer of certain virtues, but to proceed beyond and ask, "What is wrong with these virtues?," the answer would be that these are merely one set of values among many which happen to be dominant in a particular historical setting. But from the perspective of the contemporary adolescent, they are the ones which are challenged most often. The challenge is not primarily in terms of another set of values being inherently superior, but that the particular socialization process which inculcates these virtues, via family and school, makes it difficult to be able to criticize or appraise these virtues if one really wished to join the system. This is the precise conflict verbalized by many adolescents in therapy. While the psychodynamic features in the individual adolescent will not be pursued here, this type of societal double bind elicits great rage and protest in the vulnerable. On the social and vocational level, the conflict is between the professional ideology of schooling and work and the de facto mission of most public education: to ensure the maintenance and operation of a socio-economic system in which recalcitrance is required to be minimal. If a personal price has to be paid by some in terms of individualized neurotic suffering, this is the price for civilization.

Most crucial to the production of an orderly society is the renunciation of overt aggressive displays. To do this requires aim-inhibition for drives or sublimation. Explanatory hypotheses may be offered that in the presence of a shift toward less inhibition in child-rearing practices and in the cultural atmosphere there will be fewer restrictions on aggressive displays by adolescents. There will then be less guilt for what have been viewed as transgressions in the past, and consequently less remorse to renounce such desires.

ATHLETICS

The preoccupation in the United States with sports is not unrelated to the preceding sections devoted to the development of character structure, achievement, and work. Not only have different types of athletes grown in popularity over the decades, but an affluent economy has permitted many more spectators to pursue sports and pay enormous salaries to stars. Television has brought to America the visual presence of many athletic events. While many hypotheses may be raised about cultural change and continuity through the dimension of sports, there are many factors which have led to this shift.

Relationship to Play.   While simplifications tend to distort accuracy, they do contain some truth by way of introduction to the meaning athletics has for some adolescents. It is not that athletics is merely a later form of play, since multiple factors enter into why and how a given adolescent participates in sports. Yet, developmentally, there is significant continuity from play to athletics. While the meaning of play varies widely, covering activities from football to sexual seduction, there is a theme of diversion from the serious or intense preoccupation with reality that is present in sports. A working definition regards play as something done voluntarily, within limits of time and place, according to rules which are binding but sufficient unto themselves.[155] Play has accompanying feelings of tension and joy, with a conscious sense of the activity being different from the rest of life. This means that play has three requirements: (1) freedom to choose to participate or not (which excludes physical education required in schools), (2) a restriction to a given time and place, and (3) rules which take precedence during the course of play.

This is similar to the ideas of Erikson in his reflections on what should be considered play. "When man plays he must intermingle with things and people in a similarly uninvolved and light fashion. He must do something which he has chosen to do without being compelled by urgent interests or impelled by strong passions; he must feel entertained and free of any fear or hope of serious consequences. He is on vacation from social and economic reality or, as is most commonly emphasized, he *does not work*. It is this opposition to work which gives play a number of connotations. . . . Let a player forget that such play must remain his free choice, let him become possessed by the demon of gambling, and playfulness vanishes again."[156]

Theories of play abound. Early writers were interested in playing games as expressing drives. These theories tended to limit themselves to the obvious, such as play using up energy. There was a teleological reduction in reasoning that the purpose of play must be physiological. There is a quality of inadequacy in explanations which hold that play occurs to reduce tension. Without elaborating, the following theories of play, compiled by Groos at the turn of the century, are still relevant:[157]

Physiological

1. Play as a necessary discharge of superabundant energy not needed for vital processes
2. A contrary theory that play affords relaxation and conserves energy
3. Play recaptures a pleasurable stimulus or a state of relaxation in exhaustion that follows a reaction to a stimulus

Biological

1. Play as instinctual in origin
2. Play derives out of biological needs to obtain food and sustenance and arises when the vital function is fulfilled

Psychological

1. Play is a pleasurable activity, the conscious or unconscious copying of youthful pursuits, a reproduction of pleasure with a non-serious aim

2. Playful experimentation precedes play, but it is not play; it becomes play when it is repetitive, conscious, and accompanied by tension and enjoyment. The joy of being in an active cause, physical or mental, adds its creative aspect

3. Play has a dream quality

4. The pleasure derived from play comes from the satisfaction of inborn impulses

5. Some play is not psychological at all; psychological play involves self-deception

6. The pleasure from play derives from pleasure in a stimulus, agreeable, and in its intensity

7. The pleasure from play is a feeling of freedom, creativity and mastery

Aesthetic

The pleasure of play can lead to aesthetics in art. The skills in artistic endeavor resemble those in games and play

Sociological

The cheering and harmonizing effect of play strengthens social ties. Communication is aided

Pedagogic

While some hold that play weakens character and should be forbidden, others have held it has educational value. It can be used as a method of instruction or converted to teaching in a systematic way. There may be a playful quality in the most serious work, which is seen in the highest and noblest forms of work being pleasurable

To a great extent, many of these theories are still viable. What they lack is sophistication in two senses: developmental and psychodynamic. The cognitive implications of exploration, curiosity, sensory-motor stages, the use of logic, and so on, were not available to early theorists, nor were id and ego aspects in terms of the unconscious meaning of play, overdetermination, the principle of multiple function, and defensive operations. Questions as to the motivation for playing games are always able to stir argument. Most pervasive is the dualistic element in which an attempt is made to distinguish play with a functional component (such as that involved in development-resolving conflict), from that which is supposedly pleasurable in its own right. The latter is viewed theoretically as under the aegis of the conflict-free part of ego functioning and not primarily id-bound. However, such arguments often end in some form of the conundrum dealing with whether meaningless play or activity is not functional in some sense.

Although Waelder differentiated between functional pleasure and mastery, he presented a developmental schema indicating the pervasive role of conflict in play.[158] He saw play as having elements of mastery, wish-fulfillment, assimilation of anxious experiences by way of repetition, transformation of passivity to activity, acting out of fantasies about real objects, and gaining distance from both the demands of reality and the superego.

Aggressive derivatives occupy conspicuous roles in games of all types. Again, caution is needed in reductionistic explanations of play being nothing but a vehicle for aggressive discharge. It should not be assumed that all aggression is somehow drained to start another day anew. Even the most civilized of games, such as chess or Monopoly, have elements of sublimated aggression. In some play the cathartic element is conspicuous. There is play that requires less of a veneer of friendliness, with little need for dignity or grown-up-ness. Many hurts and grievances are relieved through such consciously employed fantasies as capturing a piece of carved wood, called a king, on a chess board. Even loss is still only play. As Menninger explained, "With the aim of magic, all the dreams of fairy tales can be realized in play: giants slain, treasures discovered, kingdoms acquired, distances annihilated, dragons destroyed."[159]

While words used in competitive games are those connected with naked aggression (kill, beat, attack, annihilate), there is even less concealment in the open encouragement that coaches and fans give to play against the enemy. This expression of aggression essentially promotes success and victory in athletic contests at any price. The confusion, begun in the pre-oedipal child between athletic teams and countries at war, persists into adolescence.

Developmental Lines Involving Play. Anna Freud described a developmental line involving three sequences: (1) egocentricity to companionship, (2) body to toys, and (3) play to work.[160] In the first there is a transition from a narcissistic view of an object world to one where objects are given cognizance; later, other children become temporary help-mates governed by the duration of a task, followed by a level where mixed feelings toward others predominate. Going from a body to a toy involves a shift from playing with one's own body—that of the mother—to a transitional object such as a soft, first plaything. Various toys are selectively chosen after that, with an extension to things, such as those used for filling up or opening or shutting, then on to moveable toys, to toys that can be broken or destroyed, and finally to toys connected with sex-typing in a masculine or feminine manner. From these, pleasures in achievement and mastery occur.

Advances in ego development and impulse control are needed to change from the ability to play to an ability to work. Modification of impulses is needed not to use things in an aggressive manner or destroy them. Ability to carry out preconceived play with delay to attain a distant outcome is needed which requires the dominance of the reality principle. Games, as distinguished from play, are seen in this developmental framework as taking origin from derivatives in which masculine and feminine trends can be expressed. Symbolic and formalized expressions of aggressive attack, defense, and competition then take place.

Ego development must proceed to the point where reality testing and adaptation are operative. Equipment used in games may serve many symbolic needs valued by the child. In competitive games the child's body and skills are the symbol and tool. An intact body, with a functioning motor component, an investment in the body, peer relationships, attachments and companionship, ability to tolerate frustration, and to utilize controlled aggression, are all necessary for participation in games.

Since games involve rule-following, as well as understanding the reality of the game, superego development must have proceeded sufficiently so that cheating is minimized. To cheat is to play unfairly. While being a poor loser is being a poor sport, winning unfairly is dishonest. To play fairly has overtones of not taking undue advantage of an opponent, a remnant of the child's underdog feeling of not having things equal. In some settings, an honorable defeat may be chosen by an individual to an inglorious victory, which is a means of tempering the unbridled aggression which leads to a victory at any price.[161] The breakdown of the rules of the game, seen in some American troops in Vietnam who shot unarmed women and children, elicits a feeling of unfairness in those who were not there. Winning that way is seen as having too high a price.[162]

Conversely, the adolescent who is caught up with excessive concern about driving home an aggressive advantage will be the athletic underachiever. Yet, in many of the contact sports a set of values develops to win first, and congratulations are given for laying an opponent out. This is inherent in the condonation of socially accepted violence and also in the covert, if not overt, realization that softening an opponent is likely to enhance the chance for victory. Does this type of social sanction lead to a superego development which accepts these norms? Or does the use of violence by those in positions of authority and respect lead to adolescents internalizing this as approved behavior?

Sports as Equivalent to Play. During adolescence, sports become the equivalent of play. This includes contact sports as well as participation in activities which have elements of mastery and competitiveness, even with the self.[163] Physically aggressive sports are increasing for girls, in keeping with the changing sex-role standard. As part of reality testing, the aggressive element in sports provides the adolescent with a confirmatory test of his own abilities, and also a test of how much aggression it is safe to release.

Competitiveness can be seen in may areas besides sports, where more direct evidence of winning is lacking. Ego-ideal components, the developmental precursors of being brave, strong, and fearless, are seen in adolescent forms as well. While athletics may be a way of mastering earlier fears, some adolescents overcompensate so that bravado becomes a dominating characterological trait. Self-esteem is intimately connected with being able to conform according to the standards of the ego-ideal. By this measure, the connection is seen between work and sexuality in terms of adequate or inadequate performance. The particular athletic vehicle chosen by an adolescent to confirm his capabilities varies according to antecedents in his own personality.

The risk of physical injury permits indulgence if a victory occurs. The threat of a retaliatory punishment is ever-present, but after one has conquered and taken risks exultation can occur. The punishment was forthcoming during the event, and after it is over one can relax and feel secure in having met his own ego-ideal standards. However, repetition enters in for periodic needs either to bolster self-esteem or meet the internalized demands again. While individual symbolic features may operate, a culture shares a sufficient number so that most adolescents are able to operate within a common core of meaning. Any one act is seen as serving multiple functions to offer the opportunity of resolving conflicts with authority figures. In the absence of this cure for many adolescents, the game is likely to continue by way of trying to compete and best authority representatives through antisocial acts in which police and the system are the opponents. In this way, inhibitions or work avoidances are dealt with. This is especially so when the pure nature of a sport is prominent, which carries a continual impact in the alteration of feelings in other areas of life apart from sports. To be able to endure physically, to tolerate delay and gratification, to accept defeat, endure frustration, and work long hours, are more than just play. For some these qualities may become part of their work life, but during adolescence many components of the personality are being handled in this manner.

Intensely competitive sports have a developmental role for adolescents who do not directly participate. From the mixture of chaos, fun, aggression, and playing which comprise latency contact sports, a few boys with good coordination, personal needs to succeed in this area, prominence of fantasies of glory by such a route, and peer approval, gain ascendancy. One or both parents become identified with the success of the child in the particular sport. This is portrayed in the cartoon of a Little League baseball game where an eleven-year-old batter is talking to a twelve-year-old catcher while four umbrella-wielding mothers are beating the umpire over the head. One is saying to the other, "Ya know, I'd give up this darn game if it wasn't such a healthy outlet for my parents' frustrations." One study of a thousand athletes in football, baseball, basketball, and track evaluated 150 different personality dimensions.[164] The following comprised the athletic profile: greater achievement orientation, greater aggressive tendencies, more willingness to pay the physical and emotional price for success, more realization of the reality demands of life, a more open and trusting personality, and a definite lack of extroversion in the form of showboating. The latter is interesting from the inherent exhibitionistic element in athletic performance, but corresponds to the sublimation of these interests. This becomes clear when the inability to perform, or hence sublimate, is impaired.

The family psychodynamics of athletic achievement are intriguing, as is any other area of psychopathology when there are manifestations of under- or overachievement. The need of a family for a star can result in overreaching analogous to academic overachievement. Given a setting in which early success can be had, there is little preparation for the disappointments when a boy may not make the team and has few other talents.

> A nineteen-year-old was first seen following his discharge from the armed forces for neuro-psychiatric reasons. He had been groomed to achieve success as a boxer—his father's frustrated ambition—since beginning school. During latency and adolescence, he achieved some success in amateur participation and Golden Glove boxing, but at that point his luck ran out. He was finally told that no future awaited him in that career now that he was grown up. Upon finishing high school with a mediocre record, he joined the Marines and enjoyed boot camp. However, while overseas he began to feel isolated and had feelings that others regarded him as a coward. Frank paranoid psychotic material emerged and he was eventually discharged.

Fathers and Sons. The father whose need for success stands or falls by that of his son indicates many unresolved conflicts. Explanations vary from the father's self-esteem being regulated by the accomplishments of his children to acting out repressed aggression or other antisocial impulses through them. In some cases the father may overtly act out conflicts with his own superego by way of criticizing a coach for the way he is handling his children or for mistakes in using the wrong players or the wrong strategy. These mechanisms permeate a good deal of the passive participant syndrome of spending hours before a television set observing the physical aggression of others. When it is realized that this commences with the five- to six-year-old, a significant impact on personality development would occur if this variable was lacking. A dramatic situation of a father whose potency, maleness, and success were tied up with the athletic performance of his son to a pathological degree is seen in the following case:[165]

> Louis, a thirty-eight-year-old father, was seen because of his inability to control rage towards his sixteen-year-old son, Richard. The boy was in the eleventh grade, a popular football star in his school. For two years, the boy excelled in sports, yet the father continued outbursts of rage and assaultive behavior toward the boy.
>
> The inappropriate outbursts were triggered by minor incidents, such as the boy coming in fifteen minutes late from a date. During two of these episodes, the father was jailed. One occurred after his running up and down the sidelines in a hotly contested high school football game before thousands of spectators as he yelled obscenities toward his son. This was after he made a bad play, in a game in which he otherwise starred.

Existing side by side with this extreme and inappropriate behavior was a sort of hero worship for the son. The father would go out of his way to do favors for his son and he expressed a keen interest in his son's development. In time, the father began wearing his son's football jersey and spent hours pouring over newspaper stories of his son's achievements. He wanted to share the intimacies of the boy's life, was excited by fantasies of his son's life, and wanted to double-date with his son.

He organized his seven other children into a cheering section to greet Richard when he came home from games. When rebuffed by the son who wanted to live his own life, the father became depressed and rageful. He concluded that Richard was ungrateful for the sacrifices he made. Louis began to confront Richard with choices such as, "Would you prefer to be with me or your girl friend?" He attempted in subtle ways to sabotage his son's relationship with his girl friend.

The involvement with his son was very intense. During this time, the father's sexual interest in his wife began to wane, and he resorted to masturbation, during which he often had thoughts of Richard and his girl friend. He became jealous when his son danced with his mother; at the same time he began leaving himself out of family affairs, turning more and more of his responsibility over to Richard.

When the boy finally went to college, the father moved into his room and intensified his identification. He again had fantasies of Richard winning the Heisman Trophy as outstanding football star of the country. Presentation of honors would spotlight Louis, in his fantasies, as the father of the winner. In spite of these inappropriate feelings and behavior, Louis was able to hold a good job and do excellent work.

If a boy is successful at athletics, his phallic and narcissistic gains are temporarily immense. Not only do peers give him at least some type of acclaim, despite a few who oppose sports, but those younger and older do so as well. This is an area in which his family and friends can express admiration as well as temper early rivalries. In an oedipal sense, the boy secures gratification, with his father now admiring the powerful and aggressive son. Athletic success is totally congruent with the sex-role standard, and the high school athletic star rates high in the hierarchy of securing desirable girls and social mobility. How can any adolescent boy give this up and become just another one of those struggling for mundane vocational success later?

Some needs are overtly aggressive in terms of physical contact. One professional football player related picturing his brother's face behind the faceguard of an opponent to throw a successful block. In some cases, the physical contact of the game is eroticized, as in the piles of twisting bodies. Many types of gratification may be involved: the ties from membership in a group with common goals; opportunities in the locker and shower room for exhibitionism; voyeurism; phallic curiosity; sexualized horseplay; and joking.[166]

Ego devices which regulate self-esteem, and superego sanctions for these activities, must be given up if the successful athlete is to find his way elsewhere. If athletic activity is used as a source of self-mastery, with the aggression being ego-syntonic, the transition to other techniques for esteem is easier.

Difficulties may be perpetuated in later life with work or vocational problems. Those for whom athletics served as a rather direct outlet for unneutralized aggression may find it difficult to handle aggression. Some resort to antisocial or illegal acts in the absence of a sport which socially sanctions aggression. Others act out their impulses in various characterological maneuvers. Nor can the consequences of ungratified wishes on the family unit be ignored in terms of marital disharmony, as well as the subtle but definite impact on siblings.

> A former successful athlete became just as successful coaching in a highly competitive high school football conference. During his winning years, there was apparently little disturbance. Due to a combination of personal and situational factors, his winning seasons began to dwindle to the point where he was asked to resign. Over the period of the next few years, efforts to deal with his depressed state by himself had had only transient effects. His eleven-year-old son was the one who forced the issue after all efforts to deal with his encopresis had failed. The symptom had its onset the year of his father's dismissal as head coach.

REFERENCES

1. C. E. Bowerman and J. W. Kinch, Changes in family and peer orientation of children between the fourth and tenth grades, *Social Forces* 37(1959):206-211.
2. M. Gold, *Status Forces in Delinquent Boys* (Ann Arbor: Institute for Social Research, 1963).
3. R. J. Peck and R. J. Havighurst, *The Psychology of Character Development* (New York: Wiley, 1960).
4. M. J. Rosenthal, M. Finkelstein, E. Ni, and R. E. Robertson, A study of mother-child relationships in the emotional disorder of children, *Genetic Psychology Monographs* 60(1959):65-116

5. A. Bandura and R. H. Walter, *Adolescent Aggression* (New York: Ronald Press, 1959).

6. M. J. Rosenthal, E. Ni, M. Finkelstein, and G. K. Berkwitz, Father-child relationships and children's problems, *Archives of General Psychiatry* 7(1962):360-373.

7. W. McCord and J. McCord, *Origins of Crime: A New Evaluation of the Cambridge-Somerville Youth Study* (New York: Columbia University Press, 1959).

8. R. M. Counts, Family crises and the impulsive adolescent, *Archives of General Psychiatry* 17(1967):64-71.

9. N. Ackerman, *The Psychodynamics of Family Life* (New York: Basic Books, 1958).

10. M. Schofield, *The Sexual Behavior of Young People* (Boston: Little, Brown, and Co., 1965).

11. D.R. Miller and G.E. Swanson, *Inner Conflicts and Defense* (New York: Henry Holt, 1960).

12. E. Douvan and J. Adelson, *The Adolescent Experience* (New York: Wiley, 1966).

13. G. Glueck and E. Glueck, *Family Environment and Delinquency* (Boston: Houghton Mifflin, 1962).

14. A. Freud, Adolescence as a developmental disturbance, *Adolescence: Psychosocial Perspectives*, ed. G. Caplan and S. Lebovici, pp. 5-10 (New York: Basic Books, 1969).

15. S. Freud, On the universal tendency to debasement in the sphere of love, *Standard Edition* 11(1957):177-190.

16. R. D. Laing, *The Divided Self* (London: Tavistock, 1960).

17. L. C. Wynne, The study of intrafamilial alignments and splits in exploratory family therapy, *Exploring the Base for Family Therapy*, ed. N. Ackerman, F. L. Beatman, and S. N. Sherman, (New York: Family Service Association of America, 1967).

18. R. D. Laing, Mystification, confusion, and conflict, *Intensive Family Therapy* ed. I. Boszormenyi-Nagy and J. L. Framo, pp. 343-363 (New York: Harper, 1965).

19. J. Anthony, The reactions of adults to adolescents and their behavior, *Adolescence: Psychosocial Perspectives*, ed. G. Caplan and S. Lebovici, pp. 54-78 (New York: Basic Books, 1969).

20. T. Szasz, *The Myth of Mental Illness* (New York: Harper, 1966).

21. T. J. Scheff, *Being Mentally Ill* (Chicago: Aldine, 1966).

22. C. Rycroft, ed., *Psychoanalysis Observed* (London: Constable, 1966).

23. J. C. Little, The athlete's neurosis—a deprivation crisis, *Acta Psychiatrica Scandinavica* 45(1969):187-197.

24. H. Deutsch, Menstruation, *Psychology of Women*, vol. I, pp. 149-184 (New York: Grune and Straton, 1944).

25. J. S. Kestenberg, Menarche, *Adolescents*, ed. S. Lorand and H. I. Schneer, pp. 19-50, (New York: Paul B. Hoeber, 1961).

26. T. Benedek, *Studies in Psychosomatic Medicine: Psychosexual Functions in Women* (New York: Ronald, 1952).

27. S. Freud, The economic problems of masochism, *Standard Edition* 19(1961):159-170.

28. R. J. Stoller, Symbiosis anxiety and the development of masculinity, *Archives of General Psychiatry* 30(1974):164-172.

29. R. Moulton, Women with double lives, *Contemporary Psychoanalysis* 13(1977):64-84.

30. Group for the Advancement of Psychiatry, *Normal Adolescence* (New York: GAP, 1966).

31. R. Redl, Adolescents—just how do they react?, *Adolescence: Psychosocial Perspectives*, ed. B. Caplan and S. Lebovici, pp. 79-99 (New York: Basic Books, 1969).

32. A. Freud, On certain difficulties in the preadolescent's relation to his parents, *Indications for Child Analysis and Other Papers—1945-1956*, pp. 95-106 (London: Hogarth, 1969).

33. S. Isaacs, The nature and function of phantasy, *International Journal of Psycho-Analysis*, 29(1948):73-97.

34. L. Peller, Daydreams and children's favorite books, *Psychoanalytic Study of the Child* 14(1959):414-433.

35. P. Blos, *On Adolescence* (New York: Free Press, 1962).

36. A. Frank, *The Diary of a Young Girl* (New York: Doubleday, 1952).

37. E. Weiss, *Principles of Psychodynamics* (New York: Grune and Stratton, 1950).

38. J. L. Freedman and A. N. Doob, *Deviancy: The Psychology of Being Different* (New York: Academic Press, 1968).

39. R. J. Stoller, A contribution to the study of gender identity, *International Journal of Psycho-Analysis* 45(1964):220-226.

40. A. Freud, *Normality and Pathology in Childhood* (New York: International Universities Press, 1965).

41. C. W. Socarides, *The Overt Homosexual* (New York: Grune and Stratton, 1968).

42. S. H. Fraiberg, Homosexual conflicts, *Adolescents: Psychoanalytic Approach to Problems and Therapy* (New York: Harper, 1962).

43. P. Federn, *Ego Psychology and the Psychoses* (New York: Basic Books, 1952).

44. K. Kenniston, Developmental aspects of psychosocial disturbances, *Journal of the American Academy of Psychoanalysis* 1(1973):23-38.

45. E. Kris, On preconscious mental processes, *Psychoanalytic Explorations in Art*, pp. 303-318 (New York: International Universities Press, 1952).

46. W. Hoffer, Mouth, hand, and ego formation, *Psychoanalytic Study of the Child* 3/4(1949):49-56.

47. H. Hartman, *Ego Psychology and the Problem of Adaptation* (New York: International Universities Press, 1958).
48. P. Blos, Character formation in adolescence, *Psychoanalytic Study of the Child* 23(1968):245-263.
49. E. Kris, Laughter as an expressive process, *Psychoanalytic Explorations in Art* (New York: International Universities Press, 1952).
50. L. A. Spiegel, Comments on the psychoanalytic psychology of adolescence, *Psychoanalytic Study of the Child* 13(1958):296-308.
51. P. Blos, *The Young Adolescent* (New York: The Free Press, 1970).
52. E. Jacobson, Normal and pathological moods: their nature and functions, *Psychoanalytic Study of the Child* 12(1957):73-113.
53. S. Freud, Analysis terminable and interminable, *Standard Edition* 23(1964):211-223).
54. H. Hartmann, Mutual influences in the development of ego and id, *Psychoanalytic Study of the Child* 7(1952):9-41.
55. J. Piaget, *The Child's Conception of the World* (New York: Humanities Press, 1951).
56. B. Inhelder and J. Piaget, *The Growth of Logical Thinking from Childhood to Adolescence* (New York: Basic Books, 1958).
57. D. Elkind, Egocentrism in adolescence, *Child Development* 38(1967):1025-1034.
58. D. Beres, Clinical notes on aggression in children, *Psychoanalytic Study of the Child* 7(1952):241-263.
59. A. H. Modell, *Object Love and Reality* (New York: International Universities Press, 1968).
60. H. Hartmann, Comments on the psychoanalytic theory of the ego, *Psychoanalytic Study of the Child* 5(1950):74-96.
61. H. Nunberg, The psychology of the ego, *Principles of Psychoanalysis*, pp. 114-177 (New York: International Universities Press, 1955).
62. D. Hume, *An Enquiry Concerning Human Understanding* (Chicago: Philosophical Classics, 1935).
63. J. Piaget, *Judgment and Reasoning in the Child* (New York: Harcourt Brace and World, 1926).
64. D. Beres, Ego deviation and the concept of schizophrenia, *Psychoanalytic Study of the Child* 11(1956):164-235.
65. A. Freud, Adolescence, *Psychoanalytic Study of the Child* 13(1958):255-278.
66. A. Freud, Studies in passivity, *Indications for Child Analysis and Other Papers—1945-1956*, pp. 245-259 (London: Hogarth, 1969).
67. P. Blos, op. cit., 35.
68. K. Abraham, The influence of oral erotism on character-formation, *On Character and Libido Development*, pp. 151-164 (New York: Norton, 1966).
69. K. Abraham, Character in formation on the genital level of libido, *On Character and Libido Development*, pp. 188-198 (New York: Norton, 1966).

70. W. Reich, On character analysis, *The Psychoanalytic Reader*, ed. R. Fliess, pp. 129-247 (New York: International Universities Press, 1948).

71. M. Gitelson, Character synthesis: the psychotherapeutic problem of adolescence, *American Journal of Orthopsychiatry* 18(1948):422-431.

72. P. Blos, Character formation in adolescence, *Psychoanalytic Study of the Child* 23(1968):245-263.

73. M. S. Mahler, On human symbiosis and the vicissitudes of individuation, *Journal of the American Psychoanalytic Association* 15(1967):740-763.

74. M. S. Mahler, On the significance of the normal separation individuation phase, *Drives, Affects, Behavior*, vol. 2, pp. 161-169, ed. M. Schur, (New York: International Universities Press, 1965).

75. P. Blos, The second individuation process of adolescence, *Psychoanalytic Study of the Child* 22(1967):162-186.

76. H. F. Waldhorn and B. D. Fine, *Trauma and Symbolism* (New York: International Universities Press, 1974).

77. K. M. Williams, Jr., *American Society*, 2nd Ed. (New York: Knopf, 1960).

78. T. Roszak, *The Making of a Counterculture* (New York: Doubleday, 1969).

79. B. C. Rosen, H. J. Crockett, Jr., and C. Z. Nunn, eds., *Achievement in American Society* (Cambridge, Mass.: Schenkman, 1969).

80. L. M. Terman and M. H. Oden, *The Gifted Child Grows Up: Twenty-Five Years Follow-Up of a Superior Group* (Stanford: Stanford University Press, 1947).

81. D. C. McClelland, et al., *The Achievement Motive* (New York: Appleton-Century-Crofts, 1953).

82. R. D. Hess, High school antecedents of young adult achievement, *Studies in Adolescence*, ed. R. E. Grinder, pp. 401-414 (New York: Macmillan, 1963).

83. D. E. Lavin, *The Prediction of Academic Performance* (New York: Russell Sage Foundation, 1965).

84. R. H. Turner, *The Social Context of Ambition* (San Francisco: Chandler, 1964).

85. E. Klinger, Fantasy need achievement as a motivational construct, *Psychological Bulletin* 66(1966):291-308.

86. A. Skolnick, Motivational imagery and behavior over twenty years, *Journal of Consulting Psychology* 30(1966):463-478.

87. J. S. Coleman, *The Adolescent Society* (New York: Free Press, 1966).

88. E. Douvan and J. Adelson, op. cit.

89. J. K. Myers and B. H. Roberts, *Family and Class Dynamics in Mental Illness* (New York: Wiley, 1959).

90. B. C. Rosen, The achievement syndrome: a psycho-cultural dimension of social stratification, *American Sociological Review* 21(1956):203-211.

91. A. Davis, Socialization and adolescent personality, *Adolescence: 43rd Yearbook of the National Society for Studies in Education*, ed. N. B. Henry, pp. 189-216 (Chicago: University of Chicago Press, 1964).

92. K. T. Hill and S. B. Sarason, *The Relation of Test Anxiety and Defensiveness to Test and School Performance Over the Elementary-School Year: A Further Longitudinal Study* (*Monograph of the Society for Research in Child Development*, vol. 31, no. 2, NC. 104, 1966).

93. J. Shelton and J. P. Hill, The effects on cheating of achievement anxiety and knowledge of peer performance, *Developmental Psychology* 1(1969):449-455.

94. J. P. Hill and R. A. Kochendorfer, Knowledge of peer scores and risk of detection as determinants of cheating in a resistance to temptation situation, *Developmental Psychology* 1(1969):231-238.

95. T. Parsons, Age and sex in the social structure of the United States, *Personality in Nature, Society, and Culture*, ed. C. Kluckhohn and H. A. Murray, pp. 269-281 (New York: Knopf, 1953).

96. Coleman, op. cit.

97. E. Janeway, *Man's World, Woman's Place* (New York: William Morrow, 1971).

98. Lavin, op. cit.

99. W. H. Sewell and V. P Shal, Socioeconomic status, intelligence and the attainment of higher education, *Sociological Education* 40(1967):1-23.

100. G. H. Elder, Jr., Adolescent socialization and development, *Handbook of Personality Theory and Research*, ed. E. F. Borgatta and W. W. Lambert, pp. 239-364 (Chicago: Rand-McNally, 1968).

101. M. Winterbottom, The relation of need for achievement to learning experiences in independence and mastery, *Motives in Fantasy, Action and Society*, ed. J. W. Atkinson, pp. 445-479 (New York: Van Nostrand, 1958).

102. B. C. Rosen, Race, ethnicity, and the achievement syndrome, *American Sociological Review* 24(1959):47-60.

103. J. Kagan and H. A. Moss, *Birth to Maturity* (New York: Wiley, 1962.)

104. B. C. Rosen, Socialization and achievement maturation in Brazil, *American Sociological Review* 27(1962):612-624.

105. D. C. McClelland, *The Achieving Society* (New York: Van Nostrand, 1961).

106. J. S. Coleman, et al., *Equality of Educational Opportunity* (Washington, D.C.: U.S. Government Printing Office, 1966).

107. H. Beilin, The pattern of postponability and its relation to social class malulity, *Journal of Social Psychology* 44(1956):33-48.

108. R. H. Ellis and W. C. Lane, Structural supports for upward malulity, *American Social Review* 28(1963):743-756.

109. E. Y. McDill and J. Coleman, Family and peer influence in college plans of high school students, *Sociological Review* 38(1965):112-126.

110. J. Calusen, Family Structure, socialization, and personality, *Review of Child Development Research*, ed. by L. W. Hoffman and M. L. Hoffman, vol. 2, pp. 1-53 (New York: Russell Sage Foundation, 1966).

111. J. H. S. Bossard and E. Boll, *The Large Family System* (Philadelphia: University of Pennsylvania Press, 1956).

112. J. K. Lasko, Parent behavior toward first and second children, *Genetic Psychological Monograph* 49(1954):96-137.
113. C. McArthur, Personality of first and second children, *Psychiatry* 19(1956):47-54.
114. W. H. Sewell and J. M. Armer, Neighborhood context and college plans, *American Sociological Review* 31(1966):707-712.
115. Coleman, op.cit.
116. Coleman et al., op. cit.
117. T. R. Sizer, *The Metropolitan Enigma: Inquiries Into the Nature of America's "Urban Crisis"* (Washington, D. C.: U.S. Government Printing Office, 1967).
118. J. Coombs and W. W. Cooley, Dropouts, in high school and after high school, *American Education Research Journal* 5(1968):343-363.
119. D. Schreiber, ed., *Profile of the School Dropout* (New York: Vintage Books, 1968).
120. S. R. Hathaway, P. C. Reynolds and E. D. Monachesi, Follow-up of the later career and lives of 1,000 boys who dropped out of high school, *Journal of Consulting Clinical Psychology* 33(1969):370-380.
121. S. R. Hathaway, P. C. Reynolds and E. D. Monachesi, Follow-up of 812 girls 10 years after high school dropout, *Journal of Consulting Clinical Psychology* 33(1969):333-390.
122. L.E. Datta, E. Schaefer and M. Davis, Sex and scholastic aptitude as variables in teachers' ratings of the adjustment and classroom behavior of negro and other seventh-grade students, *Journal of Educational Psychology* 59(1968):94-101.
123. D.A. Payne and W.W. Farquhar, The dimensions of an objective measure of academic self concept, *Journal of Educational Psychology* 53(1962):187-192.
124. T.A. Ringness, Identification patterns, motivation, and school achievement of bright junior high school boys, *Journal of Educational Psychology* 58(1967):93-102.
125. H. D. Carter, The development of interest in vocations, *Adolescence, 43rd Yearbook of the National Society for Studies in Education*, ed. N. B. Henry (Chicago: University of Chicago, 1964).
126. H. Borow, Development of occupational motives and roles, *Review of Child Development Research*, ed. L. W. Hoffman and M. L. Hoffman, vol. 2, pp. 373-422 (New York: Russell Sage Foundation, 1966).
127. E. Ginzberg, et al., *Occupational Choice* (New York: Columbia University Press, 1951).
128. D. E. Super, R. Starishevsky, H. Matlin and J. P. Jordaan, eds., *Career Development: Self-Concept Theory* (Princeton: College Entrance Examination Board, 1963).
129. Elder, op. cit.
130. A. Roe, *The Psychology of Occupations* (New York: Wiley, 1956).
131. A. Roe, Early determinants of vocational choice, *Journal of Counseling Psychology* 4(1957):212-217.

132. A. Roe, Personality structure and occupational behavior, *Man in a World at Work*, ed. H. Borow, pp. 196-214 (Boston: Houghton Mifflin, 1964).

133. W. W. Cooley, Current research on the career development of scientists, *Journal of Counseling Psychology* 11(1964):88-93.

134. J. W. Trent and LV. L. Medsker, *Beyond High School: A Psychosocial Study of 10,000 High School Graduates* (San Francisco: Jossey-Bass, 1968).

135. N. C. Morse and R. S. Weiss, The function and meaning of work and the job, *Vocational ehavior: Readings in Theory and Research*, ed. D. G. Zytowski (New York: Holt, Rinehart and Winston, 1968).

136. S. L. Wollbein, Labor trends, manpower, and automation, *Man in A World at Work*, ed. by H. Borow, pp. 155-173 (Boston: Houghton Mifflin, 1964).

137. S. H. Osipow, *Theories of Career Development* (New York: Appleton-Century-Crofts, 1968).

138. Elder, op. cit., 100., p. 348.

139. B. Nachman, Childhood experience in vocational choice in law, dentistry, and social work, *Journal of Counseling Psychology* 7(1960):243-250.

140. S. J. Segal, Psychoanalytic analysis of personality factors in vocational choice, *Journal of Counseling Psychology* 8(1961):202-210.

141. S. Freud, Civilization and its discontents, *Standard Edition* 12(1961):101.

142. R. W. White, Motivation reconsidered: the concept of competence, *Psychoanalytic Review* 66(1959):297-333.

143. I. Hendrick, Work and the pleasure principle, *Psychoanalytic Quarterly* 12(1943):311-329.

144. B. Lantes, Work and the instincts, *International Journal of Psycho-Analysis* 24(1943):114-119.

145. K. A. Menninger, Work as a sublimation, *Bulletin of the Menninger Clinic*, 6(1952):170-182.

146. C. P. Oberndorf, Psychopathology of work, *Bulletin of the Menninger Clinic* 15(1951):77-84.

147. E. H. Erikson, *Childhood and Society*, 2nd Ed. (New York: Norton, 1963).

148. W. S. Neff, *Work and Human Behavior* (New York: Atherton, 1968).

149. D. C. Miller, Industry and the worker, *Man in A World at Work*, ed. H. Borow, pp. 96-124 (Boston: Houghton Mifflin, 1964).

150. R. W. Hodge, P. M. Siegel and P. H. Rossi, Occupational prestige in the United States, 1925-1963, *Vocational Behavior*, ed. D. G. Zytowski, pp. 86-95 (New York: Holt, Rinehart and Winston, 1968).

151. P. M. Blau, et al., Occupational choice: a conceptual framework, *Vocational Behavior: Readings in Theory and Research*, ed. D. G. Zytowski, pp. 358-370 (New York: Holt, Rinehart and Winston, 1968).

152. M. B. Katz, *The Irony of Early School Reform* (Cambridge: Harvard University Press, 1969).

153. T. Caplow, *The Sociology of Work* (Minneapolis: University of Minnesota Press, 1954), p. 216.

154. P. Lauter and F. Howe, *The Conspiracy of the Young* (New York: World Publishing, 1970).

155. R. E. Harron and B. Sutton-Smith, *Child's Play* (New York: Wiley, 1971).

156. Erikson, op. cit., 147., pp. 212-213.

157. K. Groos, *The Play of Man*, trans. E. L. Baldwin (New York: Appleton, 1913)

158. R. Waelder, The psychoanalytic theory of play, *Psychoanalytic Quarterly* 2(1933):208-224.

159. K. Menninger, *Love Against Hate* (New York: Harcourt, 1942).

160. A. Freud, *Normality and Pathology in Childhood* (New York: International Universities Press, 1965).

161. N. Evans, The passing of the gentleman, *Psychoanalytic Quarterly* 18(1949):19-43.

162. S. M. Hersch, *My Lai 4* (New York: Random House, 1970).

163. R. T. Porter, Sports and adolescence, *Motivations in Play, Games and Sports*, ed. R. Slovenko and J. A. Knight, pp. 73-90 (Springfield: Charles C Thomas, 1967).

164. J. P. Dolan, Parents of athletes, Ibid, Slovenko and Knight, pp. 299-306.

165. J. Lupo, Case study of a father of an athlete, Ibid, Slovenko and Knight, pp. 325-328.

166. A. A. Stone, Football, Ibid, Slovenko and Knight, pp. 419-434.

Chapter Two

The Youth Period

The vastly expanded impact of social factors is one reason the determination of early, mid, and late adolescence varies widely. Operationally, late adolescence is used as equivalent to the youth period, and as a rule, is thought of as commencing in the post-high school years, although for some individuals it continues up to age twenty-five and even beyond. The onset of adolescence is generally agreed to be coterminous with the physiological changes of puberty, but no set criteria exist for the endpoint. Past investigations have been preoccupied with the social concomitants of early adolescence, but the current scene is one of confusion about when adolescence ends—if it ever does. Events of the decade of the 1960s (campus uprisings, protest groups focused on civil rights, anti-draft movements, anti-war activities, and the emergence of militant minorities), in many ways stand in stark contrast to the lethargic skepticism of the 1970s.

Youth as a stage is conceptualized as a state of tension and hesitancy between the late adolescent and his society, a curious mixture of efforts to solidify the personality structure, so that diverse needs can be met within an integrated self. A sense of purpose can give rise to a dedication to a worthy social cause, if the cause touches earlier roots and needs. If the behavior is ego-syntonic with the pursuit of ideals, a gradual sense of finding the self emerges. The cause can vary from VISTA, or the Peace Corps, to working with Nader's Raiders or the Young Republicans. In some cases political causes—which vary from the radical right to the radical left—are embraced. In any case the youth feels a sense of believing that he has gradually been able to determine what really counts. While some of these causes temporarily serve a particular purpose, and subsequently subside, others remain part of a process of continuity. What seems significant is that particular causes come and go, as though they are part of the self-therapy administered by late adolescents to themselves.

Some youths can tolerate a good deal of ambiguity and anxiety with respect to delay of commitment or the perseverance needed for pursuing long-range goals. Others begin to demonstrate signs of conflict as this developmental phase drags on. The hypothesis is that an optimal degree of anxiety for functioning is needed. This is related to formulations regarding the need for maintaining some degree of tension or disequilibrium to avoid the lassitude which becomes too comfortable to promote striving. All preceding conflict—maladaptive patterns, defenses, ego deformations, and regressive tendencies—can be placed under greater strain in late adolescence. The ego strength that has evolved, with its particular set of tolerances, will be called upon to deal with the crises attendant upon finally abandoning adolescence. When this leaving is unusually prolonged or never attained, it requires an examination of the conflicts which have not been mastered, and which have left the late adolescent prone to developmental problems.

Problems cluster around the failure to consolidate earlier crises in the personality: (1) the failure to attain a stable hierarchy of ego functions which reflect permissible individual differences, (2) limitations in conflict-free ego functioning which handicap the emergence of secondary autonomy (basically a freedom from interfering neurotic conflict), (3) a sexual position which has not solidified in the sense of object choice or preferred expression of sexual impulses, (4) an unstable image of the self and other object representations, and (5) an unpredictability involving aspects of psychological functioning which leave the organism vulnerable to external and internal threats.[1]

RESOLUTION OF PAST CONFLICTS

A major struggle confronting youth is the need to work through earlier conflicts which have remained dormant. Similar to unresolved conflicts in latency, dormant conflicts during the course of adolescence come to the fore. While the original situations, or interpersonal relationships, are often mastered by way of internalization, during late adolescence these old threats are re-externalized.

Rather than remaining with old threats, resolution is sought with whatever objects or institutions are currently available. The quality of repetition is striking.

Two points of caution are required. Late adolescence is not just a recapitulation of themes which occurred earlier in life, although certain types of unresolved conflicts, in which a high anxiety level is attached, retain a pathogenic potential which may be continuously recreated. Secondly, the vulnerability of those adults or institutions who—at a particular historical moment—are duped into the role of foil for particular adolescents must be made clear. Foils fill the bill so conveniently that they are taken as the epitome of conformism and authority. As such, many adolescents easily fall into the role of expecting privileges and authority based on their accepted position, rather than their actual accomplishments. It is precisely in this area of earning respect that adolescents have usually been nurtured. Many are chagrined to find that respect is not necessarily earned in this world, but that power accomplishes things more readily.

Institutions with more authoritarian trends are extremely vulnerable and have demonstrated this by their repeated problems with youth. Churches, the military, and colleges and universities are prime examples. In many ways they have been sitting ducks for the recrudescence and re-externalization of conflicts present in youths. These institutions, or more specifically the individuals representing them, may be used in attempts to resolve authority conflicts. To the extent that the institutional representatives have carved out their niche based on identifying themselves with powerful institutions without having sufficiently worked out their own needs to gain security in this manner, they are easily used as targets for youthful critics. Their own defenses remain rigid, and prevent a resilient bending and springing back from the onslaught of the late adolescent age group. In time, some youths resolve their own dilemmas and terminate their period of youth by joining the establishment and gaining their security by seeking out their own niche to defend. For others, the struggle for freedom from within continues throughout life according to what seems like a ceaseless attempt at working through authority problems.

By late adolescence a solidification of character structure is usually present. Unresolved and debatable questions about the extent to which character has become relatively fixed still exist. What appears less debatable is the extent to which the devices for dealing with impulses are still in flux. The indecisiveness and fluctuating state of selecting and relating love objects is one prominent example. This is not to say that by age nineteen or twenty a degree of commitment to certain object relations is not made. In fact, nineteen appears to be a crucial age with respect to realization and self-acceptance of perverse or deviant practices as a prominent part of sexuality.[2]

Preference for certain activities at this period is under superego and ego-ideal direction to a great extent. Some preferences have become reactive to exaggerated types of defenses which have emerged. Unresolved conflicts manifest themselves in continuous reactivations under the most adverse environmental situations. These press for resolution by repeatedly enacting events which are not resolved, or by striking characterological distortions. The greater mastery which occurs, the more conflicts are absorbed into the character structure so that they become ego-syntonic. In this way the self-esteem system of youths is enhanced so that they do not continue to experience a personal discrepancy between their ideals and wishes. The self-image then becomes congruent with the idealized part of this self-image.

As channelized and sublimatory activities become possible in late adolescence, the free-flowing play characteristic of earlier adolescence subsides. In part this is due to the ascendancy of cognitive operations in contrast to the type of indulgence in introspection seen earlier. The value of abstract thought processes is accentuated once the capacity for this type of thought has been achieved. If development proceeds without too many regressive components, commitments to specific types of love, work, and play can be made without reliance on aims tinged with grandiosity. Earlier preoccupations manifest themselves by interferences with superego functions, such as unrealistic self-appraisal. Common examples are gross narcissistic, voyeuristic, or exhibitionistic components dominating relationships and involvements. If this takes place, only the youth who is particularly gifted in some particular area will remain comfortable. This is one antecedent situation giving rise to conflicts about identity discussed in chapter 6. Rather than a dominance of the synthetic function of the ego, a persistence of intrasystemic conflicts persist. Narrowing of ego interests corresponds to a gradual realization that the number of options that are realistically possible are limited. In turn, this is a reflection of ego processes solidifying in terms of differentiating means and goals.[3]

Throughout the course of adolescence many aspects of superego functioning have undergone a progressive specialization. In a parallel process, the ego-ideal has also been undergoing a series of changes. When identity problems enter in, ego-ideal change is a broader problem involving structural elements of the id, ego, and superego—as well as that of the entire self. In earlier adolescence, more blatant conflicts between superego prohibitions and ideals have been perpetuated. This is seen in alternatives between a behavior which abruptly shifts from one extreme to another.

> A seventeen-year-old boy presented with a history of assaultive episodes when intoxicated. He would stagger, bleeding and intoxicated, into a church and pray for forgiveness. Seen after this behavior continued for some time, he felt deep remorse about his behavior, despite its repetitious quality. His ideal was that of a kind and gentle person who would help people in distress. Balanced against this when he was sober was a set of inhibitions which permitted only minimal aggressive displays, accompanied by a deep-set frown and self-effacing manner. On follow-up at age thirty-two, he was a full-fledged alcoholic, culminating in his working as a counselor in an alcoholic treatment center.

These types of episodic aggressive displays illustrate the fluctuating nature of youthful aggression as well as sexuality. Filled with hate and self-loathing for various sexual thoughts and acts, a youth may discharge his hate in an outburst of violence against some neutral object. Dissociative episodes result from the degree of aggression directed toward the self or others in which there is a failure of internalized controls and ideals.

> A sixteen-year-old girl from an upper-middle-class background resorted to periodic episodes of running away from home. On one of these, she tried prostitution. When home, she was contrite and self-effacing. At home she described herself in a religious framework, heavily emphasized by her family, as being evil. In fact, she described different dissociative states, without amnesia, in which during one of her bad self states, she would drink, use profanity, and act out prostitution themes. While in one of these states and without experiencing affect, she described her participation with a pimp in the knifing of a fellow prostitute. While fully aware, in a cognitive sense, of what she had done, the correlative emotion never appeared.

ROLE OF THE EGO-IDEAL

The ego-ideal is regarded by some as a more mature form of development than the superego itself. In fact, the issue of whether the ego-ideal is more accurately regarded as evolving through ego development is still germane.[4] Although precursors of the ego-ideal originate in identifications with idealized parental figures, it is insufficient to regard this as the whole story of the evolvement of ego-ideals. The influence of the autonomous ego, as well as the personal and conscious values and ideals to which an adolescent is exposed, prominently influence the behavior of a youth. Ideally, these influences modify the exaggerated fears induced by shame and inferiority as a basis of control which actually stifle ideals.

By the end of adolescence the choice of idealized models based on id-dominated desires, hates, and power strivings still persists in some form. The model chosen is not always based on exaggerated virtues such as overzealousness, humility, or chastity. Searching for an extreme model to emulate as the ideal is more involved with resolution of narcissistic conflicts, loss of a loved person, or disillusionment with a cause, and the effect is to lower moral esteem and self-esteem. This is connected with identity loss related to disappointments and disillusionments, with choices of various adult models to emulate which have not solidified into a single coherent self.

Related to unresolved narcissistic conflicts is the inability to assume responsibility for adverse environmental circumstances. This does not mean that the adolescent must rely on a blithe optimism, where the defense of denial is used to excess and everything is viewed as turning out for the best. The danger lies in the persistence of hopes that others—people, something in the environment, or situations—will guarantee a state of optimal bliss. This is an extension of the rescue fantasy, whereby dependency gratification is sought in the enlarged world of the post-adolescent. Hope remains that luck or special circumstances will intervene to save one from a rather humdrum existence in which effort is required merely to stand still. Attempts to eliminate a feeling of personal helplessness by rescuing others from predicaments is one variety of rescue fantasy. This is seen in such phenomena as groups of adolescents who run drug-centers to help those addicted to drugs. In many types of rescue operations the need for self-rescue is apparent.[5] As long as one can focus on the problems of others, the threat of exposing one's own inner life is minimized.

The contribution of such rescue fantasies to vocational choices has been mentioned in connection with service-oriented occupations reflecting ego-ideal influences. It is perhaps less clear that types of object choices related to friendship or marriage obey the same principlee. Saving others may be a response, in a selfish way, to wishes for possession of another who in turn becomes indebted.

Thus, saving may correspond to a denial or an unconscious wish to destroy or injure. The close relationship between the two is seen in the reaction of a rescuer whose efforts to help are rejected.

Reactions of outraged betrayal by ungrateful wretches are common. Alternating with attempts at rescuing others, these youths are likely to say, "If only so and so had happened," or "It might have been different if," or "If that had only not occurred to me." Hope continues that self-realization will come from chance circumstances. A variety of outcomes are possible. Periodic depressive episodes connected with impulsive acts to secure coercive or magical gratification are connected with threats to the denial mechanism. Masochistic phenomena appear, in which the feeling is transparently clear that someone or something is withholding rescue. In these cases the overall context of disappointed hopes for wish-fulfillment or rescue are often in the background. These impairments in superego and ego-ideal development in youths often persist into adulthood.

THE MAJOR THEMES OF YOUTH

Several themes dominate the daily pattern of most youths. These are not isolated, but function in a recurrent pattern which is detectable in clinical situations. Some questions involve vocational or marital choice, others the relationship to society and its institutions, or to various social roles and life-styles. Obviously, in any given youth they present in different ways.

Problems with Authority. Many youths continue to have problems with authority even in contemporary settings where authority seems undermined. That this has always been present to some extent tells us that the problem is not one peculiar to a given historical period. For some youths there is a continuance of authority difficulties from earlier adolescence, while for others a new twist is added. The new twist may be that while previously intrafamilial conflicts were the paradigm for authority problems, a transformation has occurred whereby the family is seen more as a reflection of the larger problems existing in society.

Hence, a youth becomes preoccupied with trying to change society. However, some writers continue to perceive the family as the ongoing and continuing center of conflict throughout all age ranges.[6] Categorization of a given adolescent as a conformist, rebel, or jock becomes superficially easier if we use external criteria. What is more important is the congruence or incongruence between the identity and integrity adolescents have achieved and the demands made by society. Of course, the limits for opportunities are relevant. Solutions for confrontation with society are helpful. Those who take their places in the ranks are often referred to by adolescents in the peer group as having copped out. This is conceptualized in terms of participating in a relatively meaningless and automotized role in the system. A place in society is thereby achieved at the expense of self-realization. What will happen to the vulnerable who conform but eventually fail to find a niche is problematic.

A polar opposite is the youth who continues to battle with society in the form of its representatives and institutions. This need not take the extreme form of delinquent or criminal behavior, but it can appear in its opposite form where a youth attempts to live his life outside the system. While he preserves his personal integrity and values in this manner, he loses the effectiveness to attain goals within a given social system. Pushed to the extreme, this position maintains that the format of society as it now exists is not worth the effort, and one can only maintain self-respect only by living outside the system. The difference from earlier is that we are not now simply talking about the verbalizations of someone in mid-adolescence, but rather someone with many contemporaries who have moved into the system at some level and are committed to vocational and marital goals, but who feel they are living out a life with little self-respect. Indeed, psychiatrists, such as R. D. Laing, support the degrading effects of trying to act sane in an insane world.[7]

While college, graduate, and professional schools permit an extended deferment of commitments, conflict is manifested in the delay given by preoccupations with the corrupt system in which time is spent without fulfillment or gratification. The popularity of books emphasizing how to win in life by dirty tricks or putting oneself first is in striking contrast to the emphasis of the 1960s on freedom outside the system.[8] The latter mercilessly exposed the bourgeoisie mentality with its emphasis on domestic order, security, moderation and diligence, coupled with its parallel devotion to nationalism, aggressiveness, and institutionalized religion. Such writers, past and present, appear to perform a function for many anguished American youths.

Shifting to An Independent Status. Achieving independence acquires a meaning beyond asserting a desire for autonomy. While development of the capacity for independent functioning is not separate from the issues just discussed regarding relationships to authority, independence is often experienced as meaningless unless the youth is economically self-supporting. While that criterion may be employed, another is the degree of ego-autonomy achieved. Without the latter, a series of rebellious patterns reflect the outcome of earlier and persistent psychological conflicts.

Antecedent patterns of family problems contribute to striving for autonomy in ego functioning. Strivings in some form are indispensable if late adolescents are to take responsibility for their own lives. Overt effort may bear an exaggerated quality for some: patterns of unresolved ambivalence, neurotic ties based on guilt about separation, and sado-masochistic patterns are examples. Related to these struggles is the situation where youths feel that whatever they do is supposed to aggrandize their parents or family. The use of athletics in this manner was discussed in chapter 1. While a strict set of controls may have accomplished this dedication when younger, it does not auger well for the future when it is continued. For some youths, distress is seen when the parent for whom one has been an extension is no longer on the scene. When forced to struggle on their own, or to evolve their own goals, confusion or a form of apathy sets in. Not until the period of youth does it appear that parents are accepted as individuals in their own right and with their own private neuroses, loves, hates, and ambitions, based on their personal life histories. There is then the encounter with the need to expand and perhaps be free from the constraints of a particular family tradition.

It is too gross a simplification to presume that ambivalence must necessarily lead to visible protest. Other outs are utilized more frequently in an effort to bypass personal discomfort. Psychotherapy may be tried, especially by youths from the affluent sector who are seeking a way to come to terms with their ambivalence toward authority. Sundry group experiences may also provide temporary release from the struggle: hallucinogens, retreats into asceticism, meditation, prayer, and experimentation with different religions or group experiences are all possibilities. Part of these experiences involve a self-probing to seek out the limits of the youth's strength, weakness, vulnerability, and resiliency. These appear related to tests of the capacities a person has to withstand the demands of outside authorities and to use what is available.[9] The probings of youth fall somewhere between the fluctuating contacts of the adolescent and the more irreversible commitments of the adult. While this period may last from months to years, the aging process itself changes the status of the probing. Some probings become solidified in terms of ongoing and permanent commitments, but most appear to subside when the youths commit themselves elsewhere, and the scene shifts to new challenges.

The search for a partner goes beyond casual relationships. Preoccupation with sexual fantasies and masturbation shifts to a desire for more regularized intimacies with someone to whom there is a deeper attachment. This implies a cognitive capacity that permits friendship and emotional closeness. From an egocentrism in which others are seen as having value from their similarities to the self ("He's more like me than I am myself"), progress is made in perceiving others as equals though different.

The next step is the capability of feeling emotional warmth toward those perceived as different. A final stage of mutuality is a positiveness for others when they are seen as unique but as deserving concern without regard for immediate gain. This raises complex issues about altruism as a psychological and philosophical phenomena.[10] Is altruism mainly a hypothetical state or is it related to gratification and security? Some continue to believe in the possibility of pure altruism, even though rare.

Traditional Views on Partner Choice. Romanticized versions— even on a sociological level—of how partners are chosen are surely insufficient from a psychodynamic viewpoint. Narrowing to one person has an implication of something special rarely attained to the same degree with any other person. While selective attachments occur among humans as well as other mammals, cultural and historical patterns rarely permit free mate selection. Wishes of parents and relatives are influential, as are money, social class, power, and privilege.

Note that relevant psychodynamic and unconscious factors have not been mentioned in this obvious list. A fascinating study of how searching for a partner occurred in Ireland over the last century revealed that in reality a match was not for companionship, children, or sex. Searching for a partner arose when a plot of land "needed a woman," perhaps the epitome of woman as economic and sexual object.[11] When a man's mother became too old to carry out household functions, a replacement was needed. The result was a mean age at marriage of thirty-eight years for the male. If one criterion used for the passing of the youth is that of choosing a mate, the age in this example has been pushed far beyond the usually accepted. When such stark economic factors are not so controlling, much greater freedom of choice is given to youths to stake out relationships subject to existing psychological or social ties to his family and conventional morality. The freedom of choice then is less correlated with social class. American youths would feel quite oppressed if they could not choose a partner based on at least some basis of feeling companionship and of being in love.

A plethora of sociological works on marriage exist. These emphasize such topics as family and social class in marriage, parental influences, choice of a partner, socialization practices in families of origin regarding marriage, peer influences, and courtship patterns. All of these are relevant to the theme of choosing a mate among youths, but the following discussion focuses on the intricacies of sexuality and choice from the psychological perspective of youths.

The main impetus toward forming a more intense heterosexual attachment in late adolescence appears to be an alteration in the personality structures of two people. A commitment to new forms of intimacy—extending beyond copulatory acts per se—exerts an influence on the egos of both parties. Influence on the superego occurs by way of new models and directives which are available from the partner.

But situations of increased intimacy cannot ignore the possibility of reactivating neurotic conflicts which have remained dormant. The demands for closeness, not just in the context of randomized sexual release, frequently resurrect childhood anxieties. (These should be distinguished from anxieties which arise subsequently and secondarily to the marriage in which a youth establishes a legalized relationship. Here, closeness poses a threat for a need for a commitment.) Preceding experiences with controlling female figures raise threats for males. For girls the fear of exploitative males who will use and abandon them is a frequently encountered theme. When the anxiety mounts, psychopathology in diverse forms emerges.

Terminating Relationships. The majority of cases resolve themselves by three alternatives:

1. Terminating a relationship which permits other, less threatening, partners to be sought. Themes along this line are not only seen in clinical contexts but are the source for novels and short stories.

2. Development of a series of medical or psycho-physiological

complaints leads to a postponement or avoidance of intimacy. Some
of these pertain to sexual performance, such as premature ejaculation or dyspareunia. Others involve physical complaints such as
headache, backache, leg cramp, or dizziness which lead to many
organic evaluations. In some youths, the emergence of psychosomatic illnesses are precipitated after the termination of a relationship. Ulcerative colitis or regional enteritis are two possibilities from
a diathesis to deal with losses.

3. Entering into a marriage accentuates the problems existing
during the preliminary period of attachment. The peak year for
divorce during the second year of marriage indicates pre-existing
problems that were not resolvable or capable of denial.[12] The
decision to divorce is common during the first year of marriage since
it often takes some time to secure a divorce. The majority of these
couples are childless and overall figures indicate three-quarters of
the people who divorce remarry within five years.

Theoretically social phenomena such as mixed parties and going
steady during adolescence are presumed to prepare an adolescent for
later intense attachments. Divorce rates are one indication of the
extent to which these devices fail. If more exacting criteria are used,
such as the extent of personal, marital, or sexual disharmony
despite perpetuation of the marriage, the degree of disability to the
partners and offspring seem almost incalculable. Once this is
realized, such topics as dating and going steady as socialization
processes in preparation for marriage seem grossly deficient. While
such processes have some relevance for the overall processes of
socialization, such as trying out roles or playacting, they do not
accomplish the mission of identifying which couples are most likely
to have enduring and contented relationships. To achieve this goal,
more complex variables would need assessment.

The Engagement.   The engagement process, either as a formal
commitment or as a primitive agreement, is still a crisis period for
many youths. Even for couples who use the engagement for
experimental marriage which may not terminate in legalization, it
changes the nature of the relationship and adds stress.

Several formal functions are included in descriptions of engagements:

1. An engagement is seen as a period of delay in which an
intensified preparation for marriage takes place. This is usually a
focused preparation to seek advice about marriage from those who
supposedly possess the expertise to advise. In recent years both the

qualifications of those doing such counseling and the content of their message have come under increasing challenge. The preparatory period of delay is supposed to permit a separation from families, giving up other potential partners, and establishing relationships with friends of the same sex in a new light.

2. Engagements are an opportunity for a couple to achieve an identity in a joint partnership. This is partly a result of the shared intimacy of the couple when previous secrets or data about their past lives, families, property, and formal state are shared. It permits the couple to try out their unity as a couple with others. For some, this role-playing is a rehearsal for marriage which aids later adaptation. For others, the major function might be to realize the warning signs in the relationship during rehearsal. Unfortunately, the warning signs are not taken seriously. Trial marriages are seen as a preventive step to cut down later mismatches.

3. Sexual release is cited as one of the fringe benefits of an engagement. Over twenty years ago in the staid 1950s, the figure of 40 percent of engaged couples engaging in sexual intercourse was given.[13] Kinsey's 1948 study of male sexual behavior indicated 85 percent of men had engaged in premarital intercourse.[14] College students now become anxious when they do not feel ready to have intercourse.[15] This has been at least constant since 1948, if not vastly increased, according to survey material. If earlier articles which suggested that premarital intercourse gives rise to more unstable marriages are accurate, the divorce rate is likely to increase. Valid data on the incidence of intercourse, circumstances thereof, frequency, and other variables, need determination.

4. The engagement period is to taper the insecurities based on earlier, more formal relationships. Yet this is more relevant to an earlier historical period than the model of experimenting with various people carried out by contemporary youths.

What clinicians can help shed light on are the covert and depth factors operating at the time a youth selects a partner. Reference has been made to the phenomena of falling in love. Surveys among youths would undoubtedly cite falling in love as the prime reason for choosing a partner. Factors such as security for the girl or gratification of sexual needs for the boy rarely would be listed first. However, additional factors make the marital choice one of the most complicated in the life span.

What about the question of personal attractiveness? Once beyond some generally recognized cultural component of personal beauty, we enter the area of preceding attachments throughout the course of development and the affective associations a potential partner arouses. This includes gross perceptual and sensory experiences which stimulate. Individual factors operate, such as the need for physical contact and comfort, depressive-proneness seeking object closeness, and the need for reassurance as a male or female. The most important influence of these contributors is their lack of association with what will make a secure marriage. For some youths attraction is based on neurotic components. The frequent overestimation of the loved person supports this, but ideally neurotic components are either minimal or complementary. The latter pave the way for fused character traits in the partners.

A late adolescent remaining in the parental home becomes incongruous. The function of the family of origin in terms of child-rearing, nurturance, dependency gratification, and achieving a modicum of socialization has been reached by late adolescence. If these processes have been successful, the center of a youth's life shifts from the family. If the center of activity persists in the family matrix, it is indicative of difficulties resolving earlier attachments. As long as these attachments remain prominent, commitments to a partner outside the family is difficult if not impossible without ambivalence and guilt. Divided loyalty precludes the possibility of freedom to give primary emotional attachments elsewhere.

As young adulthood is entered it is no longer possible to achieve self-esteem by the techniques available at an earlier age. The youth period is used for the game of playing the field with a mixture of adventure, excitement, and final solidification of gender identity. In fact, a major impetus toward selecting a partner is by way of gender solidification in which traits and attitudes that have evolved as part of the core gender identity achieve more lasting integration. Such things as cognitive styles, diverse ways of relating to the opposite sex, interest patterns, and a host of culturally sanctioned gender behavior obtain fullest development in the intimacy achieved in heterosexual youthful unions. This means that the fears and anxieties attendant upon such unions are not sufficient to prohibit sexual activity. Common interferences are seen in impairments to carry out sexual intercourse: impotency, premature ejaculation, a lack of interest in intercourse in boys or a pleasureless, anesthetized experience in girls.

Repetition of Old Patterns.   Another source of difficulties in late adolescence is the repetition of conflicts experienced earlier within the family of origin. The attachments and stages of object relationships through which the human has matured—with all their affective components—are major factors leading to seeking out deeper attachments, in contrast to relationships which serve functional needs such as sex or procreation. In this sense the attachment during this culminating phase of biological and psychological maturation is partially regressive in nature, with all the affect of past nostalgias and pleasures.

The wish to recapture experiences from childhood lurks as a primary motivator. Resolved and unresolved oedipal ties, with repressed and sublimated components, give further impetus to seeking out a member of the opposite sex. This determines selective components which take the form of direct displacement or reaction formations against similarities which are too dangerous. The choice of a partner diametrically opposed in certain ways to a parent is a common example. Coalescence of all these factors permits a given object choice to occur which will enhance self-esteem. It is a choice in which the lovers feel they have advanced themselves as a result of loving and being loved.

Conflicts throughout adolescence within—with parents or siblings—can lead to a flight from home. There are a variety of people and locations to run to. Another cause of early marriage is increasing anxiety about sexual performance. For example, the threat of homosexuality may hasten the need to portray oneself as the opposite. For some, sexual anxiety is associated with guilt over masturbation, seen as having adverse consequences in selecting a marriage partner. Needs for security and dependency gratification have been mentioned.

The pressure toward one intense relationship, or the security of one sexual partner, should be contrasted with experimentation. The latter may become a burden in contrast to the ease of arranging more permanent contacts. For girls the same components can lead to painful outcomes. Illegitimate births are one possibility, but more frequent are masochistic relationships in which the girl is treated badly. Upward social mobility is another factor, especially with girls (who tend to marry upward more often than do boys). Revenge motives against ex-boyfriends or girlfriends may prompt a rush into new attachments. Spite or the need to show a parent is a generational theme. In other cases complementary sado-masochistic impulses come to the fore when a partner who can meet these needs appears on the scene, and is perceived as attractive based on a mixture of conscious and unconscious reasons.

TOLERATION OF AN UNCERTAIN FUTURE

Tolerating uncertainty involves multiple developmental themes and lines. It has antecedents from preceding psychosexual and psychosocial stages involving uncertainty and ambiguity. When the period of late adolescence is reached and pervasive questions are present as to how much a person can really trust others, vulnerability is high. Yet precisely at this intersection a contemporary youth raises questions about the nature of the world and its institutions as well. To what extent is a person really duped if he goes along with the beliefs and slogans of the wider world? Youths who raise questions of this type often require skillful and sensitive appraisal.

During the earlier adolescent period it is customary to view such questions as normal behavior. It is a truism to realize that adolescents challenge authority figures and their cultures. By late adolescence, the questions have another connotation. They reflect a reality-based appraisal of the way things are. In that sense we can predict certain potentials for commitment to chronic oppositional states. This does not necessarily mean overt involvement in protest groups; it could take the form of quiet dedication, to work within a system dedicated to change. On the other hand, persistent questioning regarding the basis or irremediability in a system can reflect internal conflict being handled by externalization and procrastination. Severe disillusionment can lead to its polar opposite—withdrawal from participation.

> A nineteen-year-old asked persistent questions about the purpose of it all. Always an honor student, for the first time he began to inquire seriously into his life's ambition of receiving a Ph.D. degree. A period of involvement with various action-oriented groups ensued in which his academic pursuits became stalemated. Throughout he continued to receive a few honor grades, but he continued to express himself consistently against a system which forced him to go through such rigid programming to avoid being a beggar. By age twenty-four he was not progressing satisfactorily in his graduate work. He continued to express similar thoughts with a dry passion, but with fewer clever phrases. Much of his time is now consumed in long conversations with peers who are in similar predicaments. He also spends much time reading materials far removed from his academic ambitions. At this point he appears at a crossroads, exhibiting various symptoms of depressive and schizoid personality organization.

Tolerating Hate. To experience and tolerate periodic hostility without needing to hate persistently is the hallmark of an integrated ego. In the absence of utilizing aggression the individual is prone to denial and avoidance. These portend another type of personality limitation of equal dimension. Balance is rarely achieved among youths, or adults, as witnessed by the difficulties in these areas which many people experience. Marked ambivalence in which love and hate have not been resolved is a compromise solution. The subsequent vacillation fosters insecurity. A mixture of self-hate and contempt contribute to depressive-proneness or tendencies to paranoid projective mechanisms.

Ideally, a balance should be maintained between a complete sense of futility and withdrawal and a semblance of optimism that existence is not meaningless. Uncritical adaptation to the system can hardly be taken as the epitome of adjustment, but unfortunately, this standard is used too often. Achievement of a balance implies a degree of ego integration in which internalized images of good and bad objects can be tolerated. Too severe a degree of ambivalence toward objects, coupled with anxiety, is likely to lead to a semi-paralysis of several executive and cognitive ego functions. Rather than participation in life with a sense of responsibility, a seeking to undermine and destroy emerges.

The causes which presage difficulty in responsible participation as adults appear rooted in early infantile experiences. These have been widely written about, but an intriguing problem is to understand why some who are predisposed toward difficulties in this area become rebels while others seek to obtain their due by taking their place in the ranks. To experience a destructive desire toward an object the youth is dependent upon and still retains part of the object internally as desirable and rewarding. If an individual in the course of his development has been subjected to unpredictable experiences with these objects, it is not surprising that during late adolescence a tranquil fusion of images is difficult. What tapers the desire to destroy during the developing years is the opportunity for the child to give or take care of things and not only to hurt. This is a process of neutralization of aggression, but it is also a reparative device which saves mankind from destroying itself. How fragile a device it is is all too evident.

Affective states of guilt, irritability, or depression appear when reparation as a neutralizing device is not available. The implication is that the limitation of continued opportunities to carry out restitutive activities leads to a predominance of aggressive emotionality as well as acting-out of aggressive impulses. In terms of development, it is the ability of the child to assume responsibility in a progressive manner not only for his own impulses—which may have some rather nasty components—but to learn a way to express concern for others balanced against his own needs. In other words, we are studying how one human being develops a concern for other human beings.[16] If this is realized during the last stages of childhood development during youth, a preoccupation with aggression and its derivatives may be avoidable.

Fidelity.   Being true or loyal to somebody or something has been suggested as the basic virtue for youth. Virtues are viewed as essential to ego development and also as measures of ego strength. In terms of developmental schema, in infancy hope is the virtue; in the preschool child it is will and purposefulness; in the school-age period it is skill; in youth fidelity; in young adulthood care and concern; and in old age it is wisdom.[17] In this schema, development of fidelity could not occur before the youth period, but it must make its appearance at this stage. Fidelity manifests itself in a search to dedicate which will retain durability amidst change. In the absence of a reasonable degree of certainty that youths can live in a setting in which they sense loyalty in others and an opportunity to return it, a state of infidelity emerges. Hence, the urge to find the real self takes on an intensity not matched earlier or subsequently.

Drivenness as a Solution.   Resolution of ambiguity can take on qualities of motor restlessness. Being on the go is seen in an absorption in athletics for those with the required physique; or compulsive addiction to work; extension of restlessness to machines (such as reckless driving of cars) is another form. Absorption in cults of the day has been commented upon. The risk is to avoid the amorphousness of diversity where motion itself becomes a primary goal.

Uncertainty can be tolerated by a youth as long as there is an avoidance of a sense of stasis. Stasis is experienced as tantamount to ceasing development—perhaps even life. In essence, tolerance of uncertainty for youths becomes possible by way of a sense of history for the era in which they live. This means having a sense of being the beneficiary of the culture's tradition, the user and innovator of its technology, and a renewer of ethical strength. Many institutions contribute to a mythology offering an historical orientation: politics, religion, the arts and sciences, theater, fiction, and the press.[18] At its best, psychiatry itself may contribute to this. If these fail, in all likelihood, youth fails as well.

STABILIZATION OF SELF-ESTEEM

The Role of Disillusionment. Stabilized self-esteem systems in youth allow earlier turmoil with respect to self-appraisal to recede. Accomplishing this means that wide mood swings accompanied by regressive tendencies diminish. Persistent themes of megalomania alternating with self-abasement are evidence of instabilities. Perhaps the most pervasive problem pertaining to self-esteem in a youth is that of disillusionment.

Sources of disillusionment are multiple. In some ways disillusionment is a direct confrontation with an insight about parental disillusionments in the course of attempting to move on to individual commitments. Most challenging to the clinician is the exceptional youth. In this context the exception is one who achieves insights which he does not lose as readily as others. When this persists beyond a few years at most, it leads to a low-grade chronic depression in which there is a passionate hanging on to illusions and delusions which permit despair and humiliation to reign. Hope functions to prevent total resignation. While this keeps a youth plugging away, its long-range success may take its toll in other ways. The writings of F. Scott Fitzgerald[19] in the 1920s exemplified the despair of the youth of that generation, as did the writings of Kipling in an earlier generation:

> We have done with Hope and Honour,
> We are lost to Love and Truth,
> We are dropping down the ladder rung
> By rung;
> And the measure of our torment is the
> measure of our youth;
> God help us! For we knew the worst too young.

Environmental Contributions. Withholding, for the moment, a discussion of intrapsychic components, three environmental themes contribute to disillusionment in youths; (1) an oversell of education, (2) being burned-out, and (3) an over-responsiveness to environmental shifts.

Educational oversell inevitably catches up with youths. Years of hard work and diligence culminate for many in the realization that gratification from a given vocational choice may be minimal. Worse yet, jobs may not be available at the level they thought would be possible. Many of those who pursued the academic rat-race realize that the formal aspects of education are often shallow. For some of these youths the developmental years were spent in a parental atmosphere where goals were to pursue success. Success was presumed tantamount to happiness at a later date. Co-existing with all of this was the de facto identification with the core personality of the parents in whom the youths may have sensed a lack of self-respect and self-esteem.[20] An interesting side issue is the essential difference between those who cannot avoid the disillusionment of frustrated achievement and work during youth, and those who face disillusionment in the fourth or fifth decades of life, where a different clinical picture emerges. In all of these cases—in some decade—the realization dawns that diligence and dedication to the Puritan ethic may have been misguided. A massive self-questioning and an overwhelming sense of having been deluded then begin.

A second type of disillusionment is the experience of feeling burned-out by the time youth period is reached. Such a variety of experiences have already been encountered by then that there has been little comprehension of meaning. Some have compared this to the economic practice of obsolescence in industry in which goods are developed to be used for a certain period and then discarded. Another comparison is to the obsession to form contacts in which feelings are seldom deep, lasting, or meaningful.

Environmental disillusionment pertains to the latching-on to what, at the moment, seems like an opportunity for a deep commitment. In reality grasping is often what seems to have a sense of purpose, but may shift out of style in a short time. This is often not a commitment based on comprehension, but rather a response to a deep-felt need to overcome the superficiality present in past exposure.

These phenomena are related to the idiosyncratic depressions experienced by youths. They are experienced differently from those witnessed in the younger adolescent, the child, or the adult. While some youths show a full-blown depressive character, the most frequent picture is a type of reactive depression in response to developmental conflict. It has been held that a temporary psychotic episode in a youth which is followed by a depression, actually has a better prognostic outcome than when there is no ensuing depression.[21] The depression is an indicator of the capacity and desire to work through the despair of the present situation coupled with the need to separate from old and familiar objects, particularly when there is permanent separation from the parental home, difficulty in tolerating continuing frustrations, and conflict over sex-role behavior. Depression in this age group can signify the capacity to tolerate developmental conflict. Based on several years of learning experiences, self-esteem is contingent upon praise and approval from important people—peers or adults—and this has become an essential part of personality functioning. Earlier conflicts give rise to needs for possessiveness. In competitive situations, jealousy leaves a youth insecure in dealing with rivalries. What can occur is a reversal of idealization directly to hate.

Whatever the term applied—youthful depression, alienation, anomie, or lack of motivation syndrome—the picture of apathy, loss of effectiveness, diminished capacity for carrying out long-term work, and mastering new material are all present.[22] Attempts to deal with the feeling of flatness and anhedonia may lead to drug usage. A passive, regressive inability to initiate minimal activities raises differential diagnostic questions about such schizoidia. When threats to self-esteem are met with apathy they can take multiple forms. A common threat is the fear that if the youth is active and competitive, an injury may ensue. The injury need not be physical, although this type of anxiety is more prevalent in young males. For girls, the threat may involve loss of love or of loved things. While there is acquiescence to an environmental defeat, self-esteem is protected by denigrating efforts to work. This is the connection between the depressions of youth and the insights of disillusionment with the establishment.

There are also deeper conflicts expressed by withdrawal into passivity as a reflection of conflict over gender identity. Curiously, passivity in the young female is usually not seen as reflecting gender conflicts because her esteem in the past has not been so contingent upon expectations of being entitled to rewards for assertiveness or work. Hence an integral part of the young female's existence is tied to depressive-proneness, although this appears to be changing for many young women. One false criterion may be getting exchanged for another; feeling rejected from not being loved as a measure of well-being to a substitution by achievement in the world of work may not be progress.

SUPEREGO AND CHARACTER CHANGE

The Pervasiveness of Duplicity. Changes in character structure in youths reflect a further elaboration of complex aspects of personality growth and organization. On an empirical level the late adolescent is confronted with reconciling his high idealism with the overwhelming amount of mediocrity and indifference to which he is exposed in so much of his life. Not only are performance and standards in doubt, but the duplicity that youths sense attempts to conceal the pervasive norms of incompetency and dishonesty. Perhaps it is the realization that the intellectual inculcation of moral virtues has proven sadly insufficient to regulate behavior that gives rise to talk about a need for moral education.[23] All too frequently the continuing need for controls and ideals is by-passed (with caustic references to the failure of past efforts in this regard). This is similar to pointing out the adverse consequences of corrupt parents on superego development and then arguing for abolishing family life.

To be able to justify the beliefs which a youth arrives at independently still appears worth the effort. At best, beliefs entail a conviction that one has some type of accountability for behavior toward others. Unless certain norms and concepts, such as justice and virtue, are internalized as part of the superego system, there is likely to be a deep-seated contempt for those who attempt to live by certain values. The problem is to confront a world where virtue is often negated and may even seem adverse to self-advancement.

Limitations of the Moral Duty Approach. Exhortations to moral duty, as well as cognitive moral imperatives, show a lack of empirical and experimental confirmation for building and regulating character.[24] The highest levels of cognitive processes pertaining to morals and moral reasoning can only be attained during the period of youth. Obviously this does not mean that a majority attain such an ideal, but that if they ever do, that is the age at which it is attainable.[25] Since more detail on moral development is given in chapter 7, the reader is referred there for extensive discussion.[25]

Self-sacrifice. Innumerable religious martyrs exemplify sacrifice as an ideal. These acts cannot be explained solely on the basis of psychological conflict, or as a product of masochistic needs. Such commitments also require cognitive and affective aspects. They cannot be discarded simply by referring to psychopathology. They involve an appeal to principles which are supposedly binding for all time. The principles may merely be those which at a particular time appear paramount and in need of subscription, so that among contemporary youth appeals to the sanctity of life and the attraction of certain moral virtues (justice, honor, and truth), claim ascendency.

Youth and Political Attitudes. Before proceeding to a more microscopic look at superego development by late adolescence, an examination of how definite attitudes about law and government are arrived at and progress through the course of adolescence is relevant. Some mundane examples set the stage. What is it that leads to a cognitive appraisal of police as pigs, or a need to spit or stomp on the flag? For the adolescent of thirteen years and under, the purpose of government is primarily viewed as enforcing laws in the context of curbing wicked acts. In behavioral terms, this is equivalent to putting a restraint on the expression of impulses on a pre-moral level.

The attitude of the young adolescent appears to be that of duty to obey authority, and punishment for failure to do so. The youth believes he owes obedience, and that his rights are not paramount. He sees authority as omniscient but benign, since it operates for the common good. Rules and laws are not functional in the sense of existing for the people. Hence, however unjust or ineffective a set of rules and their operations might be, the youth is not motivated to modify or eliminate them. It is unbelievable how prevalent this viewpoint remains beyond the early adolescent years and appears to be the highest developmental achievement respecting man's legal institutions for a majority of citizens. Since it appears that most of mankind remains at this level, this constriction cannot be ascribed to intellectual limitations. The number of individuals who continue to participate in groups in which they are clearly exploited, as well as ones in which they recognize their situation as hopeless, is quite high. These attitudes toward authority were once personified in the divine right of kings as a basis for rule. For young adolescents these attitudes operate as their normative way of conceptualizing the way those who rule make and administer rules and laws.

Perhaps there is some hope in the final response to a corrupt government as exemplified by Watergate, but others do not see Watergate as an example of how well tyrants are disposed of.[27]

Adelson and Beall studied a changing perspective on law and government in four age groups (eleven, thirteen, fifteen, and eighteen years respectively), using different countries (the United States, England, and Germany).[28] While cognitive maturation appeared important across national boundaries in many respects, it was not so in all. As the years transpired, there was a shift from a primitive to a rehabilitative emphasis in dealing with crime. More understanding of the needs of the total community as against a single individual evolved. A shift from an absolutist to a pragmatic way of formulating political issues was an accompaniment.

Cross-national results emerged as well. German youths tended to continue seeing the citizen's duty as that of obeying the authority of the state. Authority was idealized because it was competent and strong while the individual was viewed as weak, dependent, and inept. Diversity in views raised fears of a potential to breed chaos and disunity with people needing to be guided.

While the English in some ways were just as authoritarian in their youth, they differed in seeing the power of the state as a necessary evil to be tolerated. The state was viewed as necessary to control self-seeking men who will take what is not theirs. Hence, government was necessary within carefully defined limits, and it was viewed as undesirable to have it extend beyond this into the private realm. While the American sample scored lowest in authoritarism, there was a preoccupation with how to balance individual freedom to achieve with the need to control rampant individualism. An emphasis of compromise and consensus often leads to an acquiescence by the majority not to rock the boat. The vulnerability of the consensus approach has become more apparent to youths who seem caught between dilemmas of challenging authority or the passivity accompanying disillusion.

THEORETICAL ISSUES ABOUT YOUTH

The diverse manifestations of youth give rise to formulations regarding differences in outcome. These are what the clinician must assess in the context of developmental norms utilizing diverse criteria.

The Integrated Ego. Youths who emerge from adolescence with the least difficulties show a relatively stable concept of the self and object representation; ego development shows satisfactory integration with minimal symptoms of identity diffusion. Little ego-splitting is in evidence, and the main defenses are repression, avoidance, or reaction formation. If neurotic conflict comes to the fore, it centers around the ego, directly limiting impulse expression. On the whole, socialization has progressed throughout antecedent stages so that object constancy is present in the form of a capacity to retain object representations and attachments. This persists even when hostilities emerge in relationships. Since the object relationship involves a total image—with the good and the bad being retained and not seen as exclusive—when losses are sustained such a youth can experience deep affect and proceed to experience mourning and guilt.

Superego Harshness. When more severe manifestations of superego psychopathology are present, the corresponding ramifications on character structure are greater. A severe and punitive superego does the most personal damage. This is even more so than it is with psychopathic character types, since personal suffering occurs less frequently in this alloplastic form of adaptation. An esoteric type of conflict appears between superego and ego-ideal components if they are separated for heuristic purposes: on the one hand are sadistic demands for moral strictness, and on the other there is an over-idealized ego-ideal system, with grandiose concepts about what it is supposed to do.[29] Three clinical manifestations are present, separately or together: (1) Contradictions in values and norms are defended rigorously even against purely intellectual insight; varying degrees of splitting of contradictory ego states occur. (2) Accentuation of mood lability from adolescence does not disappear. (3) Projections of superego prohibitions emerge as paranoid trends. These blunt feelings, where guilt could guide actions, do not elicit a feeling of wrong-doing but rather one of being unjustly accused by others.

Episodic or selective breakthroughs of impulses occur with this type of character structure. Those who emerge into youth with such handicaps show critical manifestations of disturbance in the realm of orality. Standard diagnoses such as "passive-aggressive personality" or "hysterical personality" appear to contain these structural defects in the personality. Another outcome is sado-masochistic trends in those who are reacting to the qualities listed above. Selective forms of sexual perversity can occur as a possibility of compromising a harsh control system.

If difficulties have preceded the delineation of the image of the self from others, they can be expected to continue. A variety of drive derivatives are played out, with associated affects, to integrate conflicting aspects about the same object.[30] The extreme case of youths whose differentiation of self from non-self comes into jeopardy has been written about more often than the common case, in which a youth experiences difficulties synthesizing contradictory aspects of himself and others. It is simpler to impose divisions of goodness and badness or lovable and hateful, toward others, than to deal with them as puzzling and changing mixtures within one person. To persist into adulthood with such a dichotomy handicaps the capacity to perceive accurately who others truly are.

In cases where relatively severe personality disturbances have developed, ego splitting and a tendency to use projective mechanisms arise.[31] A problem results from splitting: how to cope with an exaggerated ego-ideal system in which perfectionistic strivings for greatness gain strength? A knowledge of realistic aspirations may never emerge. This leaves a youth prone to constant feelings of dissatisfaction. Relief may be sought in taking great risks or clandestine behavior. The youth may fight against a projected part of the self that is perceived in others, as well as within the self. This struggle is against ideals for which the introjects stand. Both the objective failings of adults and the external need to see their limitations facilitates a final dethronement of the parents in terms of these ideals. If this dethronement does not occur, a tenacious but ambivalent clinging to the parents' ideals persists. This is in place of what was once a literal clinging based on a level of physical proximity. The seeking out of new objects and attachments is accordingly handicapped. Throughout these changes, if a level of development is reached where not only the image remains relatively fixed, but also part of earlier preferences, an intact and functional ego-ideal will survive.

The more severe types of impairment in superego development show severe disparities by the time the youth period is reached. Antisocial personalities belong in this group, as do impulse-ridden characters. By the youth period a recognition and acceptance of severe personality deviations on an intellectual level is reached even when capacity to change is limited. A potential for psychotic episodes exists, particularly with schizoid and paranoid characters.[32] Paranoid traits and projected identifications are conspicuous in these youths. Harsh and hostile demands on the self are projected so that youths who live with a feeling that they are amongst enemies or people who do not like them live with a great vulnerability to distortion.

A vicious cycle can occur when the hostile world is projected and later reintrojected. A variation of this is a feeling of inner divisiveness which corresponds to parts of the self being invaded. This is not merely a lack of satisfactory differentiation of self from non-self, but an intersystemic blurring between ego and superego. When this is present, any reliable basis to appraise the self is grossly impaired since how can a youth, caught in such a quandary, really appraise when he or she needs to feel guilty? Similarly, how can he or she know when to attack someone and when to temporize? Difficulties permeate necessities to distinguish between narcissistic aspects of the ego-ideal from ego strivings for admiration, power, and possessions.[33] Capacity to tolerate guilty affect is so minimal that guilt is handled by an impulsive pattern of direct drive gratification or resorting to reaction formations for control of impulses and affect. Objects are used for direct release with little accompanying empathy, without taking their place as part of a stabilized series of internalized representations.

REFERENCES

1. P. Blos, *On Adolescence References* (New York: Free Press, 1962).
2. L. A. Spiegel, Comments on the psychoanalytic psychology of adolescence, *Psychoanalytic Study of the Child* 13(1958):296-308.
3. P. Blos, op. cit., p. 189.
4. J. Bing, F. McLaughlin, and R. Marburg, The metapsychology of narcissism, *Psychoanalytic Study of the Child* 14(1959):9-28.
5. R. Seidenberg, Catcher gone awry, *International Journal of Psycho-Analysis* 51(1970):331-339.
6. D. Cooper, *The Death of the Family* (New York: Pantheon Books, 1971).
7. R. Laing and A. Esterton, *Sanity, Madness, and the Family: Families of Schizophrenics*, 2nd ed. (New York: Basic Books, 1971).
8. E. Schwarz, Herman Hesse, the american youth movement, and problems of literary evaluation, *PNILA* 85(1970):977-987.
9. K. Keniston, Youth: a new stage of life, *American Scholar* 39(1970):631-654.
10. T. Nagel, *The Possibility of Altruism* (New York: Oxford University Press, 1970).
11. K. H. Connell, Peasant marriage in Ireland: its structure and development since the famine, *Economic History Review* 14(1962):502-523.
12. W. J. Goode, Family disorganization, *Contemporary Social Problems*, ed. R. K. Merton and R. Nisbet, pp. 390-458 (New York: Harcourt, Brace and World, 1961).
13. E. W. Burgess and P. Willin, *Engagement and Marriage* (Philadelphia: Lippincott, 1953).
14. A. C. Kinsey et. al., *Sexual Behavior in the Human Male* (Philadelphia: W. B. Saunders Co., 1948).
15. Student Committee on Human Sexuality, *Sex and the Yale Student* (New Haven: Yale University Press, 1970).
16. D. W. Winnicott, The development of the capacity for concern, *Bulletin of the Menninger Clinic* 27(1963):167-176.
17. E. H. Erikson, The roots of virtue, *The Humanist Frame*, ed. J. Huxley (London: Allen and Unwin, 1961).
18. E. H. Erikson, Youth: fidelity and diversity, *Daedalus* 91(1962):5-27.
19. F. S. Fitzgerald, *The Stories*, ed. M. Cowley (New York: Scribner, 1951).
20. P. L. Giovacchini, Compulsory happiness—adolescent despair, *Archives of General Psychiatry* 18(1968):650-657.
21. F. S. Hoedemaken, Psychotic episodes and postpsychotic depression in young adults, *American Journal of Psychiatry* 127(1970):66-70.

22. P. A. Walters, Depression, *International Psychiatry Clinics* 7(1970):169-179.

23. J. R. Unwin, Depression in alienated youth, *Canadian Psychiatric Association Journal* 15(1970):83-86.

24. L. Kohlberg and E. Turiel, eds., *Recent Research in Moral Development* (New York: Holt, Rinehart and Winston, 1972).

25. L. Kohlberg, Moral development and the education of adolescents, *Adolescents and the American High School*, ed. R. F. Purnel (New York: Holt, Rinehart and Winston, 1970).

26. W. Gaylin, *In the Service of Their Country* (New York: Viking, 1970).

27. R. Woodward and C. Bernstein, *All the President's Men* (New York: Simon and Schuster, 1974).

28. J. Adelson and L. Beall, Adolescent perspectives on law and government, *Law and Society*, 4(1970):495-504.

29. H. Kohut, *The Analysis of the Self* (New York: International Universities Press, 1971).

30. Z. A. Aarons, Normality and Abnormality in Adolescence, *Psychoanalytic Study of the Child* 25(1970):309-339

31. O. F. Kernberg, Structural derivatives of object relationships, *International Journal of Psycho-Analysis* 47(1966):236-253.

32. J. Frosch, Psychoanalytic considerations of the psychotic character, *Journal of the American Psychoanalytic Association* 18(1970):24-50.

33. A. Reich, Narcissistic object choice in women, *Journal of the American Psychoanalytic Association* 1(1953):22-44.

Chapter Three

Adolescence:
The Biological Dimension

Whenever the question is raised as to what the criteria for adolescence are, confusion arises. This is due only in part to the behavior of adolescents and cultural ambiguity. A major contributing factor to the confusion is the number of disciplines concerned with this age group which lack knowledge of the other's work and perspective. This often leads to a failure to delineate basic areas which need investigation, along with a critical appraisal of the methodologies used. It seems obvious that adolescents are a group of people, most of all, who cannot be studied apart from the growth and change in their physical bodies. The various somatic alterations that occur, both grossly and physiologically, require appraisal. These physical changes will be discussed because of their meaning in the wider context of adolescent development. They provide an illustration of a significant aspect of adolescent development that is often neglected. Such knowledge, while important in its own right, also provides a groundwork which is available for appraisal of psychopathological deviations involving physical development in a primary sense, and also for secondary psychological consequences.

When considering the criteria employed for the commencement and termination of adolescence, an immediate impression is that they vary so widely that there should be substantive doubts about their reliability. Consider some of the traditional signs used as criteria for the onset of adolescence as a cultural phenomenon: entrance into a middle school or junior high school, the teens as a chronological concept, the first menstruation, and the physical changes of puberty with or without some qualifying features. Similarly, the end of adolescence involves such signs as: graduation from high school, end of the teen years, marriage, economic independence, autonomy from parents, emotional and intellectual maturity, sexual maturity, or some legal criterion such as reaching a given age (usually eighteen or twenty-one years).

Many of these definitions are patently frivolous and lack substance. However, they have a sense of meaning by virtue of their connection to tasks which individuals face at a certain age. A basic problem is the lack of physical or psychological specificity. We do not know how to evaluate independence or maturity except in terms of verbalizations employing similar abstractions. Nor do we know how to assign different weightings for the relative importance of these factors. Variations exist among these criteria contingent upon the socio-cultural setting a given adolescent is in. The confusion is believed to come closest to being allayed if a developmental approach involving biological norms is used in addition to psychological and social material.

Classifications are useful as heuristic devices. In the adolescent age period this permits grouping on a rational basis. Simple classifications of adolescents by sex characteristics have been made based on attributes associated with maleness or femaleness. An added step lists the types of activities carried out at different ages. This is based on frequency distributions, so that sampling techniques and cultural groupings must be closely examined. Gesell, Hill, and Ames drew up a classification based on the chronological age span ten through fifteen years—describing the classification as a "maturity profile" of a particular age in terms of a characteristics and traits representative of certain age zones.[1] Although their effort was not to present a psychometric average, but rather to give a picture of the currents and contours of development, these data have often been taken as normative. Maturity traits for each chronological age were presented in terms of behavior problems and symptoms in nine areas: (1) total action systems, (2) routines and self-care, (3) emotions, (4) a growing self, (5) interpersonal relationships, (6) activities and interests, (7) school life, (8) ethical sense, and (9) philosophic outlook. In addition, maturity trends were described in terms of sequences and gradients of growth.

A biological framework requires a preliminary distinction between the terms *puberty* and *nubility* as distinguished from *adolescence*. The former are regarded as biological concepts and hence are associated with physiological alterations. The common meaning given to puberty refers to it as the phase from the first appearance of secondary sexual characteristics to the inception of reproductive capacity. Nubility is the period which begins when full reproductive capacity is obtained. Puberty refers to external and visual manifestations of change which need not correspond to fertility levels. Reproductive capacity for girls is thought of in terms of menstruation, yet it may be one or two years before conception is actually possible. For boys ejaculation is taken as a criterion for puberty, yet it usually takes one to three years after the occurrence of the first ejaculation for sufficient spermatogenesis to occur for fertilization.[2] In practice, the terms puberty and nubility are often combined into pubescence, which includes the onset of secondary sexual changes as well as the period of achieving reproductive viability. In a developmental sense, the major changes in biological sexuality take place during pubescence.

Adolescence is a much broader concept than pubescence. It includes sexual development as well as the impact of socio-cultural changes upon the adolescent and in turn his impact on the culture. If puberty heralds the onset of adolescence, the prior period is that of prepuberty or prepubescence. When discussing biological concepts the appropriate phraseology is puberty or pubescence, but usage is often so careless that adolescence is referred to as having three stages: early, middle, and late, with preadolescence and postadolescence at the two outer extremes. Early adolescence corresponds to the prepubescent period in which there are the beginnings of secondary sexual characteristics. As an example, downy, pubic hair may appear. Middle adolescence corresponds to pubescence proper in which development of the secondary sexual characteristics flourishes. Menstruation for girls and seminal emissions for boys commences. Development of the primary organs of reproduction progresses at that time as well. Late adolescence is the period of postpubescence which completes the development of the secondary sexual characteristics as well as that of the primary organs. These distinctions are of importance not only for academic pedantry, but for clinical appraisal and valid research. Clinical and research findings must take developmental phenomena into account in order to sustain their overall integration as part of comprehending the particular stage of development of a given adolescent.

CRITICAL PERIODS, SENSITIVE PERIODS, AND DEVELOPMENTAL LINES

The notion of chronological age per se as a significant index for adolescence or puberty has long been surpassed by the use of developmental and physiological criteria. This is true not only for adolescence but for infancy, early childhood, and latency as well. Several concepts have evolved in this regard, with the central concern of *growth gradience*. Patterns occur for parts of the body to develop. This applies to organs, systems, and discrete physical measurements such as height and weight.

Biological concepts of development have been extended into psychological and socio-cultural theories. Thus stages of development take place sequentially in terms of organ development, and also for various periods gaining ascendancy. Embryology concerned itself with an epigenetic principle where anything growing has a ground plan or blueprint from which parts arise. Each part is viewed as having its own special time of ascendancy until all the parts coalesce to form an overall functioning unit. This principle was later borrowed by Erik Erikson in his formulation of psycho-sexual stages of development.[3]

Critical periods are based on other hypotheses. During certain periods there is an unfolding of biologically timed behaviors. A corresponding biological base is that of *sensitive periods* in which the changes or experiences must take place. The time period may vary in duration from hours to years, depending upon what is in question. The original concept of *criticalness* has a connotation of relative irreversibility. If the critical period was bypassed without a given experience occurring, it was believed impossible to compensate for at a later date. The analogy was to neurohumoral and enzymatic mechanisms operating in the embryo or fetus developing in utero. Certain effects must occur for organ development to proceed. The critical period for laying down the notochord in the embryo occurs within the time sequence of a few weeks, and this cannot—without serious adverse consequences for later physical development—be omitted or shifted to an earlier or later time period.

The formulation of sensitive periods has been applied to a host of psychological phenomena. Many functions need not take place at an exact time period with irreversible consequences of loss if they do not occur. However, similar experiences, inducers, or stimulation occurring at later periods, may have a much less noticeable effect because of the capacity to respond to special stimulation at the sensitive periods. Learning which occurs during a sensitive period has a greater tendency to persist than it would otherwise have. This does not mean that such learning cannot occur at any other period, but rather that it is more difficult than acquired additional features are to match. Perceptual ability is one illustration of this.

Sensitivity to stimuli is determined by the cognitive organization of the child rather than by the chronological age or stage of physical maturation per se. Stimuli only function as such if they are assimilable. Once cognitive structures are sensitized they are not subject to extinction in the subsequent absence of the stimulus which originally promoted it. This allows the potentiality for subsequent sensitizing experiences to remain if they are missed at a given chronological age. Some theorists are critical of the permissibility allowed. They insist a child is more sensitive to the same stimulus presented at an earlier time period than later—given a sensitizable period. Infancy presents a need for a selective range of sensitive experiences since many cannot be assimilated. Lack of the required stimulation at sensitive periods is a situation of stimulus deprivation which becomes critical during succeeding developmental periods.[4]

Sensitive period theorizing has also been applied to adolescent personality development in diverse ways such as socialization exposures to dominant social groups on the one hand, to reactions to bodily changes and peer relationships on the other. Erickson's extension of the epigenetic principle used a succession of potentialities which emerge for interaction with other individuals. Acknowledging cultural variations, Erikson held that there was a proper rate and sequence which governed the growth of a personality as well as the organism. Personality develops according to steps determined by the sensitivity of the child to be driven toward and interact within a widening social radius. Decisive changes occur within the environment in the form of particular ideas, concepts, and cohesiveness. These encounters inevitably lead to crises at different stages and in different psychological and social spheres. Each successive attempt has a potential for crisis from the accompanying radical change and perspective required.

Another example is the psychological use of *stage theory* with sensitive periods posited in the form of *developmental lines*. These formulations will be given before pursuing the biological gradients of development so that the manner in which comparative extensions to the psychological sphere occur are illustrated. The traditional psychosexual stages (oral, anal, phallic, latency, preadolescence, and achievement of genitality) had a crude approximation to chronological age. When it came to parallel manifestations of aggression, no such variation was noticed. Clinical observations sought out parallel formulations with respect to ego and superego developments as part of personality development. What is sought in terms of either stages or periods of personality development is not solely a picture of psychosexual stages, deviations, or changing ego functions, but the basic interactions between id and ego, and the respective developmental levels and age-related sequences which can be correlated with other maturational processes. Whatever level a given child reaches represents the results of interaction between drive and ego-superego development.

Developmental Lines.   There is also the reaction to environmental influences, such as between maturation, adaptation, and the structuralization processes themselves. These ideas began with the clinical need to assess the presence or absence of psychopathological development. Since the criteria used to evaluate adults has limited applicability to children, in view of symptoms appearing and disappearing in a disorderly fashion, appraisal of development and the handling of critical periods is crucial. Categories of development utilized are: (1) maturation of drives, ego, and superego functioning, (2) adaptation to the environment and establishment of object relationships, and (3) organization which involves both integration and conflicts within the structure. Harmony or disharmony along developmental lines in relationship to both the id and ego permits a developmental example to be used to illustrate the shift from dependency to emotional self-reliance and adult object relationships.[6] Consider the following steps:

1. A biological unity exists between the mother and infant which involves an extension of the mother's narcissism to the child. The child in turn includes the mother in his internal narcissistic milieu. This period may be further subdivided into the autistic, symbiotic, and separation-individuation phases which may have significant danger points for development in each phase.
2. The part-object, or need-fulfilling, anaclitic relationship is based on the urgencs of the child's bodily needs and drive derivatives. It is intermittent and fluctuating since object-ties are formed under the impact of imperative desires and withdrawn when satisfaction is achieved.
3. Object constancy enables an inner image of an object to be maintained, irrespective of either satisfactions or dissatisfactions.
4. Ambivalent relationships are characterized by ego attitudes of clinging, torturing, dominating, and controlling objects.

5. Object-centered relationships are thought of as characteristic of the phallic-oedipal phase. Such characteristics include possessiveness toward the parent of the opposite sex, jealousy and rivalry with the parent of the same sex, protectiveness, curiosity, bids for admiration, and exhibitionistic attitudes.
6. Latency shifts to a transfer of intense feelings from parental figures to contemporaries, community groups, teachers, leaders, impersonal ideals, and aim-inhibited sublimated interests. There are fantasy manifestations indicating a gradual disillusionment with parental objects.
7. A preadolescent prelude is seen in returning to earlier attitudes and behavior—especially those of a part-object, need-fulfilling, and ambivalent type.
8. Adolescent struggles center around denying, reversing, loosening, and shedding ties to infantile objects, defending against earlier pregenital strivings, and eventually establishing genital supremacy with respect to objects of the opposite sex outside the family of origin.

GROSS ASPECTS OF PHYSICAL DEVELOPMENT DURING ADOLESCENCE

The crucial question: what begins the physical changes of puberty which lead to the psycho-social ramifications of adolescence? This is a fascinating question inasmuch as it is in the nature of a first causes approach with philosophical overtones which appeals to diverse backgrounds. The first causes referred to here are not ultimate causes with a teleological base for the onset of puberty, but hormonal mechanisms which trigger the onset of puberty. Endocrinological study of special organs or ductless glands is the key. First causes are hormones and neurohumoral mechanisms that regulate internal activities and lead to the onset of the changes of puberty.

Changes associated with puberty are part of a complex series of alterations in the rate of production and secretion of hormones. What initiates these changes is unknown, although tautological explanations are given, such as stating that the changes are in the nature of the human organism, or that man is preprogrammed to have the changes which commence during the pubertal period. Besides increases in the production of hormones, there is an altered sensitivity to hormones in target organs. These begin to respond in a differential manner. However, in an ultimate sense, beyond these

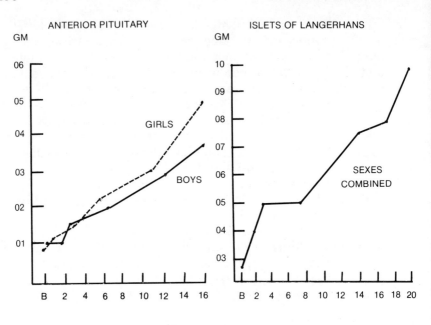

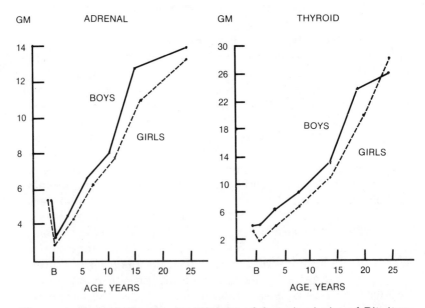

Figure 1. Growth Curves for Weight of Anterior Lobe of Pituitary, Islets of Langerhans, Adrenal, and Thyroid. Cross-sectional data. From Tanner, *Growth at Adolescence*, 1962, p. 177.

somewhat circumscribed biological answers, we do not actually know why at a certain stage the processes of puberty begin.

Changes in the size and morphology of the endocrine glands reveal some of the gross changes which occur (see Figure 1).

The Role of the Pituitary. The anterior lobe of the pituitary shows a growth spurt which is greater in girls than boys. This change persists into adult life in the form of a greater weight for the organ in females. Preceding the pubertal period a gradual shift occurs in the types of cells present in the organ. The presence of acidophil cells increases, and the percent of chromophobe cells falls. At puberty a much greater development of acidophils occurs in girls. In contrast to these changes in the anterior pituitary, the posterior or neural portion shows no specific pubertal changes.

The Adrenals. In contrast, the adrenal glands show an adolescent spurt in weight which is greater in boys than girls. However, the adrenals of adult females are larger, so that the situation during the course of adolescent development may be reversed in adulthood. The adrenals are so overdeveloped at birth that they do not attain such size again until eight or nine years. This large size at birth is due to a special group of cells which comprise the fetal cortex which some believe secretes androgens, but the evidence is unclear. The medulla, an inner layer of the adrenal, becomes similar to the adult form at one year of age and thereafter simply increases in size. There is a gradual increase in extractable adrenalin and noradrenalin from birth onward.

The thyroid glands show an additional growth spurt in weight which is the same for both sexes and this is so for the parathyroid glands as well. A change in the latter gland at puberty is the addition of new cell types in the form of oxyphil and Wasserhelle types in addition to the existing chief cells.

The Organs of Reproduction. The primary organs of reproduction undergo major changes. In the male, the primary sexual organs or characteristics are: testes, epididymus, seminal vesicles, prostate gland, penis, and urethra. In the female there are only two: uterus and ovaries. The secondary sexual characteristics are those not directly involved in reproduction. For the boy they are: pubic, axillary, and facial hair, deepening of the voice, and bone and muscle changes. For the girl the secondary sex changes are: breast growth, changes in the shape and curvature of the pelvis and hips,

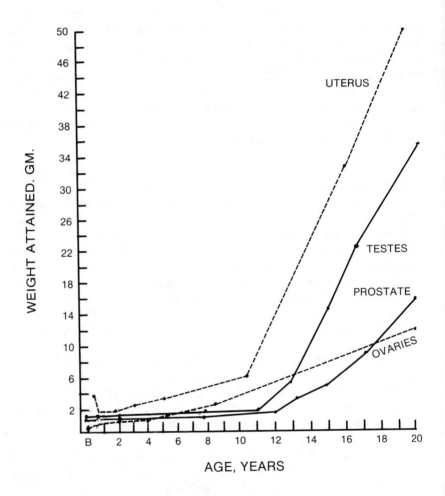

Figure 2: Growth in Weight of the Testes, Prostate, Ovaries, and Uterus. Data from autopsies. From Tanner, *Growth at Adolescence,* 1962, p. 28.

and pubic and axillary hair. Figure 2 illustrates some of the dramatic changes in size which occur at puberty.

For the boy, acceleration in growth of the testes and scrotum is one of the first changes which occur in accompaniment to a slight growth of pubic hair. At age ten there is usually an increase in the size of the seminal tubes. Undifferentiated cells called sertoli cells and primitive germ cells, spermatogosonia, become recognizable. At puberty the whole process is accelerated and spermatogenesis begins. The range for beginning growth of the testes and scrotum is from ten to thirteen and a half years. In some populations this may extend up to age fifteen. Accompanying the acceleration in height is an increase in penile length. The age range for this acceleration is from eleven to fourteen and a half years, with a mean of thirteen years. Completion of penile development occurs between thirteen and a half to seventeen years, with a mean age of fifteen years. Observe that boys who are late maturers may not have commenced this growth at the time that early-maturing boys are completing it. Boys thirteen and fourteen show a wide variability which may range from the prepubertal stage physically to complete physical maturity. By-products of these physical changes are seen in amorphous ramifications in the psychological, educational, and social spheres.

Genital development can be summarized as follows:

1. *Prepubescence:* Testes, scrotum, and penis are about the same proportional size as in early and middle childhood.
2. *Pubescence:*
    A. First changes: Enlargement of scrotum and testes. The skin of the scrotum reddens and changes in texture. There is a slight enlargement of the penis at this early stage.
    B. Further changes: Penile enlargement occurs in terms of length. There is continued growth of testes and scrotum. A close correlation exists between the acceleration in height and in the growth of the testes and penis. The height spurt and penile growth begin about a year following the testicular growth and never before it. Correlations between height and penile growth are in the range of 0.85 to 0.87.[7]
    C. Later changes: Increase in size of the penis, growth of breast tissue, and development of other glands proceeds. Scrotal skin darkens. Along with the growth of the penis, the prostate, seminal vesicles, and Bulbourethral glands enlarge and develop. The actual time for the occurrence of the first

ejaculation is determined culturally by way of social stimuli and biological readiness. It occurs about a year after accelerated penile growth.[8] The mean age for ejaculation of American boys was just under fourteen years, with 90 percent achieving this developmental stage in the range from eleven to sixteen years.

3. *Postpubescence:* Genitalia reach adult size and shape. It takes about two years to go through the changes enumerated in pubescence, and another two years to go from there to the size and shape achieved during postpubescence. Pubic hair growth commences as one of the first postpubescent signs, with axillary hair beginning about two years later. By then pubic hair resembles the adult type although the area covered is smaller and there is no spread to the medial thighs. Development of the apocrine sweat glands of the axillary area contribute to increased sweating with axillary hairgrowth. In the female sweating is believed to vary during the menstrual cycle, and be phylogenecially related to the scents used by certain animals to attract males. Facial hair growth begins about the same time as axillary hair—first at the corner of the upper lips and then spreading to the mustache area. Remaining body hair appears from the time of the first axillary hair. Enlargement of the larynx and development of the laryngel muscles is one of the more gradual changes that occur which negates its use for evaluating the progress or rate of pubertal development. The voice appears to deepen perceptibly when penile growth is nearing completion.

Secondary Sexual Characteristics. Breast development is a conspicuous secondary sexual characteristic, and it is not confined to girls. There are increases in the size of the areola in both sexes and a darkening of the skin similar to that which occurs in the scrotal sac. About one-third of boys show breast enlargement and production of an enlarged areola during midpubescence. This enlargement in boys lasts from twelve to eighteen months. For girls, breast development in the prepubescent phase is confined to elevation of the papilla. Along with an enlargement of the areola are breast buds in which a small mound protrudes. A gradual evolvement of the breast and areola occurs to the point of contours being separated. This pubescent breast enlargement is due to fat disposition in the connective tissue areas as well as the ducts, rather than to the development of breast secretory units (which occurs only with pregnancy).

In girls, the appearance of a breast bud, or pubic hair, is usually regarded as the first gross sign of puberty. The age range for the emergence of such buds is from eight to thirteen years, with an acceleration of growth in the eleven to thirteen and a half period. Pubic hair growth in the girl commences from eight to fourteen years; the growth spurt for height is from nine and a half to fourteen and a half years with acceleration most prominent from eleven and a half to thirteen and a half years. Changes in the vagina and uterus are from increases in estrogen levels thickening the epithelial cellular lining of the vagina. The cells contain glycocen, which permits bacterial flora to flourish. These bacteria produce lactic acid which shifts the chemical balance of the vagina to an acidic level. Uterine changes are: thickening of the endomentrial lining and an increase in the muscle mass of the uterus with the capacity for contractilability. These changes are associated with certain chemicals (such as actomyosin, creatine phosphate, and adenosine triphosphate). A question raised by analogy to the boy is why the onset of puberty in the girl is not heralded by an acceleration of growth in the ovaries comparable to that of the testes in the boy? The reason is that follicles develop and degenerate in the ovary from birth onward. Hence, there are less dramatic changes in ovarian development at puberty than those occurring in the testes.

THE MENARCHE

The range for the onset of the menarche is ten to sixteen and a half years, with the peak onset at thirteen. Observational studies and surveys reveal some girls finish their pubertal development and are regularly menstruating before others have even begun pubertal development. The correlation between peak velocity of stature growth and menarche is 0.93. Early menstrual cycles are often irregular and sometimes anovulatory (without shedding an ovum). This means that there may be a period of twelve to eighteen months of infertility for the female. Comparable data for the male are not available. Fertility level must be closely distinguished from the level of sexual desire as well as that of peak sexual performance. Menstrual bleeding is taken as a sign that the ovary is secreting steroid hormones. The central nervous system begins to emit cyclic neuroendocrine signals on approximately a twenty-day basis, which signals the pituitary to release the gonadotrophic hormones responsible for ovulation. Again, very little is known about what starts this specific maturational phenomenon beyond some genetic contributions and the general health and environment of a girl.

Many factors influence the age of menarche.[9] Geographical location, month of birth, socio-economic factors, diseases, and genetic influences have all been cited as significant. Geographical influences are appraised in an ecological sense of the interaction between a girl and her environment. Specific components such as latitude, longitude, altitude, temperature, humidity, and lighting are the factors needing control for valid comparisons. Old myths that sexual development is accelerated in the tropics compared to temperate zones have not been borne out. It is believed that climate per se has little or no effect on menarche. This conclusion is based on studies comparing Rome, Edinburgh, and Southern Russia; it is also confirmed by a study comparing Nigeria to Alaska. Evidence suggests that higher altitudes may contribute to delayed menarche, but in the areas studied, economic and nutritional conditions may actually be the crucial variables. Some fascinating studies describe blind girls—both those born prematurely and full term—as having a lower age for the onset of menarche. No satisfactory explanation has been given for the hypotheses that light may be a significant variable in sexual maturation. The light exposure hypothesis may be relevant to investigations of the modal months for the onset of menarche. The findings are in disagreement for the four seasons, but most find that summer is the most frequent time of onset. Studies indicate that winter is the second most common. The seasonal effect might operate by the annual cycle of changing length of day.

General socio-economic factors, although extremely difficult to appraise, are believed significant in regard to the onset of menarche. Studies indicate differential ages for puberty between whites and blacks are primarily due to income levels and their associated benefits. Those in economically privileged groups mature earlier than those in less privileged groups when race and climate are held fixed. General acceleration occurs with good nutrition, especially protein, in diverse parts of the world: Denmark, China, Japan, Mexico, and Israel. Although poor nutrition can retard the onset of puberty, an improved standard of living can lower the date of onset only to a limit where those living on adequate fare have been (i.e., there is a lower limit to the age level at which menstruation can begin).

Interesting effects are noted in the opposite direction when a girl is obese. An earlier onset of puberty occurs up to a weight level of 30 percent over the maximum expected weight for the height and somatotype. Obesity beyond this level causes a delay in menarche. Related to these metabolic exaggerations are retrospective data from diabetics which indicate an earlier age for puberty. However, most diabetics whose symptoms of diabetes commenced before the pubertal period have a delayed onset of menarche.[11]

Hereditary components contribute by a racial factor. Unfortunately, conclusions about racial differences are laden with social class variations. Family studies have concentrated on correlations between mothers and daughters as well as between siblings. Methodologic difficulties arise from the maternal data being retrospective from decades past when comparisons were made. Most lacking is a longitudinal study utilizing prospective data. Acknowledging limitations, existing reports indicate a good correlation between mothers and daughters. One study of 200 mothers and their 351 daughters had a correlation of 0.40 between their menarcheal ages.[12] Another study compared ranges of maternal menarche to mean ages for the menarche of their daughters. Mothers who had a menarcheal age in the range of eleven to thirteen years had daughters with a mean age of twelve years and ten months; mothers with a menarcheal range of fourteen to sixteen years had daughters with a mean age of thirteen years, seven months; mothers with the range of seventeen to nineteen years had a mean age in their daughters of fourteen years and eleven months. Sisters also have a close correlation in the age of menarche when compared to nonrelated girls. One study reported a difference of 2.8 months between identical twins, 12.0 months in nonidentical twins, 12.9 between sisters, and 18.6 months in pairs of unrelated women.[13]

The secular trend operates with the menarche as it has with several other physical aspects of development. Tanner cites data in support of the age of menarche declining by four months per decade in Western Europe from 1830 to 1960.[14] Some question the legitimate use of the secular trend to explain such a decline from the implication that the passage of time by itself, apart from any socioeconomic changes, accounts for the change. This has been very difficult to establish, and it is certainly not validated by studies comparing the mean menarcheal age of mothers and daughters. In fact, when generational comparisons are made in areas where little technological advances have occurred, an acceleration in menarche is not observed. No change in menarcheal age of nomadic Lapps was observed from 1870 to 1930. Nor has the age of onset shifted between mothers and daughters in an Indian population when there was no change in diet.[15]

Research studies have utilized two approaches: a prospective approach of recording the menarcheal age from a sample of girls prior to onset, and retrospective approaches of questioning girls or women subsequent to the onset of their menstruation. Results indicate that by a prospective approach in the United States between 1934 and 1966, a drop of 3.6 months per decade in menarcheal age occurred.[16] Retrospective studies showed a decline of 4.4 months per decade from 1932 to 1962.

ENDOCRINOLOGICAL ASPECTS OF ADOLESCENCE

Although all the endocrine glands participate in adolescent growth to an extent, some play a more major role. This is obviously with respect to hormones from the sex glands, adrenals, and pituitary. However, the thyroid, parathyroid, pineal, thymus, and pancreas also contribute. Gonadotropins are pituitary hormones which have a stimulating effect on the gonads. The main method for their investigation in the past has been by measuring the amount of their excretion in a twenty-four-hour urine sample. The most specific test is the direct measurement of pituitary hormone in the blood. Many gonadotropins are also measurable by sensitive radioimmunoassays.[17] Studies from the 1940s correlated the level of androgen, estrogen, and gonadotropins with secondary sexual characteristics in boys. Before the beginning of the pubertal period, gonadotropins are scarcely detectable.

Maturity groups in the tables cited are: (1) prepubescence, (2) beginning growth of penis and testes with pubic hair growth, at a mean age of thirteen, (3) mean age of fourteen, (4) mean age of fourteen and three-fourths, and (5) mean age of fifteen and one half. Gonadotropin bioassay was carried out by the increase in uterine weight that occurred in mature female mice (the "mouse-uterine weight method"). It has been found that girls from age three to twelve years excrete at most one "rat unit" in a twenty-four-hour period, while from twelve to sixteen years of age, excretion rises to twelve "rat units." In boys gonadotropin excretion is detectable at about eight years and rises to a maximum value of six "rat units" at fifteen. However, interpreting the data is still ambiguous. It remains usettled whether urinary gonadotropins represent two separate hormones (FSH—follicle-stimulating hormone, or ICSH—interstitial cell-stimulating hormone), or only one hormone whose actions vary at different levels. Thus, low levels might function as FSH while at higher levels they could function as ICSH. The study usually cited as classic is that of Nathanson, who did four determinations on the ovarian follicular response in immature mice from samples of thirteen boys and fourteen girls.[18] No FSH was detectable in boys before age thirteen and the first response in girls was during the eleventh year. FSH became detectable in girls a year before the menarche. Congruent with this data, estrogen levels increase in girls from eight to eleven years. Other studies reveal that in the prepubertal period the FSH excretion level is high and the ICSH low. At the onset of puberty, FSH secretion decreases and ICSH levels increase in greater proportions.[19] However, in girls with delayed puberty, ICSH levels remain low. In boys a striking contrast is presented since there is no evidence of an increase in ICSH at puberty.

Estrogen excretion remains relatively constant in boys and girls from age three to seven years, at which point it begins to rise gradually in both sexes. The intervention of puberty in girls leads to a sharp estrogen rise as well as a monthly cyclic variation which—even at its lowest—is higher than that in boys. These cycles appear to be established at the time of the growth spurt for height, and at the beginning of breast buds. Estrogen levels during the cycle continue to increase until some years after the onset of menarche.

The source of estrogens in boys is primarily the testes, with a smaller amount derived from the adrenals. Adolescent boys continue to excrete estrogens in the urine at a fairly even level. It must be kept in mind that *estrogens* refers to a group of compounds. Until 1953 it was thought that they were estroen, estriol, and estradiol. During the ensuing years seven additional compounds related to these classic estrogens were discovered. Additional unknown estrogen-like compounds continue to be discovered. Consequently it is difficult to assign any specificity to estrogens. Further, since estrogenic substances are excreted cyclically before and after the menarche, appraisal of estrogenic excretion must be based on several samples.

Progesterone is a hormone which can chemically be reduced to pregnanediol and excreted in the urine as pregnanediol glucuronide. Its value increases in the premenstrual phase which is viewed as evidence of ovulation. It is synthesized in the testes, adrenal cortex, placenta, and corpus luteum in the ovary. It acts on female genital and breast tissues. Data are sparse but suggest that the adrenal produces this compound during childhood and adolescence.

Androgenic substances have been studied in the past by bioassay of the degree of comb growth in the capon or day-old chick by urine specimens. This led to results indicating minute amounts being present in infants. Androgens are the hormones capable of stimulating secondary sexual characteristics in the male. In fact, the regulation of protein synthesis is the principal action of steroid hormones.[20] Androgen levels are believed associated with levels of 17-ketosteroids in the blood and urine. Studies have indicated a beginning increase in amounts by age seven or eight years, which rise sharply toward the end of puberty and continue to rise until eighteen or twenty years of age. A sharper rise in pubertal boys is believed due to production from the testes. The major complication in appraising the impact of androgens via neutral 17-ketosteroids is the variety of chemical precursors which can give rise to the metabolite. In turn, the 17-ketosteroids are a mixture of six compounds regularly found in adult urine. Testosterone gives rise to three: endrostrone, dehydroepiandrostrone (DHA), and etiocholanolone. Lacking knowledge of the activity of natural androgens, their metabolism, and their excretion, the precise value and meaning of 17-ketosteroids must be held in abeyance. There is a presumption that similarity in excretion levels occurring for androgens and 17-ketosteroids means similarity in substance and action. However, the correlation is imperfect. The endrostrone of the ketosteroids is the one believed to be the closest biological indicator of testicular function.

There are many unresolved questions regarding testosterone. While it has been demonstrated that there is an intranuclear binding of the hormone within the largest cells, acting to translate genetic information as with other steroid hormones, it is not known how such binding regulates genetic machinery. Another interesting problem is that testosterone influences almost all body tissues, not just the organs of reproduction. The limits of its effects on the growth of the boy's external genitalia are not known. For example, what sets limits on how far growth goes? It is now believed that testosterone is the only steroid that induces the formation in the embryo of tissues that will later serve as major targets for its action in the accessory organs of male reproduction.[21] The major influence of testosterone on the central nervous system, beyond regulating gonadotropin secretion by the hypothalamo-pituitary axis, is by way of its contribution to gender identity and other aspects of behavior. In one study of twenty-one male prisoners between ages nineteen to thirty-two years (mean age, twenty-eight years), all from a laboring class background, the ten prisoners with histories of more violent and aggressive crimes in adolescence had a significantly higher level of testosterone than did the eleven prisoners without such a history.[22]

Adrenocorticosteroids also play a physiological role in adolescence, not in terms of a spurt occurring during puberty, but in a gradual increase from birth to maturity accompanying the increase in bodily size. The significance of the adrenal cortex on sexual development is as a source of estrogens in the male and androgens in the female. Although the adrenal secretes corticoids and aldosterone continuously during childhood, there is an increase in adrenal size during puberty from an increase in sex hormone production (adrenarche). However, no spurt in corticoid excretion occurs at puberty, so that ACTH from the pituitary cannot be the initiator which increases the production of sex hormones by the adrenals. This leads to the hypothesis that other hormones or processes are responsible. The following have been offered as explanations for the increase in *androgen* production by the adrenal glands during adolescence: (1) An unknown hormone from the anterior pituitary gland is involved in stimulating androgen and/or estrogen production by way of the adrenal cortex. (2) ACTH may effect the adrenals in a different manner at puberty due to the action of some other sensitizing hormone. (3) Luteinizing hormone, or ICSH, may stimulate the adrenals to produce androgen. (4) Gonadotropins, or sex hormones themselves, may modify the adrenal response. *Estrogen* production by the adrenal also increases in both sexes although this is less prominent. Why estrogen and androgen production increase is unknown.

VARIATIONS IN RATES OF PHYSICAL DEVELOPMENT

Variations in rates of physical development are discussed in terms of physical and sexual development. Where there is some idiosyncrasy in physical development, there are concommitant changes in the body-image. However, not all disturbances in body-image are due to physical alterations.

Ordinarily, there is an impression that it is more desirable to be large rather than small compared to the peer group. This has been confirmed, provided an extreme degree of size is not reached too rapidly. If the rate of attaining some physical characteristic has a prominent acceleration, social disadvantages may ensue. It is difficult to doubt that in a society so dominated by norms and ideals of male physical prowess, small size is a definite handicap for boys. This is demonstrated by athletics, movies, in strong feelings of identification with groups where dominance is on a physical level, and the association of sexual attractiveness with themes of physical domination.

Other physical factors contribute to a boy's advantage beside size, such as gross and fine coordination, speed, and reflex abilities. Of course, the obvious benefits of such attributes as intelligence, ambition, and diligence as reflecting personality and cognitive traits may dominate any purely physical dimension. Analogous benefits accrue to girls who have a social advantage from earlier physical and sexual development. Physical advantages for girls are not evaluated solely in terms of height and weight, but in the accelerated social development that accompanies physical development.

Questions have long been raised about the relationship between rates of physical maturity and mental ability. The principal question is the extent to which intellectual and emotional development are related to developmental rather than chronological age. Does a child whose development occurs earlier have an intellectual advantage? In fact, developmental age is rarely considered in most institutional approaches to children, such as in medicine and education, which are guided predominantly by the norms of chronological age. In almost all studies, children who are physically advanced for their age score higher on mental tests than do the less mature of the same chronological age.[23] Differences are not great but consistent, and hold for all ages studied commencing at six-and-one-half years. Post-menarcheal girls score higher on intelligence tests than pre-menarcheal girls of the same age. One nationwide study from Great Britain assessed maturity by degrees of secondary sexual characteristics present at age fourteen. The early maturers were a group who had gained a greater proportion of entry into secondary schools by age eleven.

Group results indicate that children who were larger overall in terms of height and weight scored higher on tests. Bayley found a correlation of 0.40 between IQ and stature, calculated within yearly groups for ages seven, ten, twelve, fourteen, and sixteen although the small numbers gave a 95 percent confidence level of 0.10 to 0.70.[24] There is usually an assumption that by age twenty the intelligence test score differences between early and late maturers phase out, but there is little evidence to support this. The assumption is that as growth status advances or slows there will be a parallel shift in mental development. Social variables intrude and complicate matters as does the chromosomal contribution to human potentiality.[25] If bodily size and rate of maturation are correlated positively with social class, as they appear to be from a number of related variables, and there are further correlations with intelligence test scores, it may be invalid to believe that these correlations magically disappear in the post-adolescent period. Whatever the alternative explanation, it would seem more logical to hold that some of these early changes persist from some type of genetic and/or environmental factors until this hypothesis is refuted.

Undesirable consequences for girls whose secondary sexual characteristics become manifest very early, compared to their peer group remain. However, even here the advantages may be capitalized upon by girls whose predisposing conflicts do not affect their confidence and ability to mingle with others. Some types of early development may proceed without adverse social consequences unless the reactions of the girl herself interfere. A not unusual variation is the early appearance of pubic hair in girls which appears to be related to increased levels of androgens. If the increase is from adrenal androgens, there might be an acceleration in height and weight as well. Excessive development of bodily hair (hursitism) is often familial and can be managed cosmetically. Anxiety associated with the hair is the biggest problem. Premature breast development can occur without accompanying development of other organs, and this is a situation of hypersensitivity of the end organ to hormonal stimulation. This same situation probably explains overdevelopment of breast tissue (virginal hyperplasia breasts).

The major difficulty for girls appears to be the presence of manifest secondary sexual characteristics which lead to other possibilities in the psychosocial and social spheres. In time this presents certain risks from adolescent males who go by what they see. However, most girls with accelerated development appear to share the same interests and social activities as do those of similar chronological age. Although these variations are usually within the curve of biological distribution in terms of being at one end of a curve, clinical evaluation is necessary in some cases to differentiate cases of endocrinopathies, adrenal or gonadal tumors, disorders of the central nervous system (hypothalamic irregularities, tumors, or cerebral damage from toxins and infections), that can lead to anomalous development. In some cases, exogenous administration of hormones during the developmental years must be detected in the history to track down the source of growth stimulation.

Contrasted with accelerated development are frequent complaints by adolescents that they have not advanced as fast as their peers in physical characteristics. This varies from a general delay in the onset of puberty to a lag of one or more characteristics. Since pubertal changes in girls commence earlier, boys as a group are in a position of anticipating growth changes. Hence, a boy with slower development has a greater potential for anxiety about his body and social relations. This pertains not only to height and muscle development, but to genital development. Teasing by other boys, and being bypassed for attention by girls for several years, contribute to internalized conflicts. The need to prove themselves can be a predisposing factor for daredevil or antisocial behavior.

Another observed alternative is to withdraw into angry brooding. In some cases, fathers as well as mothers bring their pre-pubertal sons in for examination, expressing concern about delayed genital growth and small phallic size. Eliciting the anxieties and fantasies of these parents is of interest in illustrating interlocking family anxieties. In practice, they are customarily handled by direct reassurance. Many of these boys have been consistently two to four years behind in skeletal development. Historically, a similar history is often present in the backgrounds of the fathers. Again, as with accelerated development, most of these variations are due to the biological distribution of certain traits. They are expressions of constitutional and polygenetic influences.

In selected cases, clinical signs and symptoms warrant more thorough evaluation. Some adolescents may be responding to dietary inadequacies. Other delays may be associated with severe emotional problems such as an unfolding psychotic process, or anorexia nervosa. The differential problem is to diagnose those rare cases who will remain dwarfed to some degree on the basis of genetic factors, neurological problems, or endocrinopathy involving the gonads or the pituitary, and to take appropriate steps for the medical as well as the psychological management that is often ignored. Most of these cases represent a delay in the maturation of the pituitary-gonadal-adrenal axis, as confirmed by the number of boys who eventually reach maturity without abnormality.

COMMON PHYSICAL CONCERNS DURING ADOLESCENCE

Obesity. The combination of an affluent economy, the appeal to individual oral cravings, lethargy and inactivity are all factors giving rise to obesity as a prevalent problem during adolescence. Dietary and psychogenic factors account for the overwhelming number of cases falling within this group.[26] However, general factors of constitutional predisposition reflecting genetic factors cannot be ignored. The problem of obesity is so significant for some adolescents that a section discusses it later in the chapter.

Breast Enlargement. Boys may become concerned about transient enlargements in their breast tissues. This type of gynecomastia should be differentiated from obesity or muscular overdevelopment. When breast tissue itself develops in the boy, it is usually in association with the occurrence of rapid virilization. Etiology, while not specifically established, is probably related to androgens being converted to estrogens. Prepubertal boys who show breast development have often been exposed to cosmetic creams or vitamin preparations contaminated with estrogens. Organic conditions which may cause gynecomastia are quite rare and are associated with other abnormal findings involving hormonal disturbance: liver diseases which prevent conjugation and degradation of estrogen compounds, feminizing tumors of the adrenals, and Klinefelter's Syndrome, which is associated with underdeveloped testicles (testicular dysgenesis).

Cryptochidism. Another condition of great concern to adolescent males is cryptochidism, or undescended testicles.[27] The incidence is 10 percent in boys at birth, but by one year it drops to 2 to 3 percent. By the postadolescence phase, it is down to 0.3 to 0.4 percent. In these cases the testes have not descended into the scrotal sac and have remained either in the abdomen, where they develop embryologically, or in the inguinal canal, in transit to the scrotum. A unilateral condition is four to five times more prevalent than the bilateral condition. In eunuchoidism, on the other hand, the testicles themselves are not developed. With cryptochidism, secondary sexual characteristics do develop, since hormones are produced from the testes, while in eunuchoidism this is not possible.

Apart from the psychological consequences of not having testes in the scrotal sac, the main liability of cryptorchidism is the inability of the testes in the abdomen to mature for spermatogenesis at puberty because the intra-abdominal temperature is higher than it is in the scrotal sac. Consequently, a byproduct of bilateral cryptorchidism is a sterile male.

There is controversy about the optimal age for surgical correction. Some urge surgery early to avoid damage to the testicular tubules needed for sperm production. The age recommended varies from three to puberty. Those who advocate delay note that some testes will descend in time. There is also the possibility that the testicles will atrophy following surgery. There can be psychological consequences for the boy with an anatomic lack in the genital region. In addition, surgery involving the genital area has not been dealt with in terms of mutilation or castration anxiety. Finally, the long-range consequences of not being able to reproduce raise severe problems.

Menstrual Irregularities. Menstrual irregularities are quite frequent. Failure to menstruate (amenorrhea) can reflect a delayed onset of puberty, but the wide range permissible for the onset of menstruation urges caution against impressions that something is wrong in the pituitary or ovary.

Once menstruation has occurred, a host of disturbances are possible. Dysmenorrhea (painful menstruation) rarely indicates organic disease, but rather some combination of anxiety and circumstances pending the evening-out of this biological function. Since one to two years may elapse before true ovulatory cycles are established, it is not surprising that irregularities occur. Secondary amenorrhea may develop after periods have begun. Metrorrhagia (flowing between periods) and menorrhagia (excessive flow at regular times of occurrence) are other types of irregularities. These may occur with different physical illnesses, a failure to ovulate, or emotional tension.

TABLE 2

Physical Problems of Development in Adolescence

Biological Variations in Maturation

Premature Development of Sexual Hair ("Premature Pubarche")

Hirsutism

Premature Development of Breast in Girls ("Premature Thelarche")

Virginal Hyperplasia of Breasts

Obesity and Constitutional Differences in Adiposity

Gynecomastia in Boys

Cryptorchidism and Eunuchoidism

Menstrual Irregularities

Growth. Many elements affect growth, from chromosomal to prenatal, natal, and subsequent exogenous factors. Adequate nutrition is a necessity, but related to it are metabolic disturbances or anoxia, which can stunt growth. Endocrines contribute, such as pituitary growth hormone, thyroid hormone, and androgens. Conversely growth may be inhibited by sex hormones, which can limit secretion of growth hormones or lead to premature fusion of bone epiphyses.

Dwarfism should be distinguished from other causes of growth disturbances. The variety of causes which can operate to induce growth retardation for dwarfism illustrates the complexity of factors. These are listed in Table 3.

ABNORMALITIES OF SEXUAL DEVELOPMENT

Anomalous sexual development can take place by diverse routes. Seven variables need consideration in understanding sex development: (1) chromosomal patterns, (2) gonadal sex as indicated by morphology of organ development, (3) endocrinological sex associated with secondary sexual characteristics, (4) anatomic genital organs, (5) internal accessory organs of reproduction, (6) sex assignment at birth and the consequences that follow for child-rearing practices, and (7) psychological sex-role and sex-identity.

While extreme cases are detected earlier, during adolescence many of the difficulties become overtly manifest. Three types of deviations in development are discussed: precocious sexual development, sexual infantilism, and abnormalities of sexual differentiation.

Precocious Sexual Development. Cases in which the normal sex chromosome pattern of maleness or femaleness is present but development begins at periods significantly prior to the typical broad age ranges are referred to as precocious sexual development. Certain sexual characteristics may have an accelerated growth in terms of an early onset of puberty. This may be eight to ten years for girls and ten to eleven years for boys. Onset of puberty prior to these norms is viewed as biologically deviant.

Changes associated with precocious elaboration of sex hormones arise in two ways: (1) early secretion of gonadotropic (gonad-stimulating) hormones by the pituitary resulting in complete sexual precocity, or (2) secretion of sex hormones by the gonads or adrenals resulting in incomplete sexual precocity. The result of (1) is a maturation of the gonads with accompanying gametogenesis and secretion of sex hormones at levels more typical of an adult or adolescent, and it reflects deviancy in the neuroendocrine system:

TABLE 3

Types of Dwarfism

I.   *Nutritional or Metabolic Disorders*

A. Celiac Disease and cystic fibrosis of the pancreas
B. Chronic renal diseases
C. Hepatic diseases
D. Nutritional defects
E. Chronic infections
F. Electrolyte disturbances (hypokalemia, hypercalemia, etc.)

II. *Constitutional Delayed Growth in Adolescence*

III. *Bone Diseases*

A. Chondrodystrophy, Hurler's Syndrome
B. Varieties of rickets
C. Osteogenesis imperfecta—with multiple fractures
D. Spine diseases—tuberculosis, caries

IV. *Endocrine Disorders*

A. Hypothyroidism
B. Hypopituitarism
C. Sexual precocity with early epiphysial fusion

V.   *Circulatory or Respiratory Disorders*

A. Congenital cardiac malformations
B. Chronic and extensive pulmonary disease—with anoxemia

VI. *"Primordial" or Genetic Dwarfism*

A. Familial
B. Sporadic (intrauterine dwarfing)
C. Gonadal aplasia and dwarfism syndrome
D. Autosomal chromosome anomalies (mongolism and trisomies)

VII. *Miscellaneous*

A. Progeria (Gilford-Hutchinson)
B. Cockayne's Syndrome
C. Associated with severe cerebral dysfunction

an abnormality in one of the target glands, (gonads or adrenals), excessive stimulation of these glands by pituitary hormones, or excessive activity of the pituitary by stimuli from higher brain centers, such as gonadotropin-releasing factors by the hypothalamus.

In many cases no basis can be established for the stimulation given to the pituitary. This condition is called "idiopathic sexual precocity." In others, organic lesions in the hypothalamus or other intracranial sites can be established. Cases classified under (2) above are usually due to pathology in the gonads themselves, such as a tumor in the ovaries or testes, or tumors or hyperplasia in the adrenals. Adrenal lesions may have an accompanying virilization which produces a pseudohermaphroditism or virilism in females. In these cases the tumor abnormality or overgrowth is confined to such pathology. Since the gonadotropic activities of the pituitary are not established, the gonads do not show normal maturation or gamete production. Classifications of precocious sexual development are shown in Table 4.

Data on the incidence and relative frequency of sexual pathologies are interesting. Although 80 to 90 percent of the pathologies caused by premature activation of the pituitary functions with gonadotropic production remain without specific etiology, a breakdown reveals that sexual precocity occurs twice as frequently in girls as in boys. In girls the idiopathic type accounts for 75 percent compared to 40 percent for boys. Cases with a verified etiology, such as a brain tumor, occur as frequently in boys and girls.

Sexual development can begin exceedingly early. The record case appears to be that reported by Plumb in 1897 of a girl who had enlarged breasts and pubic hair at birth and actually menstruated at six weeks. Cases of boys born with enlarged genitalia are also known. The consequences may be that ovulation begins to occur in girls and spermatogenesis in boys. Among 310 girls with a constitutional sexual precocity, seventy instances of pregnancy before fourteen years of age have been recorded, with eighteen instances between ages five and ten. These figures are a base line of validated cases—the true incidence is probably much higher. The most famous case is Lina Medina, a Peruvian girl, who menstruated at eight months and became pregnant at four years and ten months. In 1939, at five-and-one-half years, she gave birth to a six-and-one-half pound boy by Caesarean section.[28]

What are the psychological consequences of such precocious sexual development? There is no acceleration in psychological

TABLE 4

Sources of Sexual Precocity

Etiology	Lesion — Boys	Lesion — Girls	Characteristics
I. Gonadotropin Secretion from Pituitary A. Neurologically Activated	1. Brain tumor 2. Encephalitis 3. Obscure disorders of the hypothalamus	Same as for boys	1. Gonads mature normally 2. Gonads mature normally 3. Spermatogenesis or ovulation may occur
B. "Idiopathically" Activated	None found	None found	Sex hormones excreted in normal amounts for an adolescent or adult
II. Gonadotropin Secretion from Tumor	1. Hepatoma 2. Teratoma	1. Same as for boys 2. Same as for boys 3. Chorioepithelioma	Leydig cell hyperplasia of testes without spermatogenesis
III. Direct Sex Hormone Secretion A. From Gonads	1. Interstitial cell tumor of testes	1. Granulosa cell tumor or cyst of ovary 2. Luteoma or thecoma of ovary	1. Tumor usually in one gonad 2. Sex hormones sometimes excreted in excess amounts
B. From Adrenals	1. Virilizing adrenal hyperplasia 2. Virilizing tumor	1. Feminizing adrenal tumor (rare)	1. Gonads usually immature (17-ketosteroid excretion increased)

development.[29] Sexually precocious boys have an abundance of strength and energy. This leads to much boisterous activity, but of a clumsy nature, since motor skills and coordination are not proportionately advanced. Although it may be possible to educate the parents to accept the condition as one similar to a physical abnormality, the consequences of premature development appear to carry a greate burden. An oversupply of shame and avoidance in these families about sexual activities exists. Nor is the problem confined to parents and siblings, since other children who see precocious characteristics deal with their own anxieties by teasing and ridicule accompanied by other parents urging avoidance.

The problem of control of sexual behavior for these children is, in many ways, like that of control over other impulses, the obvious difference being in the need to regulate various genital activities. A common problem associated with heightened genital sensitivity is masturbation, as it is for an adolescent youth. The solution is one of learning the time and place for such activity. It is possible for psychological development to proceed without serious consequences, but the handicaps are greater. Not only are there the usual conflicts of childhood and adolescence, but superimposed ones. While the dilemmas associated with the prolonged period of adolescence in our society are acknowledged, the precociously developed child has a period of sexual maturity which does not fit any accepted mold. The difficulty which commonly arises with parents and teachers is forgetting the psychological and social level of the child's development and making excessive demands in terms of ego development.

Sexual Infantilism. A second area of anomalous sexual development is sexual infantilism. This refers to lack of secondary sexual development or maturation; it is just the opposite of precocious puberty in that there is a persistent lack of sexual development beyond the upper limit of age ranges present in most adolescents. The main causes are listed in Table 5.

Sexual infantilism is associated with disorders in hypothalamic, pituitary, and gonadal glands. In hypothalamic or pituitary cases, the gonads fail to mature and secrete sex hormones from the lack of pituitary gonadotropin. Infantilism from gonadal causes is associated with a defect or absence of the gonads. Differentiation between them is made by the assay of follicle-stimulating hormone in the urine, and the study of nuclear chromatin and chromosomal patterns.

TABLE 5

Causes of Sexual Infantilism

I. Hypothalamic Lesions (tumors, cysts, congenital defects)

  A. Sexual infantilism without obesity
  B. Sexual infantilism with obesity, diabetes insipidus
    1. Froehlich's Syndrome
    2. Laurence-Moon-Biedl Syndrome

II. Pituitary Deficiencies

  A. Generalized with dwarfism
  B. Specific gonadotropic deficiency (pituitary eunuchoidism)
  C. Specific ACTH deficiency

III. Primary Gonadal Disorders and Gonadal Dysgenesis

  A. Syndrome of gonadal aplasia and stunted growth
  B. Gonadal hypoplasia or dysplasia
  C. Primary testicular disorders
    1. Defective testes
    2. Anorchia (lack of a testis)
  D. Prepubertal castration

Hypothalamic lesions resulting in infantilism are classified as follows: those associated and those not associated with obesity may be due to tumors arising in the hypothalamic area (craniopharyngiomas, gliomas, or tumors of the hypothalamus or optic chiasm, which present with neurologic signs and symptoms). Other types of sexual infantilism with hypothalamic etiology are associated with obesity. At the turn of the century, a case of a sexually infantile fourteen-year-old boy with obesity and stunted growth was reported. He had diabetes insipidus and signs of a tumor in the hypothalamic area. Subsequently, from the expansion of discussion in medical literature, all manner of obese preadolescent and adolescent boys were seen as being similarly afflicted. The diagnosis in question was "Froehlich's Syndrome," described earlier. Confusion proceeded to the point where some advocated abandoning the diagnosis altogether, since accurate usage should have confined it to rare cases with proven hypothalamic lesions inducing a deficiency of pituitary gonadotropin. The "Laurence-Moon-Biedel Syndrome" is a genetic recessive disease. Groupings of the following occur: sexual infantilism, obesity, stunted growth, diabetes insipidus, mental defect, retinitis pigmentosa, polydactylism, and syndactylism.

Pituitary hypogonadism occurs in boys and girls without any gross lesion of the pituitary. In the prepubescent period it may be difficult to differentiate from delayed adolescence or primordial dwarfism. The features remain immature and bone epiphyses may occur. In girls, ovaries do not mature, breast development is absent, and the external genitalia remain infantile. The uterus is small and menstruation does not occur, nor do pubic or axillary hair develop. The low level of secretion in the urine of 17-ketosteroids compounds indicates androgens from the adrenals are insufficient.

In boys the testes are small and sperm is not produced. The secondary sexual characteristics fail to develop and there is a low level of 17-ketosteroids. In most cases the infantilism persists. Unfortunately, of the various pituitary functions the gonadotropic is one of the first to be affected, which contributes to the usual, although not invariable, complete lack of sexual development.

More common are situations of deficient sexual development associated with a specific lack of gonadotropic action of the pituitary, but not accompanied by dwarfism. Degrees of hypogonadism may be present. Since androgenic activity of the adrenal may not be impaired, sexual hair can develop. In fact, the secondary sexual characteristics attain moderate development with hypogonadism manifested in lack of sperm production and infertility. In girls the manifestations are associated with deficiencies in estrogen production from the diminution of pituitary gonadotropic hormone. Gradations of disturbances are possible with secondary sexual characteristics and a normal-appearing genital tract being present, but menstruation is absent or appears irregularly. Another variation is anovulatory menstruation with accompanying infertility. To further complicate matters, the gonadotropic activity of the pituitary gland is a very sensitive mechanism which can react adversely to many circumstances and temporarily impair its functioning. This has been seen in association with acute or debilitating illnesses, malnutrition, and emotional upset—the most dramatic of which is anorexia nervosa. Such upsets are noted in males and females.

A third grouping of those who lack adequate sexual development are the gonadal disorders. In contrast to those associated with hypothalamic or pituitary lesions, a greater quantity of pituitary gonadotropin is secreted in these individuals. The gonadal defect varies from a defect in the embryonic development (dysgenesis) to an impairment from injury, disease, or removal of the organ after differentiation. Deviations occurring earlier (at the stage where sex chromosomes themselves determine differentiation of primitive gonads) is discussed later.

Gonadal disorders, causing absent or incomplete sexual development, occur from a defect at the embryonic level of gonad development and are referred to as gonadal dysgenesis. Two main divisions are based on phenotypic characteristics being either male or female. For females, three gradations are designated: gonadal aplasia (complete lack of gonads), hypoplasia (rudimentary ovarian development of the cortical component), and dysplasia (rudimentary ovarian development of the medullary component).

For those with a male phenotype and testicular dysgenesis there are four gradations: Klinefelter's Syndrome, germinal aplasia, syndrome of rudimentary testes, and males with a webbed neck resembling what is called *Turner's Syndrome*. The latter was described by Turner in 1938 in studying seven girls who were not only sexually underdeveloped but had accompanying physical anomalies. They were short and appeared to have abnormalities of the neck, faces, and thorax. By 1954 it was shown that the absence of ovaries was not a sufficient explanation since most of these girls had a chromatin-negative nuclear sex pattern resembling that of normal males. It was then assumed that these girls were genetic males whose phenotypic development was due to the loss of an ovary on some basis. By 1959 methods for studying the actual chromosomal constitution in humans had developed. The Turner Syndrome was then redefined as a phenotypic female with the external and internal genitalia of a female, but the gonad was an undifferentiated streak with no true germinal or secretory elements. More detailed examination revealed that these chromatin-negative individuals had forty-five chromosomes with only a single X sex chromosome (XO), and without the XY constitution of the normal male. Something was seen as defective in the second sex chromosome in at least some of the cells. This led to work demonstrating varieties of chromatin-positive persons with abnormal sex chromosome constitutions. There have been mosaicisms of XO/XX, or XO/XX/XXX types, and structural anomalies of the X chromosomes.[30]

An association exists between conditions grouped under sexual infantilism with accompanying somatic anomalies. Many of these were contained in the first syndrome described by Turner, but they can occur separately. The most frequent somatic condition is a short stature with a webbed neck in which triangular folds of skin extend downward from the ear. Skeletal anomalies are frequent, with thinning of bones in the hands, feet, elbows, and the upper arm or thigh bones (humerus and femur). There may be skeletal peculiarities such as a broad shield-like chest, pectus excavatum (caved-in chest), or pigeon chest (pointed-outward chest). Fingernails are thin and narrow. In addition to the redundancy of neck and skin folds, there may be a webbing of the fingers, or a webbed fold of skin across the front of the armpit region and a proneness to excessive scarring (keloids). Problems in the cardiovascular system occur, such as coarctation (narrowing of the aorta), intestinal hemorrhages, hypertension, excessive accumulation of lymph secretion, and occasional kidney abnormalities. About 25 to 33 percent of these cases show a slight-to-moderate intellectual impairment. However, an occasional individual is in the superior range.

Primary disorders of the testes need sharp differentiation from hypopituitary eunuchoidism. This differentiation not only involves increased amounts of gonadotropin in the urine, but these males show normal differentiation of the external genitals with better development of the secondary sexual characteristics at puberty. Virilization is somewhat deficient, but growth is not stunted. Hence, the psychological consequences are not as severe, though later consequences with sterility may be. Klinefelter's Syndrome is when these characteristics are present along with testes that are small and do not attain adult size in the course of puberty. Before puberty these individuals are phenotypic males with no characteristic abnormality. There is generally a complete absence of spermatogenesis. In some, gynecomastia may be present. Subsequent genetic work has demonstrated that about 80 percent of these males have a positive nuclear chromatin pattern. This is most typically an XXY sex, i.e., the nuclei contain a chromatin mass which is a darkly staining clump containing Desoxyribonucleic acid (DNA)—the "Barr body" found in normal females.

The general rule is that persons with a chromatin-positive Klinefelter's Syndrome have at least two X's and one Y chromosome in their cells as the basic cytogenetic defect. Other possible karyotypes are: XXXY, XXXXY, and XXYY complexes and mosaicisms of XXYY/XY, XXY/XX, and XXX/XXXXY. Studies of prepubertal boys have been made by buccal smears performed on the basis of a higher incidence of mental retardation when small testes are present.

SEX DIFFERENTIATION PROBLEMS

The third deviation in sexual development involves abnormalities of sex differentiation. Sex refers to many things, such as the seven scientific usages pointed out. Other factors held constant, the initial determiner of sex constitution is genetic, although beginning with conception difficulties can arise. The stages of sex differentiation are given in Table 6:

TABLE 6

Stages of Sex Differentiation

Stage	*Determination by*
1. Sex chromosomal constitution (XX or XY)	1. Fertilization of X ovum by X or Y sperm
2. Gonad differentiation—ovary or testis	2. Sex chromosomal constitution
3. Duct differentiation	

At birth sex assignment is made by observation of a few characteristics of the external genitalia but this can become complicated. The most sophisticated techniques may not be able to make an unequivocal assignment of sex. Fortunately, most cases are accurately assigned.

Differentiation of gonads begins in the fourth week of gestation. In the embryos of both sexes an undifferentiated gonad appears. The inner part, or medulla, of this structure may evolve into a testes. The cortex then regresses. In the seventh to ninth week of gestation a genetic female complement begins to show differentiation of the cortex into an ovary, and the medullary portion disappears. The next step is the differentiation of internal genitalia, or ducts, which develop from separate sets of primordia that transiently coexist in both sexes. In males, Wolffian ducts give rise to the vas deferens, the seminal vesicle, and the epididymis, with the Mullerian ducts disappearing. In females, the Mullerian ducts fuse to produce the uterus, Fallopian tubes, and upper third of the vagina, while the Wolffian ducts regress. A hypothetical inducer substance is posited from the fetal testis which suppresses the Mullerian ducts and instead stimulates Wolffian development. If this inducer is absent, regardless of genetic sex, the duct system differentiates along female lines. Androgen, along with the inducer, cannot suppress Mullerian structures.

A subsequent step is the differentiation of external genitals. Again, the baseline is from primordia common to both sexes. In males, androgens act on the genital tubercule to form the phallus, and the genital folds fuse upward to move the urethral opening to the tip of the penis. Failure results in hypospadias—often a valuable clue to incomplete virilization. The final process is a mid-line fusion of genital swellings to form the scrotum. In the female, genital folds develop into the labia minora, while genital swellings form the labia majora and the genital tubercule becomes the clitoris. In contrast to internal differentiation to reproductive organs, which is a choice between Wolffian versus Mullerian pathways, transformation of the external genitalia is a continuous process. Intermediate effects with partial virilization may be seen. By the sixteenth week of gestation, differentiation of the external genitals is complete. Throughout all this, there is a possibility for both qualitative and quantitative errors.

Turner's Syndrome and Klinefelter's Syndrome have been discussed under sexual infantilism. They could also be classified as disorders of gonadogenesis with infertility. A further classification is made in Table 7.

TABLE 7

Disorders of Sex Differentiation

Disorders of gonadogenesis	*Klinefelter's syndrome* *Turner's syndrome*	Infertility without ambiguity
	True hermaphroditism Mixed gonadal dysgenesis Male pseudohermaphroditism (dysgenetic)	Infertility with ambiguity
Disorders of endocrinology: androgen deficiency in the male; androgen excess in the female	Male pseudohermaphroditism (familial)	
	Female pseudohermaphroditism —congenital adrenal hyper- plasia —others	Ambiguity without infertility

Source: *New England Journal of Medicine* 277:353, 1967.

True hermaphrodites have both ovarian and testicular tissue. Combinations are possible, such as an ovary on one side and a testicle on the other. There is usually a uterus, and at least one tube, on the ovarian side. Although most of these individuals have been raised as boys, external virilization is rarely complete. Those with significant phallic development have hypospadias and cryptorchidism. At puberty almost all of them develop gynecomastia, about two-thirds menstruate, and about half ovulate. Therefore, an occasional adolescent may be potentially fertile. Genetic studies indicate that 80 percent are chromatin-positive, and cytogenetic studies indicate a certain number of them are mosaics. The two stems have been 46/XX and 46/XY in a mixture of male and female cells. Most interesting is evidence from hemoglobin types and blood groups demonstrating a given hermaphrodite was originally destined biologically to become fraternal twins of different sex. The basic abnormality, which transpired at the time of fertilization, was a double fertilization, or dispermy. Two sperm fertilize two eggs, or one egg and its polar body. The resulting zygote, or zygotes, instead of separating and growing as twins of unlike sex, either fail to separate or fuse and develop into a true hermaphrodite. Unequal dominance of X or Y gonadal cells would account for the dominance of ovarian or testicular tissue in one person.

Another group is mixed gonadal dysgenesis. Combinations are found such as a streak gonad on one side and a testis on the other. If there were only two streaks, without either one being a clearly delineated gonad, there would ordinarily be gonadal dysgenesis or Turner's Syndrome.

TABLE 8

Types of Mixed Internal Organs

True Hermaphroditism	Testis and ovary
Gonadal Dysgenesis (Turner's Syndrome)	Streak and streak
Mixed gonadal dysgenesis	Testis and streak
Dysgenetic male pseudo-hermaphroditism	Testis and testis (defective)

In mixed gonadal dysgenesis a uterus with at least one tube is present, but external appearances vary. A spectrum of external virilization is possible. A few have appeared as normal females, while others have been females with clitoromegaly, some males with hypospadias and cryptorchidism, and a few with a male phenotype except for unilateral cryptorchidism. These cases are chromatin-negative in comparison to 80 percent of true hermaphrodites and all female pseudo-hermaphrodites who have chromatin-positive. The most common cytogenetic mosaicism is XY/XO.

Two abnormally developed testes, intra-abdominal and defective, lead to dysgenetic male pseudo-hermaphroditism. A true hermaphrodite has gonadal tissue of both sexes. A pseudo-hermaphrodite has unequivocal gonadal development—male or female—but external genital development is incomplete or discordant with the gonadal picture. They have two testes but incomplete virilization. Many show genital development similar to that in mosaic gonadal dysgenesis, and some have an XO/XY mosaicism similar to that of patients who have testes and a streak. Since both testes are developmentally abnormal, Mullerian suppression does not occur, and the result is a female or an inadequate male phenotype.

In addition to these three disorders of gonadogenesis which result in genital ambiguity—true hermaphroditism, mixed gonadal dysgenesis, and male pseudo-hermaphroditism—there are syndromes in which gonadal differentiation is normal. However, a defect in androgen production or action might develop. Androgen deficit in a genetic male leads to male pseudo-hermaphroditism; androgen excess in a genetic female leads to female pseudo-hermaphroditism. The males in the former group are examples of minimal virilization, in that they seem to be just barely virile. Data suggest they produce normal amounts of testosterone, endogenously, but do not react to it or to that administered exogenously. Female pseudo-hermaphrodites are all chromatin-positive, with uterus, tubes, and ovaries. Their external genitals are ambiguous in that they have been exposed to excessive androgen influence from some source prior to the sixteenth week of gestation. Of these abnormalities of sex differentiation, the female pseudo-hermaphrodites are the only ones capable of normal coital and reproductive functioning.

BODY-IMAGE

Developmental Aspects. The developmental background of one's body image has a fascinating history. Anlage commences at the intrauterine level with various kinesthetic and proprioceptive sensory experiences via receptors in muscles and joints. Hand-to-mouth movements commence in the uterus since some infants are born with well-sucked thumbs. Motility gives a wide assortment of tactile impressions.

By necessity, the mouth plays an important part in developing early image because of its central representation for so many tactile sensations which persist throughout development. Expansion of motor development permits the structuring of hand-to-mouth relationships, the entwining of various environmental objects, physical contact with other people, and exploration of bodily surfaces and orifices. The thumb comes to represent many objects in a symbolic sense. Initial explorations of movements over the body, contact with other bodies and objects, and kinesthetic and tactile sensations provide the basis for a postural model. In fact, these are probably the basic processes for the beginnings of self-awareness, which has had a long history of philosophical and biological debate about the origin of consciousness. From this self-awareness a sense of individual continuity related to early ego formation emerges. Self-awareness is necessary for later development of self-observation and self-appraisal as part of ego and superego development.

Not all emerging perceptions are tactile and kinesthetic. Sensations of pleasure and pain, and the classical sight, hearing, smell, and thermal sensations are relevant. However, these are secondary for the image of the body that evolves. Congenitally blind individuals develop a capacity to respond to double simultaneous presentation of cutaneous stimuli, demonstrating tactile and kinesthetic importance in subserving touch. Children who suffer an amputation prior to age five do not seem to develop a phantom extremity, nor do children born without limbs or with flapper limbs experience phantom limbs. After this age, with altered size and shape configurations, images of body parts remain as memory traces. They have the capacity to reappear at future times in states of neurological dissolution or psychological regression.

Socialization processes contribute to the character and quality of the body-image. The child perceives others' attitudes toward his body, its parts, and how it functions. Image representations of the body and its parts are apprized as good or bad, clean or dirty, pleasant or ugly, or desirable or undesirable. Cultural valuations of bodily aspects are seen with respect to the body-image components of strength and power for boys. Imagery related to powerful limbs and muscles, as well as potent genitalia, are prominent. For girls, the cultural representation is seen as the beautiful body, but this may change with the growing influence of women in athletics.

Cultural prohibitions and avoidances contribute to blocking out parts of the body. Exaggerated or caricatured representations are a variation.

Socialization processes occurring within the family cannot be ignored for individuals with an altered body configuration. The presence of a defect can be less important than the attitudes of the culture and family members. Compensatory activities are carried out when reinforced by these institutions to negate limitations.[31] Although mythologies no longer necessarily regard disease or deformity as an embodiment of punishment for sins, psychological reactions are often defensive in nature and lead to reactions of avoidance. These are not confined to certain cultures or social classes, but appear connected with responses which are reinforced within groups.

Body-image Anxiety. Anxieties about the inadequacy of some part of the body are projected. This is witnessed in children at the nursery-school-age level. Combinations of anxiety, rationalization, and projection that concern minor and prevalent bodily configurations as a high forehead (intelligence), a long nose (minority group), receding chin (weak), short and stocky build (low mentality, ape-like), pushed-in nose (athletic), or thinness in girls (sex appeal through an asexual body) are frequent. Family dynamic patterns may reveal hostility and rejection by mothers whose daughters are born with facial deformities or blemishes; for boys, an unathletic habitus when their father's hopes are to participate vicariously in their son's achievements leads to shame about their bodies.

Although one might expect a mother to be more understanding and supportive of a child whose body is deformed or disappointing, in some cases it is the opposite. An anxious and rejecting father induces supportive measures in the mother. However, mutual accusations between parents leads to complications. A parent may take a challenge to develop some overcompensatory ability in a child with a deformity. A host of factors such as marital conflict, difficulties with the in-laws, generational troubles, deaths or illnesses in a family, neurotic conflict in parents, and difficulties such as absence of peers or lack of socialization experiences are relevant.

From the perspective of the child, reactions accumulate and lead to secondary complications. Parental reactions, or teasing and ridicule by children, lead to withdrawal. They avoid looking in mirrors, attempt to conceal their defects, and develop a host of protective devices and fantasies. While some children become defensive, others attempt to joke and ridicule themselves. Parental involvement in the chosen solution is observed. There may be similar verbalizations by parent and child, or attempts to undo the defect by referring to it as an added advantage ("Think of how your limp gives you extra courage."). Although some of these children have a strong desire for achievement, many are plagued by the need never to let down the barrier. All of these responses become exaggerated in adolescence when the ability to avoid painful affect is minimized.

Comparative examinations of others' bodies are made constantly by children. It is a technique for furthering reality testing with respect to body-image. Overevaluations of prowess or beauty are subject to self-correcting processes. In those for whom security is connected to the maintenance of a distorted and unrealistic image there is a vulnerability toward regression. Besides the perception of the external body and comparison with others, the body-image contributes to how the child conceptualizes the inside of the body. This is initially gained from sensations of discomfort. Hypotheses regarding how the cognitive synthesis of internal bodily organs occurs through pain experiences, and how this may further contribute to distortions and how conflict is handled, can be generated. The influence of language used for parts of the body have been demonstrated in studies. Parts of the body which occur most in literature are linguistically the oldest and conform with our accepted personal bodily imagery.[32] Some have extended the concept of body-image to include body parts which occur in fantasy as wish-fulfillments as well as in defensive elaboration. However, where can one draw a line as to where perception ends and fantasy begins concerning one's body representation?

Theoretical Aspects of Body-image.   Theorizing about the nature of body-image has gone on, under some type of appellation, since the time when a capacity for self-reflection emerged. Some of the first written accounts by surgeons dealt with reactions to amputations. A 16th century military surgeon, Ambroise Pare, noted the occurrence of phantom limbs and advised that this should not deter the continued performance of amputations. Perhaps surgical amputation cases were so dramatic that they continued to stimulate thinking on how the body-image persisted despite the loss of a body part. This was observed not just when limbs were removed, but with any alteration from the previous bodily configuration, such as tumors in the head and neck regions, chest alterations, paralyses, or alterations from disease. Indeed, so entrenched is the body-image that phantom extremities persist even after removal of somatosensory parts of the cerebral cortex. The body-image persists after removal of terminal neuromata in stumps and subsequent to performances of rhizotomies, sympathectomies, cordotomies, alcohol injection into stumps, spinal anesthesias, anesthetic blocks of sympathetic ganglia, and prefrontal lobotomies.[33]

Sir Henry Head, an English neurologist, gave an interpretation to the body-image based on an integrative process carried out in the sensory cortex. This was seen as more than the sum of individual sensory experiences.[34] Modification of incoming sensory impressions occurred for a postural model of the body. The postural model of the body was an area of sensori-motor functioning in the central nervous system. This permitted projecting the recognition of posture, movement, and locality, to objects held which became part of the body schema.

A broader concept of the body-image was developed by Paul Schilder.[35] A tridimensional account of interpersonal, environmental, and temporal factors with a psychological investment in the body was included. Body-image is related to emotionality, curiosity, and ideals such as duty. It is a perceptive phenomenon which also involves expressive and interactional aspects. Schilder held that the ego relates to the body as an object, with percepts, thoughts, and affects. Federn further amplified this by differentiating attributes of the ego from the body-image.[36] Both a "body ego" and a "mental ego" were distinguished; there was a feeling that the mental ego was something concrete and inside the body ego. The ego only became equivalent to the body-image when the latter was completely invested with ego feeling. Conversely, the ego may be capable of complete dissolution, yet preserve its somatic functioning in perceptions. "The body-image is the changing presentation of the body in one's mind. Throughout the changes, the bodily ego is the continuous awareness of one's body."[37] A complex integration of the ego and body—with an ascendancy of the ego by mastery over the body—is postulated.

The course of development of the body-image and disturbances have been based on different sources:

1. Disruption in the physical integrity of the body, such as from surgical procedures, neurological diseases affecting parts of the sensori-motor system dealing with movement and posture,

deformities, or physical illnesses which hormonally or metaboli-
cally alter the body
2. Physiological research and theorizing pertaining to central
nervous system functioning
3. Developmental studies on changes in the body-image over time in
view of perceptual-cognitive changes
4. Clinical approaches derived from an ego psychology framework
which deals with percepts, cognitions, and feelings toward the
body (there are also reactive changes in the ego to alterations in
the body from these dimensions, which involve previous life
experiences, developmental norms, the body-image elaborated by
the ego, as well as the ego-ideal aspects of the body)
5. Studies of personality disturbances in terms of altered body-
image. Inquiries into the changed body-image of schizophrenics,
psychopaths, and those with psycho-physiological diseases have
been made. A related approach has been to discriminate healthy
from pathological responses to body alterations. Studies of body-
image in the deaf and blind are needed along with their
corresponding ego development.[38]

Significance of Adolescent Body-image. The particular significance of adolescent body-images is a product of the heightened
degree of narcissistic concern about the intactness and capability of
the body. The body-image in the adolescent encompasses the
corporeal body, the physical attributes, and the psychological
conceptualizations and feelings about these things. Conflicts prior
to entering adolescence predispose toward anxiety-proneness over
changing body-image. Given the wide variation in growth rates
which occur for most physical attributes, including the sexual, the
individual entering adolescence with other conflicts has concerns
which lead to fluctuations in self-esteem. Any conspicuous physical
deviancy, lag, or acceleration, appearing objectively, may be seized
upon and contribute to brooding. It can serve as a focus for
displacement of many other conflicts. This is a period when radical
reconstruction of the body-image is needed from the rapid changes
in size, proportion, and the emerging primary and secondary sexual
characteristics.

Impaired or inadequate virility is an ever-present threat to the
adolescent male. For the adolescent female, there is the constant
threat of loss of esteem attendant upon loss of sexual attractiveness.
These anxieties are found in nonclinical populations and may be
regarded as significant indices in normal adolescents. Stolz and

Stolz, in a group of ninety-three normal adolescents, found 7.5 percent of males still concerned about shortness, and 13 percent of adolescent girls worried about excessive height. About 27 percent of the boys were concerned about their physiques during adolescence.[39] A prominent wish among many adolescent girls is to change their physique. Concern about the body in adolescence often is a displacement from other sources of concern which arouse anxiety. Recurrent themes concerning bigness, power, and success with the body in males, and beauty, charm, and attractiveness in females are revealed in concerns directly and symbolically.

Changes in the body-image of the adolescent, for whatever reason, can be expected to lead to anxiety. A change in the body is experienced as an alteration in a part of the self. A conceptual analogy is the psychological processes related to loss of attached objects or parts of the body to the loss of the preadolescent body. A sequence of stages classified as varieties of mourning reactions are relevant.

Objective or distorted perceptions about others adversely viewing the body increase anxiety and hostility. Unconscious influences contribute, and they are modified by changing body-images. These psychological processes contribute to the depressive proneness. This is not solely a reaction to a change in the body-image, but rather related to unknown factors of what consequences ensue from the changes taking place. Hence, development of desired physical attributes may raise threats from greater competitiveness with others. This may lead to anxieties or physical complaints as a result of threats to dependency relationships. Tendencies toward periodic regression into preadolescent fantasies and behaviors may ensue. Too wide a discrepancy between an idealized body-image and the actual physical body promotes regression. A major task to be mastered during adolescence is to accept the body structure with decreasing dissonance between it and the actual body possessed.

OBESITY

Obesity is one of the main contributors to an altered body-image in the adolescent, and it merits special attention. Physical development has a range in physique and growth. Ordinary growth grids in themselves tell us little about the distribution of bodily composition. The relative differences in distribution between muscularity and adiposity is a prime example. In the absence of well-established standards, subcutaneous skin thickness is the most valuable basis for diagnosis of obesity in children. Attempts at classification have utilized genetic and environmental factors. Others focus on neurological and neurophysiological mechanisms regulating food intake. Different rates of metabolism are another consideration. Constitutional components are significant along with physique. Developmental obesity includes children who eat as much as they want and avoid physical activity. Reactive obesities, on the other hand, correspond to a pattern of eating in response to anxieties and frustrations in which overeating becomes a compensation. Excess accumulation of fatty tissue is seen from (1) genetic variations, (2) disordered regulatory mechanisms, (3) different endowment with fat cells, (4) variations in the deposition and release of fatty acids, (5) variations in metabolism or endocrine malfunctioning, (6) organic brain dysfunction, and (7) acute and chronic psychological conflicts.

Controversy reigns between clinicians who see children in offices, clinics, and hospitals, in contrast to nutritionists and physiologists who feel the psychological hypotheses are not confirmable in obese adolescents in the general population not seen by clinicians. The problem is not to eliminate formulations from clinical populations, but to test their validity in nonclinical populations of obese youths. Besides this testing, data is needed on the natural history of obese children and their fate in adolescence.

How Obesity Has Been Studied.   Approaches to studying obesity have gone through cycles.[40] Early, physique and obesity were viewed as variations of constitutional body types. In the 1930s and early 1940s the endocrine malfunction school held sway in research and clinical work. This gave way to a backlash of efforts to show the irrelevance of endocrine functioning for obese adolescents. In the early 1950s psychodynamic formulations were proposed. More recently, an effort to synthesize a more sophisticated picture of the situation has evolved. Psychological components are far too complex to be interpreted by use of one explanatory model.

Obesity can co-exist as an independent factor with almost every psychiatric diagnostic entity. In many cases, the same partial causal relationships are attributed to the psychiatric diagnosis as for obesity. Emotional disturbance can occur with or without obesity, and with or without a conflicting environment. A common pattern is the adolescent with conflicts in one realm which lead to a pattern of underactivity and accumulated nibbling. Reactive patterns of putting on weight with respect to internal or external crises need differentiation from the problem of a chronically unfolding obesity where the individual emerges from being a plump child to an obese adolescent. Emotional conflicts are also created by efforts to reduce weight.

Cultural Contributions. The most ardent advocates of a cultural approach stress that adolescents by themselves would not be concerned about obesity, or have problems, if their culture did not emphasize slimness as an ideal. This viewpoint bypasses predisposing psychological and developmental correlates connected to obesity. There can be little doubt that a culture which idealizes thinness, and emphasizes this as a moral virtue, raises anxieties and creates disappointments in adolescents. It does this directly and by secondary adverse social consequences of obesity. However, the crucial question is not whether or not these phenomena occur, but whether they are a sufficient condition for the explanation of obesity. Interpretations based on a cultural primacy are not negated with respect to their holdings, but rather their sufficiency. They do not adequately account for certain developmental experiences and family interactional patterns which contribute to overeating or inactivity.

Stereotypes. Two opposite stereotypes are difficult to dispel. One is that obesity predominates among the upper classes due to affluence and self-indulgence. Conversely, the poor should then be thin from factors operating in reverse. Another stereotype holds that youths in the upper classes, with more status consciousness, will diet to conform to their cultural ideals. How valid either of these attempts to class-generalize are is impossible to assess from studies. The Midtown (Manhattan) Study found only 5 percent of upper-class women obese in contrast to 30 percent of those in the lower classes.[41] In an earlier study Bruch cited data going back to children from lower-class homes, seen in a pediatric outpatient clinic beginning in the 1930s.[42] However, her data are incomplete and represent only approximate percentages. Her inquiries were directed to following children into adulthood. It would have been of inestimable value had there been a parallel study of children during the same years from other populations: a clinical population of obese children from private clinics in the upper-middle and upper classes, and a group of obese non-clinic children from all social classes. Bruch found that one-third of the children outgrew their obesity by adolescence, presumably by peer encouragement or by eventually being able to leave home. One-half remained obese, and only a few of these had a good adjustment. Their parents had been the least preoccupied about their children's weight. The majority of those who remained obese showed evidence of serious emotional conflict.

Psychological Conflicts. The typical psychological conflicts of the obese adolescent are not strikingly different from those in other age groups with weight problems. Body-concept and body-image formulations are relevant. One theory has held some type of combined neuropsychological signalling mechanism may be awry. Impairment is hypothesized in the discriminatory awareness of signals indicating bodily awareness or a deviancy in a statistical sense of biological variation. This leads to a misconception of not being in control of the body to the degree that people without such deviations are. Interpersonal confusion is aided and abetted.

Conflicts centering on strivings for autonomy and assertiveness can play a central role. Some give emphasis to a recapitulation of earlier conflicts characteristic of the oral period; others emphasize autonomy strivings occurring in the same period as general bodily control, such as the bowels. Yet conflicts can arise with sufficient intensity during adolescence of their own right. Asserting the self in an oppositional manner to adults may center on food intake or any other sphere wherein parental values or attempts to control can be challenged. To eat whatever one wants, whenever one wants, and without restriction, is perceived as something only an adult can do. Hence, not only periodic indulgences in food fads, but extremes of diet and indulgence in orgies of eating occur.

Psychodynamic formulations are offered to explain patterns of obesity. Food represents a symbolic equivalent for unmet needs. In the course of therapy, the pattern within an individual adolescent becomes more clear. Overindulgence in food can be associated with insatiable desires to be given to and nurtured, but overdetermination operates so that self-destructive impulses come into play as well. Similarly, overeating can be a substitute for sexual activity and at the same time serve as a punishment for condemned behavior. Exhibitionistic components in eating is another formulation. Overeating may represent a hostile dependency or an aggressive engulfing. Behind such representations the question remains as to what leads to such behavior. How does eating get used in the service of such diverse ends? In some early pattern between the infant and others who nurture him, as well as within himself, a type of biological confusion exists with respect to certain signals of bodily needs which have become entwined with eating. Inconsistency in responses to needs by others in the environment, coupled with periodic reinforcement through unpredictable responses, are prominent.

Confusion exists over which needs or impulses are from within and which imposed from without. Are impulses under the child's control or subject to that of others? A lack of separateness from others results. Responses to early signals of hunger from the infant can result in punishment, since they vary from neglect to indulgences or punitiveness. Hunger fuses with other discomforts; this is seen in situations where food is offered to the infant inappropriately for extraneous purposes, such as to quiet him, to give the mother freedom from his demands, or to satisfy parental needs of doing everything possible for their child. Such situations are conducive to peculiar cognitions of the body and its needs.

In time, it is a matter of eating without references to any specific hunger sensation or signals. One's needs are not one's own, nor can one feel that techniques of satisfying them are under one's control. These formulations have implications for understanding disordered eating in terms of the need to develop more specific control over bodily functions. Not only is this true for eating but as a general disorder of impulse regulation which, in particular situations of early development and learning, have centered on eating. Additional impulse problems are an accompaniment, or alternative reactions of an opposite nature such as excessive dieting or starvation. The extreme situation is that of the self-starving as manifested in the syndrome of anorexia nervosa, which should be seen not as a single diagnostic entity, but as a group of disorders containing syndromes of pathogenesis and varying courses.[43]

REFERENCES

1. A. Gesell; F. J. Ilg; and L. B. Ames, *Youth—The Years from Ten to Sixteen* (New York: Harper and Brothers, 1956).
2. M. F. A. Montagu, *Adolescent Sterility* (Springfield: Charles C Thomas, 1946).
3. E. H. Erikson, Identity and the life cycle, *Psychological Issues* 1(1959):52-55.
4. *Perspectives on Human Deprivation: Biological, Psychological, and Sociological* (Washington, D.C.: National Institute of Child Health and Human Development, 1968).
5. E. Pumpian-Mindlin; Anna Freud; and Erik H. Erikson, *Science and Psychoanalysis* 8(1964):1-16.
6. A. Freud, *Normality and Pathology in Childhood* (New York: International Universities Press, 1965).

7. H. R. Stolz and L. M. Stolz, *Somatic Development of Adolescent Boys* (New York: Macmillan, 1951).

8. A. C. Kinsey; W. B. Pomeroy; and C. E. Martin, *Sexual Behavior in the Human Male* (Philadelphia: W. B. Saunders, 1948).

9. F. P. Heald and W. Hung, *Adolescent Endocrinology* (New York: Appleton-Century-Crofts, 1970).

10. L. Zacharias and R. J. Wurtman, Age at menarche, *New England Journal of Medicine* 280(1969):868-875.

11. J. M. Tanner, *Growth at Adolescence*, 2nd Ed. (New York: Oxford University Press, 1962).

12. *Zacharias*, op. cit. 10. p. 873.

13. Ibid., p. 874.

14. Tanner, op. cit. 11.

15. Zacharias, op. cit. 10., p. 873.

16. Ibid., p. 873.

17. T. F. Dingman, Pituitary function, *New England Journal of Medicine* 285(1971):617-620.

18. F. P. Heald, Physiology of adolescence, *New England Journal of Medicine* 268(1963):299-307.

19. Ibid., p. 305.

20. L. Chan and B. W. O'Malley, Mechanism of action of the sex steroid hormones, *New England Journal of Medicine* 294(1976):1322-1328.

21. J. D. Wilson, Recent studies on the mechanism of action of testosterone, *New England Journal of Medicine* 287(1972):1284-1291.

22. L. E. Kreaz and R. M. Rose, Assessment of aggressive behavior and plasma testosterone in a young criminal population, *Psychosomatic Medicine* 34(1972):321-332.

23. H. J. Klausmeier; H. J. Check; and T. Feldhusen, Relationships among physical, mental, and achievement measures in children of low, average, and high intelligence, *American Journal of Mental Deficiencies* 63(1959):647-656.

24. N. Bayley, Individual patterns of development, *Child Development* 27(1956):45-74.

25. R. J. Herrnstein, *IQ in the Meritocracy* (Boston: Atlantic Monthly Press, 1973).

26. H. Bruch, *Obesity* (New York: Basic Books, 1973).

27. E. Rosenberg and C. A. Paulsen, *The Human Testis* (New York: Plenum Press, 1971).

28. L. Wilkins, *The Diagnosis and Treatment of Endocrine Disorders in Childhood and Adolescence*, 3rd Ed. (Springfield: Charles C Thomas, 1966), p. 229.

29. Ibid., p. 242.

30. E. Witschi; W. V. Nelson; and S. J. Segal, Genetic, developmental and hormonal aspects of gonadal dysgenesis and sex inversion in man, *Journal of Clinical Endocrinology* 17(1957):737-751.

31. F. C. MacGregor; T. M. Abel; A. Bryt; E. Laner; and S. Weissman, *Facial Deformities and Plastic Surgery* (Springfield: Charles C Thomas, 1953).

32. G. H. Wright, The names of the parts of the body: a linguistic approach to the study of the body-image, *Brain* 79(1956):188-210.

33. L. C. Kolb, *The Painful Phantom: Psychology, Physiology, and Treatment* (Springfield: Charles C Thomas, 1954).

34. H. Head, *Studies in Neurology* (London: Oxford University Press, 1920).

35. P. Schilder, *The Image and Appearance of the Human Body* (London: Kegan Paul, 1935).

36. P. Federn, *Ego Psychology and the Psychoses* (New York: Basic Books, 1953).

37. T. S. Szasz, *Pain and Pleasure* (New York: Basic Books, 1957).

38. S. Fraiberg, Studies in the ego development of the congenitally blind child, *Psychoanalytic Study of the Child* 19(1964):113-169.

39. Stolz and Stolz, op. cit. 7.

40. H. Bruch, *Eating Disorders* (New York: Basic Books, 1973).

41. L. Srole, et al., *Mental Health in the Metropolis: The Midtown Study* (New York: McGraw-Hill, 1962).

42. H. Bruch, *The Importance of Overweight* (New York: W. W. Norton and Co., 1957).

43. J. E. Meyer, Anorexia nervosa of adolescence, *British Journal of Psychiatry* 118(1971):539-542.

Chapter Four

Sex-Typing and Sex-Role Standards

SEX-TYPING AND SEX-ROLE IDENTITY

A proposition which may seem astounding to the uninitiated: despite chromosomal assortment, internal organs of reproduction, and external genitalia all being of a certain sex, the most important single component for the development of a sense of maleness or femaleness is the sex which happens to be assigned at birth. By the designation at birth of the label boy or girl, gender role may be determined for life. Evidence suggests that after the age of two, at the outer limit, attempts to change or reassign sex, if a mistake has been made in terms of genetics, anatomy, or hormones, will be unsuccessful and will probably lead to severe psychological conflict.[1]

Sex assignment, which is the major factor in how infants are reared, illustrates the potency of learning and parental anticipation. Its irreversibility in terms of how the developing child perceives himself by gender assignment gives a tone of determinism. Its fortuitousness is particularly striking when this crucial assignment is based on a cursory inspection of the external genitalia by a nurse or doctor, coupled with a statement to the parents: "You have a boy (or a girl)," which then fixes gender forever.

Sex-typing is the process by which a child learns the attributes culturally appropriate to whatever sex has been designated. These attributes are not restricted to overt behaviors, but include personality characteristics, emotional responses, and various attitudes and beliefs that are believed to be associated with masculinity or femininity. These are the attributes which are expected and sanctioned when performed by one sex while they are less so (and not so) for the opposite sex. There is ultimately a quantitative or qualitative assignment of differences with respect to which attributes are more or less masculine or feminine.

Sex-role is a related concept. In contrast to sex-typing, which deals with averages or differences with respect to various attributes, sex-role deals with norms or images about the traits boys and girls are expected to possess. Sex-role refers to expectations about the behaviors males or females display, and the attitudes children are supposed to have about things. There is an implicit standard governing the sex-role which permits appraisal of responses and attributes. In some respects the standard is external, in considering what composes a sex-role in terms of masculinity or femininity. In other respects sex-role has reference to the approximation to the standard by an individual in the course of his development. Great importance is attached to the standard, which has relevance for sex-typing.

Most attempts to evaluate or research the problem of sex-typing have relied on some type of sex-role standard with a goal toward appraising which attributes a child or group of children have acquired in terms of their designated sex. Here is where sociological and cultural factors enter, in addition to all the stereotypes operating within a given culture as to what is masculine or feminine. To the extent that evaluations of sex-typing processes have relied on reports of individuals about themselves, their attributes, interests, behaviors, and preferences, or the inferences of others, these studies can be no better than ratings of the relative masculinity or femininity norms existing in a given culture. The score on some measure is actually an index of how closely an individual correlates on some standard with others who are designated by a similar gender. This may be a self-rating or one made by an observer, who can vary from a peer to a teacher or a clinician. The point is that the attributes which are part of the standard exist by a majority assignment, and they involve a set of stereotypes about which attributes should be designated masculine or feminine. Related problems are those of gender relativity for different cultures and the changing norms within any given society.

Cultural Variations.   It is a truism of anthropological investigation that cultures assign different activities and personality characteristics to men and women. Further hazards are encountered when applying the sex-role standard of one culture to another. Margaret Mead long ago illustrated this in terms of three New Guinea tribes:[2] The Arapesh show characteristics of both sexes being cooperative and non-aggressive—feminine in terms of Western culture. The Mundugumors, in contrast, show both sexes being non-cooperative, aggressive, and ruthless—masculine by Western sexual standards. And the Tchambuli show the reverse from Western culture; women are dominant, impersonal, and directive, and men are emotionally dependent and assume less responsibility.

However, it has been pointed out that each culture has a core of attributes which it designates as masculine or feminine.[3] At least on the basis of prevalence, social institutions are organized more around males, and men are more aggressive and dominant. The males are assigned tasks and jobs which are physically more demanding or dangerous. In contrast, women are more often assigned to positions deferential to men. They carry out the routines of feeding and caring for others. While the role of the husband-father is instrumental (task-oriented and emotion-inhibited), the role of the wife-mother is expressive (emotional, nurturant, and responsible). Note that these sex differences are widely observed cross-culturally in children where boys more often engage in conflict and overt aggression, and girls are more cooperative, affectionate, and sociable. The argument that these roles are merely reflections of biological variables is an old and intriguing one, but its universality is belied by such empirical examples as the Tchambuli. There is also evidence from developmental deviations where biological sex has been incongruent with sex assignment. The assignment, rather than the biological component, has predominated.

Developmental Components. A large part is played in sex-role acquisitions by developmental components as the vehicle for sex-typing. The selection of which criteria to use is a crucial problem. Let us take some rather typical devices used to appraise this. A group of toys may be selected under the assumption that certain ones would be preferable to boys and others to girls. While it may be evident that a female doll would appeal more to a girl than to a boy, there may be items which would not lend themselves to such a clear distinction. If the assignment of toys is obvious (dolls and babies' dishes versus knives and soldiers) and the children are asked to select these, their preferences only confirm the obvious. A variation is the use of "IT," a sexless stick figure, to which a child is asked to designate the preferential list of objects and activities "IT" prefers.[4]

Adolescents may be given a set of statements which have been standardized by someone—the investigator or by some measure of incidence—and asked to indicate their agreement or disagreement. In contrast to these efforts at appraising masculinity or femininity, observed behaviors may be rated in a nursery-school, an elementary-school with teacher ratings, or high school teachers appraising sex-type behaviors. Again, some type of presupposition of appropriate sex-role behavior is present. A frequent approach is that of rating the frequency of aggressive behavior. This is often equated with masculinity and performed in terms of observables, such as physical assertiveness in classrooms, on playgrounds, or in structured play activities for younger children, or in time spent with a member of the same sex. Without illustrating the experimental literature at this point, the various scores or ratings obtained by this approach do not usually agree with each other and the correlations are generally low. In part this is due to different measures used for sex-typing in studies. It would appear that a more profound deficit is the simplicity of approaches which attempt to detect differences in male-female attributes by techniques which may be naively obvious. In other cases there is an avoidance of realizing how complex sex-typing processes may be, thus reducing the significance of observer rating of external behaviors. An obvious example is the late adolescent who prefers homosexual experiences but may be an outstanding performer in some athletic venture.

It is known that sex assignment appears to be a crucial and not easily reversible step. Once a sincere assignment has been made and all concerned begin reacting to the infant in terms of one gender, the process of sex-typing for practical and clinical purposes becomes irreversible within a few years. This does not appear to be by an automatic biological determinism per se, although there are genetic and hormonal mechanisms determining some types of behavior to which others react.

A series of steps transpire in the early years of an infant's life, the critical or sensitive periods. At best, by age three or four boys express a distinct preference for toys and activities a culture has labelled as masculine.[5] These processes are reinforced as time progresses. Differentiations between boys and girls reveal interesting patterns. Boys tend to show earlier and greater awareness of sex-appropriate attributes. Girls are more variable and between the ages of three and ten they show preferences for the games and activities of boys.[6]

Higher-level theoretical interpretations about this vary from those who see this as a reflection of a male-oriented culture to the resistance of latency-age girls to accept their destiny as connected with having a body with external female characteristics. Almost no studies indicate boys in that age range preferring female toys, although clinicians do witness this in their selective populations. Again, while almost all boys in a nonselective population seem to prefer friends of the same gender in that age range, the same is not so for girls. However, some older studies have indicated that girls from the lower social classes undergo sex-typing processes at an earlier age than do their middle-class counterparts, at least when six- and eight-year-olds have been compared.[7]

Explanations offered for the phenomena of sex-role development are based on different theoretical approaches. These may be classified into three approaches: (1) learning theory approaches emphasizing parental modeling, imitation, reward and punishment in terms of affection and acceptance and avoidance of social rejection; (2) cognitive-developmental approaches, and (3) sex-typing as related to some type of identification process.

Learning Theory Explanations. Developmental psychologists have favored social learning theory approaches, which employ principles familiar from learning theory. This coalesces with implicit assumptions of laymen and professional people alike that a child learns behaviors characteristic of males and females in a given culture. Some well-known principles are employed: rewards and punishments, generalization, mediation, imitation, vicarious reinforcement, and modeling. There is the presumption that responses which are sex-appropriate in a given culture and social class will be rewarded (reinforced) most specifically within the family matrix, while those considered inappropriate will be punished and diminish in strength and frequency, leading to eventual extinction.

It is not that the principles of learning themselves come under criticism by those who see this explanation as insufficient, but rather that such common sense assumptions that mothers and fathers naturally reward sex-appropriate responses and punish those which are inappropriate may not altogether be true. While these assumptions may hold for many children and parents, there are still variations with respect to attributes which provide—at least in part—a differential distribution of male-female attributes even apart from the psychopathological. Certainly, a methodological approach to such a theory based on attributes fathers want to see in their sons, such as aptitude in athletics, tolerance of pain, predominance of activity over passivity, and good school performance, would tell us little about the more subtle processes to which a boy is reacting. They do tell us what his father has learned about how to classify attributes of his social group into those which are more or less masculine and which are the correct responses.

A further problem is that sex-typing processes begin very early in infancy. A social learning theory model would have to establish that necessary steps were taken by parents in the first two to three years to ensure the reinforcement of sex-type behaviors. However, evidence is lacking that such differential handling of boys and girls actually follows the formulations of social learning theory that should make the crucial difference.[8] The evidence becomes more persuasive with respect to broad traits such as aggression and dependency. Patterns of differential rewards for boys and girls, modeling influences, and the peer group, begin to assert their influence in terms of physically aggressive behavior and less acceptance of dependent behaviors for boys. A boy rewarded for striking back at home and with children in the neighborhood becomes more likely to do so at nursery school and subsequently in his development. Such processes are related to types of parental disciplinary techniques. This is congruent with longitudinal findings in which behaviors conforming to the sex-role standard are stable over the long run.[9]

In a permissive home atmosphere a child of either sex is rewarded for aggressive activity in the sense of curiosity and exploration. There is a correlation between this orientation and masculine preferences. A restrictive home atmosphere in a child of either sex secures rewards for obedience, passivity, and the inhibition of strong responses about anything which may be considered feminine. More subtle combinations of permissiveness-restrictiveness, such as with parental warmth or hostility, complicate the picture even on a conscious level. Sex-type responses of a model may be acquired without the child having to imitate them or receive reinforcement at the time. Of course, direct advice and encouragement to act like daddy may occur with a host of constant exposures to aggressive displays by fathers.

Cognitive Theory Explanations. Cognitive theories of sexual development use sex-typing as an accompaniment to cognitive development and maturation apart from learning experiences. Piagetian psychology has exerted a strong influence but other trends, such as an interest in exploratory behaviors, curiosity, and competence, have also contributed. The cognitive position holds that, along with other areas, the child organizes his social world along sex-role dimensions.[10] This occurs by processes of cognitive growth in which the child's modes of thinking change. His perceptions of the physical and social world change, and include both himself and his sex-role. Learning is viewed as secondary to the selection and structuring of perceptions. This gives a cross-cultural emphasis for patterns of cognitive structuring which presumably is not confined to one culture. Rather, they are natural components of patterning from being rooted in the child's conception of physical things, including his own body and those of others. "Rather than biological instinct, it is the child's cognitive organization of social role concepts around universal physical dimensions that accounts for the existence of universals in sex-role attributes."[11]

Imitation of sex-typing occurs through a process of labelling which corresponds to hearing words boy and girl and learning their meaning. By age three the child knows which category he has been assigned, and this self-concept preserves a stable and positive self-image. The sexual self-concept of the child becomes an organizer and determinant of behaviors and attitudes. Cognitive theory approaches emphasize initial steps by which a child says, "I am a boy or girl," which then directs attitudes he takes. Cultural stereotypes are developed (such as males being aggressive), not primarily from parental behaviors but rather from perception of sex differences in body configuration and functioning. The sexual self-concept is viewed as stabilized by age five or six, paralleling the understanding of the principle of conservation by which physical properties, such as mass, number, and weight become stable and invariant.

Kohlberg listed five mechanisms by which sex-role concepts are translated into masculine-feminine values.

1. Assimilation processes permit the child to respond to new activities and interests consistent with earlier ones. Since sex differences in personality traits and interests are present at two to three years, consistent new activities are assimilated while discrepant ones are not.

2. The promotion of masculine or feminine sex-role is further encouraged by the egocentrism of the child who places a higher value on things like himself or develops from his own interests.

3. Sex-role stereotyping accrues which gives motivation toward one role or another.

4. A moral factor enters since the child views his gender as normative for certain values and behaviors. To deviate from these is then a moral wrong.

5. Identification is viewed as something that develops subsequent to sex-typing processes. Identification does not lead to sex-typing of attributes but rather is a result of sex-typing. Therefore, from the cognitive structuring which has occurred with masculine or feminine interests and values, modeling can proceed from those who are viewed as similar. The identification of the boy with his father is assimilated to general stereotypes of masculine roles which are not based on the individual role of the father and his idiosyncracies. Once begun, identification can extend in diverse ways.

Limitations of the cognitive approach to sexual development involve limitations of our understanding of cognitive development. There is an unexplained, or circular, element to positing innate cognitive structures which somehow function to determine many of the activities, values, and attributes which are specifically related to sex. Even if this is so, and even if it could be proved by empirical investigation and confirmation, it is an unsatisfactory theory because it ignores causally related antecedents, which, if included, might account for the wide variations in individual sex-typing processes that exist.

There is a more subtle question that has reference to the stress put on labelling by words as the process which initiates sex-typing. This comes close to the Sapir-Whorf hypothesis for sex-typing.[12] Stress is placed on how a language subtly molds the way people conceive their world. The culture at large, with its particular language, determines the view a child has of himself, and, more specifically for this discussion, the view a child has as masculine or feminine. Whorf, who was a chemical engineer and fire-insurance executive, as well as a gifted amateur linguist, pointed out that a limit is imposed on what we are able to think about, and how we think about things, based on the concepts and relationships of our language. Once language is established, we are limited in the ways we can think about ourselves. These formulations have validity for the difficulties that can ensue when there are errors of sex assignment or anatomical mixtures, yet Whorf's view is a hypothesis rather than an explanation. Its validation remains elusive. If one wished to argue that the child is actually reacting to differences in perception or cognition which he then labels with a word, language would not play such a determing role. This may be what the cognitive theorists are hypothesizing by a cognitive explanation, yet the stress on labelling is burdensome.

Identification Processes. Identification theories provide a major way of conceptualizing the development of sex-role. Identification is basically a view that a same-sexed parent serves as a model to facilitate the acquisition of sex-type attributes. Inherent in this theory are all of the unresolved dilemmas and vagaries associated with the development and meaning of identification. It is used by some experimentalists in a restricted sense equivalent to imitation, which in turn is defined as the occurrence of matching responses.[13]

In this sense it is difficult to distinguish such formulations from those learning theories discussed earlier.

> The diversity in the definitions of imitation and identification also springs in part from the fact that some writers apply these terms primarily to response-defined variables, others apply them to antecedent or process variables which are stimulus-defined, while still others assign to imitation the status of a dependent variable and treat identification as an independent variable, and vice versa. It is possible to draw distinctions between these and other related terms—for example, introjection and incorporation—based on certain stimulus, mediating, or terminal-response variables. However, one might question whether it is meaningful to do so, since essentially the same learning process is involved regardless of the content of what is learned, the object from whom it is learned, or the stimulus situations in which the relevant behavior is emitted. Therefore, it is in the interest of clarity, precision, and parsimony to employ the single term, imitation, to refer to the occurrence of matching responses.[14]

Before discussing usages of identification which extend beyond this, other types of identification have been utilized in studies. These have been classified as follows: (1) aggressive identification; (2) dependent or developmental identification, and (3) role theory formulations. A model cited is that associated with one of Freud's earliest formulations of the oedipal situation. The boy, engaged in a competitive struggle with his father for the maternal object, was believed to forsake his erotic attachment on a conscious level and identify instead with the aggressor—his father. In giving up his longings, he would become like the father with respect to paternal attributes. Many misinterpretations made about identification have been based on the theory that this oedipal formulation is the sole, or at least the primary, source of identification in its literal sense, without conceptualizing the whole realm of envious and competitive strivings for which the oedipal may only be one of the most ultimate of competitive situations.

Developmental identification stresses the dependency context in which children are nurtured as the prime mover of identification. This varies from the child wanting to imitate, please, or be like the nurturer, as well as to do this in remembrance of the nurturing object when it is absent. There is the difficulty of explaining how boys identify with mothers or girls with fathers. Efforts have not been entirely satisfactory beyond the circular level of saying that children, regardless of sex, identify with nurturers. It has been postulated that the boy does not identify in this type of identification model with his mother as a female but with an undifferentiated human being.[15] Recent work, such as that of the Hampsons cited above, disproves the existence of an undifferentiated period for the development of sex-role. There is also the problem of the parent who is a hostile nurturer at best, with whom the child continues to identify. This requires more explanation than merely a postulate that a child identifies with someone who nurtures him. Sociological perspectives on the disorganized family structure must be taken into account for its impact on identifying with those who nurture.

Role Theories. Although some formulations border on the naive (for example, the child playing the role of father to become like him as an adult), sophisticated theorists note that role playing is based on the nature of interacting variables with a model. A child, like any person who is exposed to another in an intense and repetitive manner, is going to interact and respond to that person. To the extent that the model is in a position to control many aspects of the child's behavior, the model can give both rewards and punishments, whether nurturing or threatening.

Parsons elaborated this theory of parental power as the primary basis for the identification of a child with a parent.[16] He presumes that children identify with the most powerful parent. In this theory, the role of the father is instrumental in terms of performance of tasks, while that of the mother is expressive. It is therefore the mother from whom the child learns expressive behavior patterns. The difficulty with such a formulation is the dichotomous quality of it. Not all fathers are instrumental nor all mothers expressive. Most parents are a mixture of both and it becomes a relative matter in different family configurations. Not to recognize this leads to the postulation that mothers do not respond differentially to children by sex at all, but fathers do. Therefore, fathers would be of more importance than mothers in sex-typing of both sexes.[17]

Appraisal of Studies. The masculine or feminine attributes which children acquire can be divided into the following: physical qualities, behaviors, personality traits, emotionality, attitudes, and beliefs. These are related to the emergence of a cognitive differentiation of people by the child into classes of male and female. Although the process of acquiring sex-typed characteristics is begun early, and indeed may be irreversible by age two to three, the discrimination of others into one or another sex is evident by age three and certainly by the time children begin school.[18]

In terms of physical attributes, maleness and femaleness are subject to enormous and probably dispositive influence from the mass media in contemporary Western civilization. A child of eight to ten years may view an attractive face as a sex-type attribute for girls and a tall, muscular physique as a sex-type attribute for boys. By preadolescence the most culturally approved characteristics for girls in terms of sex-role are those of an attractive face, hairless body, small frame, and moderately sized breasts; for boys the characteristics are those of height, large muscle mass, and facial and bodily hair.[19]

Behaviors are classified by sex-role standards as well. Aggressive displays are primary. For girls an inhibition of verbal and physical aggression is preferred, while for boys aggression, at least when threatened or attacked, can be expressed. Studies confirm that the sex-role standard operates in this manner in almost every investigation. It is noted in nursery school age groups, in the elementary years, in games children play, in their fantasies concerning themselves, and in stories. Adult males are perceived as more aggressive, dangerous, and punitive. More parents expect their boys to be aggressive. A triad of sex-type behaviors continues to appear: dependency, passivity, and conformity are present in girls, and far less so in boys, throughout childhood, adolescence, and adulthood. Boys are expected to inhibit these behaviors. Children of both sexes expect to receive more gratification of their dependency needs, passive behavior, and obtaining nurturance from females rather than from males. During adolescence, submissiveness to males, inhibition of overt sexual desires, and cultivation of domestic skills are added to the sex-type pattern of girls. For boys during adolescence, independence, interpersonal dominance of both sexes, sexual conquests, and acquisition of power become sex-typed.

The games children play are often used as an index of sex-typing behaviors. Work has been directed to confirming the differential factors operating within a culture between the toys children prefer. Boys choose objects related to aggression and power, such as those involving sports, war, or mechanical aspects. Girls choose objects in terms of maternal activities, personal attractiveness, or a vocational position subordinate to males, such as nurses or secretaries. The "IT" test, already mentioned, will be discussed further.[20] It reveals an approach with serious methodological limitations. A sexless figure, "IT" is presented to children together with a collection of toys, clothes, objects, or activities. The child is required to select toys or activities "IT" wants to do, with the presumption that this reveals their preferences, and that "IT" will tell us something about sex-typing processes.

The test is not used merely to classify toys, for some investigators have extended it in an attempt to evaluate other hypotheses. An attempt was made with a group of five-year-old boys to evaluate the relative importance of their fathers to confirm one of the three main theories of identification which were noted above (the aggressive, dependent, or role theory models).[21] The masculinity scores of the "IT" were related to the perception of fathers. Relevant hypotheses were: Do boys who score highly masculine view their fathers as nurturant (dependency theory)? As punitive and threatening? Or as power figures who dispense rewards and punishments (role theory)? In the particular study cited, the more masculine boys perceived their father as nurturant and rewarding, although at the same time as punitive. However, there is also support for the thesis that boys who rank high on masculinity on the "IT" rank higher in father power in terms of the degree to which the latter has power over them.

As in so many of these studies, the test results indicate support for all three theories of identification and masculinity and none of them are disconfirmed. While some would say that the dependency theory of identification has more impressive results from a greater degree of statistical correlation, all three theories continue to be viable. In fact, some studies fail to find significant correlations between the degree of parental nurturance or power and the sex-role behavior of nursery school children.[22] An endless series of nuisance variables begin to intrude on such studies. Ad hoc hypotheses are introduced, in that children may not have been from the same age or social class, which would account for the lack of similar findings. There is also the problem of evaluating the validity of superficial tests, such as the "IT," and basing the sex-role development on a compilation of toys children use.

Extensions of this approach complete doll-play stories, or parents are given questionnaires or asked to compile lists of activities and games their children prefer, or which ones the parents themselves would encourage or discourage. The conclusions must be viewed as tentative and obvious in many cases, although they may go along with some of the more usual beliefs about sex-typing differentiation. These studies conclude that from age three boys are cognitively aware of which activities and objects are masculine, although for girls preferences are more variable up to nine or ten years. We have noted it is unusual for a boy to prefer feminine activities up to age ten, but many girls prefer masculine activities. This parallels the greater number of girls in this age group who express a desire to be a boy compared to boys who express a desire to be a girl. Again the methodological limitation of giving such opinions, based on overt responses for boys in a culture which reacts in a highly adverse manner to such opinions, must be acknowledged.

Two other factors must be noted in studies. Changing patterns of games that might be acceptable with the sex-role for girls at present, compared to boys, have evolved over several decades. Further, a social class difference operates with respect to the games children play. Choices of both boys and girls in the lower social classes conform to traditional sex-type standards rather than the choices of middle-class children. The conclusion is that sex-role differentiation is sharper in lower-class families. In support of this is a study that lower-class mothers encourage sex-typing more consistently than do middle-class mothers. However, middle-class girls have greater freedom to indulge in the games and activities of boys than their middle-class, male counterparts do.[23]

Covert attributes of sex-role refer to personality characteristics, emotional responses, attitudes, motives, and beliefs. For females these appear to be: the ability to gratify a love object, to elicit sexual arousal in a male, the desire to be a wife and mother, and the related desires to nurture a child and give affection to a love object, and the capacity for emotion. For males these are: a pragmatic attitude, an ability to gratify a love object, the ability to suppress fear, and the capacity to control expression of strong emotion under stress. This division of core attributes is consistent with the instrumental-versus-expressive dichotomy. An interesting problem is the extent to which covert attributes are changing for a sex-role standard. Are they changing so rapidly that they lack contemporary validity? Much publicity about the changing scene makes this question relevant, yet studies based on clinical approaches and ratings of self and others do not seem to indicate a divergence from these attributes. In fact, it may be that these attributes have become more accentuated so that there is a greater differential. This could occur by the bombardment of imagery from the media of what masculinity represents in terms of aggression in its various forms. In turn, the sexually appealing female is one presented in terms of an attractive woman who controls her emotional display while remaining nurturant.

The freedom of a female to become more overt in her sexual displays, and to not be as tied to her home, would be in the direction of making her more clearly differentiated from males. But if the sex-role standard for femininity is defined in terms of remaining at home (so that its opposite is masculine), there is an obvious change by definition. Similarly, is working in the service of becoming less feminine or rather to assist the family financially? These questions about covert attributes demonstrate that motives need full exploration.

SEX-ROLE IDENTITY

Sex-role identity is a component of overall identity or self-concept. The identity of an individual is a composite of many interlocking beliefs and aspirations. If the sex-role standard refers to an abstract concept of what attributes an ideal male or female, within a given culture, should possess, sex-role identity refers to how an individual views himself in terms of this standard. While a man may view himself as more or less masculine, with variability on different overt and covert attributes, it is the degree to which he believes he possesses certain sex-typed traits which is important.

A number of problems exist in appraising the sex-role identity of an individual. Many of the attributes, feelings, and personality traits which compose an individual's belief about his degree of masculinity (or femininity) are not entirely conscious. This is an inherent limitation in any concept based on a degree of belief. The most effete of males may regard himself as the most masculine of creatures, yet he may be highly feminine in overt attributes. In a less obvious way, there is an imperfect correlation between sex-role identity and possession of the sex-role standard in terms of cultural norms, in that sex-role identity may not be congruent with the attributes a culture says are masculine or feminine.

Importance of Sex-role Identity. What is the importance of sex-role identity for the development of the individual child? It is believed to have psychological significance in three areas:[24] (1) stability of behavior over time, (2) differential mastery of academic skills, and (3) sexuality and behavior with love objects. In a theoretical and practical sense, it would be desirable to know the sensitive periods with respect to various components of sex-role identity and their stability. The irreversibility of sex assignment after age two to three has been noted, but to what extent are the attributes which comprise sex-role identity modifiable or reversible? This involves important prediction questions in which attributes may remain stable or fixed over time, both in the developmental sense and from therapeutic attempts at modification.

One of the important studies in this regard was conducted at the Fels Research Institute.[25] This longitudinal study utilized middle-class subjects who were independently rated at four developmental periods: birth to three years, three to six years, six to ten years, and ten to fourteen years. The ratings were based on observations in the home, in nursery schools, in camps, in public schools, and on interviews. Behavioral variables evaluated included aggression, dependency, passivity, intellectual achievement, social anxiety, heterosexual behavior, and sex-typed activities. Between the ages of twenty and thirty, interviews were conducted for an independent set of data. An important was the behavioral stability of responses at age six to ten with adulthood when the response was congruent with sex-role standards. There was a minimal amount of behavioral continuity when the sex-role standard decried inhibition. A girl who exhibited passive and dependent behaviors would usually continue to do so as an adult, since this was congruent with the female sex-role standard. This did not hold for boys, in which influences operated for him to cease demonstrating such behaviors during adolescence and adulthood. A latency-age boy with high aggressivity and heterosexual behavior, both congruent with the sex-role standard, permitted a fair prediction of anger arousal and sexual behavior of an assertive nature as an adult, a prediction which did not hold for girls. Correlations between the practice of sex-appropriate activities from six to ten years and adulthood was 0.63 for men and 0.44 for women.

Problems arise in studies regarding the more subtle character changes that accompany development. To say that an overt behavior, congruent with a sex-role standard, remains in evidence, while others do not, leaves unanswered the question of what happens to sex-typed attributes. To say they are inhibited seems insufficient. They most probably continue to influence behavior and feelings in covertly manners or through characterological devices. A passive and conforming boy in the elementary school years who has become aggressive during adolescence has not lost these attributes, which are seen in displays of dependency longings which may not be recognized as such by his social group. In fact they may not be recognized by him, as in the case of the previously passive and effeminate child who has handled these strivings in adolescence by a reaction formation of bullying and attacking behaviors.

The prevalence of these demonstrations in adolescence may constitute modeling, but also be defensive. Continuance of these techniques into adulthood is amply demonstrated by general observations and clinical work. Examples from literature, drama, and biography abound. The schoolmaster in *Tea and Sympathy*, who is punitive to his passive charges, illustrates the theme. The unresolved dependencies, feelings of masculine inadequacy, and homosexual strivings between two star football players in *Cat On A Hot Tin Roof* is another example. An autobiography of a former pro football player illustrates his identity conflicts.[26]

Academic Skills and Sex-role Identity. Mastery of academic skills has a relationship to sex-role identity. To what extent is intellectual mastery a sex-typed behavior? The question involves not only developmental differentials in skills, which includes differences in fine and gross motor coordination between males and females, but the influence of the sex-role standard. It is interesting to speculate on the extent to which skills involving spatial and mechanical reasoning are determined by different factors. Investigations tell us that boys perform in a superior manner in these skills, but is this primarily a result of genetic factors or rather the gradual accumulation of superior skills due to the sex-role standard?

At least in the past adolescent males obtained higher scores than their female counterparts in mathematical or geometrical reasoning.[27] Females who reject traditional feminine interests perform better on mathematical and geometrical problems than do girls with more feminine interests. A point in favor of the sex-role standard is seen when verbal problems dealing with feminine content, such as cooking, but requiring the same logical steps and computations as problems involving more masculine contents such as guns or money, reveal girls obtain higher scores. Motivation to solve a feminine problem is involved. Conversely, this may operate in some girls who do not want to appear unfeminine by performing too well on tasks on which males are supposed to do well.

Two other areas are cited as illustrative of the significance of the sex-role identity of a child related to academic mastery: autonomy strivings, and the sex-role identity of the female as more dependent on maintaining love relationships than academic excellence. Autonomy is manifested in greater persistence to solve a task as well as boys utilizing more techniques of analysis and reflection. These differences appear quite early in childhood and the discrepancy is widened by adolescence to the point where some believe girls feel inadequate when confronted with problems which require analysis and reasoning. Whether this reflects an actual difference in intellectual ability, or rather a culturally influenced abandonment of this type of thought process, is difficult to assess. The need for acceptance in girls may be related to their working for approval in contrast to boys who sense the need for vocational success to achieve a sex-role identity congruent with the sex-role standard. Yet, to hold that boys do not work for the approval of surrogate parental figures appears unwarranted.

Further evidence for the impact of the sex-role is seen in the changing configuration of academic performance from the elementary years to high school. Through fourth grade, the evidence is overwhelming that girls excel in every academic area. Clinical evidence on learning disorders or reading disabilities shows boys outnumber girls—often by a ratio of five or ten to one.[28] Explanations for the shift in academic proficiency after fourth grade have usually been in terms of girls sensing the competitive and aggressive aspects of academic success as part of the male sex-role. In turn, boys sense a greater realization that male sex-typing means vocational success, in part based on academic performance. There is also the matter of school itself having a female sex-typed quality in the early years from female teachers who stress female interests. Emphasis on control of motor activities, and inhibition of aggressive displays is indicative of school as a female operation. By adolescence, not only do male teachers begin to appear, but the pragmatic and instrumental aspects of the male sex-role standard are introduced in certain subjects. This is often used as a contributory explanation for why certain scientific subjects begin to appeal to the boy, while subjects emphasizing language and ideas remain preferential for girls.

What is lacking in such an analysis? The explanations are not entirely inaccurate. Many children and adolescents experience sex differentials to school, yet gaping questions remain. The failure of boys in the lower social classes to have scientific interests during their adolescent years is one example. Many other variables must be considered: the impoverished quality of many schools, disorganized homes, and other detrimental influences which adversely affect educational achievement prior to the adolescent years. These limitations hold apart from genetic arguments concerning the nature of intelligence. For example, language and ideational subjects rarely appeal to the lower-class, adolescent girl who is plagued by hardships. Even though girls in such circumstances may evince more interest than boys in these subjects, their performance is governed more by other factors.

Behavior with Love Objects. Heterosexual object relations is a third area influenced by sex-role identity. In a normative fashion through the sex-role standard, boys are supposed to take the initiative, being attracted to girls, and dominant, while girls are supposed to be passive, attractive, and conceal sexual feelings. Without discussing developmental deviations or gross areas of psychopathology, the variations within these norms are quite wide and getting wider. It would be difficult to sustain a position that adolescents who do not live up to these norms will experience anxiety, let alone develop symptoms. Perhaps it is more accurate to view the norms as mythologies which individuals may parrot but do not necessarily feel constrained to achieve. Perception of physical attractiveness to the adolescent has a great deal of confirmation through social experiences as well as from exposure to the mass media. Apart from grossly disfiguring physical defects on the one hand, and great aesthetic beauty on the other, much leeway is permitted in styles of dress, mannerisms, and social poise in terms of self-appraisal of attractiveness. A subtle relationship operates between external performance in heterosexual life and sex-role identity.

If belief in one's relative masculinity or femininity is affected by practices and conquests, we would expect that practice makes perfect. The plaguing question is the relationship between such practices and the components which enter into a sex-role identity. It is absurd to say that sexual intercourse is a necessity for consolidating the sex-role identity of every adolescent boy. It would be difficult to defend a position that adolescents who have sexual intercourse during adolescence have their sex-role identity necessarily affected in a more masculine or feminine direction. The personality structure and conflicts of a particular adolescent would need appraisal. Social factors may have influence by leading to questioning identity if they do not partake, but more important in terms of psychological development is self-evaluation if they do perform sexually.

It would seem an oversimplification to think that a boy who has conflicts and inadequacies regarding masculinity would not continue to have them even if he has sexual intercourse. In some cases, the doubts merely shift to ruminations on the adequacy of his performance—something not unusual in girls as well. Similarly, it is not just the reinforcing social effect of others on an adolescent who does not date that is determinative, but rather the developmental lags or conflicts which have led to a lack of heterosexual interests and pursuits. Nor is it the perception of deviance from an ideal that is a necessary antecedent either, for this is a reflection of pre-existing difficulties. The significant antecedents are the neurophysiological and psychosocial characteristics that have led to what may be an accurate perception of one being skewed from the sex-role standard.

VARIATIONS AND VALIDITY OF IDENTIFICATION THEORIES

Identification has been used as one of the explanations for acquiring sex-typed behaviors. In addition, it has many implications for the entire development of self-identity. In this section identification is explored with reference to these areas. Later, some of the clinical contributions to identification processes and identity will be examined.

Difficulties in the Identification Construct. Two basic difficulties remain with identification: lack of agreement on the meaning of the term, and insufficient explanations for the development and maintenance of identification processes. Various meanings are used between and among different disciplines. As noted, some use the concept as equivalent to imitation. A "dust bowl empiricism" approach does not extend the usage beyond the level of observable behaviors and it eschews hypothetical constructs. Since this definition is so appealing to large numbers of behavioral scientists trained in a tradition which has interpreted empiricism as equivalent only to observables, its validity will be explored.

Such a restrictive position has long been abandoned by those working in the area of the philosophy of science dealing with theory construction. It was a position advocated by operationists who were particularly influential in the philosophy of science in the 1920s and 1930s. Historical reasons can be given for the appeal this purifying approach had when introduced. However, it was then and is now more of a fiction than a sufficient theory, since no theory is based on nothing but observations. Further, historians of science have been able to see that scientific knowledge in hard sciences, such as physics and chemistry, was never able to operate within the limits of observables.[29] [30] [31]

To point out these theoretical and historical facts is not to invoke a stricture against using ad hoc operational approaches in their experimental or clinical work. Many investigators and clinicians utilize approaches based on discreet measurements and observations of externals. They should not be discouraged or abandoned. But no one should assume that a justification from the philosophy of science dealing with theory formation, or from the history of science, is available for such a position. It is a matter of preference for the type of work one wishes to engage in. For those with hypothesis phobias, who abjure the risks of theory, working life must be confined to observables. Nor does the greater ease of confirmation or discomfirmation of a discreet, external situation, and the difficulty in doing this in such soft fields as clinical research, mean that only the latter should be given the pejorative label of unscientific.

These comments are raised in the context of the meaning and validity of identification, since several alternatives are used apart from those of matching externals for identification. Identification has been used by some psychologists and psychiatrists to refer to (1) processes by which certain behaviors are acquired, (2) motives which lead a child and adult to want to engage in such processes, or (3) a set of beliefs about oneself. These alternative formulations all refer to an inner process or event. The main difficulty appears to be acquiring knowledge about the postulated inner processes. The attendant vagueness thereby introduced is an unsettling situation for the empirically inclined. To obviate this one would need a list of the relevant state-variables and know that the list is complete. This would eliminate the continuous injection of new state-variables to account for newer behaviors not satisfactorily explained by existing theory. An exhaustive index of internal variables and also an index to know how these variables themselves are operating would then be needed. However, as Skinner pointed out long ago, even such pure responses as the strength of a reflex in the lowly white rat is an ambiguous fact.[32]

To determine if a response is due to a drive, emotion, or conditioning process requires the elimination of various hypotheses. With respect to eating or not eating, the response of the organism may be governed by conditioning, fear, or extinguishment alone, or various combinations of strength. Surely, more complicated classes of operations are contributing to something like imitation or matching behaviors. What seems straightforward on the surface involves extremely complex variables—even when confining analysis to observables. Of course, one may choose not to inquire beyond correlation of externals which anyone can see. This in itself does not resolve the problem, even for one who avoids invoking hypothetical constructs or nonobservable entities, since the problem of classifying variables, which includes responses, remains a fallible process. Nor is it logical or sufficient to maintain that we need not inquire or take account of such processes. But a need exists for relating the external, such as talking like one's father, with the determining magnitude of an inner state. It does not matter how this is done—be it by qualitative observation of similarity or some mathematical formulation—since the relationship is what is evaluated. Nor can it be assumed that the determining inner states do not vary from one individual to another or within one individual at different times or different physiological states.

Perception and Identification. Having raised some of the theoretical difficulties with the concept of identification, difficulties of a psychological nature will be explored. In many respects, the development of identification implies that perceptual processes eventuate in identification. If identification involves a belief in the congruence between some attributes of a model and the self, these similarities must be perceived. This operates in three ways for identification to proceed; a model must be perceived as (1) similar in overt or covert attributes to oneself, (2) as nurturant, and (3) as in control of certain things the child views as important, such as power, obtaining love from others, or competency in activities which he would like to achieve.[33] There is an additional need for cognitive operations, so that the child classifies objects that appear similar in some respects as being unalike in others.

Yet one might question if the child believes this, or is rather acting in response to other dispositions such as a wish to share in the power or competency of the model. It could be hypothesized that a child behaves like a model to please, to receive affection, or to avoid anger. This is an extension of the old identification with the aggressor model. It leads us back to the unresolved problem of determining the inner state of the rat who emits a certain response. Again, the solution would not appear to lie in the position that only the emission is responsible, but the slow process of determining in a probabilistic manner which states lead to identification operations.

PARENTAL MODELS

If perception of a model is a significant part of identification, the qualities of the model will have a specific impact. In the presence of other variables being constant, what differences have been found if a boy is exposed to a father whose sex-typed attributes are minimally male versus one in which they are maximally male? What if no male model is available in the family of rearing? What are the most significant attributes in the parent which promote sex-typing identification processes in a girl? Several studies indicate that parental warmth and nurturance promote identification. This was seen in high school boys who demonstrated the most sex-typed masculine behaviors and attributes.[34] It has also been noted in studies involving both boys and girls in which warmth in parents facilitates sex-typing of the same sex-typed parent.[35] Many studies of this kind rely on behavioral ratings of children done by observers, such as in schools, ratings in doll play, or completing stories. Parental appraisal is made by ratings or some psychometric device such as the "femininity" and "self-acceptance" scale of the California Psychological Inventory. The "F" scale is held to measure femininity of interests and attitudes while the "S-A" measures a set of personal worth, self-acceptance, and independence in thinking and action variables. As the validity of these measures goes, so goes the validity of conclusions made on sex-typing by their children.

Dominance appears frequently in studies as one of the critical variables for boys identifying with fathers. Boys from father-dominant homes display more sex-role preferences according to the masculine sex-role standard and are more identified with fathers than are boys from mother-dominant families.[36] This holds for the late adolescent in the college population as well.[37] Explanations for the significant impact of dominant fathers on boys are: (1) A dominant father facilitates a shift in identification from the nurturant mother to the father if the latter is viewed as the possessor and bestower of desirables. (2) A dominant father is more congruent with the culturally determined sex-role standard and available for continued reinforcement of such behaviors when they occur in the boy. (3) Identification with the aggressor may be used more easily in response to a dominant male figure. (4) Less discrepancy will be perceived between other males outside the home and the dominant father in the home, which eliminates cognitive disonance between a model, who may be idealized, and the sex-role standard in the community. There would be less disharmony in the boy's attributes and those of his peers in a situation which permits easier entrance into the peer group in contrast to teasing and possible ostracism.

Nor is the father insignificant for girls. He plays an important part in the development of femininity. Girls who identify with maternal figures displaying feminine attributes, such as an inhibition of aggression, nurturance, relative submissiveness with boys, cultivation of personal attractiveness, and an interest in domestic activities, have the advantage and disadvantage of more easily acquiring these sex-typed attributes. Until recently this identification was seen as desirable, but empirical evidence now raises serious questions about whether identification of the girl with her mother and her sex-role are not negatively related to self-esteem and adjustment.[38]

FATHERS: THE SIGNIFICANCE OF ABSENCES

Since fathers are important, as well as mothers, what are the consequences of their absence in terms of sex-typing and sex-role standard? Such commonly encountered situations as the presence of family disturbance, deprivation, parental emotional conflict, or marital disharmony themselves can produce developmental alterations and complicate any evaluation of the one variable of father absence. The reason for the absence needs to be distinguished, such as a culturally sanctioned absence from custom, war, or occupation, in contrast to a parental desertion or divorce. Permanent or temporary absence, the duration of absence, and the age of the child are all relevant. Absence of the father has been assessed in both a correlational and causal manner with respect to acting out, delinquency and depressions.

Much of the literature has relevance to the development of sex-role identification. Prediction of outcome is difficult from the number of variables involved and the complexities of interaction possible over the years. Two overall approaches are: (1) *clinical interviews*, which involve appraisal of the child at the time of upset or disturbance and the techniques of handling feelings and impulses with behavioral manifestations, and (2) *ratings or developmental observations* of children in naturalistic or non-clinical settings. A general and tentative conclusion is that boys with an absent father, seen in clinical interview approaches, appear to have difficulties in the realm of sex-role identity, while studies appraising this from groups of children in naturalistic settings by some specific appraisal technique, such as ratings of play patterns, do not necessarily show consistent findings at all age levels.

Clinical Insights.   Until recently, a great deal of the clinical work concerned with the impact of an absent father was focused on children who were most likely to be candidates for therapy. Of course, studies on attachment behaviors and deprivation abounded, but typically dealt with mothers. A scarcity of studies in the preschool age-group existed with the exception of the few nursery schools which had clinically trained observers. In their widely cited war-time studies of English nursery school children, Anna Freud and Dorothy Burlingham noted that young boys could identify with male figures in the absence of their own fathers.[39] They did this via fantasy operations in which strong attachments resulted in an idealized male who functioned as an identification object.

Perhaps the situation of a total absence of male objects, which would be desirable experimentally, cannot be obtained in reality due to the multiplicity of male figures available either for direct or brief contact. Consider the impact of mass media and literature. Only a mad scientist type of situation, which could raise a child in isolation from any physical exposure to males, or verbal references thereto, could answer the question. Even then, the role of fantasy could not be omitted. Children create in fantasy what is absent in reality.

August Aichhorn, based on clinical work with delinquent boys, believed that the fatherless, delinquent boy was prone to have deficit in the ego ideal.[40] Nunberg saw such children utilizing an idealized fantasy of a missing father as a device to form attachments to real men, while others appear to have superego deficits and live out a pattern of taking ruthless revenge on the world for depriving them of a father.[41] The story of Lee Harvey Oswald, the alleged assassin of President John F. Kennedy, is an example of this.[42]

Early clinical work was concerned with the impact of paternal absence in terms of maternal dominance on the boy. It also focused on the consequences for sexual development and deviation. As early as the *Three Essays on the Theory of Sexuality*, Freud stated, "Early loss of one of their parents, whether by death, divorce, or separation, with the result that the remaining parent absorbs the whole of the child's love, determines the sex of the person who is later to be chosen as a sexual object, and may thus open the way to permanent inversion."[43] Ferenczi emphasized the fixation on a lost father from an absence of the usual unavoidable conflicts between fathers and sons, which had a detrimental effect.[44] In the absence of such conflict, there seemed to be a predisposing background toward male homosexuality. Isaacs stressed the negative oedipal complex when competition occurred between the mother and son for the fantasized image of the absent father.[45] Fenichel added complications pursuant to guilt from having achieved an oedipal victory from the absence of the same-sexed parent, and the simultaneous consequence of a grossly over-idealized father image that was not resolved.[46]

The idealization of the absent father may serve as a defense against maternal seductiveness, leading to later difficulties in heterosexual object choice. In turn, a hostile yet stimulating maternal object can lead to a flight from females as well as hopes for an idealized father to serve as a protector from women.[47] Castration threats in the shape of direct challenges, observations, or injuries have consequences dependent on the time they occur and their coincidence with things such as phallic masturbation, passive-feminine wishes toward the father, or guilt from some source. "Where the father is absent owing to divorce, desertion, or death, there is the lack of a restraining oedipal rival, a circumstance which intensifies anxiety and guilt in the phallic phase and promotes unmanliness. In this situation, the boy's fantasy that the father has been removed by the mother as a punishment for masculine aggression acts as a disturbance to the boy's normal heterosexual wishes."[48]

Girls Who Lose Fathers. Girls who experience a paternal loss suffer different consequences in terms of sex-role identification. An intensified attachment to the maternal object results in repressed aggression. During the phallic phase the girl experiences her mother as a threatening figure. She defends herself by identification with the absent father who can please mother and permit her to retain the love of her mother. This is one mechanism for establishing a propensity for later homosexual bonds. Unresolved conflicts of oral dependence and defense, and aggression can result in an orally punitive superego structure.[49]

In some cases there is an explicit, and implicit, expectation that the girl will take her dead father's place. The danger is that the child may invest much effort in identifying with objects that exist in fantasy, and stable identification with nonsexual qualities of other individuals is not attained. The combination of a sexualized, ideal father with early identifications leads to a sadistic superego structure which is difficult to please.[50] Failure to desexualize the original oedipal attachment persists and becomes manifest in adolescence.[51]

In the past, emphasis was placed on mother-girl relationships or the psychosexual changes occurring in the girl herself. Minimal emphasis was given to the availability of a father, let alone qualitative differences in available paternal figures. The classic psychoanalytic position was put best by Freud:

> The effects of the castration complex in little girls are more uniform and no less profound. A female child has, of course, no need to fear the loss of a penis; she must, however, react to the fact of not having received one. From the very first she envies boys its possession; her whole development may be said to take place under the colors of envy for the penis. She begins by making vain attempts to do the same as boys and later, with greater success, makes efforts to compensate for her defect—efforts which may lead in the end to a normal feminine attitude. If during the phallic phase she tries to get pleasure like a boy by the manual stimulation of her genitals, it often happens that she fails to obtain sufficient satisfaction and extends her judgment of inferiority from her stunted penis to her whole self. As a rule, she soon gives up masturbating, since she has no wish to be reminded of the superiority of her brother or playmate, and turns away from sexuality altogether.[52]

Even when attempts were made to see ramifications of such psychosexual development on relationships with others, few specifics of the father-daughter attachments were given. Recent emphases on family psychodynamics and family therapy have involved family configurations rather than those between father and daughter specifically. Many interesting elucidations have been postulated, especially with disturbed families or one member is presented as the one in distress. However, in the course of the girl's development, it may be that there are periods when her need for a paternal object is greater than at others.

The above quotation by Freud stresses the significance of the oedipal, yet participation by the father and the quality of his contribution is important. The preadolescent period, extending into adolescence, may be a significantly sensitive period. Unless a girl obtains the reassurance from her father that he sees her as an emerging woman, her confidence suffers in terms of sex-role identity. As noted in discussions of the impact of absent father on boys, the father who is totally lost appears to exert an influence by remaining as an idealized image. Fathers who remain fleetingly and unpredictably present in their daughters' lives contribute to feelings of paternal aloofness and rejection which impair self-esteem with respect to sex-role identity. This is related to the paternal figure manifesting little, if any, interest in the girl. The real father may remain unknown with a confused mixture of objective perception blending with fantasized distortions. Why should this matter to the development and sex-role identity of a girl? It is clear that such difficulties contribute to the problem of reality testing and appraisal. There is also the absence of a situation in which the girl is placed in a competitive situation with her mother. Without this competition, the driving force to relinquish the earlier type of attachment to her mother is absent.

Another variation for girls is the father who expresses little interest in the budding feminine sex-type attributes of his daughter. While being a tomboy during the latency period may not be a severe handicap at that time, continuance of boylike activities during adolescence creates difficulties in sex-role identity. In an interpersonal sense, the rewards for tomboyishness, which may have been present from both mother and father, no longer secure praise. Although the adolescent girl may continue trying to please her father by being a boy, the psychological and sociological complications for the adult woman in this role are immense.

Some fathers who appear indifferent to their daughter's femininity may in reality be using this as a defensive measure in their own right.[53] The result may appear to be the same as when the father is genuinely aloof. A pattern of retaliation may come to fruition in adolescence by which provocative behaviors in a girl succeed in eliciting counter-retaliation from parents and other authority figures. Acting-out behaviors may be one manifestation. Disregard for parental, and especially paternal, authority is the vengeance for the years of seeming aloofness. If the parental aloofness was defensive, the acting out is even more provocative to the father, who is presented with a greater need to maintain his own controls. The aloof figure may then be pressed into an overt authoritarian mold as well.

Fathers who are overtly seductive with their daughters may lead them to reject many sex-typed behaviors as too dangerous. In turn, this may lead to a girl struggling to emancipate herself by precipitation of arguments which lead to recurrent patterns of separation and remorse. Role-reversal is a not infrequent theme, handicapping the girl in achieving many of her adolescent sex-typed behaviors. This is seen in the paternal expectation that a daughter will nurture or care for a father in the future. Examples

from literature as well as clinical work demonstrate this. King
Lear's expectations of Cordelia would be an example.[54] These
influences continue to exert their presence in the vocational and
marital choices of the girl as well as her general character structure
throughout life.

Neubauer notes that the early loss of one parent and pathological
pre-oedipal relationship to the other parent predominate.

> The data do not permit etiological classification between the effect of the
> parent's absence and the pathology of the remaining parent. Other significant
> variables in the oedipal development of children with only one parent are the
> timing of the loss, and the relationship of the child's sex to the sex of the
> missing parent. Fantasy objects, immensely idealized or endowed with terribly
> sadistic attributes, replacing an absent parent are nearly ubiquitous; their
> frequent occurrence in dynamically very different situations underlines their
> significance in the development of object relations.[55]

Child Development Research on Absent Fathers. Developmental
studies on the consequences of paternal absence have attempted
assessment of externally observed personality variables. Early
studies During World War II assessed personality by projective doll
play and found less aggressive doll play in boys whose fathers were
gone.[56] Stoltz observed more overt feminine behaviors and fantasies
when fathers had been absent during the first year of their lives. On
the return of the father, the children showed greated aggression in
doll-play experiments.[57] These studies are interpreted in terms of the
absence of a father who would display dominant and aggressive
behavior as a model.

A widely cited study was done on preadolescent Norwegian
children, aged eight to nine-and-one-half, by Lynn and Sawrey.[58]
The children were those of sailors periodically absent on voyages.
This is a situation similar to a pattern in American society where
fathers travel frequently, such as salesmen. The Norwegian
children were compared to children from intact families. The sailors'
children were more immature and insecure in identification with
their fathers and had difficulties in peer relationships. Deficiencies
in the development of masculine skills, or over-compensatory
masculinity led to peer rejection. Girls in the study were more
dependent on their mothers, perhaps in response to the mothers
being more protective and authoritarian in their child-rearing
practices. A crucial factor is the intermittent presence of the father
with its uncertainties and promotion of types of differential

fantasies. A straightforward explanation of the difference between a father being unavailable most of the time in contrast to the continuity of a paternal presence may spell the difference. In the presence of longer periods of absences, reactions to the reappearance of the absent father complicate the situation. This has been noted in fathers returning from military service with the competitive overtones and new family alignment required.

Burton and Whiting reviewed cross-cultural data and found evidence that boys reared in societies where the father was absent during infancy, together with a lack of males available as identification models, have conflicts in sex-role identity.[59] Feminine identification may result in compensatory male sex-role behaviors. Clinical studies as well as sociological investigations of delinquent subcultures confirm this. However, Andry failed to find a significant relationship between father-absence during early childhood and later delinquent behavior.[60] There was a suggestion that disturbances in the relationship between fathers and sons were operating. This illustrates the need to delineate why the father may have been absent. Situations of permanent loss cannot be equated with temporary loss, where the father, whatever his sex-typed behaviors may be, is present to some extent.

One study of permanent father-absence in broken homes found that there were no differences in dependency needs between boys and those where the father was present. In fact, those from broken homes were more aggressive.[61] When fathers leave home after the child is age five, sex-typed behaviors remain similar to those from homes in which the father remains when preadolescent males are investigated.[62] In contrast, if the father left during the first four years of life, considerable disruption of sex-typing behaviors occurs. The father-absent boys appear more dependent on peers than do the father-present boys. Differences between white and black boys were negligible, except that black boys participated more in competitive activities involving force.

Fathers: General Significance. Fathers are influential in sex-role development beyond the significance that accrues from absence. Nor do they play a nothing but role of instrumentation in which the son benefits by accompanying his learning how to do something. It is not confirmed that fathers are the only ones who deal with the environment and actively seek accommodation with it. Nor can it be said that fathers are not oriented toward various feelings and attitudes of others. The dichotomy between instrumental-expressive, meaning male-female, appears to be an imposition of a convenient functional distinction onto the sex differentials which is not validated. This is especially so when changing economic conditions have altered family relationships so that the father is available a great deal more of the time in the home and mothers spend time working outside the home. The impact of industrialization led, until very recently,. to the disruption of families working together for survival, so that the father worked long hours away from home. By necessity, the mother was required to rear the children. The recent freeing up of fathers, permitting them to have time to be affectionate and nurturant toward children, may result in the weakening of the instrumental part they play in the sex-role standard.

In some groups the father as instrumental patriarch persists, but it should be emphasized how change has permitted them to function expressively without negative sanctions. More specifically, many males can now accept and pursue these activities without pretense, so that developmental factors in themselves will contribute toward the type of family interactional processes in which more fathers react expressively with their children.

Some interesting by-products of this shift are seen in efforts to demonstrate that the father may be even more significant with respect to sex-role, and other aspects development, than are mothers. Goodenough maintained that the father is most significant in determining the quality of the child's sex-role since he more distinctly differentiates his responses to daughters and sons.[63] An extension is a proposition that identification with fathers involves an internalization of reciprocal role relationships. Girls learn their sex-role in part from identifying with the role of a cross-sex parent at different periods of development. After infantile dependency, where identification is not viewed as sex-typed, the father is seen as differentiating his role toward opposite-sex children while the mother does not. This radical position does not deny that mothers are aware of sex-type differences in their culture. Rather, this view postulates that, "She neither plays wife to her son nor does she urge her daughter to 'buck up and get in there and be a woman,' but thinks of both sexes as 'children' whom she treats in the light of her general nurturant and supportive role in the family."[64] Others believe that paternal influence is what establishes a sound basis for cognitive development as well as creativity.[65]

PARENTAL INTEGRATION AND SEX-ROLE IDENTITY

Trends not only reinstate fathers by placing them in a far more significant social role than mothers, but may represent as one-sided a position as mother-oriented formulations. However, there is probably little need for worry since many of the factors which emphasize mothers still operate:

1. For most families the mother is primarily the nurturer for young ages, although not in such an undiluted manner as in earlier historical periods.

2. The heavy emphasis on infancy in much research in child development, as well as clinical scrutiny for early diagnostic insights, means that mothers will continue to occupy much attention along with their infants. This is seen in work on cognitive sensori-motor development, attachment and dependency behaviors, and early developmental deviations.[66]

3. Emphasis on studying families has not meant a discreet investigation of the fathers and their roles and relationships with sons and daughters, nor has it involved the differential effects of the ordinal position of the child, the effective sibling rank of a child as well as the parent, and personality attributes in the father. There has rather been a view of the family as an integral unit in which the father is one contributor.[67]

4. A pragmatic reason which operates for studying mothers more frequently is their easy accessibility compared to fathers. This holds for schools as well as clinical studies. Rarely is there access to the upper-middle classes who may not mind being discussed anonymously in certain clinical reports, but are rarely available for much else. However, even at the lower socio-economic levels, there is little knowledge or mention of the impact of paternal deprivation. Bowlby's classic study, *Maternal Care and Mental Health*, dealt with mothers.[68] Subsequent work has followed this path. In *Deprivation of Maternal Care*,[69] one of six articles included reference to paternal and maternal roles in delinquency. An almost endless bibliography dealing with maternal deprivation could be given. Those whose work has placed them in direct contact with children, whose difficulties were often seen to be involved with paternal absence or paternal conflicts, sensed the omissions. Until recently these were often social workers recounting their impressions. By adolescence, the presence of an adult male with particular attributes has an influence on boys and girls which both builds on earlier patterns and deviations and makes contributions in its own right.

Nash has provided an exhaustive and excellent review of the father in contemporary culture as portrayed in current psychological and sociological literature.[70] He notes that a sizable proportion of those writing have been sociologists and anthropologists. His view, unfortunately, has a paucity of clinical literature that is relevant. Most of the literature is observational in nature rather than experimental or theoretical. A review of 19th century American literature on child-rearing found unanimous agreement on the primacy of the mother's role.[71] Few would question child care in Western culture, and most especially in the United States, as child-centered. The center of the child's universe is usually that of the mother in her manifest activities as well as in her personality and its relationships to the child. Commentators about the mother-centered nature of American family life have varied from popular writers, such as Philip Wiley's "momism" in *Generation of Vipers* to anthropologists such as Clyde Kluckhohn stating that in the absence of domestic chores, the American woman had little to do but pamper her children.[72] [73]

To a certain extent the attacks have capitalized on an unavoidable situation. So great a significance has been placed on child-rearing capacities as a source for all developmental difficulties that ad-hoc explanations have been offered for every biological and sociological deviation in addition to the psychosocial. By virtue of the position of the mother with the child, clinicians have become aware of the impact on personality formation from the mother, in terms of her background and marital life, which contribute equally to her maternal role. This has led to a ludicrous search for books, lectures, counselors, and pseudo-therapists, from whom mothers avidly seek to be told what is correct in child-rearing practices. As in most historical periods, there seems to be little effect on the incidence of disturbances in families or the individuals in them. Only the fads which are currently in vogue seem to vary.

While there have been references to the biological qualities of mothering, minimal mention of correlative qualities in males exists. This has been a product of the view of fatherhood as a social role which not only debiologizes it, but depsychologizes it as well. However, note the tenacity with which the law in England and the United States, both in its common law and legislative aspects, held to the paternal blood tie as crucial for many legal rights. Few boys during the course of development have a guiding image of themselves as potential fathers.[74] In part the sex-role standard operates, since fatherliness is not recognized as part of the norm for masculinity in the way that nurturance is for femininity. As noted above, a concerned and tender father may be regarded as effeminate. As a result, tender affectivity is ascribed to the mother even though the boy may experience it from his father as well as in himself. "To fulfill his biological heritage of being a man, he must repress that which he has experienced chiefly in his relationships to women. One of his chief struggles is identifying with a masculine figure as the apparent necessity to abandon his similarity to a woman."[75] A changing sex-role standard is involved, such as finding it less censorious for the father to change a diaper, but perhaps more important are the attitude and affect in the male for the relationship and nurturance pleasure in response to less concealed feminine desires of his own. When Freud posed the question as to what his experience had shown to be the mental structures least accessible to change in male patients, he said it would be the feminine attitude in the man toward his own sex.[76] If so, changing sex-role standards give permission for expression of this aspect of man's nature.

FATHER ROLES IN PSYCHOPATHOLOGY

Fathers are often singled out as attaining significance when juvenile disturbances arise. Again, lack of specificity plagues studies. Early impressionistic positions attributed delinquency to "faulty identification" Q.E.D. In other cases the delinquent was seen as identifying with an antisocial father. One way or another, identification was to be inclusive. Many studies continue to ignore fathers by emphasizing maternal absence or separation as the crucial factor unless the absence of the father, or his failure to be a good provider, secondarily affected the mother. Andry's study of eighty delinquent boys, matched with eighty nondelinquent boys, aged eleven to fifteen, found a greater degree of paternal than maternal rejection.[77]

METHODOLOGICAL PROBLEMS

Many hypotheses involve partial confirmations including some evidence for psychopathological development apart from delinquency being attributed to personal conflicts. Some hypotheses refer to the effects of paternal absence, while others stress the maternal response. These studies have dealt with schizophrenia, the consequences of maternal overprotection, all types of perversions, the relationship of father-absence to sensitive periods, and consequences in peer relationships. The most important thing to evaluate in the studies is the methodology. Several times conclusions are drawn and perpetuated in the literature from data gathering or case selections which have little validity. The following limitations appear most prominent:

1. Some studies offer conclusions based on significant differences with respect to conditions or attributes being appraised, and then infer that the significant variable producing this was what was being investigated. A common example is research which appraises the significance of paternal absence on sex-typing, sex-role identity, or delinquency. A logical control group is one where the father has not been absent. If a significant difference is found, the conclusion is offered that paternal absence is causal. No such conclusion can justifiably be made. Earlier, reference was made to criteria for matching groups, and also the need to appraise specifics of the groups, such as the age of the child at the time of the parental loss, and if the loss was a complete or partial one.

2. Even more serious are conclusions made about paternal or maternal loss when parental insufficiency or inadequacy are present. It is then not the literal loss of the parent which is pathological, but the response of the remaining one. Rarely have there been attempts to make this differentiation.

3. Cross-sexed indicia are badly needed. It is obvious that a boy may react differently to a paternal loss than his sister, and he may also react differently at various developmental stages; this also holds for a maternal loss.

4. Studies and conclusions based on retrospective use of charts or clinical files should be suspect. The quality of the examiner and his data collection may be inadequate and often inaccurate as well. Only the most elementary of hypotheses seem testable with any confidence by such data.

5. The difficulties in ascribing more or less masculinity or femininity to ratings based primarily on overt sex-role attributes are enormous. Only the most naive or conflicted children fail to learn the adverse consequences of not being one of the boys. This is perhaps why ratings of these attributes are most useful with nursery-school-age children and have little validity beyond that.

6. Behavioral sophistication of the interviewer or rater needs appraisal. All too often these ratings may be done by students or trainees with unreliability unknown. The absence of some type of control over this, such as a Q-Sort measure, makes conclusions

suspect. Even with this, there are problems of appraising traits by externals.

7. Unscreened populations of children investigated for sex-typing behaviors or sex-role identity, as well as their use as control populations, cannot ipso facto be considered normal controls. This means that using children from normal schools or volunteers in the absence of psychological assessment raises questions about comparative differences which are found. The presence of pre-existing social pathology or psychopathology is always relevant. This is not an argument to exclude groups who are believed deviant, but rather to give acknowledgment to this when drawing conclusions about significant differences. As an example, concluding that children in in-patient psychiatric populations do not significantly differ in terms of the incidence of psychiatric symptoms from those in a normal school is invalid unless one has acknowledged the baseline of psychiatric symptoms in the school. Further investigation would have to be done with respect to many variables, one of the most prominent of which would be an appraisal of what led to the hospitalization when carried out.

8. The follow-up of variables by longitudinal investigation for differences that may arise, or internal differences that phase out, is rarely done.

9. Socio-economic and ethnic data must be available and accounted for before causality is assigned to some type of parental deviation or absence.

By way of illustration, some 400 studies dealing with fatherless homes have been appraised.[78] Our lack of knowledge becomes significant when it is realized that 6,000,000 children are growing up in homes without fathers. A goal of this review was to determine how many studies reported adverse consequences from fatherless homes versus the absence of adverse consequences. To do this, the studies were appraised as to methodology in terms of soundness. A core of fifty-nine studies was so appraised. There were three conclusions: (1) Existing data do not permit a decisive answer as to the effect of fatherlessness. It would not appear that dramatic differences will be found from fatherlessness per se. (2) Investigations need to be broadened to include knowledge about families, individual roles, and family interactions. The fatherless family itself merits study as an intact unit rather than being approached as defective by definition. There are suggestions that fatherless boys, especially those in low-income families, may not lack readily available male models. Most in need of investigation are the differences in the attributes of mothers who differ in the respect to which their boys or girls achieve their sex-role identities. What are the personality structures which permit this to occur or interfere with it? The number of relevant variables is large, but not unresearchable. In addition to maternal personality structure, data are needed on how mothers cope with their children, how they portray the absent father, and the effect of this on sex-role identification. Types of disciplinary patterns the mother uses, her transmitted ideals and values, and the contribution of environmental support from friends, family, and community may all be significant. (3) Focusing on a single variable is insufficient for conclusions. There is rather a cluster of interacting factors. These and their interactions are what bear on the isolated variable of father absence.

REFERENCES

1. J. L. Hampson, Determinants of psychosexual orientation, *Sex and Behavior*, ed. by F. A. Beach, pp. 108-132 (New York: John Wiley, 1965).
2. M. Mead, *Sex and Temperament in Three Primitive Societies* (New York: Morrow, 1935).
3. R. G. D'Andrade, Cross-cultural studies of sex differences in behavior, *The Development of Sex Differences*, ed. by E. Maccoby, pp. 174-204 (Stanford: Stanford University Press, 1966).
4. M. Rabban, Sex-role identification in young children in two diverse social groups, *Genetic Psychology Monograph* 42(1950):81-158.
5. W. W. Hartup and E. A. Zook, Sex-role preferences in three and four-year-old children, *Journal of Consulting Psychology* 24(1960):420-426.
6. D. G. Brown, Sex-role preferences in young children, *Psychology Monographs,* 70(1956):1-19.
7. Rabban, op. cit., 4.
8. W. A. Mischel, A social learning view of sex differences in behavior, *The Development of Sex Differences*, ed. by E. Maccoby, pp. 56-81.
9. J. Kagan and H. A. Moss, *Birth to Maturity* (New York: John Wiley, 1962).
10. L. A. Kohlberg, A cognitive developmental analysis of children's sex-role concepts and attitudes, *The Development of Sex Differences*, ed. by E. Maccoby, pp. 82-173 (Stanford: Stanford University Press, 1966).
11. Ibid., p. 82.
12. E. Sapir, *Language* (New York: Harcourt, Brace, 1939).
13. A. Bandura and R. H. Walters, *Social Learning and Personality Development* (New York: Holt, Rinehart, and Winston, 1963).
14. Ibid., p. 82.
15. O. H. Mowrer, *Learning Theory and Personality Dynamics* (New York: Ronald Press, 1950).

16. T. Parsons, Family structure and the socialization of the child, *Family Socialization and Interaction Process*, ed. by T. Parsons and R. J. Bales, pp. 35-131 (New York: Free Press, 1955).

17. M. M. Johnson, Sex-role learning in the nuclear family, *Child Development* 34(1963):319-333.

18. Hartup and Zook, op. cit., p. 426.

19. H. Y. Cobb, Role wishes and general wishes of children and adolescents, *Child Development* 25(1954):161-171.

20. D. G. Brown, Masculinity-femininity development in children, *Journal of Consulting Psychology* 21(1957):197-202.

21. P. H. Mussen, and L. Distler, Masculinity, identification, and father-son relationships, *Journal of Abnormal and Social Psychology* 59(1961):350-356.

22. R. R. Sears, Development of gender role, *Sex and Behavior*, ed. by J. A. Beach, pp. 133-163 (New York: John Wiley, 1965).

23. Kagan and Moss, op. cit., 9.

24. J. Kagan, Acquisition and significance of sex-typing and sex-role identity, *Review of Child Development Research*, vol. 1, pp. 137-167 (New York: Russell Sage Foundation, 1964).

25. Kagan and Moss, op. cit., 9.

26. D. Kopay, *The David Kopay Story* (New York: Arbour House, 1977).

27. G. A. Milton, Five studies of the relation between sex-role identification and achievement in problem solving, Technical Report No. 3, Dept. of Industrial Admn., Dept. of Psychology, Yale University, 1958.

28. J. Hellmuth, ed., *Learning Disorders*, vol. 3 (Seattle: Special Child Publications, 1968).

29. I. Lakatos, Changes in the problem of inductive logic, *The Problem of Inductive Logic*, pp. 315-417, ed. by I. Lakatos (Amsterdam: North-Holland Publishing Co., 1968).

30. C. G. Hempel, *Aspects of Scientific Explanation* (New York: Free Press, 1965).

31. H. Feigel and G. Maxwell, *Scientific Explanation, Space and Time* (Minneapolis: University of Minnesota Press, 1962).

32. B. F. Skinner, *The Behavior of Organisms: An Experimental Analysis* (New York: Appleton-Century-Crofts, 1938).

33. J. Kagan, The concept of identification, *Psychology Review* 65(1958):296-305.

34. D. E. Payne and P. H. Mussen, Parent-child relations and father identification among adolescent boys, *Journal of Abnormal and Social Psychology* 52(1956):358-362.

35. P. Mussen and E. Rutherford, Parent-child relations and parental personality in relation to young children's sex-role preferences, *Child Development* 34(1963):589-607.

36. E. M. Hetherington and G. Frankie, Effects of parental dominance, warmth, and conflict of imitation in children, *Journal of Personality and Social Psychology* 6(1967):119-125.

37. R. W. Moulton; E. Burnstein; P. G. Liberty; and N. Altucher, Patterning of parental affection and disciplinary dominance as a determinant of guilt and sex-typing, *Journal of Personality and Social Psychology* 4(1966):356-363.

38. G. K. Baruch and R. C. Barnett, Implications and Applications of Recent Research on Feminine Development, *Psychiatry* 38(1975):318-327.

39. A. Freud and D. Burlingham, *Infants Without Families* (New York: International Universities Press, 1944).

40. A. Aichhorn, *Delinquency and Child Guidance: Selective Papers* (New York: International Universities Press, 1965).

41. H. Nunberg, *Principles of Psychoanalysis* (New York: International Universities Press, 1955).

42. R. Hartogs and L. Freeman, *The Two Assassins* (New York: Crowell, 1965).

43. S. Freud, Three essays on the theory of sexuality, *Standard Edition* 7(1905)125-245.

44. S. Ferenczi, The nosology of male homosexuality (homoerotism), *Sex in Psychoanalysis* (New York: Basic Books, 1950).

45. S. Isaacs, Fatherless children, (1945) *Childhood and After* (New York: International Universities Press, 1949).

46. O. Fenichel, The pregenital antecedents of the oedipus complex, *The Collected Papers of Otto Fenichel*, vol. 1, 181:203 (New York: Norton, 1954).

47. I. Bennett and I. Hellmann, Psychoanalytic material related to observating in early development, *Psychoanalytic Study of the Child* 6(1951):307-324.

48. A. Freud, *Normality and Pathology in Childhood* (New York: International Universities Press, 1965), p. 194.

49. A. Eisendorfer, The clinical significance of the single parent relationship in women, *Psychoanalytic Quarterly* 12(1943):223-239.

50. A. Reich, Early identifications as archieve elements in the superego, *Journal of the American Psychoanalytic Association* 2(1954):218-238.

51. S. Keiser, A manifest oedipal complex in an adolescent girl, *Psychoanalytic Study of the Child* 8(1953):99-107.

52. S. Freud, An outline of psycho-analysis, *Standard Edition* 23(1964):193-194.

53. M. R. Leonard, Father and daughters, *International Journal of Psycho-Analysis* 47(1966):325-334.

54. R. Seidenberg and E. Papathomopoulos, Daughters who tend their fathers, *Psychoanalytic Study of Society* 2(1962):135-160.

55. P. B. Neubauer, The one-parent child and his oedipal development, *Psychoanalytic Study of the Child* 15(1960):286-309.

56. G. R. Bach, Father-fantasies and father-typing in father-separated children, *Child Development* 17(1946):63-80.

57. L. M. Stolz, et al., *Father Relations of War-Born Children* (Stanford: Stanford University Press, 1954).

58. D. Lynn and W. L. Sawrey, The effects of father-absence on Norwegian boys and girls, *Journal of Abnormal and Social Psychology* 64(1962):361-369.

59. R. V. Burton and J. W. M. Whiting, The absent father and cross-sex identity, *Merrill-Palmer Quarterly* 7(1961):85-95.

60. R. G. Andry, Paternal and maternal role and delinquency, *Deprivation of Maternal Care*, pp. 31-44 (Geneva: World Health Organization, 1962).

61. J. McCord, W. McCord and E. Thurber, Some effects of paternal absence on male children, *Journal of Abnormal and Social Psychology* 64(1962):361-369.

62. E. M. Hetherington, Effects of paternal absence on sex-typed behavior in negro and white preadolescent males, *Journal of Personality and Social Psychology* 4(1961):87-91.

63. F. W. Goodenough, Parenal identification in young children, *Genetic Psychology Monograph* 55(1957):287-323.

64. M. M. Johnson, Sex-role learning in the nuclear family, *Child Development* 34(1963):319-333.

65. L. Carlsmith, Effect of early father absence on scholastic aptitude, *Harvard Educational Review* 34(1964):3-21.

66. J. Hellmuth, ed., *Exceptional Infant* (Seattle: Special Child Publications, 1967).

67. R. Hill, Status of research about the family, *Marriage and Family Counseling*, ed. by J. C. Peterson, pp. 19-43 (New York: Association Press, 1968).

68. J. Bowlby, *Maternal Care and Mental Health*, 2nd ed. (Geneva: World Health Organization, 1952).

69. *The Significance of the Father* (New York: Family Service Association of America, 1959).

70. J. Nash, The father in contemporary culture and current psychological literature, *Child Development* 36(1965):261-297.

71. R. Sanley, Early nineteenth-century American literature on child-rearing, *Childhood in Contemporary Cultures*, ed. by M. Mead and M. Wolfenstein, pp. 150-167 (Chicago: University of Chicago Press, 1955).

72. P. Wylie, *Generation of Vipers* (New York: Farrar and Rinehart, 1942).

73. C. Kluckhohn, *Mirror for Man* (New York: McGraw-Hill, 1949).

74. R. E. Hartley; L. K. Frank; and R. M. Goldensen, *Understanding Children's Play* (New York: Columbia University Press, 1952).

75. I. M. Josselyn, Cultural forces, motherliness and fatherliness, *American Journal of Orthopsychiatry* 26(1956):264-271.

76. S. Freud, op. cit., 52, p. 194.

77. Andry, op. cit., 60.

78. E. Herzog and C. E. Sudia, Fatherless homes—a review of research, *Children* 15(1968):177-182.

Chapter Five

The Psychopathology of Adolescent Sexuality

THE DEVELOPMENT OF ADOLESCENT SEXUALITY

Contemporary viewpoints on sexuality emphasize a broad grasp of the factors entering into this area of behavior. Initial distintions are needed, including an examination of the differences between *legal* canons about sexual behavior and *clinical* appraisals of personal psychopathology. In this connection developmental antecedents, which are connected with psycho-sexual and psycho-social development, are relevant. Another distinction is between *psychological theory* about the nature of infantile and childhood sexuality in contrast to *empirical observations* on the diffuse manifestations of sexuality which commence in infancy and continue in diverse forms until the pubertal period. In turn, all these phenomena must be distinguished from *sociological* and *cultural* orientations on what, if anything, is considered deviant sexuality.

Variations by social class, locale, subcultural norms, role, status group, and age, contribute to variant sexual behavior in adolescence. Finally, judicial and statutory definitions of sexual offenses, which categorize adolescents as "sexual delinquents" must be differentiated from developmental and psychodynamic formulations regarding the meaning and significance of sexual behaviors. The adolescent suffers a double endemnity: behaviors considered as sexual offenses for adults are considered offenses for the adolescent, but he may also be condemned for a miscellany of sexual behaviors viewed as unacceptable, be these fornication or promiscuity.

Adolescent Sexual Behavior. A few points concerning adolescent sexual behavior need clarification. Many behaviors in the latency-age child may be seen as thinly concealed sexual fantasies. A common example is that of the sexualized play activities, such as the twisting, turning, purring, and thematic content which accompany seemingly asexual tasks as telephoning between those of the same sex.[1]

This background is relevant to the topic of the ongoing debate on the changing nature of sexual mores as they pertain to adolescents. Although the concept of latency construed in terms of a relative lack of genital sexuality has few contemporary adherents, it is generally accepted that during the preadolescent period, changes in sexual life occur. This corresponds to neuro-humoral alterations accompanying the striving for puberty with an accompanying adaptation to the peer culture. Given these biological wellsprings, the pattern of activity chosen and the objects used for gratification vary. The entire background of prior development, with operant and respondent situations, enters into what type of sexual sensitivities an individual will cultivate. Factors such as identification, imitative or modeling behavior, sex-typing, level of drive intensity, family conflicts, superego functioning with respect to inhibition, controls over impulse life, guilt or shame over sexual strivings, phallic narcissism, and idealization of certain objects or causes are relevant to the final outcome.

The Female Adolescent. Questions about the variation of the emergence of sexual activity at puberty are relevant to criteria for perversions. If sexual performance is defined in terms of frequency of ejaculation or orgasm, most studies indicate the male achieves his peak at sixteen or seventeen years of age, while the female's peak occurs several years later.[2][3][4] However, caution must be exercised in terms of explanations offered for this phenomenon. Biological, cultural, and experiential factors may be dispositive in different cases. In determining when an adolescent has become a sexual being in terms of behavior, sexualized components are confusing.

Conflicts for the adolescent female within this framework exist between a way to secure self-esteem by being attractive to males in a seductive manner, but also by not actually participating in intercourse. Only through marriage, so the norms held, were girls to have the social security and consequent psychological freedom to enjoy intercourse. Demonstrations of the absence of this security or freedom for large numbers of women had relatively little impact until recently. Whether there has been an actual increase in adolescent sexual practice is difficult to assess methodologically— once conjecture or opinion is bypassed. While an adolescent girl who dabbles in intercourse for experimental purposes may be rare outside of clinical settings, this does appear to be part of sex-role identity for the adolescent boy. The mass media would seem to promote such a change but also to reflect it.

Arguments that the pill has changed the position of the adolescent female so that she may now pursue her sexual life with freedom and abandon ignore the fact that relatively secure contraceptive devices have been available for some time for those possessed of minimal intellectual abilities, funds, and, most important, a desire to use prevention. To expect an immediate abandonment of psychological inhibitions and controls by the ego would be a gross oversimplification of ego development.

Keeping the limitations of interview and questionnaire techniques in mind, it appears that little actual increase in coital experience in late adolescent college girls has occurred (the figure has been estimated as staying at about 20 percent).[5] Acknowledging the social class bias of studies, note that Kinsey's study of volunteers showed no increase in girls having intercourse before marriage from 1910 to the 1950s.[6] A greater number of girls who are psychiatric patients have had sexual relationships premaritally.[7] This raises interesting questions of a cause-effect nature not satisfactorily resolvable. Is sexual permissiveness a contributory factor in a greater vulnerability toward emotional disorder in girls who do not stand against the tide?

Propositions relating to permissiveness have been summarized by Reiss.[8] The less sexually permissive a group is, the more likely it is that new social forces will lead its members to become more permissive. If there has been greater permissiveness in the lower social classes, the members will be relatively more immune from the shifting social climate with respect to sexual standards. Secondly, a group which views itself as liberal in such fields as religion or politics is more prone to shift toward sexual permissiveness with the changing social climate. Sexual differences are operative in that romantic involvement is more conducive to female permissiveness (this is not so for the male). Sexual equality also promotes tolerance, as do parental values which intellectually and affectively transmit permissiveness. Those more vulnerable to the influence of their peer group rather than parents are more subject to permissive sexual behavior, as are those having the least responsibility for the other members of a family group. Only children in a family have the greatest permissiveness.

These are merely some of the social variables which bear on decision-making processes for the adolescent. Although it is still debatable whether there is more overt coital activity compared to earlier decades when social class and rates were controlled, greater freedom for discussion and toleration of sexual deviance is present. Change in the cultural and intellectual atmosphere has left the adolescent still having to synthesize various conflicting demands in adapting, or maladapting, to this culture.

The Male Adolescent. Sexuality for the adolescent male has a different connotation. He is not solely interested in drive gratification, but is similarly burdened with a psychological and cultural heritage that sexual activity with a "good" girl should be for procreative purposes. Problems of impotency and frigidity often stem from this in adolescence.[9] Sexual activity during adolescence revolves about masturbation, or its equivalent, through random sexual acts. In these the component of tender attachment and affectivity is often lacking, and conquests become demonstrations of masculine prowess. The number of makes are chalked up and compared—often on a level of gross exaggeration and bravado. Lack of involvement fosters a means-focusing on the girl as a vehicle wherein the object is masturbator-equivalent.

Individual conflicts and patterns of sexual activity do not seem easily disposed of immediately after a marriage ceremony. What must also be considered are factors of anxiety, guilt, shame, and other adverse affects to sexual experiences once they commence in adolescence. Nor can a contrary pattern of psychopathology be ignored where a semi-permanent attachment, or marriage, impairs sexual pleasure and performance. Earlier psycho-sexual conflicts contribute to this diathesis, which leads to a series of acting-out maneuvers or neurotic suffering. Practices such as mate-swapping, or married males seeking a relatively consistent pattern of extra-marital mates while "mother" tends the house, are not merely adolescent creations, but rather a widespread continuation of patterns of adolescent sexuality. If best-selling novels and plays are any index of a society's desires and behavior, in addition to therapy and studies with selected clinical populations, such themes are pervasive. These guides to the American family are used paradigmatically by adolescents who in turn are utilized by adults in the form of overtly condemning adolescent promiscuity.

Social Factors. The proposition that social class and cu'ture provide a groundwork for the degree and type of sexual activity sanctioned during a particular historical period elicits little controversy. What remains difficult is the degree of acting upon these ideas. Frank discussions of topics that were previously avoided, must somehow be assimilated. This makes conscious denial more difficult for sexual subjects and allusions.

Perhaps one of the earlier contributions to openness was the publicized sexualization of psychoanalysis which permited more open joking about sexuality in discussions.[10] The gross misunderstanding that was often present is beside the point. Instead, this began a progressive exposure over the decades to an enormous amount of data, devices, and techniques, so that a contemporary adolescent who reads Freud is struck by his old-world conservatism. Influences from the Kinsey reports of 1945 and 1953, with their attendant publicity and dissemination of sexual data, and the more recent reports of observers who recorded physiological alterations in the female genitalia during intercourse or self-stimulation have followed a pathway of openness. This is not a judgment of the validity of Kinsey's findings, nor of the desirability of sexual experimentation utilizing human subjects, but an illustration that exposure to such information via mass media changes the milieu for sexual conversations long before puberty.

Further, an emphasis on information about contraceptive techniques, the ease of obtaining such materials, and facilitation of abortion if needed, promote opportunities to experiment, if desired, with less chance of irreversible consequences. The duplicity in our culture for the adolescent is as striking as that with respect to cigarette smoking or alcohol. Handling of juvenile girls who are promiscuous, with its vagaries, needs reappraisal. While intervention was originally seen as a need to save the wayward girl from sin, what is most apparent now is the widespread prevalence of such behavior among many nonjuveniles in our society. The condemnation of such behavior is understandably seen as oppressive by the juvenile.

To prohibit sexual activity while offering contraceptive devices ad libitum over-the-counter is one hypocrisy fanning adolescent anger. There is suggestive data that the age of women seeking abortion is dropping. In Sweden the highest incidence from 1964 to 1966 was the twenty to twenty-four year age group, but second was the fifteen to nineteen year age group, most of whom would be considered minors in the United States.[11] With increasing equal rights for females, and demands for adolescent equality as well, will abortion be available to young females on the same basis as it is to their older counterparts?

Questions on the efficacy of sex education courses in the schools are many and varied. Goals are vague and unclarified, but if the main goal is to decrease subsequent sexual acting-out or experimentation, it is not successful. If the goal is to impart knowledge about sex, analogous to a segment of a course in biology, begining in the early elementary grades, little could be challenged except by way of the adequacy of the teaching, as with any subject. There seems to be a hopeful assumption by some that undefined goals, such as providing the child with a healthy attitude toward sex will reduce sexual conflicts in adolescence and subsequently in marriage, yet evidence appears extremely tenuous. Teachers have a multitude of attitudes and personality configurations, like those in any other profession.

ADOLESCENT SEXUAL CONFLICTS

The phase-specific developmental sequence is another perspective to keep in mind. Perhaps at no other period is it so clear that sexual behavior is not autonomous from the remainder of the personality but rather an integral part of a diverse system of drives, intersystemic changes, and attempts at adaptation to the peer culture. An impulse-ridden youth approaching adolescence, who may be primarily motivated by immediate gratification, reflects this in his sexualized activities, just as another with marked dependency needs or a wish to be taken care of reflects these trends in the sexual sphere. The difference at adolescence is that sexual drives cannot be ignored or repressed with as much ease. Earlier types of fantasies and urges are now too obvious and lead to various kinds of sexual activity or defensive maneuvers. The latter may be flights into asceticism or intellectualization, provocative challenges, or defiance of authority which seemingly have little to do with sexuality per se.

Wide alternations occur within individuals as well as groups. Greater anxiety and turbulence elicit stronger defensive efforts. Some delay in adolescent capacity to integrate sexual drives with the remaining parts of the personality results in a developmental lag. Others overtly regress in the sexual sphere, producing stages of profound disorganization or transient psychotic episodes in which florid sexual acting out occurs. The need to integrate contradictory masculine-feminine strivings accentuates this. For some, pregenital impulses reemerge and lead to sexually perverse *behaviors*—which must be distinguished from clinical diagnoses of perversions, not only because such diagnoses carry adverse social consequences but because of the different psychological implications in transient behaviors as opposed to the relatively fixed patterns in an adult. This distinction about perverse acts in adolescence has significance for both legal and treatment approaches. Once the legal classification of sexual deviancy has been made, we may be confirming this identity for the adolescent in his own eyes as well as in the eyes of his contemporaries. There is a similar danger in treatment approaches which focus on acts rather than having an accurate perception of their meaning within the context of adolescent development. Particularly can this occur with girls.[12]

Specific Adolescent Anxieties. Within this framework the typical adolescent experiences anxieties in response to emerging sexuality. Feelings of guilt from earlier prohibited sexuality may still be operative, and the prohibitions and strivings generalize to sexualized areas, such as in searches for power, status, or money. Demands to perform heterosexually can specifically stimulate anxieties varying from fear of genital injury to more complex and symbolic derivatives. Demands to establish attachments outside the home with other objects may require too great a relinquishment of dependency and sexualized gratification presently existing within the home and lead to conflict. Group experimentation of a homosexual or heterosexual nature function to permit the safety of groups, since the intensity of a one-to-one attachment can be overwhelming. Experimentation can vary from mutual masturbation to several boys indulging themselves sexually with one girl. The latter is often a regressive manifestation to a latency group experience transposed to the sexual now that biological puberty has arrived. Threats to heterosexual capability give rise to flights into homosexual activity used defensively to counteract anxiety. At times, variations of pseudo-masochistic behavior toward the opposite sex emerge, indicating some of the earlier sexual components have temporarily gained ascendancy. Again, homosexual behavior and not homosexuality is the key distinction.

The Struggle for Control. Adolescence may be viewed as a struggle for control as much as the oft-quoted quest for identity. Perhaps the recurrent theme of protesting against insufficient freedom betrays the ambivalence which adolescents have toward accepting freedom. While continuously demanding freedom and more license, they are at the mercy of their impulses in many respects. The concept of freedom can have meaning only in terms which extend beyond lack of restraint. If the focus is shifted to self-control, the individual adolescent can choose to exert control over how he wishes to express his impulse life.

These usages of freedom often confuse the issue and lead to endless and unresolvable arguments. Sexual gratification, like other types of gratification, is contingent upon the ego having developed a capacity to delay pleasure. This is a consequence of learning that impulsivity is a defect which makes one prone to anxieties contingent upon the failure to have developed sufficient inhibitory mechanisms. The rationalized nature for much of what some adolescents call strength becomes apparent when it is used to refer to brooking no delay in obtaining their demands, sexual or otherwise. These concepts have direct bearing on the capacity of the adolescent to choose sexual behavior rather than feeling driven to perform by intrapsychic or social pressures. This means that the developing ego must have a relative independence not just from drives, but from the multifarious stimulations of the external environment.

While sexual impulses are one main determiner of development, they are subject to control by ego and superego influences. The entire role of developmental precursors to the superego then becomes relevant, such as identification with authority figures, internalization processes, appraisal of behavior and desires, and the integration of cultural norms. Theoretically, the role of ego development has been well summarized in the following quote about how the ego of the adolescent deals with sexuality:[13]

> Man has developed an anticipatory apparatus which is far more effective than any other animal's. This apparatus is very effective for outside events and fairly effective (anxiety and other affect signals) for internal events. These events play a causal role in behavior. But man himself (and every organism to some degree) is a source of causes. Man's anticipatory apparatus is a particularly effective mobilizer of man's own causal role. Man isn't freed from internal and external causes by means of his anticipatory apparatus, that is, by dint of his being also a source of causes. But he certainly can within limits avoid, evade, cushion, and counteract causes which would determine his behavior. Some of these causes he is less adept at avoiding or cushioning (instinctual drives)—but to the extent that he has a relatively autonomous ego,

he can do even some of that. Instinctual drives are causes and motives; other causes of the same sort (neutralized to various degrees) he can cushion better.... Assuming the capacity of the ego to adapt its operations and reactions to the environment and its realities, we can expect that the ego can be purposefully influenced by reality factors. Thus, specifically the reality fact that traditionally, conventionally, and tacitly every individual is considered to be responsible for his acts by the society in which he lives, and that this is inculcated in the child through the educational and rearing process, constitutes a powerful reality factor to which the ego has to adapt itself and is capable of adapting itself. The established standard provides the environmental setting to which the adaptable ego responds.

JUSTIFICATIONS ADVANCED FOR
LEGAL APPROACHES TO SEXUAL BEHAVIOR

What are the justifications for treating certain non-aggressive sexual behaviors as criminal or delinquent offenses? The question is raised here for its validity, the goal sought, and the impact on the adolescent from this approach to changing behavior—whatever the specific means employed. An additional point is that the degree of developmental advancement or retardation need not, and often does not, correspond to the ages set for handling an adolescent as a juvenile or adult offender. Statutory provisions for juvenile jurisdiction set at sixteen or eighteen years is more of an arbitrary device for convenience than one with validity. There is an initial assumption that the behavior is offensive to a majority of the community. This may be judged as morally wrong, or something in need of correctional, educational, or psychiatric tinkering.

Types of Sexual Offenses. A distinction is made between two types of sexual offenses. One involves an act of violence against a person, such as a sexual assault upon a woman or coercively carrying out a pedophilic act. The second group, offenses against morals, includes a variety of sexual acts such as fornication, adultery, sodomy, incest, and prostitution, as well as perverse acts such as exhibitionism, voyeurism, transvestism, fetishism, and homosexual conduct. The comments which follow consider the implications of the latter group which lack a component of violent physical aggression. Such behaviors are viewed as requiring moral censure because of their opprobriousness, which is the basis for viewing them as delinquent or criminal acts. Morals offenses are not such from their relationship to morality in general but from an absence of ordinary justifications for punishment by a non-theocratic state for such conduct.[14] To view such sexual behavior as unoffensive means it would either have to be seen as a desirable expression of sexual life—a position most do not adopt—or as something that should be handled outside the realm of the legal system, analogous to the disposition of individuals who become personally troubled by their desires or behavior for a variety of reasons. Part of the public nature of such behavior contributes to labeling it as deviant. Thus, if an individual makes his hallucinations known, it may be discomforting to those around him, but it does not lead to the stigma of criminality. Hence, there must be some additional distinguishable points to justify the separate categorizing of deviant behavior.

The degree of tolerance for deviancy is what leads to decisions to intervene by the state or to ignore individual idiosyncrasies. Where, then, short of acts involving violence, does tolerance stop? The basic social justification appears to be that behavior is unacceptable to the majority being imposed upon an individual who does not conform to judicial, political, and legislative processes. In terms of the customary justifications given for criminal punishment for wrong-doing, deterrence of such behavior in an individual in the future, or general deterrence of others who may be tempted to try such behavior, discomfort arises about handling non-aggressive sexual conduct by such a route. The repetitive nature of sexual perversions, with or without punishment, is a primary consideration. Contrariwise, if the act was sporadic or transient, what purpose is served by the delinquent or criminal approach? Rehabilitative goals for perversion have not been realizable in many cases either for a multitude of reasons which vary from insufficient rehabilitative efforts to the complexity of the behavior eluding the approaches available.

Justifying Arguments.   What are the legal and social arguments to justify approaches to emergent patterns of sexual deviation? The usual arguments for criminal or delinquent sanctions, such as punishment, preservation of public order, or community protection, as noted, have little relevance to non-violent behaviors. There is no overt threat to public safety, persons, or property. Indeed, constitutional questions have been raised about whether "morals legislation" contravenes certain individual liberties, such as the right to do what one pleases without the religious or moral beliefs of the majority being imposed upon an individual who does not conform to these beliefs. This issue was raised long ago with respect to polygamy and practices of Mormons, and the reasoning of the Supreme Court in 1890 on this matter has not appeared to change.[15]

> Bigamy and polygamy are crimes by the laws of all civilized and Christian countries. They are crimes by the laws of the United States, and they are crimes by the laws of Idaho. They tend to destroy the purity of the marriage relation, to disturb the peace of families, to degrade woman and to debase man. Few crimes are more pernicious to the best interests of society and receive more general or more deserved punishment, for such crimes would be to shock the moral judgment of the community. To call their advocacy a tenet of religion is to offend the common sense of mankind.

The opinion went on to cite the legal and social problems which arise if certain sexual practices are to be considered part of a given religion. As such, they would *not* be subject to criminal sanction, while anyone else engaging in such practices *would* be subject to criminal sanction: "Suppose one believed that human sacrifices were a necessary part of religious worship. Would it be seriously contended that the civil government under which he lived could not interfere to prevent a sacrifice? Or, if a wife religiously believed that it was her duty to burn herself upon the funeral pyre of her dead husband, would it be beyond the power of civil government to prevent her carrying her belief into practice? ... To permit this would be to make the professed doctrines of religious belief superior to the law of the land, and in effect to permit every citizen to become a law unto himself." On this basis certain practices—sexual, religious, and social—are prohibited by the state. For juveniles the mandate extends not only to certain designated statutory sexual offenses, but sexual mores as well.

For some "offenses against morals," individual and vested community interests may prosper rather than the community suffer by their occurrence. It would be difficult to establish that greater suffering arises by tolerance of morally condemned behavior as prostitution, polygamy, or polyandry. Nor can one establish that communities have specifically benefited, nor their young, by prohibiting exposure to forms of literature covered by pornographic statutes. There is little causal evidence to demonstrate that the flourishing of homosexuality in a culture has led to the decline of the society; on the contrary, there is much evidence that in societies which employ criminal sanctions against homosexuality a great deal of individual suffering is induced by scapegoating effects, as well as the promotion of secondary criminal activity such as blackmail. A fortiori, the utilization of police and probation officers, as well as the criminal courts, to deal with such matters may lead to a wasteful use of our resources which might be more profitably devoted to other problems.

What, then, is the justification from criminal codes applied to offenses against morals? Several lines of defense are commonly offered. In many of the acts regarded legally as sexual deviations there is a presumption that the psychological welfare of individuals may be protected by such an approach. It is felt that the psychological development of the child and the adolescent, as well as the family, are best protected and nurtured by lessening the probability of such behavior occurring or limiting the risks of exposure. This is tantamount to an attempt at primary prevention—to eliminate noxious exposures which could later lead to a disease. How valid this rationale is raises a crucial question. Its validity is primarily on the level of a belief at this point. This is a type of reasoning from what are presupposed to be the results of traumatic experiences, such as the exposure to an exhibitionist. The sensibilities of a community include such diverse moral areas as prohibiting public lewdness, open purchasing of pornography, spitting on the flag, and certain sexual practices deemed harmful to the young or the community at large.

Various assumptions and moral sentiments are implicit in much of this. Attempts to justify such legislation on psychological grounds open up historical and cross-cultural anthropological analyses. The well-known fact that homosexuality flourished at the peak of the history of Greece does not require elaboration. Civilizations continue to flourish in the Pacific, where unmarried adolescents engage in sexual relations, even though some become pregnant, without incurring community disapproval. Similarly, a position of historical and cultural relativism shows that some behaviors are considered morals offenses only at particular times and places. In colonial New England blasphemy was so treated. Divorce and contraception have been so treated in contemporary theocratic Catholic countries. Confusion, from the blend of morals and legislation pertaining to sexual behavior, leads to efforts to give a justification for morals offenses based on a utilitarian argument.

The utilitarian position is that certain behaviors need to be controlled since greater harm will result to more people in the community if they are not, and this justifies their legal prohibition. A specific illustration is the postulation that exposure of adolescents to movies with sexually prurient themes risks increased promiscuity. Hence, it is possible that the community will have to assume care for pregnant teenagers and their offspring, and later the tax burden of AFDC payments—all risks which can be controlled. Better, then, to stop the disease at its source by controlling exposure to prurient movies, literature, or pictures.

Another example is controlling the exposure of adolescents to homosexual experiences on the basis that homosexual experience increases the chances of forsaking heterosexuality. The community believes it is better off with guarantees of marriage, family units, and procreation than with homosexual ties. Although several steps in such reasoning can be questioned empirically, the utilitarian bases for the measures employ *social* justifications. The pragmatic interests of the state are held to justify the penal handling of homosexual behavior. The goals of promoting future marriages, substantiating the basis for marriage, preventing illegitimacy or disease, promoting healthy individual psychological development, and injecting the overriding interest of the state where it is believed relevant, become the bases for legal sanctions applied to sexual deviations as offenses. The basic question, often begged, is whether the above goals are actually promoted by handling sexual deviations as offenses.

A devious justification for handling sexual delinquency under penal sanctions is seen in arguments that such regulations permit agencies or courts to control the commercialization of vice. It is held that when offenses, such as inducing young males or females into prostitution, are controlled, racketeering and other types of organized crime also become more subject to prosecution. This is not an argument for control on the basis of immorality, psychological development, or even a purely secular justification, but a means of preventing a type of criminal group behavior organized to exploit behaviors for which an individual is either developmentally vulnerable or psychologically predisposed. Again, is this the most efficacious or desirable means of controlling such activities? Instead of dealing directly with the underworld itself, the onus is placed on individuals who respond to the enticements.

A more fundamental problem is why such business continues to flourish while the burden is placed on the sexual behavior of the individual. Overtones are present for the continuance of an ethic of individual responsibility carried into the sexual realm, while what is more essential—a system of social corruption—is ignored. Sporadic adjudication of sexual delinquency, the low risks of being caught, the pleasurable reinforcements of most sexual acts on a direct or derivative level, all raise questions about handling sexual conflicts of a nonaggressive type in this manner. Exploitation of individuals makes them vulnerable to practices such as, scapegoating or being used sadistically. A byproduct is to foster secrecy by those adolescents who may be concerned about seeking help for some aspect of their sexual life, since the risk of adverse consequences is quite high in comparison to the chances of obtaining assistance.

LEGAL PROVISIONS REGARDING SEXUALITY

Legal provisions are discussed to illustrate the following: (1) They exemplify a mode of approach with the maximum of coercive sanctions. (2) Changing trends can be followed by way of evolving statutes. (3) Juvenile sex offenders may be caught up in a juvenile court or in higher courts over a stated age—whatever their developmental level. At first glance the legal approach seems straighforward. Espousing values of protecting the bodily integrity of individuals from unwanted sexual or aggressive use seems a goal to codify in terms of acts which are prohibited. Within this schema, fornication or homosexual behavior are classified as harmful or unpleasant to a majority of the public to justify restrictions. Although this is not customarily done for private acts at the present time, it illustrates one approach for unacceptable sexual behavior. However, disposition of individuals prone to sexual acting out is an extremely complex subject.

This is not simply a matter of classification. It is not a matter of psychiatrists differing among themselves on the nature of deviancy. Psychodynamic formulations may perceive that some delinquency of the psychopathological type has elements of the sexually perverse. Legal classifications of delinquencies, governed by values implicit in judicial institutions, do not necessarily correspond to what may be the appropriate treatment requirements for an individual. While in part this is due to inadequate diagnostic assessment, involving lack of developmental knowledge of sexual psychopathology, the tendency to rely on rote approaches or mass treatments applied to entire populations negates optimism.

After a series of commitments to correctional faciliites for breaking and entering which began at thirteen, an evaluation at seventeen years revealed the boy had begun this compulsive activity seeking women's undergarments. He would find them, masturbate, and leave. This fetishistic behavior was usually pursued alone, but it was complicated when he was caught in the apartment. To make it appear that the intent was to take money, he would take some, although he would leave hidden amounts or 'drop' some on exiting since 'I really didn't need it.' During the course of his several commitments the sexual nature of his offense was never discovered. A ten-year follow-up revealed that he continued his behavior to the point of having spent time in a state prison as a burglar.

THE AMERICAN HERITAGE

Early Origins. In the traditions of the Anglo-American legal system, the English ecclesiastical courts exercised a wide jurisdiction over matters pertaining to morals and the family. Church courts took over jurisdiction from primitive approaches which severely punished offenders. Apart from offenses that were punished by the common law, the church assumed jurisdiction for the offenses involving sexuality.[16] The upper classes in England availed themselves of a second approach to family matters by an administrative body, the Court of High Commission, which dealt with unusual practices from 1558 until 1640. Offenses such as adultery, assault with intent to ravish, incest, bigamy, immorality, swearing desperate oaths, or blasphemy, were handled by these two parallel approaches, depending on economic and social rank.

By the time of Puritan ascendancy and the English civil war, which abolished the English monarchy in the mid-seventeenth century, the ecclesiastical jurisdiction and the High Commission fell into decay. Although the former was restored with the monarchy, a period of existence without these devices occurred. Over the centuries, common-law courts took charge of offenses within the domain of marital and sexual matters. Even in the reign of Henry VIII (1507-1547), a specific statute dealt with "unnatural offenses," and in 1603 bigamy became a crime. However, the lingering influence of ecclesiastical courts is seen in their retention of divorce jurisdiction until 1857 when divorce courts were created.

The transmission of these standards to the United States is seen in the handling of sex offenses in colonial Massachusetts during the seventeenth century. Fornication and "lewd, lascivious, or wanton" behaviors were the most prominent punishable offenses. These words had no fixed meaning at the time, but could best be summed up as representing various activities considered sexually unclean, such as prostitution, abduction, or other types of sexual dalliance. "Bodily punishment" was the cure. It appears that ideas of punishment for such sexual transgressions fused with deterrence as the rationale. It is estimated that half the public whippings in the market place were for sexual behavior. Within the group of sexual transgressors, about three-fourths were for fornication, usually young people in the adolescence group.[17]

This preoccupation with fornication as a sexual offense reflects the mores of the colony and what types of sexual offenses predominated. The contemporary version of this practice is the adjudication of adolescent females as delinquent for sexual activity through the juvenile process although males are almost never prosecuted for such activity. Not every fornicator was whipped in colonial Massachusetts, since those in the upper social classes could often pay a fine or at times have marriage enjoined if it was feasible. When the whippings occurred, they were not paltry affairs, but were carried out with the stern conviction that a reformative treatment was being administered.

Punishment by whipping was the favorite disciplinary technique for non-capital offenses from Biblical times. To set limits to sadistic involvements, specific injunctions were directed to this aspect of the treatment so that no one who was "cruel or barbarous" could be the administrator of whippings. Similarly, the number of lashes laid on was limited—usually to fifteen or twenty, and even a destestable offense did not get more than the Biblical thirty-nine. This was based on Paul's Second Letter to the Corinthians which stated, "Of the Jews five times received a forty stripes save one." Whipping was also the chosen treatment for adultery and for girls delivering illegitimate children. As such it was one of the accepted practices for changing behavior—sexual or otherwise—in houses of correction.

Eighteenth Century Massachusetts.   The provincial government of Massachusetts lessened the punishment but did not change its character. *Fornication* with a single female could be punished with ten stripes or a fine of five pounds. *Adultery* was regarded as a capital offense in colonial times, punishable by death if with a married woman, with both parties put to death. From 1692 to 1780, the offense became punishable by forty lashes and sitting in the gallows for one hour with a rope around the neck to enforce the deadly seriousness of the behavior. Thereafter, adulterers were required to wear the letter "A," two inches high, upon their clothing for the rest of their lives, subject to fifteen lashes for failure to wear the badge. *Incestuous marriages* carried the same penalty as adultery except that the letter "I" was to be worn for life.

Transvestite behavior in men was punished by corporal punishment or a fine up to five pounds.

Following the common law, *rape* was punished by death as a capital offense. An obstacle to this in colonial Massachusetts was the inability to find a warrant for this in the Bible. The most severe penalties short of death were originally meted out if the victim was a minor. This might be the maximum number of whippings, or an order to have the nostrils slit and to wander about thereafter with a halter about the neck. Subsequently, statutes were enacted making statutory rape punishable by death, although lives were usually spared. Other rapists, were rarely executed but instead given whippings and the humiliation of standing in the gallows with a rope about eh neck for an hour. During the nineteenth century, rape of a woman or *carnal knowledge* of a child under ten years of age continued to be punishable by death. Sodomy and bestiality, viewed as acting "contrary to the light of nature," again relying on a Biblical definition as "mankinde lyeth with mankinde," was punishable by death unless the perpetrator was under the age of fourteen; by 1805, these were removed from the list of capital offenses.

Other Developments. Colonies on the frontier varied in their handling of sex offenses. Throughout the nineteenth and into the twentieth centuries states developed laws superceding the original common law practices. As criminal codes evolved, sexual offenses were included. There was no movement to codify or handle sexual offenses separately. Some of the offenders might be found incompetent to stand trial or could plead insanity, as with any criminal indictment. Minors were handled through juvenile court processes as sexual delinquents, once these courts were established.

The first state law to be upheld as constitutional was the 1939 Minnesota Psychopathic Personality Law. "Psychopathic personality" was "the existence in any person of such conditions of emotional instability, or impulsiveness of behavior, or lack of customary standards of good judgment, or failure to appreciate the consequences of his acts, or a combination of such conditions as to render such a person irresponsible for his conduct with respect to sexual matters and thereby dangerous to other persons."[18] As defined, this is similar to a combination of irresistible impulse and the American Law Institute formulations of rules for insanity. However, such psychopathic personality statutes are not a substitution for an insanity defense applied to sexual crimes. Most startling about the Minnesota Law was the lack of any need for a criminal conviction for commitment since all that was required was to allege that an individual fulfilled the behavioral requirement for a "sexual psychopath." One forty-two-year-old married man with six children was committed by his wife as a sexual psychopath on the basis of his "uncontrollable craving for sexual intercourse and self-abuse," which was upheld by the State Supreme Court.[20]

PROBLEMS POSED

Community Concerns. The concerns that gave rise to such a legislative approach will be noted. Community anxiety about sex crimes with violent overtones, or those involving children, set the atmosphere for passage of such legislation. There is also great exposure by the public to brutal offenses from the mass media in the last forty years. It appears that sexual legislation, like most other legislation, attempts to appease many conflicting interests. The attempt to define a psychopathic personality legally is an example. In one sense the hope is for public protection from the behavior of sexually disturbed individuals who would presumably be treated while confined. Pessimism about the deterring effects of incarceration per se gave way to complications attendant upon inadequate or ineffective treatment. An unjustified optimism was seen in views that psychiatry could identify and predict who would behave in a sexually dangerous manner.

The assumption of treatment availability by-passed many complex problems. Myriad forms of sexual maldevelopment and associated conflicts exist. Methodological handicaps which permeate much of the research in this area make conclusions about treatment tentative. Studies done on those in detention, the difficulty in determining who is handled as a sexual delinquent in contrast to ignoring this behavior due to some other offense (such as robbery), social class variations, the zealotry associated with certain treatment programs, short-term follow-ups with little overall personality assessment, make what is a seemingly simple approach to sexual psychopathy a cure that may be worse than the disease.

Conflict occurs, on theoretical levels and in administrative decisions in dealing with the sexual psychopath. Consider a statute providing that anyone convicted of a certain sex crime, such as rape, aggravated rape, sodomy, sexual intercourse with a child, indecent liberties, or incest, should have a pre-sentence social, physical, and mental examination.

The examination may recommend various possibilities, few of

which are likely to be carried out with any aplomb. If no treatment is recommended, he is sentenced on the criminal charge for which he was convicted; if some type of specialized treatment (usually unspecified) is recommended, other options are presented: placement on probation for in-patient or out-patient treatment under the control and supervision of some state agency, such as a welfare department, or commitment of the defendant to a facility for sex deviates are two possibilities.

Debatable Questions. Questions arise: Does the defendant have the right to contest the findings of an examiner that he be committed as a sex psychopath? One case held that to be classified on the basis of an uncontestable and unanswerable determination by a welfare department was a violation of due process.[21] In one case, not only was the defendant held to have the right to a hearing on the matter with examiners being cross-examined, but also the right to an examination by a doctor or psychiatrist of his own choosing and the right to counsel.

Other questions pertain to clinical evaluation. What types of qualifications should be expected of examiners? Does any type of mental health personnel suffice? Need the examiner be a psychiatrist? Should a juvenile, who is to be handled as a sexual offender, be entitled to an examination by a child psychiatrist? Do trainees in teaching centers suffice?

> In one case a fourteen-year-old who had strangled a much younger child in a fit of homosexual frenzy was certified to adult court and routinely evaluated at a facility dealing with adult offenders. The evaluation consisted of conclusionary answers to competency and responsibility questions related to a homicide indictment with no appraisal of the sexual conflicts.

What are the bases for recommendations? Are the recommendations that an individual be handled as a sex offender based primarily on the independent variable that he has been convicted of an offense labelled as a sex offense, or has there been an additional independent basis for determination of why he should be handled other than as a convicted criminal and sentenced accordingly? To what extent have issues of treatability been explored? What type of treatment will be available in an institution? Has the issue of dangerousness actually been dispositive in terms of a recommendation that an individual be committed as a sex offender? How reliable are statements predicting dangerousness?

Other questions concern policy with respect to administrative practices. To what extent should decisions regarding disposition of convicted of sex offenders be handled by administrative machinery whose workings remain largely invisible, i.e., not brought out clearly for argument and dispute? To what extent should be public, via the judicial system interfere in the workings of departments of welfare or corrections? The risk of public involvement is that correctional facilities may become subject to greater public pressure. They can be criticized as being too permissive or soft on sex offenders, as well as required to justify less-publicized—and frequently harsh—practices. Should legislatures spell out the criteria to be followed for the requirements for the commitment of sex offenders? Or should this be left to the idiosyncrasies of personnel working in hospitals, clinics, and correctional facilities— subject to a case-by-case determination? Who should determine what treatment, how much of it, and who is entitled to give it?

Should the clinician be confined to giving an opinion about whether a certain defendant is dangerous, or should he in addition determine the criteria of dangerousness to be employed? For example, exhibiting oneself might be viewed as dangerous to the public in a social or moral sense, but not in a psychological sense. Is "dangerous" to be viewed as a clinical or a non-clinical concept? Is there any validity to the concept, "sexually dangerous"? Is the combined legal and psychiatric machinery for handling those alleged to be sexually dangerous merely an aborted form of preventive detention? To what extent are concepts of criminal responsibility infused into decisions for the determination of sexual psychopathy, such as a finding that at the time of committing a rape a person would not have been able to act otherwise, or that the act was the product of his sexual psychopathy? If such criteria are used by clinicians and administrators, are they bypassing the insanity defense at the trial level and using these rules of responsibility as a means of deciding between prison or a security hospital? What are the criteria which will determine eventual parole or release? Are many of the decisions being made primarily on a level of countertransference judgments?

SPECIAL PROBLEMS OF DISPOSITION AND TREATMENT

Problems in Application. What are some of the problems in applying such a special mechanism for dealing with individuals whose sexual behavior violates criminal statutes? At present more than half of our states have sexual psychopathic statutes. Some define a *sexual psychopath* broadly as someone unable to control his sexual impulses or as having propensities to commit a sexual crime.[22] A glaring problem from such statutes is the meaning of sexual psychopath. Although legislatures may use words any way they please, the multiple goals sought by such legislation lead to pseudo-psychiatric nomenclature. Since no psychiatric diagnosis of sexual psychopath is equivalent to those from other professions or disciplines legislative definition must interpret it the best way they can. Most frequent is a definition of sexual psychopathy based on the commission or conviction of a certain offense specified as a sex offense, such as rape, sodomy, etc.

Missing in this approach is a set of independent diagnostic criteria which would permit clinicians or courts to decide whether someone should be subject to special handling as a sexual offender. In effect a dilemma is created. Either it is assumed that the factual occurrence of a given sexual transgression makes one a sexual offender by definition, thereby making an independent appraisal by any standards redundant, or the meaning of the concept is so vague and subject to idiosyncratic interpretation that disposition becomes arbitrary. It is reckless to identify what a statute specifies as a sexual offense as indicative of disturbed sexuality in a clinical sense. The varieties of conflicts and developmental phenomena that may give rise to homosexual acts illustrate this discrepancy. Conversely, it is not valid to equate the existence of sexual psychopathy in a population as equivalent to a group of adjudicated sex offenders. In fact, the discrepancy between these two groups promotes a feeling of injustice.

Some hope that the severely disturbed who commit sexual offenses will qualify as legally insane. If the aberration has involved sexually offending behavior, the category of criminal insanity should not to be superseded. A schizophrenic adolescent who kills while raping would be an example. However, the converse is specifically excluded as well, i.e., sexual psychopathy is not to be taken as negating criminal responsibility. This is seen in jurisdictions where sexual psychopaths civilly committed to a hospital upon discharge stand trial for the criminal offense. In some jurisdictions, once a finding of guilt for a sexual offense is made, and psychiatric treatment recommended, the offender is sentenced to a treating hospital. Any given sexual act raises the necessity for differential diagnoses varying from neurotic conflict, psychosis, a reactive response in a crisis situation, multiple developmental arrests, and conflicts.

Another group is composed of those who have had a mode of sexual behavior heavily reinforced so that it has become the preferred manner of sexual life. Contributing factors of mental retardation or organic brain syndromes are excluded. The closest approach in psychiatric terms to a sexual psychopath might be someone categorized as a general sociopath in which the criteria in terms of asocialization and impulse control have taken on a specific form pertaining to sexual impulsivity. However, this is again to be distinguished from the random predatory activity of the sociopath whose exploitations are not confined to sex, although an act of impulsivity specifically involving sex may result in his classification as a sexual offender.

It is deceptive to believe that much has been accomplished by holding sexual psychopathy is a restricted form of psychopathy pertaining to sexual behavior. This merely the problem back one step to the unresolved basis for the development of psychopathy in general about which vociferous arguments continue. Problems arise such as a need to explain individual variations from peeping Toms to sadistic sexual murderers, both having prominent psychopathic trends. Few clinicians would be willing to conflate these categories diagnostically, and an even worse sin is to fuse them for treatment.

Special Studies. Ellis and Brancale studied 500 convicted sex offenders in New Jersey.[23] The first 300 examined revealed only 3 percent with a diagnosis of sexual psychopathy. The remainder was spread out as follows: 35 percent severely neurotic; 29 percent mildly neurotic; 14 percent psychologically normal; 8 percent borderline psychotic; 2 percent psychotic; 5 percent brain-injured; and 4 percent mentally deficient. The investigators then shifted from diagnosis in an attempt to predict who would continue to commit dangerous acts. They concluded that sex offenders who use force and duress may not be the ones who need help most, nor are they necessarily "sexually deviant." Those who committed minor legal offenses were more often severely disturbed. Without clinical intervention they were seen as more likely to get into serious trouble.

Other studies use varying criteria for dangerousness with different types of follow-ups. It is extremely difficult to generalize on the incidence of dangerousness and who is most likely to be included in such a category. This question has serious consequences in some cases and illustrates how complex outcome predictions can be.

At thirteen years a pattern of exhibitionism caused little concern to one boy's family since it seemed harmless. Occasionally a neighbor would complain, which led to an adaptation of moving to different neighborhoods. The pattern was to stand in a clump of bushes and as a woman—of no particular age—passed, to expose himself. At age sixteen, an eight-year-old girl rode by his concealed location on her bicycle. For the first time in hundreds of exposures, he ran out, knocked the girl off her bicycle, hit her several times, dragged her into the bushes, and removed her underpants. After a period of prolonged staring at her genitals, during which he lost his erection, he left without acting further.

A study at Sing-Sing prison evaluated those convicted of serious sexual offenses, such as rape, sodomy, carnal abuse of minors, and assault with intent to commit these offenses.[24] Although every one of 102 inmates studied evidenced some type of mental or emotional disorder, they were not viewed originally as sufficiently psychotic to be committed as mentally ill. Although none of the men examined before trial or sentencing were diagnosed as psychotic, on admission to prison four were found overtly psychotic and one mentally retarded. More significant was the failure to find more than a few superficial diagnostic characteristics of the psychopath although most of them had been given this diagnosis. Utilizing Cleckley's sixteen characteristics of the psychopathic personality, they found only five present in these sex offenders. In four of the five (pathological egocentricity and incapacity for love, poverty and major affective reactions, unresponsiveness in general interpersonal relations, and a sex life that was impersonal, trivial, and poorly integrated) the common denominator was a disturbance in affective capacity. Impoverished emotional relationships and withdrawal were an integral part of this personality picture. Rarely did the sex offender have a complete disintegration which persisted. Rather, a facade of external normality was maintained which was mistaken for psychopathy when a sex offense was committed. Rather than viewing them as psychopaths in the sexual realm, they were appraised diagnostically along a continuum of schizotypic personality organization, with a few presenting more overt, demonstrable schizophrenic psychoses.

Relevance of Diagnostic Studies. These diagnostic problems are relevant to several issues. Proceedings in different states to determine whether an individual is a sexual psychopath come at two main points: (a) prior to the conviction of a given criminal offense, or (b) at a post-conviction level either for a specific sex crime or some criminal offense. The former may require that an alleged offender be charged with some crime or a sex crime, or only that a county attorney—if he is satisfied good cause exists—prepare a petition alleging a man is a psychopath. These suffice to initiate the machinery for subsequent commitment as a sexual psychopath. At that point there is usually provision for an examination. Some jurisdictions merely specify a medical examination while others request a mental examination. In no jurisdictions are professional qualifications as to the examiner set forth beyond such phrases as *qualified*, referring to medical licensure for some. Illinois appears to be the most specific in precisely stating that a qualified psychiatrist be a "reputable physician who has specialized in the diagnosis and treatment of mental and nervous disorders."[25] Some states specify the examination be done in one of the mental hospitals maintained by the state or by the staff of a state public health department. The report is subsequently returned to the referring court. As indicated above, questions arise as to the mandatory acceptance by courts of the findings of a state agency that someone is a sexual psychopath.

Other rights, such as presentation of evidence, subpoenaing witnesses, cross-examination of lay and medical witnesses, right to counsel, jury trial, and appeal, varies from state to state. The question of a psychiatric examination by a psychiatrist of one's own choosing is of great personal, psychiatric, and legal significance, and will probably become even more so. This is most important when juveniles are being appraised for behavior which is allegedly deviant sexually—be it in a juvenile or adult court. The routine examination often done with adults is most inappropriate in the assessment of an adolescent, and the disposition made may have serious and adverse consequences for the individual and society. Ten states make no provision for a hearing.[26] A finding of sexual psychopathy results either in an order for out-patient treatment, or what is held to be a civil commitment which results in an indeterminate confinement in some type of state hospital, or a special unit of a state penitentiary designated as a treatment unit.

Constitutional Questions. Attacks have been made on these commitment processes, based on the contention that such statutes deny due process and equal protection of the laws under the Fourteenth Amendment to the Constitution, and that they result in cruel and unusual punishment under the Eighth Amendment. Other allegations are that the right to jury trial is impaired, as well as privilege against self-incrimination if a person cooperates in a medical examination which may lead to an opinion that he is a sex offender and in need of segregated handling for the treatment the state offers. A refusal to cooperate in the medical examination raises the danger of contempt of court.

Courts have not usually found the statutes unconstitutional. One exception was a 1938 Michigan statute which required an examination of a person convicted of a sex offense prior to his release from a penal institution.[27] If he was found to be a sexual deviate, he would be hospitalized instead of released from prison. The court felt this exercise of the police power to keep a person confined was not a civil proceeding, and was therefore unconstitutional. However, the next year the Minnesota statute referred to above was passed and held constitutional by the United States Supreme Court in 1940. That paved the way for succeeding states to develop such legislation.[28] This key case held that provisions of the statute for determination of a psychopathic personality were not too vague to be held unconstitutional, and that the standard of required proof of a habitual course of sexual misconduct with a lack of power to control sexual impulses which was likely to lead to "injury, loss, pain, or other evil on the objects of their uncontrollable desire," was sufficient. Alabama's sexual psychopath law was declared unconstitutional since commitment was not in lieu of a sentence for a conviction which could also be carried out.[29]

Clinical Problems. Diagnostic confusion about the sexual psychopath is relevant to constitutional attacks made on these statutes. Are due process and equal protection being violated if improper or inadequate classifications of behavior are being employed for dispositions based on the assumption that an individual will receive treatment? Concepts employed in the statutes are largely meaningless by medical or legal criteria. Looseness of the classification system results in discretion being permitted to judges, juries, examining physicians, and administrative bodies to classify someone as a sexual psychopath based on all manner of subjective moral, social, cultural, and accidental factors not clearly articulated. The problem is not only a failure to diagnose by a standardized set of signs and symptoms, but the lumping of a heterogeneous group of problems together. The infusion of questions of social dangerousness as the determinative motivation further contributes to issues becoming clouded, since if this becomes one governing principle—cloaked under a guise of treatment—a form of disguised preventive detention is being practiced which itself is not being appraised for its effectiveness. If it is in fact the dangerous sexual psychopath for whom confinement is desired, the issue should be directly faced.

Clinical approaches can only point out the difficulties of making predictions and their lack of reliable base rates which need correlation with many variables, such as the type of behavior, developmental fixations, socio-economic factors, intelligence, and so on. A statement that "dangerousness" is being used as a social policy cannot ultimately escape the question of whether the concept has any predictive reliability. Balancing of social values occurs in the application of all statutes. In the sexual realm this is seen in problems such as evaluating whether a compulsive voyeur creates a sufficient degree of public annoyance that he should be indeterminately confined in an institution. Does an offense such as sodomy, defined by statute as carnally knowing any person by the anus or mouth, lead to the possibility of abuse of the law? Should sodomous behavior be considered evidence of psychopathy in and of itself, or only if the behavior is coercively imposed on another?

Should sexual intercourse with a child under eighteen be considered sexual psychopathy? What if the sexual development of a fourteen-year-old girl places her in the category of an eighteen-year-old girl? Should indecent liberties with one not his spouse be so labelled when the phrase is left vague and undefined? What about the situation where an adult female is charged with sexual activities with minor males? This is the equivalent of statutory rape on an underage female applied to underage males and adult females. A Michigan statute prohibiting females over fifteen from inducing a boy under fifteen to engage in intercourse was construed as requiring actual knowledge that the boy is under the statutory age.[30] Should proven incest be handled by labelling the perpetrator as a sexual offender from what is known of the family psychopathology in these cases? Although we have come a long way since colonial Massachusetts required the lifelong wearing of an "I," we still appear to handle these cases in psychologically and socially unwise ways.

One position is that there is no reason to dispose of sexual offenders differently from those convicted of any criminal offense. In practice this is what results anyhow, since sexual-offender provisions are not used nearly as frequently as they might be. From the consequences of these procedures—and the largely unfulfilled promise of treatment—there is strong motivation to avoid their use. Some other type of charge may be preferred to avoid a sexual offense (such as simple assault or vagrancy for minor offenses, and aggravated assault instead of aggravated rape). Other dispositions, such as incompetency for trial or civil commitment, are options. The argument is that a sex offender should have the right to be treated like any other offender, and that criteria to distinguish him from other criminals are insufficient and unreasonable. A classification of *arsonist psychopaths* or *stealing psychopaths*, with separate dispositional procedures for each, is seen as equivalent to the procedures for *sexual psychopaths*.

Motivations which become involved in sexual activities are almost endless. They depend upon biological variables and psychosocial-sexual development. Manifest needs for material conquest and advantage, securing financial advantage, gaining vocational promotion, obtaining revenge, seeking pity, providing relief for anxiety, expiatory or restitutive acts, may all serve sexual needs. A possibility permits these needs to be handled in sexualized activities which are seen as having perverse elements. While some of these are illegal, the great majority are not. Pregenital components persist in some personalities and need not necessarily interfere with an otherwise satisfactory ability to perform sexually. Whether the need to handle sexual impulses partially in these diverse ways tapers the degree of sexual gratification is another matter.[31]

Problems from Special Categorizing. It is often held that the only valid justification for singling out a group of offenders as "sexual" is for treatment purposes. To argue that it is primarily to protect society from dangerous people, or to practice a form of preventive detention, raises serious constitutional questions as well as concern for those committed. Right and adequacy of treatment for patients civilly committed as mentally ill, and for those held after a successful plea of not guilty by reason of insanity, have relevance for those detained as sexual offenders. Distinguishing a confinement process that is treatment oriented from one whose de facto operation is custodial, or penal, may be extremely difficult. Maintenance of an individual in an institution which is basically a security facility for people considered dangerous with perfunctory rehabilitative measures hardly meets medical, ethical, or legal norms for treatment. Constitutional arguments are relevant if detailed examination and testimony on the facilities, staff, and number of inmates are examined. This is even more so when a statute creates a right to treatment for persons incarcerated under a state's sex-offender statute, as in New York.[32] The same holds for commitments of sexual psychopaths when no treatment facilities are provided, which invalidates the commitment although not the statute.[33]

In states where adjudication of a sexual psychopath is possible
without conviction of a crime, it would be difficult to justify
detention on a penal basis since no crime has been committed. But
detention for treatment is also difficult to justify if it is inadequate or
unavailable. We are forced back to issues of potential dangerousness
or preventive detention. An individual committed as a sexual
psychopath to a hospital for the criminally insane who continues to
deny his guilt and proves recalcitrant to treatment cannot
justifiably be transferred to a prison to make him more amenable to
treatment.[34] Such processes result in imprisonment without conviction. For juveniles not certified to adult courts, there are rarely
separate institutions maintained for sexual delinquents. This
means that adolescents are handled in the mainstream with all
other delinquents. The solution is a treatment predicated upon the
types of conflicts and stresses that exist for a given individual, and
not the facade of special handling as a sexual psychopath, or
lumping offenders with other delinquents to receive whatever
treatment is in vogue at a particular time.

RELEASE

When to Release.   Release is obtained on different bases. Legal
questions pertaining to evidentiary or procedural questions, which
can form a basis for appeal, rehearing, or release, are one basis. The
indeterminate nature of the commitment process, for sex offenders,
accentuates efforts for those with knowledge, determination, or
resources to secure release. Questions pertain to when such terms as
"cured," "fully cured and not dangerous," or "no menace to society"
are satisfied. These are used on the erroneous assumption that
problems of sexual perversion are analogous to physical illness.
Although surgical treatments (such as castration), or surgical
procedures to transform the external genitalia on transsexuals, may
give the impression of a set of medical procedures which are
available, for most cases this treatment model is misleading.

For the overwhelming number of sexual offenders no such
procedures are available. The dilemma is that criteria to permit
discharge are predicated upon institutional personnel being willing
to state that an individual is cured or no longer dangerous. The
clinical judgment for discharge is based on a series of factors, often
poorly articulated, that the individual will not repeat the behavior
which resulted in his incarceration. Development of adequate norms
for discharge based on different treatments, different treaters, as

well as combinations of treatments for different problems, the frequency of such behaviors, utilization of behavior under certain environmental precipitants, differences which occur when out of a corrective institution, would be needed to meet any semblance of objective release standards. This is attained for very few.

Is There A Special Treatment? Some propose that only those who could benefit from treatment should be committed as sexual psychopaths. However, this presupposes a greater degree of knowledge about these conditions, as well as therapeutic efficacy, than we possess even under optimal conditions. Few contemporary facilities would qualify, even by minimum objective standards, as treatment institutions as now constituted. If this is the situation, there is little justification for using sexual psychopath statutes in preference to other procedures which involve the use of probation, probation plus treatment, criminal sentence, or regular civil commitment, and for a few, disposition by way of insanity pleadings.

It does not help to limit sexual offender statutes to the sexually dangerous. This solution raises all the same unresolved questions concerning dangerousness that are present with other types of behavior, such as aggressive outbursts or recidivism. Problems of determining dangerousness for those called "mentally ill and dangerous" or those legally insane raise analogous issues. While court estimates as to dangerousness function as the operational criteria for detaining many individuals, this practice is loaded with personal, psychiatric, and legal handicaps. We do not have techniques or devices to tell us which sexual offenders will be dangerous, even if the term is defined in terms of recidivism. However, most of the time the standard and its application remain vague, perhaps intentionally so from the multiple motives and goals operating. In order to develop accurate base rates for the prediction of dangerousness a convicted rapist would have to be released without confinement. Subtypes might be needed to correspond to types of acting out rapists. Since such is not likely to occur, individuals will continue to be handled by educated guesses at best, and on some occasions by a continued presumption of dangerousness on the basis that an act once occurred.

SEXUAL OFFENSES AMONG JUVENILES

General Theory. There is a partial coalescence between sexual offenses committed by adolescents and the various nosological entities assessed by clinicians. The major types of sexual conflicts among adolescents are seen in terms of developmental antecedents and meaning. This requires a general theory of the development of the diathesis toward sexual perversions. Without this, one is unable to progress beyond recounting and classifying what the performed acts have been. We are then confined to the level of description performed by Krafft-Ebing and Havelock Ellis at the turn of the century.[35] [36] Caution is needed for the wide variation among individuals in sexual behavior, particularly during adolescence. Not only are there cultural differences, but inter-individual and intra-individual differences. The major contributions of descriptive studies by Kinsey, and more recent physiological work of Masters and Johnson, are the recognition of widespread differences in sexual behavior and ways of obtaining sexual gratification.

The ultimate connection between childhood and adult sexuality is seen in the viewpoint that perversion represents the persistence beyond childhood of earlier or infantile sexuality. "Preferred" is the key word, since transient elements of perversity exist, and under conducive circumstances they may become dominant. Situations in schools where students are of one sex during adolescence, or similar situations in correctional facilities, are examples. The pattern of development during adolescence is crucial for during this transitional period we begin to witness the emergence and solidification of certain patterns of sexual activity and object choices.

Habitual patterns may not phase out. Perverse sexual development then becomes, by definition, the persistence into adult life of these elements of childhood sexuality. It is a failure of polymorphous perverse elements to undergo transition and to be subsumed under the striving for a heterosexual object with coitus the goal. This does not imply a teleological explanation based on non-heterosexual activities being perverse by reason of their adverse effect on reproduction and family life. It is rather an explanation of the psychological development of the individual in which psychopathology is defined in terms of two hallmarks: the habitual or repetitive quality of certain behaviors, and tendencies to replace a tender relationship involving sex with a member of the opposite sex with some other activity.

Neither historical inquiry into civilization's past, nor developmental inquiry into individual pasts, can hold the position that only a life of heterosexual coital activity can sustain a civilization or the development of an individual. Civilizations giving rein to sexual expressions of diverse types have attained great intellectual or artistic achievement. This is also true for individuals, regardless of their sexual choices and activities, unless this is part of a regressive and chaotic clinical picture. Multiple functions are served by sexuality. The unanswerable elements of the psychosexual stages that remain involved in sexual activity permit many earlier experiences to persist. The primacy of seeking a discharge experience cannot be totally superseded by seeking a relationship with another based on tenderness. This lends insight into certain patterns of sexual behavior, labelled perverse by some, and existing without impairment of other ego functions. Eissler hypothesized an ego function of sexual discharge which would permit an impairment in this function but not necessarily in others. [37]

In contrast to insights about sexual development and deviation with sexuality seen as an antecedent for most psychological development, it can be viewed as a significant antecedent. The theoretical difference is that implied by human development as more complex than just instinctual unfolding. It is the theoretical position of ego development as relatively independent, and not just a consequence of sexual development. Hartmann, among others, emphasized not only the importance of aggression, but the independent functions of the ego as well. [38] What also results is a viewpoint of human development more complex than that defined primarily in terms of a certain object relationships—the heterosexual—and the coital activity performed with this object. Superego components need consideration, as do psychosocial components, and the role of aggression. The concept of genital primacy as a criterion for normal sexuality does not have meaning unless it is considered in the light of these other factors. As an example, consider the impact on sexual functioning of identity problems during adolescence and subsequent stages when a narcissistic threat may arise. [39]

The existence of sexual feelings in parts of the body provides the groundwork for diverse sexual activities. While there are specifically erogenous zones, such as the mouth and genital organs, there is also the potential for almost any part of the body to become erotized in association with learning experiences. This is particularly so for experiences which are gratifying, and hence provide impulse gratification but at the same time give reassurances against anxiety or other types of painful affect. This is, in essence, a security device which builds in a double reinforcing effect that makes change difficult. The zone of erogenous interest does not disappear, but continues along with other zones that emerge.

What results are fixations in two dimensions: method and object. Fixation as to method leads to actions to obtain gratification or security, such as sucking. Fixation as to object refers to the vehicle that is used for gratification, such as a member of the same sex or a younger child. During adolescence, when elements of childhood sexuality are phasing into adult heterosexual methods and objects, the possibility exists for the transformation not to occur or for earlier patterns to reemerge by way of regression. Rather than defensive operations of the ego creating a neurosis, some perversions are closer to direct expression of infantile sexuality in certain modes. This is what is meant when reference is made to perversion formation being essentially an id phenomenon. This corresponds to other aspects of adolescence which also my be id-dominated.

It is fallacious assume that sexual development which tends toward perversion is characterized by the absence of ego involvement. Not only is there an involvement in the sense of defenses, but a certain ego deformation is associated with the ontogenesis of perversion. It is vivid in youths in which all manner of defenses are employed against sexual strivings. This was discovered early when certain sado-masochistic fantasies were unravelled and seen to be a defense against oedipal conflicts.[40] Developmental techniques to deal with anxieties—castration and otherwise—were also understood to operate with neuroses and perversions. Glover once suggested that perversions were a developmental series reflecting stages of overcoming anxiety about eh body or external objects.[41] Perversions were seen on the level of primitive defenses on an introjective-projective level, related to the maintenance of a sense of reality. Hence, perversions could be related to psychoses as well.

Clinical observations reveal that not only do neurotic symptom-pictures exist in some who have perverse symptoms, but intermittent alternations occur. Hence, there is no sharp dichotomy between the two, but rather a difference in the degree to which a wishful fantasy might be acceptable to the ego. While in neuroses the wishes are unacceptable and internalized conflict results in neurotic symptom formation, in perversions the wish is more acceptable and hence ego syntonic. The difference in ego acceptability is what makes the difference. For perversion formation a particular component of infantile sexuality remains visible and unrepressed, while a greater amount of infantile sexuality stays repressed.[42] This is then a pars pro toto operation.

Added to these factors are insights related to superego functioning dealing with the ramifications of guilt. While the neurotic struggles and devises ways to handle guilt, perversions also must do so. Insights into the role of ego and superego functioning have been extended in terms of parental conflicts regarding sexuality that could emerge in the form of perversion expression during adolescence. This might be by way of chronic exposure during the developmental years through modeling and identification processes. In other situations the adolescent becomes the vehicle for the expression of the unconscious perverse desires of the parents. Parental pleasure is experienced in patterns such as leniency, mixed with occasional exaggerated outbursts of condemnation, regarding the perverse activities of the child.[43] These parental conflicts are transmitted and internalized as part of the superego of the adolescent whose parentally influenced superego permits such development to take place. Not only does this permit the behavior to emerge, but it allows it to do so with a tolerable amount of anxiety or guilt.

Specific Syndromes: Homosexuality. Homosexuality is the behavior which receives most publicity both among and about adolescents. If we exclude autoerotic practices like masturbation, it is the most prevalent sexual behavior causing concern to the adolescent and others in terms of quantitative incidence. Homosexual behavior will be used as a paradigm for describing the developmental approach to sexual activities in the adolescent.

Uncertainty permeates attempts to define who should be included within any grouping of perversity among adolescents. This is especially so in discussing homosexual activity or sexual activity not involving physically assaultive behavior on others. There is an inherent uncertainty as to when a set of behaviors can be considered a preferred mode of sexual activity. Couple with this the potential reversibility of what may be preferred activities during the whole of adolescence.

Attempts to predict adult personality characteristics from those in childhood present even more difficult problems when adult sexual behavior is predicted on the basis of *adolescent* sexual behavior. Throughout childhood various attachments and intense relationships have taken place with people of both sexes. Even apart from the theory of bisexuality, these relationships are based more on function than anything else. Included are a host of cognitive-affective components. The young child has usually undergone homosexual attachments by virtue of relationships based on intense emotionality. In most there has not been the availability of a specific genital gratification. During the intense love-life of the oedipal period, many positive and negative strivings exert a lasting influence. All of the following have been hypothesized as operating influences which foreshadow the future sexual inclinations of an individual:[44] sex-role identity of the parents, identification processes, fixations to sadistic or aggressive trends, tendencies to passivity, or fears of anal rape. While a heavy emphasis was placed upon the triangular relationships of the phallic oedipal period, recent work has emphasized pre-oedipal components which contribute to perverse development. These take on significance not only for sexual development, but for general personality traits.

When the post-oedipal period ensues, there is a return to attachments based on a seeming indifference to the sex of the attachee. Again, personality variables such as warmth, criticism, dependency gratification, guilt-inducement, anxiety-alleviating patterns—regardless of sex—predominate and elicit patterns of attachment or rejection.

The normal pattern is accepted in terms of boys preferring male companions and saying so, and only a jokester refers to this as implying homosexual trends. Only in cases of neurotically conflicted children is there concern about their continuing to seek out relationships with children of the opposite sex during the latency period. For girls, the preference for boys comes into the tomboy classification, and is based on components such as envy rather than wishes for a heterosexual relationship. With the onset of preadolescence, a plethora of diverse homosexual manifestations may ensue which include fantasies, voyeuristic and exhibitionistic trends, intense attachments, mutual masturbation within a peer group, and sometimes overt homosexual relationships with older members of the same sex.

The narcissistic bases for these choices have been discussed elsewhere. Components of the idealized self are involved, which the young adolescent loves, as well as regressive backing from heterosexual opportunities. Whatever particular basis exists for homosexual development in a given case, we can never say beforehand, with any degree of certainty, whether or not it will occur. Many outcomes are possible from a given set of childhood factors which appear significant in retrospect when dealing with a confirmed, adult homosexual. The reason is that an enormous number of variables intervene over the course of development, especially during adolescence when we are talking of sexual deviation, and these alter a given sexual object or activity.

The following have all been considered as independent variables favoring homosexual development:

1. Individual variation in genetic or constitutional tendencies toward a bisexual orientation, or toward sex of opposite gender
2. Narcissistic factors leading to object choices in self-image
3. Fixations in the oral or anal stages
4. Phallic overestimation which dominates love relationships to possess the highly desired object, and/or possess someone with desired attributes
5. Extreme dependency on either parent, which is a generalized personality attribute of dependency
6. Hostility to a parent
7. The impact of traumatic experiences, such as excessive and easily provoked sexual stimulation from adults in the course of development (in some cases this takes the form of great fear in the boy of the female genitals)
8. Envy of the female body
9. Intense sibling jealousy which is handled by developing love relationships with sibling substitutes in the future, and
10. A pattern of homosexual experiences which are repetitively reinforced once puberty has commenced

Having emphasized the postdictive nature of reconstructions which assign causal significance, and our weak predictive capacity even from known childhood situations, there are, nevertheless, some behaviors in adolescence which raise clinical concern about which direction development is taking:[45]

1. One is the emergence and continuance of homosexual behavior which occurs with comparatively little anxiety or guilt. When this occurs, with the addition of periodic excursions to polymorphous activities coupled with minimal anxiety, it raises the probability for a given pathway being chosen.

2. Absence of masturbation, or its delayed onset, especially without fantasies, may be a sign of conflict. While this may portend a course of development leading toward perverse preferences, it is seen in those with massive sexual inhibitions or schizotypic conflicts as well. Many fantasies have a theme of personal degradation or contain the malign influence or control of another in fantasy who may excrete, tie up, beat, or subject the fantasizer to experiences where control over aggression is lost or someone is

forced to be cruel. In some, minor acts of cruelty are elicited from others while inflicted upon the self, such as structuring situations of rebuff or asking friends to touch the dreamer with lit matches or pins. Self-pity permeates fantasies of overtly structured situations.

3. Strong feminine identifications which persist throughout adolescence, coupled with the absence of exposure to triangular oedipal relationships from an absent or withdrawing father, lend another weighting to what may be a difficulty in forming heterosexual attachments. The absence of an effective male figure, coupled with a female who is domineering, punitive, and harsh in her maternal attributes, creates a doubly damaging situation. In the absence of previous oedipal strivings—or if an abandonment of such struggles has taken place—there is an established pattern of retreat into isolation, sexual abstinence, or perversion. Not having mastered earlier conflicts involving sexuality, the temptation to maintain early and constricted life patterns is tempting.

4. Heterosexual fears may inhibit taking the risk for such activities. At least in the American middle-class culture, heterosexual taboos have been greater than homosexual ones.[46] These fears may be the result of anxieties about the opposite sex which involve genital fears or the fears of a castrating personality. Once adolescence arrives, there may be little conscious desire for any sexual experiences. This is latent homosexuality in a strict sense, defined as an absence of desire for sexual activity. In this land of sexual absence, sexuality is confined to nocturnal emissions during sleep or an occasional dream with a disguised sexual theme, often with a fearful content.

5. A deep and persistent attachment to an older person of the same sex, which is beyond the transiency of a crush and has taken on the coloration of exclusivity associated with a love relationship, is an adverse prognostic sign. Ramifications of this type of adolescent socialization go far beyond the realm of sexuality, with the consequent impairment this has for heterosexual development. An intense relationship with an adult of the same sex is seen as a regression to an object toward which the adult originally had a tie based on homosexual feelings.[47]

6. An adolescent who presents with a sincere, conscious, and firm conviction that he or she is a homosexual should be taken seriously in terms of the solidification this may represent in sexual identity. Once this conviction is present, it may lead to a homosexual surrender in which the passive childhood desires toward an older person are given in to. While this of presenting complaint tells us

nothing about ontogenesis, it must be evaluated for the degree of ego-syntonicity that already may be present. *Boys* may use primitive defenses such as a general denial of their masculinity, or specifically the reality of their genitals. Dependency needs are revealed in incorporation fantasies, or the acting out of fellatio, which provides love and nourishment. Ego-splitting is seen in the confused identity of a boy who sometimes experiences himself as a male and sometimes as a female. If earlier patterns of massive denial have existed, the adolescent has actually made the full transition to an absence of feelings or identity that he is a male at all—the transsexual phenomenon. For *girls* the mechanism may take the form of an outright denial of any genital differences in the sexes. Milder versions have the girl avoiding the sight of the female body, if not being repulsed by it. Substitutive and symbolic fantasies are usually fully developed by adolescence, such as the girl's whole body being perceived not only as a narcissistic and beautiful thing, but as a precious phallus.[48] There may be hallucinatory episodes involving the possession of a penis. Projection of fears and hatred onto older women may take place with two frequently observed patterns: a repetition of themes of rejection and being left out by a cruel and rejecting mother-figure, or an overcompensatory obsequiousness and little-girlishness toward older women. Adolescent girls with deep attachments to their fathers, and aggression toward their mothers, may attempt to demonstrate their guiltlessness by way of homosexual attachments. This carries the meaning of, "See how uninterested I am in all men." For some, this may be a bid to the maternal object or other older women to continue a nurturing relationship.

Problems and Application of Legal Codes to Sexual Deviation. In view of the prevalence, concern, and confusion within communities and decision-making bodies about the sexual behaviors of juveniles, a brief digression into the problems arising when juveniles are alleged to have committed sexual offenses is important. An accusation gets them official recognition, in which a process of bestowing status occurs. Problems inherent in the vagueness attendant upon definitions of delinquency mean that juvenile delinquency may encompasses *anything* listed under adult offenses, in addition to what offends the current mores of the community as interpreted by its officials. While some statutes specify that delinquency involves violation by a minor of any federal or state law, violations of city and village ordinances are usually included as well. In more recent decades, provisions defining juveniles "in need of supervision" encompass the remainder of behaviors seen as incorrigible, unfit, or beyond the lawful control of parents or other lawful authority.[49] In some states there is merely a provision for delinquency to include a minor who so deports himself as to injure or endanger the morals or health of himself or others.[50]

This is the type of predicament which leads some to feel adolescents are being scapegoated for the sexual conflict and ambiguity present in adults. Apart from sexual behaviors involving the physical exploitation of another—adult or minor—few legal sanctions are applied to the sexual behavior of adults. Yet, despite this, adult authorities continue to re-enact a tableau of sexual morality where the adolescent is held accountable for sexual acts in a manner which no adult is. Adolescents are bound to the professed adult norms which adult society and courts have long in practice regarded as an empty set of rules.

Within this framework the adolescent is held accountable his sexual behavior based on different combinations of circumstances:[51]

1. The social visibility of the *offense* is one factor determining disposition. While few states enforce the provisions which make it a crime to encourage masturbation, juveniles engaged in group masturbation in a conspicuous manner may be chastised. The more exhibitionistic the behavior, the more likely the juvenile is to have sexual sanctions applied. Similarly, when fornication is performed privately and does not result in a pregnancy, or does not become involved in family patterns of conflict where there is a need to flaunt the behavior in front of parents, the behavior is likely to be ignored.

2. The social visibility of the *offender* is a second factor. An adolescent boy who persists in dressing like a girl, or who insists to all who will listen that he really is a girl, increases the probabilities of being officially handled as a sexually deviant delinquent. An official adjudication proffer solutions subject to even more vagaries than are property offenses.

3. The extent to which *behaviors* deviate from sex-typed standards further contributes to accountability. An effeminate adolescent boy who is a passive but willing participant in homosexual activity is more likely to incur legal sanctions than a mesomorph who is a local jock. On a family level, incest illustrates the deviation of several family members from the expected sex-typed role, which frequently brings condemnation to the juvenile alone. An interesting dilemma confronts the system of juvenile justice for sexual

activity in contemporary adolescent females, where the girl may be the active solicitor. This is contrary to the sex-typed behavior based on middle-class norms which in the past was seen as a justification for intervening and inculcating these norms into transgressing lower-class girls. However, when the middle-class girl herself adopts a norm of sexual behavior in which she is not a victim, but an aggressive seeker, even more severe sanctions may be applied since she is supposed to know better.

4. Related to sex-typed behaviors is the degree to which the boy is viewed as using sex for an *end in itself*. In contrast, a girl is supposed to use sex as a *means*, such as for achieving security or dependency gratification. While a group of teen-age boys who frequent a house of prostitution or use a girl for a gang-bang are not seen as sick or bad, the girl who uses a relationship for sexual pleasure may be condemned as both sick *and* bad.

5. The *further behavior deviates from the norm* of heterosexuality, the more likely it is to secure official condemnation. Certain acts, like oral sodomy, are less likely to incure official scrutiny if they have a heterosexual base rather than homosexual. Autoerotic practices with low visibility will similarly incur less wrath than those which take place with younger children or animals. It is a striking paradox that adolescent boys and girls manifesting such sexual trends are often sent to facilities which actually foster the behavior. The single-sex atmosphere of delinquent correctional facilities is well-known for fostering homosexual proclivities. These reinforcements cannot always be viewed as merely transitory experiences which disappear once the juvenile is released. A similar stricture applies to in-patient units or residential treatment facilities if the opportunity for heterosexual experiences is severely limited or restricted. This is even more impressive when discussions raise questions about the desirability for adults confined in penal institutions to have conjugal visits either in the institution or at home.[52] In contrast, juvenile socialization processes are not seen as requiring this even on the basis of heterosexual mingling.

Another point which needs examination is the extent to which multiple and extraneous factors determine to whom sanctions are applied. Especially is this so for the selective discrimination processes operating for sexual offenses among all ages. Resistance to this categorization is massive and determined by the five factors listed above. The fact is that no one really knows what the true incidence or prevalence for sexual offenses as a generic grouping, or even for specific sexual offenses of an aggressive type—such as aggravated rape—might be. If law enforcement were diligent, Kinsey estimated that 85 percent of the younger male population would be convicted as sexual offenders.[53]

Two fallacies are present throughout the mythology associated with sex offenses: the first is that adolescent girls are exploited and used and are therefore victims; the second is that adolescents who are involved in sexually offensive behavior are victims of the sexual aggressions of others, primarily adults. While the former myth seems to be yielding to the onslaught of the efforts of the liberated female adolescent herself, the latter can only yield to facts which demonstrate the high drive level of the adolescent himself regarding both aggression and sexuality. While quantitatively the majority of sexual acts involving adolescents—of a homosexual or heterosexual nature—are between those within a few years of age-range of each other, and while even those which involve a relationship with an older person are performed on the basis of each obtaining something from the other, the myth of exploitation continues. Of course, pedophilic behaviors *do* occur, in which an adolescent sexually molests a young child, and there are always some physically assaultive acts which are disposed of by incapacitating the juvenile. Relationships between adolescent males and adult male homosexuals have contractual quid pro quo. The adult receives sexual gratification based on his own needs, a preference for an adolescent male with the preferred activities of fellatio or masturbation. The young male receives his payment, usually a direct amount in cash, or being maintained economically like a mistress. To counter this argument requires resort to moral arguments about the corruptibility of such practices, such as adolescents not developing a sense of doing gainful work for money. This takes the argument far afield into interesting but nonresolvable questions about moral character. From a psychiatric standpoint, the question about factors that promote adolescent homosexuality have some validity in reinforcing this mode of sexual activity. For girls, the relationship with an older male is often one that has a mutual element. Short of a physically assaultive act, a sexual liaison serves diverse and overdetermined components in the life of the adolescent girl. A more firm attachment to an older male fulfills gratifications in terms of her own predisposing personality. To perceive this as a statutory rape for an adolescent girl often misses the psychological components.

In many situations if the attachment is transient, it often involves a family friend or relative. These types of contractual relationships for boys and girls come to the attention of the clinician, by way of other presenting complaints. These may be depressive symptoms, acting out not confined to the realm of sexuality, or psychophysiological problems. The relationship with an older person may have begun in their teens and been present for years with earlier conflicts remaining nascent. In some cases a lover's quarrel—homo- or heterosexual—precipitates an emotional crisis and brings the parties to the clinician's office or some mental health facility. Where an element of public disturbance is created through an argument or physical violence, the police, or juvenile and adult courts, may became involved, but these are a small percent of the cases.

It is not unusual for an ex post facto exploitative presentation to be attempted by one of the parties. The past relationship is then portrayed as one of victimization. Dramatic blow-ups seem to be one way of terminating these relationships in a manner analogous to the way some marriages utilize this as a step toward dissolution. Whatever approach is used (dismissal, referral, probation, or a fine for the adult) it is wisest not to pursue the matter further by remanding the juveniles to an institution. The juvenile will become more confused by such a solution in contrast to having options to begin anew in the community. Unless the adult has clearly been physically abusive, little is gained by his removal. By casting an adverse judgment on the cases that come before agencies or courts, the moral sense of the community is maintained as well as the community's sense of doing something.

Fetishism. As with homosexuality, the diagnosis of fetishism as a perversion should be made with great caution during adolescence. Fetishistic behaviors, using inanimate objects for sensory experiences of smell, taste, or sound, are transiently used as displaced objects of sexual excitement. Early theories of fetishism, regarded it primarily as a chance phenomenon, but were unable to go beyond this explanation. Binet in 1887 proposed such a theory.[54] The difficulty of explaining why some adolescents seem not only to be excited by certain sexual objects—much in the way that commercial advertising involving sex does—but why some begin to acquire a certain object as the sine qua non for sex release, was seen as a quantitative extension. Missing was the realization that many of these polymorphous activities continue to operate as excitants and forerunners, and for the adolescent they occupy a foremost place for a period.

Exactly how many who have a passing interest in some fetishistic article end up with it as the preferred sexual object is impossible to predict. The valid question for a longitudinal investigation is: "What are the conditions which favor the continuance of these trends?" Behavioral similarity in acts confuses two things. In some cases the fetish becomes a preferred object for sexual gratification instead of seeking genital union while for others the fetish becomes a defensive effort at mastery. Rather than a fetishistic object serving only one purpose as the sexual object, a variety of meanings and purposes may be attached to it. Theoretically, temporary fetishism serves different developmental meanings as well as structural ones in terms of id or ego. These differences have confused those not versed in clinical aspects of child psychiatry who confuse and label a transitional object as a fetish when its purposes are rather to achieve separation and object constancy. Developmentally, the same object may serve as something bearing the brunt of many tender and hateful feelings during the anal stage. During the phallic stage, it comes closer to a phallic representation. All of these are present when puberty commences, and no one knows to what extent they are antecedents for fetishistic behavior in adolescence or later perverse formation.

Clinical evidence about fetishism comes from two sources. One is based on *retrospective work with adult fetishists* in which they date the onset of their behavior to early adolescence. The behavior is often connected with what seems like a chance occurrence, such as sexual arousal upon seeing a mother or sister undressing, or observing their undergarments. What this misses is the cogency of why these always-available experiences take on significance at that *particular* time. In some cases an article, such as a shoe, a glove, a piece of hair, a sound or smell, take on fetishistic meaning.

What are the criteria for when a fetish is established in a perverse sense? One group considers the presence of one of the following three to suffice: (1) obtaining definite and reasonably strong sexual arousal from the fetish alone in terms of tumescence, (2) disregarding an attractive sexual partner who lacks the fetish in preference to an unattractive one who possesses the item, and (3) beginning a collection of fetishistic items.[55]

While all three of these may be present, the first two are vague. Many fetishistic items give rise to an erection for men which would meet the first criterion. The second is complicated by the subjective criterion of what is attractive. The third is significant when present, but not essential for fetishistic development.

Those who work directly with children provide a second source of clinical data about the development of fetishism. Apart from direct clinical observation utilizing knowledge of how children use fetishistic objects, adolescents present first-hand accounts during therapy.

> A fifteen-year-old reported he began to peek into the girls' locker room at his high school and become sexually excited. This continued as a pattern wherein he would peek and masturbate. When a janitor caught him and warned him, he stopped but then began to masturbate at home, using his mother's undergarments. This phase lasted only a few months, following which he became a 'fetish thief,' taking women's undergarments off clothes lines in a state of great sexual excitement. He would masturbate while holding garments and then discard them. What determined that this boy not confine his activities to voyeurism but switch to fetishistic thievery? The common pattern of an easily available object—such as his mother's undergarments—not sufficing is common. Nor did creating a collection of garments suffice, for a 'fresh start' was needed each time.

An intriguing aspect of fetishism is in its close relationship to the development of normal sexuality. Since a sexual choice based on nothing but a set of genitalia is insufficient, a pervasive displacement operates in what begins to make a love object appealing. While somatic factors operate, so do all of the elements associated with such things as clothes, smell, or sounds. In fetishism, a further split occurs between the body and its accouterments. The female body per se and coition with it recede as choices in preference to the accouterments.

Freud postulated that the genesis of this split was due to the inability of the boy to accept the anatomical differences between the sexes. The cognitive awareness of such a state induces a fear that this lack could happen to him. This was held to result in his having little attraction to such an object. By way of a fetishistic object, the boy masters his castration anxiety. Denial operates to negate the cognitive impression that the fetish was merely a symbolic equivalent for what the female lacked. Again, the question arises of whether or not to pursue a homosexual course of development, with an attraction to a male as germane, and this remains as a possibility. The fetish functions by way of a defensive split in the ego to deny what is perceived. Identification with females is pervasive in this course of development as it is with certain types of homosexuality and transvestism. With the boy teetering on the brink of fetishism for his sexual activity, there is both the fear of being a woman and identification with her, together with an effort to nullify it.

Sometimes the boy identifies himself with the phallic mother and sometimes with the nonphallic one, corresponding to the ego split.[56]

In some boys sado-masochistic trends come to the fore and are acted out:

> By age thirteen, a boy had become aware of the sexually stimulating aspects of his mother's undergarments, but he had done nothing about this except fantasize while he masturbated. An added step was the use of his mother's shoes as a sexual object during masturbation. This progressed to stealing women's shoes wherever and whenever he could find them and keeping them in a trunk under his bed. A dangerous twist was added by the age of sixteen, when he fantasized a need to keep women confined under his control. The essential element was that they were under his power and unable to leave. This fantasy began to be acted out. He had no desire to harm any of these girls physically, nor was genital activity attempted. Some were tied up while he talked to them gently. The essential was that girls be frightened of him while at the same time he masochistically identified with their helpless plight. In their state of helplessness he would ask them to remove their shoes and try on a pair which he provided. He would profusely apologize to the girl and tell her how sorry he was for what he had done. This boy had never heard of John Fowles' work, *The Collector*, at the time of his therapy.[57]

Boys who are acting out a sado-masochistic theme with a fetish may literally bind themselves with rope. For some this goes to the extent of a counterphobic simulation of hanging. In some cases the simulation becomes reality, and self-strangulation results. The fear of being harmed is coupled with the desire to harm. Hence, the object the boy has identified with is placed in a position of helplessness at the same time that it is treated gently and comforted. But it is even safer for all concerned in such a predicament to use an inanimate object. The danger is when the maintenance of the displacement breaks down and the shoe must be tried to see if it fits, in a literal as well as a metaphorical sense.

Transvestism. A desire to masquerade in the clothing of the opposite sex touches many practices of childhood. When this is confined to childhood games of dressing up like others and trying out these various roles, it is considered part of the experimental trying out of different identities. The illusion created is part of testing reality by way of temporarily playing the imposter. Observe how cross-dressing can be carried out by adults in different cultures if it is done during a period of festivities or for fun at a party.

These dressing ups serve additional functions. They confirm a given sex-role identity, permit the trying out of different roles which vary from high to low status, and allow the pretended use of sex symbols. Consider the girl whose physical appearance and demeanor show a boyish preference. These may be part of her exploration of roles, imitation of boys she admires, male identification, and reacting to a perception of the social disadvantages of being a female. These acts do not have the same meaning as those of an adult female with transvestite perversion problems in which dressing like a male is a direct manifestation of sexual fantasies and excitation.

Being able to predict which early childhood traits, family interactions, and genetic loadings lead to transvestite behavior in adolescence and later to this as a perverse activity raise the old prediction question. There is the difficulty, even in retrospect, of hypotheses from work with adults, in differentiating why a specific developmental pathway was taken. During the phallic stage of development, between the ages of three and five, some boys manifest a feminine behavior in contrast to phallic narcissism and intrusiveness. This may show up by trying on female clothes and expressing a preference for wearing these clothes, which may include females garments, jewels, ornaments and frilly undergarments.

Girls' toys may be chosen along with girl playmates. Verbalizations of wishes to be a girl and to be given a girl's name are all part of this picture. Demands can be made openly or detected in covert behaviors where the clothing is hidden and the boy feels humiliated and tearful when his behavior exposed. In these cases, conflict about sex-role identities exist within the family. These will be discussed in the section on transsexualism, since at this time we do not have sufficient differentiating features in the family interactions of potential transvestites or transsexuals at ages three to five to separate them.

During adolescence many transvestite behaviors occur:

1. The pretend quality may exist in the form of put ons at parties. Although this may be the expression of transvestite derivatives, it will usually not interfere with the solidification of a masculine identity during adolescence.

2. Those with a theatrical bent may take on jobs or roles which require the activities of a member of the opposite sex or their impersonation.

3. Dressing like another permits one to attract homosexual companions more easily. In some cases this extends to the point of fooling an older person of the same sex who does not catch on.

4. Emergence of transvestite impulses may not merely be for acting purposes, but can take on direct sexual gratification. Lack of emerging heterosexual interests is a warning sign of fixation. In some, homosexual impulses begin to come to the fore as well. The activity then becomes a major form of sexual gratification although this need not imply a fixity.

One difficulty in formulations about the solidification of transvestite impulses during adolescence is the paucity of investigations. Psychodynamic formulations categorize transvestism as a combination of homosexuality and fetishism. Classical formulations add the castration anxiety threat for the boy and penis envy for the girl, who is denying her femininity as essential components. The theoretical difficulty is the lack of specificity. Given that castration anxiety and penis envy may be involved as antecedents, there is no possibility of any point predictions regarding the developmental course being toward transvestism rather than other possible outcomes. There is also a lack of homogeneity with the group of behaviors called "transvestite."

One division of transvestism is between an exhibitionistic versus a non-exhibitionistic form.[58] The *exhibitionistic form*—for males or females—reveals a need to be viewed in the clothes of the opposite sex coupled with a minimum of autoerotic masturbatory gratification. Some of these adolescent transvestites are expressing a confused sexuality as part of a schizophrenic syndrome. In others there is a homosexual conflict which lies concealed beneath a transvestite commitment. In reality this is another version of the "as if" character who acts like a member of the opposite sex while his homosexual conflicts remain unconscious. When an adolescent becomes too flamboyant in his cross-dress, he is likely to come to public attention from creating a public nuisance, or from provocative elements in his feminine mannerisms leading to assaults from other adolescents whose masculinity is threatened by such an open display.

The *non-exhibitionistic forms* of transvestism are more akin to neurotic character problems. Cross-dressing is done in secrecy and with shame. Needs for possession of characteristics of the opposite sex reveal impulses analogous to those of taking property in neurotic characters. In some there is a periodic recourse to dressing in clothes of the opposite sex when under stress. A precipitating crisis need not be sexual, but like much acting out can be a defense against depression or deflated self-esteem.

To dress like a member of the opposite sex can provide reassurance by way of the presence of the characteristics of the comforting female that is mimicked. For the girl, masculine power is deceptively achieved. As such, these are restitutive maneuvers. Some girls are referred for therapy, or appear in juvenile court, as a result of their engaging in burglaries or thefts. This may have begun during a tomboy stage when such activities made her one of the boys. Thievery may have fetishistic qualities; consider the high frequency of thieving impulses and behavior in lesbians. Kleptomania has been regarded as the female counterpart to fetishism in males.[59]

Transsexualism. The transsexual condition is one in which an individual, through a deep identification with a member of the opposite sex, chooses to live his life as a member of that sex.[60] There is usually one major additional qualification: the person is a biologically normal member of that sex in terms of anatomy and chromosomes, and then not only has the desire to be a member of the opposite sex but there is a conviction or feeling he is. Some question whether the feeling or conviction is actually a delusional belief and thus what we are really dealing with is a psychotic individual. The counterargument is that since individuals are cognitively able to distinguish themselves as anatomically either male or female, they are not really delusional.

From there the debate takes on vehemence, particularly when the individuals seek out sex transformation procedures—often beginning during the adolescent years. These procedures are either to remove the male genitalia and construct an artificial vagina, or to compose a phallus for the woman. For the male, the procedure consists of a penile amputation, shelling the testes out of the scrotum, and creating a vaginal space between the fascial planes. Surgical debate involves whether the new vagina should be lined with skin processed from the penis and testes, grafted intestine, or a new skin graft. Such surgical issues will not be pursued, nor will the difficulties which can occur post-surgically such as urinary system problems concerned with creation of a new urethral meatus, or genito-urinary infections. Adjunctive procedures—used with or without the surgery—are electrolysis to remove facial and bodily hair, administration of estrogens to induce female secondary sexual characteristics, and surgical thinning of the larynx.

For the female, the effort to create a plastic penis, has difficulties beyond surgery—the main one being the inability to construct an erectile penis. To accomplish the desire to go beyond dressing like a man and anatomically alter the body to look like a male, females usually obtain hysterectomies, bilateral mastectomies, and androgen hormones to induce male secondary sexual characteristics. Studies reporting the usefulness of sex transformation procedures are largely impressionistic since the follow-ups are few and of short duration. Careful measurements of the psychological state before and following surgery are not done consistently, and outcome criteria as to success are not specific.

Beyond the psychiatric question of whether these individuals are de facto psychotic with respect to this area of their life, and the attendant medical and surgical problems, the debate centers around the validity of the diagnostic concept of transsexualism. Diagnostic criteria are vague and vary. In some cases the criterion is no more than the expression by a patient that he feels like a member of the opposite sex. The subtleties of any grouping are seen when it is realized that some individuals are seeking a change of their external appearance, but wish to retain their own sex identity as a male and rather only imitate a woman. What confuses the issue is that the outcome is evaluated on the level of a person's expression that he is now content or living more satisfactorily than before.

In the absence of specific criteria, assessment becomes very difficult as does comparative study of different approaches. The subtleties and necessities for diagnosis are summed up by Stoller:[61]

1. Some people requesting sex transformation are borderline or overt psychotics, and it may be hazardous to change their bodies to a radical degree.

2. Some are quite depressed. Are they depressed solely because they cannot stand living the wrong sex-role or for other reasons?

3. Some are primarily homosexual or fetishistic transvestites. For them, the genitals are essential to maintain this level of functioning and any surgical alteration would affect their pleasure.

4. Some are homosexual and wish the operation to facilitate prostitution.

Implicit in these points is the unresolved question of the degree to which a change in bodily configuration resolves internalized psychological problems. More specifically, if a change occurs in personality functioning, is it on a conscious, preconscious, or unconscious level? To appraise this requires clinical expertise of the highest order and a good deal of time. The complexity and spectrum of human motives belies any simple answer that could be given on a few brief contacts. The predominance of males seeking this change—four or five males to one female—raises developmental questions.[62]

Envy in boys of the woman's ability to procreate has long been known in clinical work.[63] While the child who consistently expresses a preference to be of the opposite sex indicates a confusion in gender identity, at what point is an assessment of psychopathology made? Taken from a slightly different tack, while all degrees of cross-identity are exhibited given a sufficiently large population, it would seem unwise to view them as merely part of a normal distribution curve with one end expressing an overt desire to be of the opposite sex. A corollary is that when an adolescent or young adult expresses such a preference, even if other overt aspects of his mental functioning seem intact, we cannot presume ipso facto that this desire is free of psychopathological determinants. The interlacing network of ego functioning can leave a circumscribed area of conflict. However, when an individual, in the course of development, has powerful needs emerging with a compulsive urge to do something about changing his overt sexual characteristics, he is least likely to wish to cooperate in exploring the degree to which this may be an expression of neurotic or psychotic needs.

Explanations for the phenomenon of transsexualism are subject to all of the above limitations regarding who is within and who is outside such a diagnosis. Hypotheses offered include: (1) biological isomorphism influenced by reinforcing factors in the course of development; (2) genetic predispositions which are not operating in terms of detectable chromosomal aberrations, but rather the genetic contributions which tend toward effeminate or masculine traits; (3) childhood rearing practices which are relatively neutral or ambiguous with respect to sexual identity, so that the onset of puberty permits a cross-sexed identity to occur; (4) a family atmosphere in which the child is victimized by a parent into behaving in the manner of the opposite sex; (5) alteration in their internal or external sex organs which predispose toward a confused sexual identity. All manner of development is possible and the end result is contingent upon when a child is made aware of discrepancies between the sex-role identity he has been assigned and some incongruent biological fact.

There have been attempts to identify children who are potential transsexuals by retrospective approches. The same troublesome diagnostic and predictive questions pervade here. If children are manifesting behaviors—sexual and otherwise—similar to those which adult transsexuals report they once manifested as children, there are enormous variables operating to preclude reliable predictive statements as to whether these children will become adult transsexuals. As in much clinical psychopathology, the few children who have been investigated in this manner are those coming to clinics or hospitals, which is quite different from a sample of a general population of children who exhibit similar behaviors. If the children coming to clinics are treated, this alters the possible consequences for the emergence of different sexual behaviors once adolescence is reached. Hence, we do not really know if the group of children who display transsexual behaviors are in fact from the same generic cloth as those who are later designated "transsexuals." With this limitation in mind, some of the observations of children supposed to have this personality disorder will be discussed.

Alleged childhood cases of transsexualism are often viewed as separate from those with organic or chromosomal anomalies, such as the adrenogenital syndrome. Primate research indicates that prenatal sex hormone levels are significant in subsequent sex-role orientation, but no applications or confirmations of this work with humans has developed.[64] The diagnosis of childhood transsexualism is thus behavioral, and the overwhelming observations have been done with boys rather than girls. For boys, parents give a history of effeminate behavior commencing in the first few years of life and almost always prior to any oedipal stage being attained. Behavior is observed in boys wanting to dress in women's clothing whenever possible—at home, at neighbors' houses, or at nursery school. If such clothes are not available, they may be created out of towels, blankets, or improvised, with a degree of artistic talent, from anything convenient. Not only is this desire to cross-dress seen with major garments, but with undergarments and accessories such as using perfume or wearing jewelry. A profound feminine identification is present whereby these little boys walk and talk with a feminine demeanor, and their gestures as they talk and recline convey femininity. These boys appear not to have learned to stand and urinate, but rather sit as girls. As cognitive abilities develop, their content of conversation is geared toward topics which girls or adult women like to hear. Their unfolding peer relationships are confined almost exclusively to girls. When they play house, they assume the role of mother or sister.

The sine qua non of transsexual development is a fixed belief that they are girls and will grow up with anatomical characteristics of women. In this sense there is a slight difference from adult male transsexuals who have given up the hope of growing up like women and instead seek surgical transformations. The internal feeling of being different from those designated of the same sex is present; this begins in these boys at age three or four and remains. All of this is congruent with data indicating the relative fixity of gender identity in the first few years of life, and that whatever induces confusion in gender is likely to remain and not be outgrown. While gender assignment at birth has been correct in terms of anatomical correlates, something in the first few years of life, when sex-role preferences are developing, has gone awry. A host of studies document the emergence of differences in the frequency of sex-type behaviors for boys and girls, particularly with respect to aggression, dependency, cognitive, and intellectual functioning. Such matters have been discussed in an earlier chapter and a specific review can be found in Oetzel.[65]

For the transsexual boy the sex-type behaviors which develop are those of the opposite sex. It appears that a cognitive awareness of two sexes begins to emerge during these same early few years in terms of role preferences. At age four, most children can correctly identify a male and female doll as well as their own sex.[66] Nursery school children as young as two years of age are likely to prefer classmates of their own sex.[67] By five years of age, personal preferences and beliefs about the activities their mothers and fathers prefer for boys and girls are known in terms of parental preferences.[68] A variety of microscopic, or subliminal, yet very potent, reinforcement practices go on from the earliest months between parent and child. This operates not only with behaviors, but with different situations, expectations, and fantasies. Vicarious reinforcement, observation learning, and imitation operate as well.

Peer influences and social models outside the family are minimal at this young age. Cognitive processes are important since once a self-categorization of gender commences, a striving for consistency and reduction of dissonance begins. Given an atmosphere in which the experiences favor femininity, elimination of discrepancies among cognitions will proceed. The self-categorized gender is one of the basic determiners of sex-role attitudes and behavior. Cognitions and self-concepts come to occupy the role of an independent variable with respect to the development of sex-typing behaviors.[69] While not all theorists give this much weight to cognitive processes—some emphasizing the role of reinforcing agents—the role as one critical variable cannot be ignored.

Young transsexual boys do not engage in feminine behavior in a haphazard or playful manner. Their behavior is an inherent part of their sexual identity which has begun to crystallize, but with discordant notes when they are exposed to influences outside their homes. While their mothers were consciously aware of the feminine behaviors, and on occasion attempted temporarily to distract them, usually no consistent effort in this direction was made. Mothers do not tell their sons they wish they had daughters, or that their wish was for a girl instead of a boy. It is more that the mothers perceive their sons as beautiful objects and encourage them in feminine behaviors. Some of these children, by the time they are seen in clinics at age seven or eight, are praying to God to be changed into a girl.[70] By that time their preference for girls' clothing, wearing high-heeled shoes, and using feminine mannerisms is conspicuous. In fact, it is usually someone outside the immediate family who presses the issue that something is unusual and that a psychiatric evaluation is indicated. So much has this become a part of them at that time that they do not look grotesque in their feminine garb but rather stylish and appealing. Creative precocity in their artistic endeavors is witnessed in painting, decorating, designing, story-telling, and music. In one study, ten of twenty-three boys with symptoms of marked effeminacy expressed a keen interest in stage-acting and role-taking.[71]

Stoller formulates the dynamics of these families as based on *mothers* who are dissatisfied with a loveless marriage and unsure of their femininity.[72] They lead a sterile affectionate and sexual life in their marriages in which they are feminine in a boyish manner. While many of these mothers looked and acted like boys during their own latency period, none of them were transsexual in feeling they were boys or would grow up to be men. As adults, they appear depressed under a bright but brittle veneer. Accompanying this is a sense of emptiness or incompleteness.

Fathers of these boys are literally absent from home a great deal, and when there they are often silent and uncommunicative. They express even less concern about their son's overt femininity and cross-dressing than do their wives. There is a literal difficulty in these mothers to let their sons separate from their bodies in the father's withdrawal. By fostering body contact to a degree beyond that required by children of comparable ages, a blurring of ego boundaries in the boy results. Maintenance of bodily contact for several hours a day promotes an atmosphere of infantile contact, intimacy, and indulgence. Conversely, a sense of privacy for the intimacies of the mother's own bodily functions does not develop. Coupled with the lack of restriction for mutual bodily exploration is the lack of awareness of anger toward the young child by the mother. Keep in mind that these boys do not experience a threat to their masculinity or their anatomy which has to be protected by defensive operations, such as in transvestism. The transsexual boy gets no pleasure by covert attempts to secrete a penis beneath female garb. Instead, the penis seems to be regarded as unnecessary, if not undesirable. The transsexual seeks to give up his male organs and sex-role, in contrast to the value put on them by homosexual males or transvestites.

While these developments continue during latency, providing the demands of the peer culture and other socializing agents outside of the family are not too great, by adolescence crisis-time has arrived. Attempts to adapt to a homosexual way of life are unsatisfactory since this identifies them as a male. The sense of femaleness is even more difficult to live with when secondary sexual characteristics make their appearance. The need to confront a female body-image with the overt changes now developing poses another conflict.

Some of these adolescents become depressed or suicidal. This appears to be related to efforts to play the role of a male—much like an adolescent with heterosexual desires would feel if coerced into acting "as if" he was a female and had to fool others into believing it. There is much hesitancy and confusion about therapeutic management for the adolescent boy who appears to be transsexual. While psychotherapy for the young boy and family are recommended, the results in terms of longitudinal follow-through when the boy attains adolescence are largely unknown. Reversal of the transsexual femaleness when the adolescent initially is seen is a difficult, if not impossible, task. Some advocate aiding the adolescent to live out and accept his cross-sexed identity and for the therapist to accept this and sanction it on an experimental basis.[73]

A word is needed on the paucity of observations on transsexual development in girls. Perhaps this lack is due to the wider latitude for sex-typed behaviors permitted girls. The result is that fewer girls are seen in clinics because of style of dress, mimicry of boy's behavior, or expressions of wishes or ambitions to be a boy. Even overt statements by the little girl that she is a boy, or will grow up to be one, are treated with a degree of benign acceptance as though this was a natural desire. After all, evidence to buttress this viewpoint was once put forth by psychoanalytic theorists as representing the natural state of envious little girls. During latency, tomboyishness may be viewed with pride by parents or tolerated with an air of humor. How many of the overall generic group contain a potential transsexual girl is impossible to know. Not until adolescence do a few emerge with an uncompromisable feeling of being a male who wish to behave in accordance with these feelings.

In childhood the girls show no female sex-typed interests. Rather they were tomboys and prone to fight with boys. Although their pattern of erotic arousal in adolescence corresponds to the female pattern of responsiveness to touch, rather than visual or verbal erotic stimuli, the imagery of arousal conform to masculine content. Hatred of breasts accompanies an intolerance of vaginal penetration.[74] Their interests in children have a paternal quality. As with boys but in reverse, a masculine psychosexual identity differentiates quite early, but predictions from childhood are few and unreliable.

Pedophilic Behaviors. When considering the sexual activities of adolescents with younger children, distinctions from adult pedophiles are needed. With an adult sexual gratification from touching or engaging in sexual play with a child is considered molestation. If the behavior falls short of intercourse, it is legally classified as "indecent liberties with a child" or some offense such as sodomy, impairing the morals of a minor, carnal abuse, or lewd and lascivious conduct; in some cases, the offense is shifted into non-sexual categories, such as simple assault. If actual intercourse has been carried out, even with the consent of the child, the offense designated as "sexual intercourse with a child," or "carnal knowledge of a juvenile" may be used. Severity of the offense varies by the age of the child. The acts may amount to rape, regardless of any consent.

These distinctions are those of the adult criminal law which covers many adolescents, depending on the age of majority in a given state or if waiver is accomplished. Behavioral distinctions are important for the clinician in assessment. While a minor female may be defined as someone under eighteen years of age, there is a great deal of difference developmentally if the adolescent boy is attracted to the five-, ten-, or fifteen-year-old girl. There is a different kind of significance if the child with whom sexual activities are carried out is of the same sex. A variation which clinicians are aware of, but which is rarely handled as a sex offense, is the sexual play of the adolescent girl with a prepubertal boy. All of this points up the need for careful delineation in discussions of pedophilic behaviors.

Descriptive approaches to classification combine some of the etiological bases grafted onto categories from the standard nomenclature. One group is composed of those with intellectual or

cognitive defects. While some of these adolescents may be organically impaired in the sense of cerebral dysfunction, or intellectually
retarded, their biological drive level is post-pubertal. Some of them
are manifesting patterns of impulsivity and poor controls as a result
of slow ego development. The difficulty with any explanation of
these adolescents using smaller children of either sex for erotic
activity is that a majority with such handicaps do not proceed to
deal with their sexual impulses in such a manner. Hence, these
limitations contribute, but the main factor would still result in some
type of developmental pathway which retards heterosexual interests with someone of a comparable age. Incidence of pedophilic
behaviors is almost impossible to determine with any age, since the
behaviors vary from something just shy of intercourse to fondling,
onanism, voyeurism, exhibitionism, use of pornographic materials,
or obscene words with a juvenile. One report does state that two-
thirds of all sexual offenses are committed against children.[75]

A second group is viewed as having sexual interest in young
children on the basis of neurotic conflict or personality disorder.
Appraisal is difficult without resorting to psychodynamic hypotheses. This need not be a chronic pattern in an adolescent, since it
can be an episodic phenomenon in response to a variety of adverse
circumstances, whether environmental or intrapsychic shifts in
self-esteem. Many psychiatric, social, and legal dilemmas are raised
with individuals who utilize such behaviors every few years, but
then vehemently resist attempts by anyone to intervene (as well as
denying the acts).

The adolescent boy who feels inadequate heterosexually may
resort to a younger and less threatening object choice. In some cases,
this behavior is a response to attempts at sexual activity which fail,
such as impotency. The naivete of the younger child will conceal
inadequacies. In some cases, the pedophilic activity, like other
acting out, may be a defense to ward off depressive states.
Regressive processes facilitate the seeking out of old childhood
wishes and gratifications, such as peeking, exposing, smelling,
touching, tickling, hugging, and playing doctor. Such play may
occur in adolescents and provide a good deal of infantile gratification so it becomes difficult to relinquish. Many object choices in the
homosexual realm operate with the added ingredient of the childlike
quality of the object. Generalized regressive tendencies—sexual and
otherwise—can be part of a schizophrenic process.

A third group are those with severe character disturbances. Some
of these youths are hedonistic and impulse-ridden. In terms of

descriptive nosology, they are given diagnoses of antisocial personality or, in some cases, their socialization has been in a setting where predatory behavior is acceptable and the diagnosis that of dyssocial behavior. Nothing in the internalized norms of these groups prohibits getting it where you can. Hence, they are not pedophilic in the perverse sense of having this object choice as a preferred means of gratification. Given the availability of an attractive adolescent girl, or older woman, she will be chosen. In her absence, what is available is used. Nor are these behaviors a source of distress to these youths since they are ego-syntonic. While some of these pedophilic behaviors occur under the influence of alcohol or drugs, this is only a requirement for those with more prominent neurotic character problems who need this to rationalize or permit such acting out. The following is a working classification of pedophilia on a descriptive level:

1. Intellectual or cognitive defects
2. Pedophilic gratification on the basis of neurotic conflicts, or which involve forerunners of pedophilia as a perversion
3. Predatory use of children in severe personality disturbances

For each of these categories a further dimension may be added in terms of the following:

1. Use of physical force or threats with a child
2. The sex of the child—the same or different
3. If the child was prepubertal or beyond puberty
4. If the child is a relative or not, which raises the question of incestuous behaviors
5. If the behavior is episodic in occurrence or rather the result of preference

Although it may be academic to make distinctions between the use of physical coercion or its absence, sexual overtures or advances to a prepubertal child contain different degrees of coercion. Given the disparity in size, strength, and status, there is always some type of coercion. However, physical force need not always be used. Nor should the differences in predisposing factors in degree of interest or cooperation in children be ignored. Particularly with adolescents involved with prepubertal children, regressive behaviors under the influence of neurotic conflict, alcohol, or drugs, may permit the acts to occur.

In some cases, the adolescent is reacting to his fright at attempted intercourse with a girl his own age or an older woman. The most likely source of reassurance is the younger child, who is someone in the neighborhood or a relative, with whom this type of relationship is formed. The desire for object-contact, a reassurance against loneliness, may be satisfied with fondling and petting techniques or mouth-genital activity. A threat to the phallic narcissism of the adolescent may lead to attempts at intercourse with a younger girl. In one study dealing with adult pedophilic sex offenders, only 6 percent had actually attempted coitus.[76]

In some cases, it is the narcissistic identification with the younger child as a precursor that could evolve into a persistence of this type of sexual preference during adolescence. Some adolescent boys still play the doctor game with younger males or females to gain reassurance about their own feelings of insecurity and sexual inadequacy. It is reassuring for some boys to explain sex to the uninitiated novice rather than perform themselves by the standards of the peer group. In one study of homosexual prisoners in a federal correctional institution—of whom 38 percent were sex offenders—a median age of eight years was given for their first homosexual experience, while the median age of their first partner in this contact was sixteen.[77]

Again, the prediction question plagues us, since these postdictive data with a group who made it into the group of adult homosexuals, as well as some achieving the designation of sexual offenders, would be a difficult base from which to make predictions. There undoubtedly is a much larger group of boys in the population who experience such contacts but do not end up in this category. Bieber found that ill health in childhood was a significant finding among later adult homosexuals and associated this with maternal overconcern for the boy.[78] Freedman reported a relationship between early autoerotic behaviors such as masturbation and homosexual pedophilic development.[79] Another interesting finding involves juvenile court records. For those who later comprise a group of identified homosexual offenders against prepubertal boys, about 20 percent have had a juvenile court record.[80]

In comparison to a control group of those in prison for non-sexual offenses who had a juvenile court record of 24.3 percent, this is quite high, although not as high as those using aggression against girls in the twelve to fifteen year grouping or peepers. However, in terms of commitment to a juvenile correctional facility for longer than six months, and conviction of a juvenile sex offense, they were only exceeded by these two groupings and by 0.3 percent for the peepers.

There is also the matter of the portion of this group who may use physical force. Although the overall incidence is probably small, the difficulties in defining coercion have been noted. When a physical assault has been made, it may be handled without any reference to the sexual activity. This is not just a device to ignore the behavior, but frequently the unavailability of the history. Neither the younger boy nor the adolescent may reveal it. Lack of inclusion of the sexual nature of an offense may be seen at all levels.

> A more detailed case history of a fourteen-year-old boy who committed a homicide on a boy of nine while home from a residential treatment center on a week-end pass is contained below. It is important to note that the entire case was handled as one of murder without any reference to the sexual nature of the act despite the homicide's having occurred with the older boy in a sexually excited state, on top of the younger one and strangling him.

Those directly involved in clinical work with juveniles puzzle over the psychogenesis of the various behaviors classified as pedophilic. Psychodynamic explanations have progressed considerably from to the old trauma theory. Rather there is an emphasis on the psychological conflicts with respect to sexual impulses that operate during development. More specifically, why is there a developmental line that has attached to younger sexual objects? The factor of fear of sexual objects and activities with a heterosexual object comparable in age is one thing. There may be a great deal of anxiety about autoerotic sexual acts, such as masturbation. For some adolescents, a moralistic justification may be a rationalization, since few put their pedophilic behaviors in the context of a moral wrong.

While a sexual act with a minor may be viewed with shame and disgust, this does not seem as impressive as the degree of painful affect reported for masturbation. It is rather that almost any sexual act evokes guilt, but some have more manifest anxiety as well. For those with an emerging homosexual pedophilic bent, a striking attachment to their mothers or older adult women may be seen. For some this is on an oedipal level of avoiding girls of their own age, but for most it appears to be a general level of immaturity.

Failure of adults to regulate behaviors based on the approval or negation by superego standards is crucial. While overt antisocial or dyssocial trends do not seem prominent in the families of these boys, there does seem to be a role conflict, making modeling and identification difficult. Many passive-aggressive or extractive devices operate, accompanied by denial of the aggressiveness. This is also true of hypochondriasis or alcoholism, if they are present in these families. Although the families are intact, and the adolescent has not sustained a parental loss, ambivalence and personal isolation are prominent. A control system based more on fear and disapproval than on self-esteem has emerged. When younger, passive compliance was obtained at the price of not providing a mechanism for dealing with the anger within an ambivalent framework. If given the opportunity later to displace the hostility to a safe object, the probability for this is increased, especially if prompted by certain seductive behaviors in the child. The control system of such an adolescent, which operates mainly by needing to avoid punishment or detection by others, is then more likely to choose a minor.

For some, the fear of loss of control—in general or toward younger children as sexual objects—leads to a superego structure with a rigid system of obsessional components. Some project blame to the child. It is impressive when an intelligent sixteen-year-old boy with an obsessional control system engages in pedophilic activity with prepubertal girls and states, "She didn't do anything to stop me," indicating the gap in his usually exaggerated control system. A distortion in cognitive functioning is coupled with observations of withdrawn, timid, isolated, and over-controlled individuals who exhibit schizoid and social deterioration, much like the adolescent schizophrenic breakdown. In one study on adults confined in Sing-Sing Prison for sexual offenses, 70 percent of the pedophiles were diagnosed as schizophrenic.[81]

The final question: How harmful is sexual behavior to the child who is party to such activity? Again, valid findings should provide analysis by sex, age, and type of activity. This is rarely available. Ferenczi described why he felt such behavior would have an adverse effect on the child from the helplessness present.[82] By submission to such activities, the child identifies with the aggressor. Most important for the child is the introjection of the feelings of the other person, such as his guilt, shame, or fear of detection. Harmless play may be perceived as a punishable thing. Anger for being used in such a manner, as a helpless victim, may also be present. Ignoring the effects of victimization upon the child is prevalent within a context of focusing on the offender. We are still at a disadvantage in knowing what the consequences in the immediate period or the long run will be. While child psychiatrists encounter patients who report these experiences, they are not great in numbers. More are seen through court systems, but there is more likelihood of the offender being seen than the child.

Complex emotional forces operate when a psychiatric assessment of the child is not pursued. The avoidance is often under the guise that "He has been through enough already." The reluctance by parents to report molestations is similar to the mechanisms operating with the offender. He often insists nothing harmful has occurred, and since the victim was a child there is a denial of any harmful effect. This is not avoiding the possible adverse consequences from pretrial interrogation of a child, or their use as witnesses in court settings. However, the remedy would seem to lie in protecting the child by special procedures for taking his testimony.[83]

In addition to the need for clarification by stage of development and gender, variables such as previous problems need consideration. This must be within the context of the individual child and family relationships. There is the further limitation of evaluation done by mere statements that the child is "doing OK," or performing satisfactorily academically. Certain children may be in high risk categories to begin with, such as those from deprived backgrounds or parental neglect. To be fondled, held, or used for fellatio or pederasty may seem desirable to these children. It may be difficult for them to give up these comforts. These activities may be sought out in a compulsive manner from the blending of attention, affection, dependency gratification, physical pleasure, and comfort.

Long-range consequences are often ignored. In a German investigation of sixty-two children—fifty girls and twelve boys— there was a follow-up at a minimum of fifteen years.[84] For girls, the offense was in terms of handling the body or genitals when younger, cunnilingus, or fellatio performed by the girl (actions akin to coitus had occurred in twenty-four, and actual coitus in nineteen). For boys the acts were masturbation. About 10 percent of the children on follow-up had emotional injury of a lasting kind. Four conclusions were offered: (1) children from a good environment and family seemed to suffer less injury; (2) children from the lower social classes are in greater danger of sexual assault from being left by themselves more often; (3) sexual offenses repeated over a long period of time are more apt to cause lasting injury, and (4) the age age which the offense occurred did not seem to be a significant factor.

Other studies with girls have observed the pattern of promiscuity developing from antecedents of sexual activity which the girl uses as payment for nurturance.

Incestuous Behaviors. Incest includes many combinations, but it is simply defined as sexual intercourse between two individuals too closely related by blood or affinity to be married. It does not matter whether they actually are married, since the norm is defined in degrees of consanguinity. Incest legally may or may not cover the situation where there has been lack of knowledge, depending on the particular state. All the intricacies of victimization and intrafamilial conflict operate in these situations. A further legal element is that penetration must be proved, although emission need not. Variations in the age of the child are not an essential component, since the incestuous relationship is the sine qua non. However, some states— with the thought of an increased biological risk if offspring result— propose to make intercourse with a blood relative, regardless of age, different from that which occurs with another member of a family unit.[85] Hence, if a stepdaughter or adopted daughter were involved, an upper age limit, such as eighteen, might be fixed. The rationale in the latter is that of upholding the family structure, whose authority is seen as threatened by incestuous activity during the course of a child's developmental years.

A classification should include the data in Table 9:

TABLE 9

Data for Incest Investigations

I. Type of relationship

    A. Blood relative
       1. Father-daughter
       2. Mother-son
       3. Brother-sister—whole or half blood
       4. Grandparent
       5. Homosexual
         a) Father-son
         b) Mother-daughter
         c) Siblings

    B. Non-blood relatives
       1. Stepchild
       2. Adopted child

II. Type of Activity

    A. Intercourse
    B. Other types of sexual behavior

III. Age of the child

    A. Prepubertal
    B. Pubertal
    C. Adult

This table illustrates how scarce our substantive knowledge about the variations of incest really is.

One result of socio-medico-legal confusion about incest regarding dispositional variation is that while an adult male can be prosecuted in some states, and if convicted as a sexual offender be sentenced from one to twenty years, in practice the variation is conspicuous. Some fathers may not be prosecuted at all; in some cases, the father is convicted and then handled separately as a sexual offender at a security hospital. A brother-sister type of incest, or that of a homosexual type, may be handled as a routine juvenile offense for a minor resulting in an adjudication as a delinquent. Probation or a correctional facility may be the result. Where serious physical coercion has been evident, or recidivism, the juvenile court may be waived and a conviction in adult criminal court may result in prison or a security hospital. Another paradox is the adolescent girl involved in incestuous activity who is adjudicated delinquent. Probation may be granted, but commitment to a girls' correctional facility is also possible. Hence, there is a risk to an adolescent reporting what goes on within the family. A social-class bias tends to operate in that girls in the middle class or above might be referred for treatment.

The major limitation of any conclusions is not merely the haphazard or inconsistent patterns of disposition, but the probability that most incestuous relationships occur in the privacy of the family, so that we do not have a means for detecting the valid incidence or consequences of these behaviors.

Incestuous strivings, and the correlative prohibitions against them, are regarded as universal in different cultures. The taboos reflect social and legal sanctions against literally acting upon these wishes. There has been debate about the universality of both the incest taboo and the related oedipal complex. If the two are defined in terms of requiring an exact replica of the manifestations of different societies and historical periods, there is no question that such universality has not been present. However, to phrase the question in such a manner is to answer it in the negative. If sexual feelings of those living in a close relationship are universal, there is evidence for both oedipal strivings and a taboo on direct expression. Classical mythology, folk tales, and children's literature abound in these themes.

If we acknowledge that most societies prohibit overt incest through moral or social norms, a logical question to ask is, Why? Pragmatic answers are: the need to populate, the difficulty of supporting a family where a pattern of intrafamilial mating occurs, the heightening of rivalrous tensions and competition within a family, impairment of children forming liaisons outside the family, and complications of inheritance. Yet pragmatic answers do not sufficiently account for the intensity of prohibiting such behaviors, and the consequent internalization by the offspring of prohibitions. What is the reason for prohibiting such a pleasurable desire which emerges so naturally in the course of family life? Psychoanalytic theory proposed the oedipal stage and its consequences. From these strivings, death wishes toward the rival parent of the same sex coexisted with the incestuous wishes toward the parent of the opposite sex. However, these two motives become repressed, and are experienced as fleeting, conscious fantasies even by the three- to six-year-old.

Differentiating a specific sex-typed identity is related to the identification with the frustrating adult of the same sex who prohibits sexual indulgence with his mate. In children, conflicted adults pose a problem of differentiating the affectionate, tender components of a relationship from the literally sexual ones. A further complication is the unconscious sexual attitude of the parents, sensed by the child and reacted to in a literal manner.[86] Not only conflicted parents experience sexual feelings toward their offspring. Many parents encounter this on special occasions; holidays, parties, or in states of altered controls, such as intoxication. In one case, both the father and his seventeen-year-old daughter were aware of their desires when the daughter commented to her father, "Wouldn't it be nice if we could do what we can't do because we are father and daughter?" Such strivings may be aroused under many conditions, but quickly suppressed in the usual course of affairs. During intensive therapy with adolescents such past feelings, desires, and memories are often reawakened.

Psychoanalytic theory uses castration anxiety theory as an additional explanation for why iscent is prohibited. Freud groped for a more basic explanation via an inherited incest taboo rooted in the eons of time during which the father was killed by a parricidal act and the sons possessed his women, which led not only to myths but institutionalized tribal acts of undoing.[87] Freud's groping reflected his intellectual puzzlement about how such a seemingly universal situation occurred. Its capacity for long-lasting psychological effects in the individual, as well as in the culture, led him to propose an ingenious solution, although it is rarely accepted today in the sense of inherited guilt.

Historically, there have been major exceptions to the incest taboo. Practical exigencies existed not only to permit, but at times sanction, incestuous ties when they were historical necessities. Matriarchal influences in ancient Egypt are cited as the main contributing influence for the incestuous activity between siblings. Since property was inherited through the female, a strong motivation to retain wealth and estates within a family existed. A brother-sister marriage permitted the family inheritance to be retained, as it would then be passed on from the mother to the daughter. There was also the motivation among the nobility to preserve the royal blood without contamination, which could be secured by incestuous offspring.[88]

However, such evasions against incest were not tolerated in ancient Israel, which set the stage for the moral and family rules of Western civilization. The "Law" consistently prohibited "uncovering the nakedness" of a female, which was the exclusive right of a husband. This is illustrated in the following rules laid down in Leviticus:[89]

> No man shall approach a blood-relation for intercourse. I am the Lord. You shall not bring shame on your father by intercourse with your mother: she is your mother; you shall not bring shame upon her. You shall not have intercourse with your father's wife: that is to bring shame upon your father. You shall not have intercourse with your sister, your father's daughter, or your mother's daughter, whether brought up in the family or in another home; you shall not bring shame upon them.

Despite all these prohibitions, no specific restriction of a father-and-daughter relationship was made. This is in line with contemporary statistics which reflect a much higher incidence of father-daughter incest than mother-son. Even in Biblical Israel, under conditions such as continuance of the race, incest could occur. When Lot and his two daughters survived the destruction of Sodom and Gomorrah, and the mother was destroyed for violating the injunction not to look back, the daughters pondered their problem: "There is not a man on earth to come into us after the manner of all the earth."[90] The sisters connived to intoxicate their father with wine to secure impregnation. Even here a denial mechanism operated in not acknowledging their sexual desires for their father, but rather stressing the need for biological propagation.

Historically, incest was considered primarily a spiritual matter to be handled by theological rules. In Anglo-Saxon jurisdictions it was not made a statutory offense until quite late, and it was never a common law crime. Only during the brief period of Cromwell's Puritan reign in England (circa 1650) was it made a statutory offense, and not again in England until 1968. A similarly broad situation operated in the United States. There were several reasons for this omission. Reference to sexual activity as the province of religion has been mentioned. It was only necessary for the law to specify the conditions under which people could or could not marry, without resort to criminal laws for sexual behavior within families. Until recent times the pragmatic reason given in Leviticus may have operated, such as on the Western frontier of the United States, or when longevity was limited and partners needed.

The same conflicts and societal needs appear to operate at present. Sociologists analyze the incest situation as one where the status and role ascribed to the participants as members of society proscribes such activities between family members. The pervasiveness of the incest taboo is taken as one sign that the nuclear family is not complete, but a subsystem of the larger society which requires preservation. Malinowski emphasized the function of the incest taboo in preserving the stability of the family.[91] This operates to protect the integrative family unit by means of role differentiation. Although marriages between mother and son or father and daughter seem prohibited by law, custom, or moral sanction in Western civilization, tribes are reported where unions between parents and children occur. Marriages between mother and son have been reported among the Caribs, Eskimo, Pioje, and Tinne in America; the Minahassa in Celebes; the Kalong in Java; the New Caledonians, and the Banyoro in Africa. Unions between father and daughter are reported from the Minahassa in Celebes; the Karene in Burma, and in the Solomon, Marshall, and Plew Islands and Hawaii, as well as with ancient Irish families, within the royal Inca line, and in Egypt.[92]

The role of the older male is part of a complex system that evolves from multiple nuclear families, rather than solely from roles available between individuals in a single nuclear family. Erotic attachments within the nuclear family are more easily repressed.

They are only permitted to become conscious as fleeting thoughts or symbolic derivatives, primarily outside the nuclear family. The association of sensual arousal and infantile dependency carry the potential for fixation and easy revival of such patterns when a safe, nonincestuous, heterosexual object choice is available. All varieties of eroticized dependency may be detected clinically from the deliberate sexualized sporting activity of a parent to deliberate seduction. The former is illustrated in a situation where a thirteen-year-old male, living in a single-room apartment with his divorced mother, is reported by school personnel to be "hyperactive and climbing the walls." Although no overt sexual behavior in the form of intercourse is present, the boy is privy to the mother's bedroom.

In more overt extensions the mother and boy share a common bed, although never explicitly confronting their sexual feelings unless they happen to enter therapy. A subtype of the latter is the teasing, yet denying, mother who jokingly refers to her boy's erections in the morning. Another is the boy with a blinking tic whom the mother describes jokingly as not being able to take his eyes off her as she dresses. Since the superego is in a vulnerable state of development, structuralized controls are vulnerable. In addition, there has not yet been sufficient social reinforcement by extrafamilial sources towards object choice outside the family or sexualized gratification in a genital sense. Social evolution has utilized psychological regression as a principal means of establishing nuclear family units, and focusing the erotic attachments of a couple on each other. Incest is thus antisocial in a sociological sense because it interferes with the formation and maintenance of transfamilial bonds in an economic, political, and religious manner. The center of authority resides within parental figures in the nuclear family who become the source of realistic and fantasied prohibitions.

This type of social theorizing has supplanted looking for one specific cause for the incest taboo. The biological need of the family for reproduction, and the maintenance of generational differences, are viewed as givens. This extension involves psycho-social characteristics of members of family units. Characteristics of small groups are present, such as status and power, and a differentiation along what Parsons calls "instrumental" and "expressive" lines related to sex-role differentiation.[93] The instrumental function is concerned with adaptation to external circumstances while the expressive function is concerned with the internal harmony or solidarity of the group.

Genital erotism is restricted to the marital pair, while pregenital erotism is permitted within the parent-child tie. Overt erotism between post-oedipal children is a taboo, with the exception of private or disguised acts. The gratifying parental object is also the frustrating object, which is the mechanism for the socialization of the child. Conversely, an erotic attachment exists between the parent and child which fosters an eroticized relationship, since the parents also receive pleasure from this. Their own ego and superego controls customarily function to keep these activities within circumscribed limits, unless psychopathological conflicts are present.

Even in Sophocles' classic play the parental impulses are dominant: the parents and the gods determine the destiny which a man must unwittingly live out. In early versions as well, Oedipus is made to kill his father in self-defense against a homosexual assault.[94] What is significant is the perpetuation among generations of the intimacies of the processes of family and cultural education. Guilt is a byproduct which restricts the expression of impulses in a young child, and which permits society to perpetuate by an outward extension of the nuclear family. Among sex offenders, the incest group is the most guilt-ridden and within prisons and hospitals they are the most socially ostracized.[95]

Incest is now a criminal offense in all fifty states, although the degree of sanctions vary depending on the degree of relatedness. Incidence of incestuous activity is believed far greater than the statistics of criminal indictments. Karpman cited a figure for incest of to 2.4 to 6.3 percent of the total number of sexual offenses.[96] Another writer estimated that approximately 15 percent of female delinquents in a correctional setting had incestuous activity.[97] The actual incidence is probably much higher.

This is especially true among adolescent girls and their fathers or stepfathers in which hugging, patting, fondling, coyness, and general seductive behavior regularly occur. What the law prohibits is intercourse in the literal sense of penetration. Although the clinician is impressed by a chronic atmosphere of seductive interplay, legal inquiry focuses on the literal question as to whether "penetration" has occurred. Legal involvement takes place in a situation where resentments or unfulfilled wishes can lead to accusations of overt sexual acts against her father, adult males, or boys in the neighborhood. In some cases, this may be based on spite and vengeance, but in other cases it is associated with hysterical and depersonalized neurotic components.

There are occasional exhortations for society to stop condemning incestuous contacts. These are based on the presumption that if society stops condemning an act, personal guilt and anguish associated with it will disappear. One writer, in discussing mother-son incest, states that "The grotesque notion that it is everyone's business what two people do with their bodies in the privacy of their homes results in countless tragedies, incalculable suffering ... society is damaged—as innumerable individuals are damaged—by anti-sexual measures taken against persons whose behavior is innocuous."[98]

Other reports have stressed that the consequences of incestuous activity may not always be viewed as pathological.[99] Whatever the merit of these contentions, there is clinical documentation for the deleterious psychological and social consequences for some incestuous behavior. There also appears to be a psychological naivete that changing a legal or social edict, such as making incest permissible, would remove the psychological consequences of an act. This bypasses the tenacity of attachments and taboos which exist. What we do not know, because of the inherent limitation on researching the problem, is what the consequences may have been for individuals who never contact a clinician. With this limitation in mind, some family psychodynamic patterns are presented.

Incest-prone families appear to operate overwhelmingly along the axis of a male relative and daughter, although occasional reports of mother-son incest appear.[100] The majority of girls involved are in the adolescent age group with the father figure in his late thirties or forties. Within this age grouping, the girl has attained puberty, and marital problems, death, or separation may have intervened with the parents. Some report a greater detrimental influence if the incest occurs with the adolescent girl rather than during her latency on the basis of subsequent promiscuity and unstable behavior patterns.[101] In most cases sexual activity has been taking place for some time—perhaps years.

Rarely does a family or child present at an office or clinic with a chief complaint of incest. Rather, an agency, school, or person refers the case after the girl has revealed her activity, often in anger. The mother may lodge a complaint against the father, precipitated by some intrafamilial shift. There are cases where a clergyman brings the case to public attention by urging the mother to file a complaint against the father at the district attorney's office after she, or the daughter, has revealed the situation to him. The behavior may have existed for years, but an altered set of circumstances has upset the family equilibrium. In other cases, knowledge of incest may be made known in the course of therapeutic work for other presenting problems.

A variety of symptoms occur in girls besides the overt sexual act. Acting out may be an accompaniment, such as petty pilfering or truancy. Absenting from home may eventuate in being sent to a correctional institution. A charge of incorrigibility may be filed by the parents for these behaviors without any reference to the incest. In many cases, absenting by a girl appears to be a costly attempt at solving a personal and family predicament. Somatization frequently occurs, such as gastrointestinal complaints, (anorexia, abdominal pain, or nausea and vomiting), dizziness and fainting. One fifteen-year-old girl experienced hysterical dissociative episodes as well as periodic attacks of the grand hysterie which gave the clinician a hypothesis to work on. More subtle organic symptomatology may develop and present continuing diagnostic puzzles to medical and non-medical personnel. Recurrent urinary retention is a pattern associated with past incestuous activity in some girls.[102]

In one case a seventeen-year-old nursing student presented with a history of unresolved gastric complaints of abdominal bloating which had been thoroughly investigated by an internist without revealing organic pathology. When her girth continued to expand there were increasing complaints and psychiatric consultation was requested. The girl always appeared for her interviews in a loose-hanging sack dress which she said was more comfortable, but it also concealed her progressively enlarging abdomen. Her symptoms had begun shortly after entering nurses' training, where one of her first clinical assignments had been the obstetrics ward. She sensed, in an intellectual way, some connection with her symptoms and the beginning of her training but passed this off as 'foolishness.' During the course of her treatment a pattern of incestuous behavior with her father was revealed. The behavior had ceased a year earlier when she had begun to date a boy regularly. The behavior originated with the father and daughter alternately 'massaging' each other's backs while straddled across the posterior thighs. During these massages, intercouse would occur vis a tergo as part of the routine with never a word mentioned between them as to what was occurring. During this period she had first experienced milder degrees of intermittent pseudocyestic symptoms prior to her 'pregnancy.'

Parental dynamics reveal a marriage in which sexual activity between the parents has been displaced to the child. A pattern of estrangement with the outward semblance of an intact family occurs in which a collusion between all family members is maintained. The crucial step is the mother's simultaneous knowledge of the father-daughter relationship, coupled with a denial mechanism.[103] This family secret solidifies family relations and is one variable responsible for permitting these relationships to continue. The non-participation of the mother may be viewed as a withdrawal, but it is also an abandonment of the girl.[104] This may be a welcome relief from what has been experienced as a burden.

The sexual part of being a woman is isolated from the caretaking part and the latter is viewed asexually. Such mothers may be tied to a pain-dependent relationship with their own mothers in which they were selected in their own families of origin as the one who could never please their mother. They spend a lifetime courting their mothers. This is a more compelling need than establishing their own autonomy as a mother-wife in a new family. Their capacity to function sexually on a genital level appears grossly inadequate. Isolation is present, with the daughter viewed as the "bad me" part of the mother. The resulting confusion and identification involves the psychological identification of the daughter with the paternal grandmother. Role reversal permits the mother to be daughter and hence not a sexual object, while the daughter in turn functions as mother and carries on sexually within the family. The father again seeks the young woman he once looked for and who is now represented in his daughter.[105]

The abandonment by the maternal object is viewed as one basis for acting out by the adolescent girl. The acting out is a defense against the anxiety from abandonment. It leads to a host of depressive equivalents with a high degree of ambivalence. Some girls appear pseudo-mature or preoccupied on the basis of their daily activity. They regress easily and may have outbursts of rage. Transient psychotic episodes may intervene in which a variety of antisocial behavior occurs. At times, a pattern of repetitive and compulsive promiscuity ensues to capture endless, unattainable males, which provokes more anxiety and defensive maneuvers.

The pattern of incest is often terminated on the basis of a discovery. This upsets the incestuous pattern in a majority of cases. At times this may be precipitated on the basis of a pregnancy (about whose paternity no inquiry is made), or the girl reveals the story to her physician or a counselor. The increased incidence of congenital defects from inbreeding is another byproduct of these events.[106] Another possibility in the natural history of incest is a younger sister who blossoms into puberty and enters the competition. For a period, one or more sisters may be sexually used by the father with acquiescence by one and jealousy in the other. Such a situation provokes the rejected older daughter to reveal the family secret. Since one of the functions of incest is to maintain a family unit, a revelation of the behavior disrupts the status quo. A typical response of the mother is to act horrified about the dirty old man. Neighbors may help the martyred mother by giving her donations of money or rallying to her support. In one case a neighborhood auction was held for the mother's benefit.

Daughters who have been pawns in this game do not fare well. They have been receiving some impulse gratification as well as displacing their mothers in what seems like a triumph, but other consequences intervene. This is especially so when guilt for their father's imprisonment is on their shoulders. The participation of the mother in the activity has been kept well-repressed, and she can continue to displace her feelings onto the "mother-daughter" child.

One escape hatch is to categorize the father as sick—that he did not know what he was doing, or that he should be in a hospital, and so on. This device may be an out for the participants, but it has the consequences of labelling the father as "criminally insane," or a "sexual psychopath," with the personal and social consequences this entails. The family dynamics are rarely presented to a court. Assessment of responsibility is made primarily on the basis of the father's act, and his cognitive awareness that he was having intercourse. If such social and legal sanctions are to be applied, there is little psychological basis for applying solely punitive measures to the father. This may be a device for helping such repressed impulses stay in check, but this approach completely ignores the personal motives and multiple parties involved.

As with pedophilic victims, children of incest rarely receive therapeutic assistance. In some cases where the father is criminally charged, his attorney may prevent the psychiatrist from seeing the child. If the father is removed, the mother may not wish to permit exploration of what has taken place within the family. But in the cases where therapy has been initiated for other complaints, the material is frequently revealed so it can be handled. The impact on personality functioning during the course of adolescence for girls who have been involved incestuously is difficult to assess. Some of these girls unwittingly provoke punishment in a masochistic manner. Others have become compliant and subservient to older women in an appeasement gesture. Some, by compulsive promiscuity, see the lost father and attempt to bring him back.[107]

Although there is the general impression that father or stepfather incest with a daughter is the most prevalent type, we do not really know. Sibling incest between brother and sister may, in fact, be just as prevalent. In one study designed to test hypotheses about sibling incest, the conclusion was that the likelihood of sexual engagement between postpubertal siblings is an inverse function of their degree of sexual propinquity before puberty.[108] The conclusion is that incestuous temptation in adolescence is less if siblings who have been raised together indulged in some type of sex-play in their prepubertal period.

There is suggestive evidence that the collusive attitudes of the parents, particularly the mother, are involved in sibling incest as well. This takes the form of lack of inquiry or supervision, under the guises of the children's self-sufficiency.[109] When daughters inform their parents about this type of activity, it is usually ridiculed or rejected.

Knowledge of mother-son incest is almost nonexistent. The clinical literature contains very few references. Cases that have been reported refer to one or both parties as psychotic at the time of occurrence or subsequent to the acts. An element of duplicity or deceit is mentioned such as a mother who threatens her son with homosexuality unless she provides "special training" for him.[110] A relevant question is the relationship between mother-son incest and the loss of a father from the home. It is a situation of temptation, because paternal inhibitions are absent and the interaction is intensified.

Factors relevant are: absence of a father, seductive interaction with the boy by the mother, deprivation of other sexual outlets for the adolescent boy, severe regressive emotional problems in one or more members of the family, and periodic lapses that occur due to the use of alcohol or drugs. Relationships with older women outside the family setting are much more prevalent. There are so many unanswered questions about the mother-son incest that it is impossible to offer generalizations.

Homosexual incestuous relationships are another pattern which may involve father-son or mother-daughter. Again, we are limited in reports and clinical experience. It is not unusual, in dealing with court populations, to hear of homosexual activity between a father or stepfather and an adolescent son. The amount of rage induced in the boy not only promotes acting out of various types—sexual or otherwise—but in time may lead to aggressive and assaultive behavior. In some cases, aggravated assaults or homicides may result. In a psychodynamic sense, there may be a displacement in which the adolescent boy or girl acts out impulses with an adult who is not a member of the family. In one case seen by the author, two brothers and a father were involved in incest as well as in some acts of bestiality.

Sexualized Aggressive Behaviors and Rape. A variety of acts involve an element of physically coercive behavior toward a victim. Earlier sections have made it clear that coercion can be present by imposing physical size or social status, particularly when children are involved. Situations include not only rape or dismemberment, but sado-masochistic behaviors in which the sexual element may or may not be prominent. While many relationships, within and without families, and with the same or the opposite sex, have conspicuous sado-masochistic elements, they will not be discussed as part of sexual psychopathology. Various behaviors are noted in Table 10:

TABLE 10

Overtly Aggressive Sexual Behaviors

I. *Rape*

    A. Statutory rape
    B. Both parties legally minor
    C. Homosexual rape
    D. Group rape phenomena
    E. Previous relationship with victim
       1. Victim known before
       2. Victim sought out
       3. Precipitous act with whomever was available

II. *Overt Sado-Masochistic Acts*

III. *Dismemberment*

Most definitions of rape are still based on the English common law that the act is unlawful, carnal knowledge of a woman, not one's wife, without her consent. In addition, there is a specification that force, fear, or fraud are used. A distinction may be made between aggravated rape—using force, fear, an unconscious female, or one who is mentally ill or retarded—from simple rape. The latter is where the nature of the act is concealed at first or where a female is induced into thinking the party is her husband. There may be other requirements for a rape. The boy need not ejaculate, but it is essential that penetration, however slight, be effected. Since in many states girls can legally marry during their adolescent years, statutory rape based on intercourse with a girl under a certain age, no matter what consent is given or admitted, raises problems of the congruence of these holdings with the social and physical status of the contemporary adolescent girl. *Myra Breckenridge*, stated that only boys can commit rape.[112]

Will a male be able in time to maintain that he performed the act under coercive threats and the cajolery of a woman or group of women? Could the male, by some type of implied bribe or physical threat to his self-esteem, be coerced into the act of intercourse? In some jurisdictions, statutes dealing with rape or related offenses, such as carnal knowledge of a female below a certain age, are applicable only to boys over a certain age, such as fourteen. A boy younger than the statutory age cannot legally rape. In some of these cases juvenile delinquency proceedings may be instituted, while criminal prosecution is not carried out. In many states a general statute proscribing the age under which an infant is legally incapable of committing a crime covers the situation. Some have shifted the commonlaw age of fourteen for these crimes to a prima facie presumption, subject to rebuttal by proof, that puberty has been attained by a boy under fourteen years.[113]

Related issues pertain to adolescents who present evidence of impotency, so that penetration would be impossible. This becomes a matter of factual dispute, for evidence is needed to establish the degree of impotence which might negate penetration.

Since force and fear are subject to interpretation of word or deed, questions are raised with respect to consent for the adolescent girl. At the time, she may have experienced an enormous struggle within herself as to whether to participate in the sexual act or not. In retrospect, she may perceive what happened as an overpowering of her will. Some girls have described this as a feeling state of being overwhelmed in which they were describing being overwhelmed by id forces which cooperated with an urging male. Later, their participatory element was not perceived. There is also the social norm in which protest is supposed to be made by the girl, or where a role can be played that a girl is so attractive that the male finds himself so overwhelmed by the sight of her that he forcibly overpowers her. Kinsey stated that the difference between a *rape* and a *good time* sometimes hinged on whether the girl's parents were awake when she arrived home.[114]

However, the opposite type of situation may exist in the young male. Since coercion and threats, as well as physical tussling, can be interpreted as playing the game, the boy may not perceive these as coercion. However, it is more striking when evidence is presented that a girl submitted "voluntarily" according to the boy who cites her disrobing but elements such as having a knife visible or hitting her are ignored. To what extent the description by the male that the girl was not coerced (since she enjoyed intercourse) is projected into his interpretation is difficult to pin down. Every male charged with rape evaluated by the author has reported that the woman appeared to enjoy the act, conversely every women victim interviewed denied pleasure.

Another point of interest about rape is the feeling of aversion toward it by the public. Although rape is classified as an offense against the person and not against property, it has psychological elements of taking what one wants to possess. Perhaps the reverse should be emphasized—as it is by some—that many property offenses are sexualized acts. The revulsion and repugnance against acts of rape might tap what are defenses against such impulses. The impulse in the male is to perform such an act, and in the female to be "taken." Permission to perform acts of "taking"—be these goods or women—are seen under conditions when controls are abandoned by groups, such as army troops in occupied territory. It may be a matter of degree when someone, by clever business arrangements, "takes" others, or when a clever seducer "takes" a female. Often the behavior is viewed in as envious, but not necessarily illegal.

Data on overall incidence of antisocial acts, or specifically sexual offenses, is conflicting (even acknowledging the unreliable nature of the statistics involved). Incidence varies by age, race, and income level. The incidence of forcible rape per hundred-thousand population is 91 for females aged ten to nineteen, 238 for those aged twenty to twenty-nine, 104 for thirty to thirty-nine, and 48 for those forty to forty-nine years. After that, it drops to a relative zero point.[115] By race, the incidence in non-white females, compared to white females, per hundred-thousand is 2,592 to 1,860.

One study indicates that 10 percent of men arrested for rape had been in trouble previously regarding sex, while over half had never been arrested for anything.[116] In contrast, the Kinsey Institute found 22 percent of those committing rape had been convicted of rape as adults, with mean age of 24.5 years at the time of offense, and had a record for some type of juvenile offense.[117] Five percent of these were for juvenile sexual offenses. By age twenty-six, 87 percent had been convicted of some crime. By age thirty, 96 percent had such a conviction. This is the largest percent of sex offenders with a crime conviction by age thirty. Half of these convictions were for sex offenses, which is a somewhat low percentage for the overall group of those studied in the sex-offender category. Other sex offenses were primarily those against willing or acquiescent females (27 percent), exhibitionism (21 percent), and peeping (19 percent). There appears to be a sharp dichotomy between juveniles interested in pubertal or older females and those attracted to the pedophilic group, for the latter were not part of the sex offenders involved in rape. Only 17 percent were not recidivists in this particular study.

The classification used by psychiatrists, the standard diagnostic nomenclature of the American Psychiatric Association, may be tried with those committing a rape. This seeks to differentiate the offender—once he has committed the rape—by the categories and sub-categories of psychosis, neurosis, personality disorder, organic brain syndrome, mental retardation. This is one framework in terms of broad categories, but it lacks specificity for different categories within sexual offenses. For rape, it would at best screen out those who are grossly psychotic or retarded. Psychogenesis, interpersonal difficulties, environmental precipitants, or psychodynamics are omitted in that framework. Guttmacher and Weihofen attempted a classification of rapists based on their personalities.[118] They divided their classification into three types: (1) Where a sexual assault is the explosive expression of pent-up sexual impulses, (the "true sexual offender"). (2) Sadistic rapists for whom rape is a miscarried effort to injure a victim—this is sexualized in nature, but it is the overt sadistic element that is dominant rather than a desire for sexual discharge via intercourse. (3) Aggressive, criminal types of rapists who pillage and take from those on the scene. This group is basically predatory, so that in the course of their offenses, such as burglary, they may rape as well. How well these distinctions hold up is questionable, since individual adolescents are seen who at different times display all three types of behavior. Nor does clinical work necessarily confirm the hypothesis of Reinhart that there is a progression from milder forms of sexual deviation, such as voyeurism and fetishism, to child molestation or rape.[119]

Gebhart and his co-workers have classified varieties of heterosexual aggressors, including an *assaultive variety*[120] for whom sexual activity without physical violence or threat is insufficient. Hostility in their interpersonal lives is pronounced. In fact, the violence may substitute for coitus and erectile impotence is seen as an accompaniment. The victims are unknown and their characteristics seem unimportant. A weapon may be used, as well as bizarre behavior exhibited, or unnecessary and trivial thefts performed. Sturup in Denmark reported on 38 rapists, viewed as the severest group of sexual criminals, at the Herstedvester Detention Institution.[121] In the case histories, 17 of the 38 studied gave histories of petty thefts or burglaries. Four gave histories of arson as well. Assessment of adolescents engaged in sexual offenses may reveal a history of property offenses concealing the sexual element. This does not refer to symbolic aspects such as "breaking and entering," but to overt, sexually perverse behaviors such as breaking and entering for the purpose of stealing women's undergarments (making it appear that the motive was that of money). The author has evaluated juveniles and adults who have spent time in correctional institutions or prisons on such charges without the sexual nature of their offense being revealed. The key question, which is of value to the psychopathologist, is which of the large numbers of youths engaged in larcenies or burglaries are engaging in a covert or overt sexual offense? Which of them will progress to more overt acts?

> One youth began peeking in apartment buildings at age thirteen. In time, he spread his activities far beyond his neighborhood, and proceeded to enter apartments. While in them, he would fondle women's undergarments and masturbate. By age seventeen, a pattern of great risk-taking developed, and few precautions were taken. If a woman was home, he would make a threatening gesture as though he had a gun in his pocket. Or he would take a knife from the kitchen to threaten them. Having them undress was usually the intent of these behaviors, since at that point he became impotent.

A second group is described by Gebhart as *amoral delinquents,* who pay little heed to social controls and operate on a level of egocentric hedonism. Women are seen as objects to be used for sexual gratification when desired. Force may be used if the woman is recalcitrant, but it is viewed as an instrumental act in attaining a goal. These appear to be antisocial personalities or dyssocial behavior patterns.

Drunken varieties of sexual assault occur in Gebhart's third category. These vary from mild release of sexual restraints to those with the full force of pent up hate and aggression released. In some cases, sexual assaults only occur during intoxication. A pattern of sexual release among adolescents under the influence of alcohol or drugs falls into this category. In some of the cases, a rape results.

Explosive outbursts of sexual assaultiveness constitute Gebhart's fourth group. These appear similar to explosive outbursts of affect or other types of impulses. In some of these cases laymen are surprised to find a previously conforming and law-abiding youth, strongly committed on a conscious level to opposing dissident elements in his community, performing a violent act of brutal rape or assault. Some of these individuals have adapted in a schizoid manner which shifts into a regressive psychotic episode.

Double-standard males fall into a fifth group. These men live out the pattern which dichotomously groups females into good and bad types. This is similar to Gebhart's first group, except that the behaviors appear confined to sexual aggressiveness toward provocative females. In many adolescent gangs this is the standard of machismo by which female pickups are raped. At times, the using is a group phenomenon in which the property is shared by the gang like communal property. Hell's Angel's women are a striking example. Homosexual elements are present in group activities. Subcultural sexual norms are influential as are provocative sexual behaviors by "dumb broads" who are viewed as inviting.

This raises the question of *victimology* in rape. It has been a source of jokes and humor throughout history and in the past, illustrated by suspected witches who were trussed hand and foot and thrown into a pond. If the woman floated, she was guilty and was subsequently burned. If she drowned, she was viewed as innocent. Contemporary situations are the girl faced with the choice of giving in or being allowed to walk back to town from a rural road. The underlying theme of the rapee as victim is that the woman is at least ambivalent, if not willing, about sexual overtures, and during the course of a sexual attack her protests will give way to consent. Legman sums this up in the following interplay:[122]

Boy: "I'll rape you, so help me."

Girl: "I'll help you, so rape me;" or, "But, if I help you, will it be rape?"

Victimology theory has been expanded into many areas and there has been a progression to the point where guilt is reassigned to victims for putting themselves into situations where others are unjustly tempted. A past rule of thumb for police investigations is that a woman who had not fought as hard as she was able to fight is suspect unless the alleged attacker had a knife or gun.[123] Further, a woman who had a prior social acquaintance with the man is viewed as unlikely to have been raped. The variety of rapists in related situations makes facile generalizations about victimization seem

Sociological data on 646 cases of forcible rape occurring in Philadelphia in two separate years were reported on by Amir.[124] Several myths were disproved in this study, and other significant findings were made. Interestingly, rape turned out to be primarily a crime of adolescence. The highest rates among offenders and victims were in the fifteen to nineteen year age group. Even when the offender was older, the victim was likely to be in a lower age group. Rape was also found to be an intraracial act with a higher incidence between black men and women. Blacks exceeded whites both as victims and offenders in absolute numbers as well as in terms of their proportion in the general population. Offenders and victims were at the same age level for intraracial rape events. Ninety percent of the offenders were in the lower occupational scale.

In this detailed study, 82 percent of offenders and victims lived in the same area, while 68 percent lived in a neighborhood triangle. While only one-third of all the rape events involved alcohol, in 63 percent of these involvements it was present in both parties. Fifty percent of the rapists had previous arrest records, and in some cases where there was a persistence in law violation, over 50 percent of those with adult records had records as juveniles. Contrary to a prevailing impression, 71 percent of the rapes were planned and 87 percent employed only temptation or verbal coercion to subdue the victim. In over half the rapes the victim displayed only submissive behavior; in 27 percent resistance was mild; and in 18 percent the victims put up a strong resistance against their attackers.

Instead of dealing with the psychological concept of "victim proneness," risk situations were discussed in the Amir study in terms of women entering situations which would increase the likelihood of their becoming rape victims: (1) victims and offenders of the same race and/or age; (2) victims of felony-rape (during the course of a burglary or robbery) who were at least ten years older than their assailants; (3) victims and offenders who met during the summer months, mainly on weekends, during evening hours in a place encouraging the development of an acquaintanceship; (4) alcohol present in both a white offender and white victim, or a white offender and black victim, or in a victim only if the assailant was white; (5) black victims with "a bad reputation" living in the neighborhood of the black attackers, when the rape was planned; (6) victims and offenders, both neighbors of the same age and race, or when a pattern of drinking relationships was established prior to the offense; (7) a drinking victim accosted in the street by strangers.

The concept of victim-precipitated rape was viewed in reference to cases where the victim actually—or so the offender interpreted—agreed to intercourse but later reneged or did not strongly resist. In this group were 19 percent of the sample. Significant factors were: (1) white victims; white intraracial rapes; alcohol in the rape situation, particularly in the victim or both in offender and victim; (2) victims with a bad reputation; victims who live in residential proximity to the offenders and/or the area of offense; victims who meet their offenders in a bar, at a picnic or party; (3) victims who were in primary relationships with the offenders but who were not their relatives; (4) victims who were raped outside the home or place of soujourn of the offender or victim; (5) victims subjected to sexual humiliation.

For some adolescent boys a fusion of sexuality with aggression operates so that only resistance by the woman elicits potency. While diverse contrivances may be arranged to facilitate this without the act of rape, in some cases the need for taking a female by force becomes the sine qua non to perform. The panoply of sado-masochistic relationships is a generic grouping of relationships that may be carried to the point of an overtly physical rape. In most cases, individuals plagued by this type of personality limitation reenact their acts of aggression and submission with many people with whom they become involved. For some, the sexualized aspects take on a noticeable twist in their love life when quarrels or physical fights become necessary before intercourse. Nor need a physical submissiveness operate, since placing a sexual partner in a grossly inferior or degrading role may prove adequate. This may be by performing excretory acts on a woman, and then submitting to her doing the same to him.

In other cases, the great passivity and fear of the male at the hands of a woman is handled by a transformation to placing the woman in the position of great fear of him. Although in many cases there may be no conscious intent to harm her, harm or death may result nevertheless.

For some adolescents, there is a diffuse display of poor sexual controls which manifest themselves in episodic perverse acts. Pedophilic activities, grabbing women, throwing women to the ground with or without a simulation of intercourse, touching the women's genital or breast areas are possibilities. Gang-bangs have been referred to, and these may represent the dependency of the adolescent male on both his same-sexed peer group and the female who is used in common. Homosexual impulses may seek their mutual gratification in such forays as well.

We have mentioned the need of some individuals for the experience of strong feelings and physical aggressiveness prior to intercourse. In a small minority this not only leads to rape, but to "rape-murders." This is a misleading phrase in some respects since the goal may not necessarily be murder, but rather a limited physical assault. the woman may be left injured (but some die as a result). However, for an even smaller subgroup, murder itself may be a condition of potency. These should both be distinguished from murders to prevent discovery. Allen lists five characteristics of the lust murder:[125] (1) Periodic outbreaks occur due to recurring compulsions or paroxysmal sexual desire. (2) Nearly always, cutting or stabbing, particularly on the breasts or genital area, occurs, and there is frequently sucking or licking of the wounds, biting of the skin, and sometimes a desire to drink the blood (vampirism) and eat the flesh. (3) Ejaculation may occur first, followed by violation of the victim, or no attempted intercourse at all. (4) An affective storm which clouds consciousness is possible. (5) Behavior is usually rormal until the next paroxysm. Such individuals are viewed as havirg not integrated their destructive pregenital components in their personalities. In some, a split occurs, within the realm of a developing control system between love for certain restraining figures and the internalized system of restraint.[126] What emerges is a fascinating type of love and devotion toward certain loved objects, while the full destructive fury is reserved for scapegoat victims. Upon the latter, all hostile feelings are projected. This accounts for normal-appearing intervals in these individuals, but the potential for compulsively recurring lust leaves them highly dangerous unless an attempted therapeutic intervention is made. The legendary Jack the Ripper appears to have fallen into this category, as well as the fictional Mr. Hyde.

Extremely aggressive behavior may result in necrophilia (intercourse with a dead female), dismemberment of the dead victim's body, defacing by acid, or cannibalism. Many of these perpetrators appear psychotic, and are reacting on the basis of a projected fear that they will be feminized as a result of mutilation. On the basis of this conscious and unconscious fear, the female victim is made to suffer. The anlage of this is seen in the fantasies of children, as played out in their activities or later in the jokes and humor of the adolescent, referred to as "sick." Occasional breakdowns in superego controls are seen in adolescents who break in and mutilate beds, pictures, or undergarments. Acting out these impulses may not be confined to adolescence or the period beyond, nor need it be restricted to boys.

A bright, physically charming girl of nine caused immense consternation in her neighborhood. Two neighborhood homes had been broken into and both the underclothing of men and women cut up. In addition, a wedding picture of one couple had been defaced with the word 'fuck' scribbled with lipstick over the front of it. One of the victims recalled the intense devotion of this girl, and how she had stopped coming over to visit in the week subsequent to this event—the origin of which was then unknown. The family was inhibited, pious, and strict about sex, without using any physical disciplinary techniques. Stunned amazement was expressed that their daughter could have carried out such an act, or even known such words. The deep attachment of this little girl and her envious resentment of the attachments these couples enjoyed led to a retaliatory type of acting out.

Exhibitionism. Although a commonplace definition of exhibitionism is the exposure of male genitals to a female in an intentional manner, and in an inappropriate public setting, seems simple it is complex in a psychiatric and legal sense. Hence, how public must public be? Need the act be witnessed? What makes the act inappropriate? Consider contemporary variations in styles of dress or exposure, or the license for theatrical nudity, or such phenomena as nudist camps, nude marathon groups, or streaking. These raise issues about indecency and decorum serving other goals, in contrast to exhibitionism as a perverse act. The act may or may not be handled legally as indecent exposure; it may be covered under "lewd and lascivious behavior," public indecency, disorderly conduct, or vagrancy, as well as under the generic heading of delinquency.

When the adolescent exposes his genitals in public, multiple functions are served. The behavior can be *phase-specific* as well as *reactive* to conflict. A variety of classifications have been compiled for the acts beyond the legal groupings or descriptive psychiatry. Norwood East and Hubert elaborated six groupings:[127]

1. "True exhibitionism" is when the exhibitionistic act is the preferred means of sexual activity in itself.

2. Exhibitionism with a goal of exciting or enticing a female into sexual intercourse may be an instrumental act. If this is unsuccessful, masturbation may take place. A projective identification appears present in which the male assumes—and in some cases delusionally believes—that the sight of his genitalia will excite a woman in the manner female genitals excite him.

3. As an accompaniment of impotence, exhibitionism may give relief or reassurance, especially when this occurs before a group of women.

4. Reactive exhibitionism occurs in response to stress, such as in situations of temptation, or under pre-existing stress from different conflicts. Drugs or alcohol may serve as the releasor. A combination of solicitation, acting out of puns or humor, or direct expression of aggressive impulses may occur. A fifteen-year-old, apprehended outside a leading department store in his city while urinating on the front door, expressed his relatively unconcealed impulse about the authority figures in his community.

5. Impaired intellectual or cognitive functioning may contribute to exposure.

6. At the commencement of heterosexual activity during adolescence, a variety of motives operate and lead to self-exposure.

Complex motives operate with most exhibitionistic activity. The distinction between a reactive pattern to threats about manhood, may not have yet acquired the quality of compulsiveness accompanying exposure as a preferred mode of sexual behavior. As a reactive solution it is secondary to another objective to relieve inadequacy from failures, disappointments, or deprivations. The Kinsey data indicated one-quarter of all exhibitionists suffer from impotence, and one-third of these are compulsive exposers.[128] In almost every case of compulsive exhibitionism, the activity started in childhood, and by puberty there were voyeuristic tendencies as well.[129] The difficulty with such findings is the presence of polymorphous manifestations among a large number of children and adolescents in the course of their struggles. The specificity question recurs in terms of the lack of indicators which offer greater evidence regarding which of these behaviors will have an ultimate outcome as a response to stress or a perversion.

Several mechanisms are possible. These represent a combination of situational, reactive, and psychodynamic possibilities. Situations of extreme threat to self-esteem, or loss of an object to which one is deeply attached, can precipitate exhibitionistic acts. While they are usually transient during adolescence, lack of resolution of the blow to self-esteem or reparative efforts to deal with the loss may lead to a reinforcement of the behaviors as an ego-adaptive device. There are several possibilities.[130]

1. Castration anxieties may be denied by the magical exposure of genitals. Accompanying this is a wish that the woman in turn expose herself by the powerful maneuver the man has carried out. Unconscious reassurance is obtained that women are afraid—and not the reverse—and there is hope that women in turn can show him something for reassurance purposes. Little girls may be preferred as

objects to expose to, since supposedly they will be more impressed and frightened.

2. Passive-aggressive defiance utilizes exposure to achieve separation from objects on whom one is dependent. They appear not only to be struggling with emancipation but also have a strong need to demonstrate their autonomy. As one teenage boy, engaged in compulsive exhibitionism, put it in discussing his mother and older sister with whom he lived, "I've got to show them that my cock is my own and not theirs." A plea for someone to extricate them from their intrafamilial dilemma is often detected. Youths with obsessional character structures may expose as a defiant solution against moral prohibitions. These challenges concern sexuality, but also corrupt authority figures. A more universal exposure in adolescents is present in their manner of dress to shock adults, which is merely regarded as part of the teenage culture.

3. Related to the defiance is a variety which is compensating for phallic impotence. These passive and docile boys are sesperately seeking reassurance that they have the ability to function as males. Antecedents of intense dependency and reinforcement of receiving pleasure without effort is present. The context of an intense relationship with a maternal figure is expected, and such boys are disappointed when women do not continue adoring them. Their contribution is minimal, and when put into a situation where they must compete for the attention and affection of women they become extremely anxious. Those who feel they possess bodies which should be a pleasure for anyone to observe, and have been extravagantly admired and petted in the past, are not likely candidates to compete successfully for affection. Later frotteur activities suffice for some. If fortunate, sublimatory achievements intellectually, socially, or athletically suffice. The magic of their exhibitionistic acts is seen in the need to make others irresistibly view the beauty and power of their bodies.

4. Exhibitionism as part of homosexual desires varies from an overtly conscious invitation to a male to take a look to unconscious seeking of "male" women. This appears to deny the fear of homosexuality by way of exhibitionism.

5. Displaced autoerotism is a mechanism for exhibitionism and works as a substitute for masturbation. The boy who masturbates as part of the exhibitionism may feel the exposure is a necessary antecedent to masturbation.

6. Defenses against orality operate by way of scoptophilic impulses. Their desires to be devoured, are counterbalanced by fears

of being devoured. Some feel oral fixation is the most important determinant for exhibitionism.[131] The exhibitionistic act itself is a coercive "taking in" of others. And in that sense, is a coercive exploitation of others for one's own sexual usage.

7. Sado-masochistic impulses are connected with many of the above factors. The need to insult or render a female helpless is part of the sadism. Self-destructive patterns fit into not only the compulsive repetition, but the lack of caution as to where the exhibitionistic acts occur. This is congruent with the observation that little resentment about punishment, or being placed in jail or correctional facilities, may be present. Punishment appears unlikely to stop these behaviors, but it may aid their perpetuation by way of a masochistic solution being available when needed. The punishment which the exhibitionistic person seeks may not be for exposing but rather for desires and impulses which are prohibited and never dealt with.

Voyeurism. The connection between voyeurism and exhibitionism illustrates the interrelationship between perverse activities. This is seen in other activities as well, such as frotteurism, obscene exclamations, obscene phone calls, burglaries and thefts. Two levels of usage should be distinguished. One describes actual acts, such as an individual who looks into a private home or area reserved for females in the hope of seeing them nude or partially clad. A second is theoretical in which a concept covers a diverse series of visually taking in impulses and activities. Developmentally, this includes a host of incorporative and introjective phenomena commencing in infancy with the closeness of looking and touching. Taking in experiences characterized by greed, hunger, and soothing experiences are not confined to one developmental process, but generalize.

The equation, "looking equals devouring," was formulated on the basis of an incorporative act.[132] Evidence for the equation is seen in the productions and verbalizations of children and adults. Hence, to be hoodwinked is to be taken in. The wolf in Little Red Riding Hood needed big eyes the better to see the victim, and next a big mouth the better to eat her up. To gaze can be a sadistic act, but simultaneously a fascination and intrigue for the gazer. This is the connection between the voyeur and exhibitionist on a theoretical level for, analogous to the hypnotic situation, when one is forced to gaze upon another, he becomes the compliant subject. He may then be forced to imitate what he witnesses. If the subject is forced to observe genitalia, he may carry out a similar act of exposing his own. The eye comes to function, in scoptophilia and voyeurism, as an erogenous zone.[133] To inhibit curiosity about the desire to look may result in a reaction formation device, such as pronounced shyness and avoidance.

From these developmental antecedents, it is clear that not all peeking is equivalent to a voyeuristic act. Perversion development is not present unless there is a clandestine type of looking, with the hope of seeing the genitals, not preparatory to intercourse but as a substitute activity. Peeking at someone who supposedly believes they are in a private location is essential.[134] Peeking on girlfriends or women whom one already knows in an intimate sense is not sufficient for the actual voyeur. However, the adolescent boy may peek at girls he knows, such as sisters or mothers, or from his own neighborhood or school. Solidified, male, adult peekers are solitary workers, but, in contrast, adolescents again may engage in peeking as a joint venture.

An overriding sense of disgust is present in these youths. While an occasional peeker may call attention to himself by tapping on windows, or appearing as the monster at the window, there is more frequently a desire to remain secreted. The impulse appears satisfied by the sight of forbidden aspects of the female, such as her breasts or genitals, to see her undressing or excreting, the prize catch appears to be that of coitus. The element of risk involves a gambler's instinct—much like someone who continues to play against the odds with hope of a victory. In some cases, the element of stealth and awe proceed to the point where the bizarre creeps in.

> A fifteen-year-old boy was apprehended after a series of repeated incidents over months. Complaints to police by parents were that their daughters had awakened during the night and found a strange boy standing in their room staring at them. Most of the victims were girls between the ages of five and ten. Peeking through windows had commenced a year earlier and led to entering houses in order to stare down at the young victims. He preferred these young girls be sleeping, related to his need for their helplessness, both from their age and unconscious state. They were not touched, although the boy could occasionally approach the bed and stand next to it for hours observing the sleeping child. Masturbation occurred a minority of times. When someone appeared to be entering the room, he would hide in closets and then return to his position near the bed. He had carried out a similar type of peeking in his parents' bedroom when younger, but this has ceased many years earlier. Adolescent sexuality reinvoked the traumatic "primal scene" material, which was not confined to masturbation but literally acted out.

This rare type of case raises the recurring question about the progression of certain types of sexually perverse behaviors. The question is whether the perverse acts remain fixed or seek diverse outlets. Most writers tend to emphasize that exhibitionism and voyeurism are more social nuisances than indications of a propensity toward physically violent acts.[135] This may be a statistical finding, since there is clinical material to illustrate that it progresses only in a few. Again, the difficulty is our inability to predict who will have a progressive course toward physically violent acts. This is a subquestion related to the broader one of which adolescents engaging in exhibitionistic behavior will consolidate it as a perversion.

Data from the Kinsey study raised similar disturbing questions.[136] After excluding those who were intoxicated, mentally deficient, situationally taking advantage of an opportunity, or who were socio-sexually underdeveloped, fourteen men in their subject group remained. Ten of the fourteen had been convicted of rape. They did not have distinguishing variables for the subgroup, but had the impression that those who enter homes or call attention to themselves are more likely to become rapists. Compared to the overall group of sex offenders in that study, they had the second largest group (29 percent) of previous juvenile convictions. Nor were the juvenile offenses trivial, for 80 percent of the commitments were for over six months. The percentage of peepers convicted as juvenile sex offenders is also the second largest in their subject group, at 11 percent. Some of these individuals have a strong sado-masochistic component, which is acted out. Those adolescent peepers most prudish and sly about sexuality may be a group who seek out this impersonalized contact. All of this coexists with a rather strict and puritanical notion about sexual conduct and decency which governs the remainder of their lives. Sadistic behaviors in latency toward animals is obtained in histories of some of these individuals, illustrating the breakthrough, much like the prim little girl who scrawled obscene words on her neighbor's picture.

Obscene Communicators.   Exhibitionism and voyeurism involve the visual component of sexual impulses. The auditory component appears through obscene messages or phone calls. Girls may even outrank boys in frequency. This is especially so during adolescence and when done by girls in a group. In some cases, it merges into the problem of obscenity and pornography. The difference lies in such varieties as the message being directed to one person rather than the public. In some cases, it may be directed to an individual who is known or a relative. A mixture involves sadistic and exhibitionistic components, such as the defacing of public buildings, walls, or sides of houses. In other cases, drawings of sexual organs or activities are made, or words and invitations are scribbled on walls. Graffiti in lavatories of buildings illustrate the wide prevalence of such practices.

While written communication and drawings occur among adolescents, phone calls are more prevalent beginning with the preadolescent group. The blending of voices at a distance, an unknown caller and rescuer, and the opportunity to indulge in all the obscenities usually considered taboo in other settings make this activity appealing to the young adolescent. No physical contact or confrontation is necessary, yet an awesome image may be conveyed. These random types of calls are done with excitement, giggling, and fear, and are usually phase-specific types of outlets for sexual feelings. In some cases aggressive threats to authority figures, such as teachers, principals, clergy, or special types of people such as old grannies are prevalent.

These activities must be distinguished from those which become compulsive wherein the gratification from this activity is preferred as a sexual or aggressive outlet. Prevalence of such phone calls can be gauged from a special "annoyance calls" bureau established in New York. In one nine-month period, 65,500 anonymous calls were reported to this bureau.[137] Five percent of the calls were threats, 19 percent obscene (in the sense of an obscenity used to female or male children under ten), 66 percent were harassing (in that the caller did not speak), and 10 percent were interference (so that a line was tied up or no outgoing calls could be made). Low self-esteem characterize these males, who have a striking need for reassurance. In some cases the calls occur as part of a mounting anxiety, while in others it is their self-respect which suffers most. Coupled with a low self-concept are power feelings which are not easily abandoned. The telephone becomes a perfect vehicle for the individual who feels he may be laughable or despised and hence seeks revenge without fearing loss of control.

> An oversized fifteen-year-old boy engaged in lewd calls for a year. He was apprehended after a series of calls to a forty-year-old divorced female neighbor. They had carried on these mutual calls for a period which covered six to eight calls, by her report, although the boy stated there were at least fifteen. During the course of the calls, the boy used language pertaining to intercourse

and at times propositioned her to meet him so that they might have intercourse. The calls were carried out with a tone of gaiety, according to the boy, with teasing by the woman that he was only putting her on. The end point came when a meeting was actually arranged. The police were informed by the woman and the boy apprehended.

This boy's home was overcrowded. Six siblings shared two bedrooms. The offender was the eldest boy and had an older sister who was insulting toward him in most respects. When his father consumed alcohol to any extent, which was frequent, he would taunt the boy with comments such as, 'You wouldn't know what to do with a piece if it was put in your face.' Another interesting aspect of this case, and others of this type, is the role of the female victim. The woman had registered a previous complaint a few years earlier. Many of the issues relevant to victimology operate here as well.

PORNOGRAPHY AND ADOLESCENCE

Pornography is a restricted grouping of what is more broadly the problem of obscene communications, vulgarity, or even poor taste. Two immediate issues arise: How can we determine poor taste or vulgarity? A mechanism for making such a judgment is needed for setting the criteria which will be used. The second question refers to how the criteria should be implemented. Of course, another option is to abandon the entire enterprise as impossible, but few to wish to do this. To regulate obscenity, subjective and moral criteria come to the fore as to what standards of modesty or decency should be. Close attention needs to be paid to distinctions between *community* mores, in contrast to *legal* standards. Nor need the community and legal standards agree. Both of these approaches in turn need to be distinguished from *psychological* curiosity in pornographic materials. A final problem is *psychiatric*: the use of pornographic materials as a preferred or exclusive mode of sexual outlet which enters the realm of perversion.

Origins of the Condemnation. Moral origins of the condemnation of looking at or reading forbidden things were from fear of inciting lustful acts. Giving free rein to one's impulses was fearful to the individual and the community. Being lewd and lascivious carries a connotation of moral wrongness, and the fear the individual may indulge beyond looking.

Marcus has traced the principles of pornography back to themes of the Victorian era:[138]

1. Sex and money (being "obscenely rich") are inseparable.

2. Splits develop between feelings of tenderness and sexuality.

3. Pornography has an autistic or soft-directed element.

4. Presentation of body parts as sexual tools which can be mechanically manipulated is germane to pornography.

5. Pornography is a masculine-oriented field, dominated by the fantasies of men as to a woman's expectations and behavior.

6. Fears of sexual inadequacy are related to indulgence in pornographic tastes and needs to banish the materials to an underground market. Statutes restrain people from doing what they want in the service of control over impulses. A premise operates that legislation will help people—the developing adolescent among others—to control their desires. Supposedly, state regulation is a benevolent gesture by the state to help internalized inhibitions which develop by way of an external threat. Exogenous censorship is to society as endogenous censorship is to the individual.

7. An exaggerated stress on the rational and objective components of human relationships dominates the conscious activities of individuals. Such an emphasis relegates to the unconscious, or clandestine operations, the field of pornography.

8. A search for the polymorphous sexualized pleasures of early childhood is handled through pornography.

9. A repetitive circularity occurs in a futile quest for gratification through pornographic indulgence.

Questions arise, such as how much erotism is to be sanctioned within a community in terms of open interest and expression. To what extent should sexual arousal be permitted or restricted? In a psychological sense, the question is a developmental one of at what stage and to what degree certain types of sexual behaviors should be stimulated? Consider whether there is anything pathological in owning and using pornographic materials where the materials are primarily and directly used to induce sexual arousal. What about statutes dealing with possession of these materials? Does pornography do sufficient psychological damage to make prohibition useful? If there are adverse consequences from pornography, is the remedy a legal one? Is there an adverse impact on children or adolescents from exposure to such materials?

There is a tangential question of pornography as a primary causal agent in criminality. Discussion of this controversial issue is given elsewhere. In essence, the evidence is tenuous for pornography as a major causal agent of crime except for the individual who is already vulnerable and idiosyncratic. While pornography may shift sexual values, this should be distinguished from inducing criminal acts.

Legal-Behavioral Issues. In view of the controversy surrounding the impact of pornography, a synthests of the combined legal-behavioral issues will illustrate the interface between the behavioral sciences and its legal applications. Nothing compels a citizen, court, or legislative body to pay heed to what psychiatric opinion is on the impact of pornographic materials. This is true even if there was a consensus of psychiatric opinion on pornography's adverse effects. Nor need what child psychiatrists call a perverse use of pornographic materials be related to whatever standard courts or social groups consider undesirable. Whether an individual should be viewed as a sexual offender is determined by criteria apart from whatever a particular psychiatrist's opinion is.

These issues come to the fore conspicuously when vague—yet important—issues arise on regulating distribution of what are alleged pornographic materials. Hidden assumptions accompany these stances, and the psychiatrist enters the scene by virtue of citations being made to the literature of the behavioral sciences to buttress one side or the other. Another point needing clarification is the distinction between *why* anyone believes certain visual materials require regulation from what *objectives* are sought by supporting such legislation. The latter presupposes that some type of regulation is not only desirable but necessary. Debate customarily proceeds within the framework of how much and what type of regulations should be enacted. The question of why goes to the heart of the question of what is the necessity for having regulations regarding materials alleged to be erotic, and by extension, pornographic.

Objectives to be sought by the regulation of erotic materials have been urged on different bases. Here we discuss a psychiatric perspective. A primary basis has been to prevent or curtail sexual stimulation. The reason is that pornography supposedly leads to behavior of a criminal type. In some cases a broader standard is employed in an effort to prevent behavior contrary to the moral standards or common conscience of a community. However, critical analysis of empirical studies, and the Report of the Commission on Obscenity and Pornography, indicate little basis for believing a causal relationship exists between pornography and much of anything.[139]

Utilization of sexually stimulating materials by a curious adolescent, or an inhibited male, in the privacy of his home must be distinguished from allegations about the impact on groups or populations. While a significant portion of individuals, particularly males, become sexually aroused by erotic stimuli in the form of pictures, books, or conversation, these appear to be situational response.[140] How long does such arousal last? Do overt acts result? What about induced attitudinal changes? What adverse consequences on psychological functioning result? These questions are all unresolved.

The type of experimentation carried out under the aegis of the above-mentioned Commission does not give much help. The number of influences and predisposing factors contributing to personality development are too complex for facile genralizations based on immediate pro or con situational responses. Further, would anyone really wish to argue that the world would be a better place, or psychosexual development enhanced, by the elimination of sexually arousing stimuli from the environment?

Are adolescents in need of protection from exposure to pornography and filth? Protection assumes adolescents are more vulnerable to such exposures. Little evidence exists to support the vulnerability thesis from the behavioral and clinical fields. The evidence is not clear about which aspect of adolescent development is seen as endangered. Some express fears about premature sexual activity. Sexual activity itself is usually left undefined as a grouping of diverse acts varying from masturbation to sexual intercourse, as well as fears that a host of perverse acts will result. It is pointed out that the greatest number of delinquents are those most likely to have poor reading abilities compared to the general public, or not have as ready access to books and materials considered pornographic. The point is that pornographic literature may have a limited erotic function on the American scene. Detail would be needed in terms of which pornographic materials one is taking about (books, movies, photographs). There is an inference that upper-middle-class boys, who have greater access to pornographic material by virtue of their social position and affluence, should show more adverse influences relative to lower-class boys. No data exists to substantiate this.

Would we expect a specific adverse effect on sexual development from exposing adolescents to pornography? Or would the effect be more on general personality development and configuration? The specificity issue is relevant since different types of pornographic materials, nude pictures for example, might be more available in lower-class settings. Clinicians must avoid the myopia of believing that when there is talk of the adverse consequences on adolescent development, consistency of criteria for what is considered developmental exist. Avoidance of certain sexual thoughts and attitudes in juveniles is considered a legitimate goal of child development by some. No justification need then be given that delinquency in general, or specific sexually offensive acts, show an increased incidence. All that is required is a belief that obscenity *may* be crime-promoting, or even a more general belief that obscenity promotes bad thoughts. A more sophisticated theory is that exposure to pornography is undesirable since it erodes a sense of mutually shared values in society. This amounts to a utilitarian argument that moral development is enhanced in a desired direction in as many individuals as possible for purposes of social cohesiveness.[141]

Nor can it be concluded, in the absence of persuasive clinical or empirical evidence, that obscenity regulations should or should not be abandoned. A position of advocating psychological health by way of pornography has been put forth in the "safety valve" theory, which sees exposure to pornographic materials as furthering a healthy course of development. Hence, pornography is held to function preventively to abort perverse development. Even if clinical evidence could support this semicathartic position, it will be exceedingly difficult to assess it as having more than a limited impact among the multifarious variables. A tentative conclusion is that the problem of promoting or banning pornography at this time should not be thought of as one amenable to solution by clinicians or social scientists. Other people and groups—politicians, clergy, and law enforcement officials—will continue to be far more influential in deciding what is classified as pornographic.[142]

Justifications for Control of Obscenity. Justification of obscenity legislation is not based solely on attempts to prevent stimulation of sexual behavior judged illicit. Maintenance of the moral standards of a community, and prevention of change in these standards, is an implicit guide to regulation of erotic materials by those who fear community standards are being eroded by tasting the forbidden hemlock. Related to this basis for opposition is the moral conviction that obscene materials corrupt character by stimulating thoughts best left unevoked. It is an argument based on the psychological assumption that repressive barriers are better left intact.

An extension of these themes is that of psychological altruism which argues that minors, will be better off if they do not have to deal with the feelings aroused from exposure to pornography. The "better off" is used in a moral sense, since we do not know if the person will be in a better state psychologically. Again, confusion of the moral with the utilitarian is present. The moral axiom that exposure is wrong is not equivalent to a position that undesirable consequences will necessarily follow therefrom. In this sense the altruistic position is analogous to the parens patriae position for dealing with juveniles, where the state judges what is a permissible level of exposure for such materials. A last objective is the curtailment of commercial exploitation from pornography. However, this argument is circular since the scarcity of materials is cited as the basis for creating a consumer market which can be exploited.

Varying legal standards have been applied within a constitutional framework to regulate pornography. Since this is a major topic in its own right, only the main points related to arguments based on the alleged adverse consequences on personality functioning will be discussed. Five main standards have been employed, which all have psychological assumptions:

1. Obscenity is viewed as appealing to "prurient" interests. The assumption is that it is desirable to protect individuals from exposure to such materials because they are bad for the person. The difficulty with this and almost any of the standards is the inherent vagueness and subjectivity, as well as the tacit assumption that prurience is bad.

2. Conflicts arise when an effort is made to delineate which group the standard will apply to. Is there a standard of prurience different for adolescents than for adults? If so, what is it, and how does one determine what it is? Or, is the standard actually directed to curtailing exposure to pornographic materials for a group with pre-existing perverse dispositions so as to make it more difficult for them to develop further in this direction, or indulge their perverse-prurient interests? The latter verges on the standard of obscenity which originally permitted something to be judged obscene by the effect of an isolated excerpt upon those who were susceptible.[143] Presumably, both adolescents and perverts would be lumped in the group of susceptibles.

3. The abandonment of the "most susceptible person" test of obscenity gradually eroded, and was supplanted by holding that material is obscene if the dominant theme taken as a whole appeals to the prurient interests of the group.[144] Most intriguing is the possibility of erotically stimulating materials being specifically directed to adolescents, and on that basis being ruled obscene. The result would be that materials are not available to adults as well. What emerges is a variable obscenity standard where the material is seen as not inherently obscene, but that it may be so for a special

group, such as adolescents.[145] Again, it is not clear whether the psychological presumption is that this would inspire desirable or healthy development. Is the assumption that adults can take it without becoming corrupted or perverted?

4. Another standard is an appeal to the contemporary standards of a community. Many of the same questions are relevant. What is the community standard? Is the community a locality within a larger geographical unit? Is it a political subdivision such as a state, region, or the country as a whole? If it is the latter, it amounts to defining a standard in terms of the norms of contemporary society for the whole country. Any of these approaches have the unclarified position that the individual and community unit will be better off as a result of regulation.

5. Once the community standard is introduced, references about the countervailing impact of the work having "redeeming social value" are invoked. Subtleties arise, such as ideas or expressions with social importance being entitled to expression, but since obscenity is not considered of such importance, by definition, it is not sanctioned.

Data from the Kinsey Institute was based on a sample of 2,721 convicted sex offenders. Only fourteen males in the sample had never been exposed to pornography, due to its prevalence in the social classes they came from; a sizable number reported little or no sexual arousal from pornography. Education and intelligence enter, since the better educated and intelligent are more likely to be imaginative and responsive to psychological stimuli. Those without these assets are more apt to use concrete sets of operations and respond to specific stimuli. Conversely, the homosexual group may be most responsive to pornography by virtue of loadings with respect to education and intelligence.

In a broader sense, offenders who utilize physical aggression may be manifesting poor controls over much of their impulse life. The only conlusions are that the capacity to benefit from pornography is associated with imaginativeness, ability to project, and sensitivity—which in turn correlate with education and youthfulness per se. Response to pornography, compared to utilization of fantasy about the sight of females, was rated by the Kinsey group. The results reveal three groups based on frequency of occurrence:[147] (1) The largest—one-third to one-half—report that the intensity of response to the two stimuli is the same, i.e., pornography is no better and no worse than utilization of fantasies. (2) The second group— one-quarter to one-half—have a more intense response to the sight or thought of females than to pornography. (3) The smallest number—one-eighth to one-quarter—have a stronger response to porno-graphy.

Is the Fuss Worth It? If the evidence is extremely unsettled about the adverse consequences of pornography, why the enormous investment of time, money, and feeling by individuals and groups representing law enforcement, education, churches, psychiatry, psychology, and sociology? While the developmental consequences for the adolescent at best remain uncertain, and pro and con arguments wax and wane.

Apart from a few compulsive individuals who engage in pornographomania as a compromise, pornographic materials take on significance by serving as a reinforcement for the majority of individuals who maintain their self-image as someone not defiled by sex. This is an example of the dichotomy between what is considered decent, ethical, and nonsexual with its opposite: sanctioning sexual license. It is therefore not so much a matter of maintaining self-control, but of maintaining self-esteem which has internalized norms forbidding sexual curiosity unless carried out in a restricted manner. The strength of this need can be gauged by the large number of groups who zealously feel it essential to impose their code on others. In one sense, this protects adolescents from the repressed and unresolved impulses of their elders who remain conflicted about looking without guilt. By imposing restrictions, neither the adults nor their progeny will obtain license to carry out these acts.

While an adolescent may clandestinely seek out an occasional venture involving pornographic materials, in time the majority go the way of all flesh and perpetuate the same concerns and repressions throughout their life. This is not an argument that the adolescent is necessarily better off by exposure to every type of sexual material—be it on the stage, screen, or in print—but rather that the consequences are unknown. While it might be argued that lack of knowledge argues for restriction until confirmatory knowledge is available, the presumption is that empirical findings of the consequences on development will resolve the issue. The position advocated here is not only that there is little to suggest that confirmatory psychological evidence will help, but rather that concern about pornography is actually a reflection and product of other needs and conflicts.

Nor can openness with respect to the expression of open violence be ignored. Unless one is willing to argue that the media have little influence on people (a position for which there is contrary evidence), we can operate on a pragmatic basis that writings, readings, and visual materials are likely to have some influence. They have different reactions based on age and psychological disabilities. But why are we still so concerned about the effects of sexual materials in an age when the promotion of violence and aggression are so much larger problems? We are fighting the wrong battle at the wrong time.

PROSTITUTION

Introduction. The original meaning of the word pornography was the description of the behavior and pursuits of prostitutes. In examining the psychopathology of adolescents who engage in this activity there are ramifications and perspectives which extend beyond the immediate act. Epidemiologic questions involve the incidence of prostitution by social class, ethnicity, and demographic area. Adolescent populations figure significantly, since that is when many girls commence sexual activity for pay; nor can we ignore homosexual prostitition.

Objections to classifying prostitution as sexual psychopathology may be valid, since it requires proof that the acts are a dependent result of personal psychological conflict. While many view prostitution as such, a contrary position argues that prostitution might be the result of a decision which perceives it as a preferable way to live a better life compared to available options. Girls engaging in prostitution do not present a homogeneous personality, motives or background. Personality types covers the standard variety of diagnostic entities from the organically impaired to schizophrenia, neuroses, and personality disorders. For some, prostitution is the way to obtain material things; for others, it is a way to maintain a drug habit. This leads some to emphasize the problem of prostitution as one more of socio-economic than psychiatric origin. The social class of girls engaging in prostitution varies, as does background and mode of operation, from street walker to call girl, depending on their talent, motivation, intelligence, and, from a psychiatric view, conflicts.

Historical reflection on the emergence of prostitution and the socio-legal ways of regulating it provides a cultural glimpse of the manner of regulating these behaviors. From colonial times until 1800, prostitution did not flourish. There are records of shiploads of women arriving in the colonies, but these were sent to be companions or marriage partners for the women-scarce colonists.

Even when prostitutes from Europe were included, they seemed to pair off and marry. Expansion of the frontier, coupled with industrialization, had the effect of leaving large numbers of women stranded without the opportunity to marry. Faced with factory labor of up to fifteen hours a day for survival, and living in a boarding-house with six to eight girls a room, prostitution assumed increasing appeal.[148] This socio-economic impetus to prostitution elicited an interesting response in the citizenry. The conditions giving rise to prostitution were ignored, while the girls were sporadically prosecuted as the houses of ill fame were burned or torn down. The implicit threat was that the family structure would be disturbed if such an indulgence for the men was provided.

When large waves of immigrants arrived in the nineteenth century, men began to outnumber women. A business opportunity was seen, and the growth of red-light districts to satisfy men's appetites began. These segregated areas flourished in most states. While only three states (Louisiana, Arkansas, and New Mexico) explicitly legalized red-light districts, prostitution was tolerated in almost all. A designated area became known for this purpose, which permitted officials to keep track of the groups. Regimentation was accomplished by city ordinances or de facto police regulations which provided for licensing and periodic medical examinations.

In some cities, in the early years of the twentieth century, houses of prostitution were closed if not first cleared and sanctioned through the police.[149] This version of prostitution has its modern advocates, who argue—on public health grounds—that government-regulated prostitution, with periodic examinations of the women, controls the spread of venereal disease. There is evidence that more venereal disease is spread by informal contact than through organized prostitution. Rather than requiring red-light districts at this time, premarital sexual activity between couples, currently provided with contraceptive mechanisms, appears to have cut down the functional necessity for isolated districts of prostitutes. Rather, various types of call houses, call girls, and those operating out of bars have emerged as modal.

Ways of Regulating Prostitution. These historical occurrences have led to the development of a melange of devices to regulate prostitution-type activities. How effective they are is another question. Keep in mind that legal and administrative approaches are not directed toward resolution of the motives which lead a girl to indulge in this sexual life. Instead, the assumption is that law enforcement regulates the traffic. This amounts to a form of secondary or tertiary prevention in which the disease is limited or its side effects minimized. In this context—if the acts as products of psychopathology are temporarily ignored—four approaches exist in communities to regulate prostitution: (a) criminal sanctions, (b) civil actions, (c) administrative devices, and (d) police regulation.

The variety of criminal sanctions attests to the vigilance with which state and local governments pursue regulation of sex-for-sale. This is more interesting when it is realized that prostitution was originally not a common law criminal act.[150] For the minor, there are the usual delinquency provisions dealing with promiscuity or absenting from home. Under criminal provisions, the most frequent charges are disorderly conduct, public nuisance, or status offenses such as vagrancy (soliciting, living without visible means of support, or maintenance of a house of ill fame). Not only are acts of intercourse for money regulated, but acts which may be preparatory to prostitution, such as street walking, bar or restaurant loitering, or soliciting are also illegal. Nor is regulation confined to the prostitite herself. The panderer or procurer who places girls in locations for prostitution, or supervises, also becomes subject to criminal sanctions. Pimp activities take two forms: solicitation of customers, or living off the earnings she makes. Both are subject to criminal sanctions.

In some cases, organized business operations of prostitution are run by groups of adolescents. The only adult participation may be as customers. Some of the adolescents in the operation are married to each other, while others engage in homosexual relationships. A variation is that of a parent who permits a daughter to prostitute, and this may be facilitated by the parent functioning as a pimp or procurer. Cases are seen where mothers utilize their daughters this way for heterosexual or homosexual purposes with clients or trio activities. While the adolescent may be handled under delinquency statutes, the parent may be charged under a criminal section or charged with neglect. If the girl is under the age of adulthood, the customer may be prosecuted for statutory rape.

Civil actions are limited in their abilities to deal with prostitution. This is partly from their utilization when other community authorities have been lax or uninterested. For a private citizen to maintain an action in equity, he must prove a specific injury to himself, not just that he, as a member of the general community, has been injured. The red-light abatement laws were efforts to remedy this situation.[151] These laws permitted private citizen to maintain an action to abate a house of prostitution without having to show particular injury to himself. They gave the right to a private citizen on his own initiative to bring such an action irrespective of what local police or prosecuting attorneys were doing. All that was needed was to show the existence of a nuisance, and on that evidence the court could issue an order selling the possessions in a building and sealing the premises for a stated period, such as a year. If the owner paid the cost of the proceedings and posted a bond to the value of the property, conditioned upon abatement of the nuisance, the premises was released from the order. This approach became one of the chief sources of closing down red-light areas.[152]

Administrative devices are used in two ways: licensure and public health regulations. The former is seen in the denial or revocation of liquor licenses when a person is convicted of a certain act, such as keeping a house of prostitution, pandering, or soliciting. Similar restrictions can apply to the issuance and revocation of licenses to operate employment agencies, escort services, dancing academies, or any business subject to the need of a permit. Thus, a taxi driver might forfeit his license if convicted of soliciting, pimping, or pandering. Public health regulations give health departments authority to seek out people with communicable diseases and quarantine them until cured. Some states make additional and specific provisions for control of venereal disease transmitted by prostitutes. Compulsory examination of prisoners in jails or prisons, before or after conviction, may be specified and detention continued until a final report is made.[153]

Interesting questions arise from statutes which deny a girl probation unless she agrees to undergo active treatment for her disease. Broader questions arise if the "disease" in question is not considered merely a venereal disease, but rather the personality conflicts in a girl which give rise to prostituting. Could such a girl be denied probation until the disease is remedied? What if the treatments available make the prognosis quite adverse? Conversely, what if the girl refuses probation and insists on a correlative right to treatment so that she can stop her behavior? If a judicial warrant can be obtained authorizing the examination and treatment for those who refuse it, is it unwarranted to expect that a girl might insist on treatment beyond the realm of antibiotic injections?

Police regulation is by direct arrest in some cases, but this is limited in its effectiveness. Rarely will prostitution be committed in the presence of a uniformed officer. If arrest is sought by judicial warrant, the problem of witnesses arises as to whom will testify.

Only if a patron has been robbed, cheated, or infected is he likely to cooperate with the police, since his own behavior violated the law. This leads to undercover practices by police and moral squads. Plain-clothesmen pose as prospective clients, and go along with the situation sufficiently far for purposes of effecting an arrest. Although these police practices are not technically entrapment (in which a criminal purpose is implanted in the mind of a person not otherwise predisposed to commit the crime), they have been severely criticized on the basis of the contextual setting of law enforcement which this fosters.[154]

A more common police practice is to regulate prostitute activities by harassment. In these cases, arrests are made, individuals investigated and perhaps physically examined, a check is made to see if other charges are pending, and a release given with a warning. The objective is not to prosecute, but to deter such activites. How successful the practice is is largely unknown since it may foster precautionary efforts by participants. In fact, the approach of periodic arrests with payment of fines amounts to an informal arrangement, like paying a license fee to practice.

The Pathogenesis of Prostitution.   No one explanation suffices for the diverse personalities of girls who prostitute. Situational and idiosyncratic factors require consideration, as do interpersonal factors which contribute to the development of a deviant role. Predisposing personality factors require appraisal as well as the pathways into the oldest profession. It would be valuable if data were available to explain why some girls end up as call girls and some as street walkers—as well as other variants. It cannot ipso facto be assumed that street walkers are necessarily lower in intelligence or come from lower social backgrounds. In fact, the shrewdness and adaptability required of a street walker may be more complex than that of a call girl, or at least require a different set of talents.

One study appraised the "apprenticeship" system to become a call girl.[155] The average period of training was two to three months. Entrance was through another girl working in the field who knew the other for less than a year. The apprenticeship period was served under the direction of a more experienced call girl or a pimp. The latter controlled referrals as well as a fee-splitting arrangement of up to 50 percent of the total price negotiated between the trainer and customer. The primary mission of the training period was to build up clinetele for a new girl. Only a few basics were provided during the brief months of training. These included the proprieties of consuming alcohol and drugs, physical and sexual hygiene, obtaining the fee before service, and how to telephone clients for appointments.

The girl telephoning the client was one of the most difficult things to learn, because of its lack of congruence with the sex-role standard. An implicit set of moral norms was conveyed in which the john was viewed with contempt by virtue of what he was doing in betraying the standards which he professed. Hence, there was no compunction in exploiting males. Conversely, fairness to other girls and fidelity to the pimp were inculcated, but not necessarily persisted in once training was done. Although little formal knowledge was needed, and the technical training minimal, the hallmarks of a vocation which could be quite lucrative were present. What needs explication is why this is chosen by some girls.

Additional processes operate regarding the self-definition of the girl. This coalesces with the branding mechanisms of society which operate prior to formal stigmatization by courts or social agencies. The cycle of being rejected by a normative group—built on initial predisposing factors tending toward difference—leads to further rejection by the group. Rejection operating on a cognitive level, as well as by a compulsive dedication to carry out the image of someone outside the system, is observed. Emergence of the desire to identify with deviant roles corresponds to the theory of criminal behavior developed by Glaser.[156] His differential-identification theory maintains that an inner image of deviancy, such as that of a wayward woman, develops prior to the outward tag of "prostitute." It does not tell us why this develops in a given girl.

Stigmatization theory has been applied to the genesis of prostitution.[157] A set of personal and family characteristics which convey a derogatory image are internalized by the girl. This occurs at a stage of ego-diffusion, although there are many antecedents. Some of the antecedents are a girl who occupies a conspicuous role. Besides obvious types of physical deformities, the conspicuousness might be behavioral, or personality assets that make her prominent within her family, such as beauty, a certain sibling position, or an extreme of intelligence at either end. These traits evoke an attitude in family members where the girl is perceived as objectively powerless, which is the way she feels. In early adolescence they are "other-directed," or score high on conformity. The authoritarian nature of a family generates intolerance of ambiguity, and the girl becomes the receptacle for stigmas of badness, inadequacy, and being a source of trouble.

Contributing to her ego identity are the role complementary expectations of others. A derogatory self-image is compliant with the expectations of her socializers. Acceptance of the image leads to expectations of approval as part of a "dyadic bargain." It is doomed to failure, since only the most overtly destructive parent can consciously sanction a daughter's promiscuity. Hence, an initial cognitive dissonance occurs between expectations and actual responses. If the girl tends toward the intrapunitive, she may push her behavior further. If extrapunitive accusations are made when her parents have confused her, we may see the beginning of paranoid mentation. Counter-rejection of her parents will lead to severance from her family.

Several clinical theories have been proposed relating to the development of prostitution. A distinction should be made between the promiscuous activities of an adolescent, even if to an extreme degree, and prostitution. Many promiscuous girls do not engage in sexual relationships for money. There is a paucity of information on juvenile prostitution.

The natural history of the juvenile prostitute is in need of clarification. If it is a sometime thing, engaged in sporadically throughout adolescence, or something that emerges into a relatively stable pattern, is largely unknown except in individual cases. Gibbens followed up 185 supervised cases of juvenile prostitution in England and rated only 34 percent as successes when utilizing even such broad criteria as steady employment, living under settled circumstances, and not apparently being promiscuous.[158]

Before pursuing psychodynamic models, two prominent fantasies in adolescent girls merit discussion: "rape and seduction fantasies," and "prostitution fantasies." Many fantasies of the adolescent girl reveal masochistic themes relating to rape or assault. These appear in dreams or be involved in the transient appearance of symptoms, or they may be used consciously with masturbation. Fantasies of male attackers with knives, burglars who break into houses, or thieves who take something valuable, are typical. Being attacked and overcome are erotized. Derivatives of these masochistic tendencies are seen in painful longings and desires to suffer for a lover or a noble cause. Rape fantasies appear as an extension of seduction fantasies and are related to the mendaciousness of the hysteric.

When rape fantasies are presented as actual occurrences, all manner of legal and social complications ensue. This has been the substance of many novels and theatrical productions, such as E. M.

Forster's *A Passage to India*.[159] What lends reality is that underlying the fabrications are actual impulses or repressed experiences. A variation is that of the girl caught in a triangular net in which a female forces the girl to submit to sexual acts performed by men. The girl may be subjected to all manner of abuse in the form of being tied, gagged, or held while sexual acts are performed on her. She may utilize the fantasy of being a maid or slave girl in this respect. If such fantasies are literally acted out, we enter the area of sexual perversion. They may then seek to be beaten, but more often other masochistic elements enter so that these girls remain vulnerable to exploitation in many ways.

In some girls prostitution fantasies accompany an ego-ideal which embody a great deal of self-sacrifice. Some girls are ascetic in their daily lives, while others show overt narcissistic qualities. The common thread is their conception of sexuality as something low and degrading. Sexuality assumes the form of being subjected to humiliating experiences tantamount to being a whore. While most of these girls go on to live a life of quiet desperation in a marriage in which they legally submit to intercourse, others act out the prostitution fantasy. In some cases, this leads to dissociative episodes or there are episodes of promiscuity.[160]

Many sexually conflicted fantasies can emerge as part of the prostitution theme. The adolescent girl may envision her mother as a captive of the sexual assaults of her father and seek to avoid the fate of her mother. However, to avoid such a fate means not to be respectable but to love freely as a whore would do.[161] Some girls secretly believe their mothers are prostituting, and in their identification emulate them. Similarly, a girl may reject identification with a respectable mother who bears children. Conflict with their mothers ensues and they leave home, or act out sexually in anger.

Family dynamics contribute in a direct way, especially if a girl has previously been deeply attached to her father. An anxious father may terminate the closeness at puberty which leaves the girl reenacting faithlessness to men. It is a self-degrading way for her to retaliate since it amounts to being used indiscriminately by many men. Compulsive seeking of rejection by men becomes a characterological trait. A father who is actively sadistic toward the mother appears to foster masochistic development in his daughter, which may lead to prostitution. In clinical work pseudologia is often detected. In many ways, this actualizes pubertal fantasies. Themes of being used and abandoned by cruel men, desertion by men who were once kind, wicked women who enslave one, kidnappings, and white slavery are core lies which correspond to the mutual elaboration of fantasies by the girl prostituting and the male customers. Male customers identify with the maltreated girl against those who exploit her. The naive young male is stunned when the girl does not avail herself of proposals to rescue her.

This background contributes to the conflicts which impel a girl toward prostitution. While parsimonious explanations based on economic hedonism may be offered—like economic necessity—they do not deal with the motives which lead a girl to such a commitment. Nor does it suffice to presume that most of these girls are psychotic, although the lack of investigations based on thorough methodology handicaps conclusions. Few appear blatantly psychotic since at those times their ego functioning may be so impaired as to interfere with sexual activity. These comments do not negate a schizoid adaptation in which psychotic episodes are interspersed. Evidence for this would be the withdrawal from relationships involving tender components and the utilization of a strictly businesslike exchange. Depersonalizations occur in which the girl perceives herself as being used while her real self only observes.[162] The emphasis is on the incognito partnership or a pseudo-personality which permits a fictional identity to be carried out.[163] Nor can the young girl who prostitutes while high on drugs be discounted as having a schizotypic predisposition. When maintained apart from the drugs, under a promiscuity block, she may evince ego inpairment and signs and symptoms of reality distortion.

More common are those girls with character defects. Some are impulse-ridden, while others portray defiance and rebellion against authority figures and institutions, seen as hypocritical. Unfortunately, their need to expose hypocrisy leads them to suffer far more than the brief pleasures of exposing authorities as frauds. Hysterical character problems appear in many of these girls in their abilities to fake and live a lie. Their psychopathic tendencies merge with lying and expectations. Difficulty in concept formation may impair their realization of the extent to which deception and distortion permeate their lives. Instead, the focus is on how others have wronged them or failed to understand them.

The need to denigrate or show up males is one motivational element, coupled with an exposure of the marriage relationship itself as degrading to a woman. While the girls who are blocked from sexual pleasure by frigidity appear more preoccupied with homosexual conflicts, not all of them have such conflicts.[164] Some girls have a range of feeling toward their male clients and are capable of orgastic pleasure, but try to conceal this show of affection or avoid it from fatigue.[165] While sexual pleasure is had by some, the emphasis persists of the relationship as purely for physical ends and not affection.

SEXUALIZED BEHAVIORS

Many antisocial or aggressive acts are never officially considered disturbances in the realm of sexual development. This does not refer to the myriad manifestations of disturbed sexuality which take the form of autoplastic suffering. Sexual conflicts are seen as entering into a variety of routine delinquent acts. The boundaries of the discussion remain vague, for many of the same impulses which give rise to types of sexual perversions discussed in this chapter are the common stem for general characgerological structure. For some this character development relies—periodically or to a great extent in some on sexual acts which lead to community concern.

Sexualized 'Taking''. A prominent type of behavior which may have sexualized components is taking something from others such as forms of theft, robbery, and burglary. A repetitive element is present and the degree of conscious awareness of a sexual tinge varies widely. For some, a vague sense of sexual excitement is present although others may have a total absence of any type of cognitive or affective sexual connotation. A state of sexual excitement may ensue after the act as opposed to before or as a concomitant. A sixteen-year-old male, who compulsively broke into apartments with no motive other than taking money that was conspicuously available, experienced no sexual excitement at the time. Once back in his own home he would masturbate with fantasies of the breaking in, but he was deviod of insight about the relationship between these behaviors. Examples are multiple and difficult without sophisticated clinical appraisal. Many components are routinely overlooked in processing these adolescents through the judicial system or mass rehabilitation programs.

Comment was made earlier about the frequency of robberies or burglaries in the backgrounds of rapists. Fortunately, most of the former activities do not routinely result in rape. Nor should a conclusion be made that all of these activities are really only disguised rapes. The boy who engages in compulsive grabbing of purses from unknown women may have no awareness that this act has many sexualized components. When one of them alternately, and without discrimination, describes grabbing at the breasts of women or their genital areas, he is a step closer to a cognitive appreciation of his motives. Discretion is needed to avoid the types of wild generalization which have discredited psychodynamic formulations in the past without integrating many variables.

Sexualized thefts and burglaries can be linked to depressed states in some adolescents. Periods of feeling lonely, isolated, or abandoned, are resolved by distorted sexual activities. Rather than experiencing the emptiness of a depressed state, ways are sought to come alive. This borders on an attempt to stay alive rather than continuing to experience an impoverished ego state. The spectrum of attachment and dependency needs is relevant. Seeking bodily contact, taking something of a symbolic type from a woman such as her purse (usually passed off as only seeking money), taking food or sweets from shops, or breaking into a place and aggressively taking that to which one feels entitled are common examples. An aggressive component of taking itself comes to the fore as an effort to alleviate or resolve a depressed condition.

Fusion of aggressivity with a symbolic sexual component is seen in the adolescent who brandishes knives or guns or who develops gun collections. While some paths of development lead to exhibitionistic acts, others take the form of frightening women with weapons. These may be dangerous if real guns are used, but toy guns may serve the purpose of inducing fright. Extensions are seen in slight punctures or penetrations carried out on women's bodies with knives. There are occurrences of girls being literally raped by a gun inserted into their vagina, in the absence of penile penetration. Robbing people by force, intimidation, or with a weapon to take something from them, are other illustrations.

Car thefts provide a thrill of pulling it off, only to abandon the car after it has been used and served its purpose. More overtones exist than merely a means of free transportation. There is a prominent self-defeating, yet driven quality, in the large number of adolescent males who repetitively engage in car theft in the most flamboyant manner, despite apprehension. Their lack of response to traditional correctional approaches may lie in components which do not respond to deterrence and punishment. In fact, the punishment may be a necessity to the maintenance of this behavior as a form of payment.

Boys describe a vague feeling that stealing cars represents forestalling some other act. The compulsive quality in some is the linchpin to the obsessional personality with its array of defenses. During adolescence, car theft provides an escape hatch congruent with the sex-role standard for a strict superego system. For other boys, there is an emphasis on the assertion of masculinity via the power and autonomy represented by the automobile. This is a repetitious theme on American television. Antecedent struggles with paternal figures may be in the background.[166] The car itself may function as specific symbolic equivalent for the male genital.[167]

Since the subject of stealing is far broader than that discussed under sexualized behaviors, the reader is referred elsewhere for its coverage. At this point, only a few comments are made relevant to kleptomania. This is distinguished from loose usage where any act of theft is called kleptomania. It distinguishes some acts of pathological delinquency as perversions or fetishes.[168] Compulsive stealing associated with kleptomania is more prevalent in girls and women. It is the female counterpart to male fetishism. In the true kleptomaniac, the taking has little economic significance, nor need the object be something of economic value. The girl who compulsively takes trinkets or pens—only never to use them or to throw them away—is manifesting a behavior similar to the boy who compulsively steals women's undergarments from clotheslines. While the sexual component is more obvious in the latter case, the addictive qualities are similar. Affection-seeking is fused with expressions of resentment or revenge. Winnicott saw pseudologia fantastica and stealing as bridging an experiential gap with respect to a transitional object.[169] Hallmarks for kleptomaniac development appear when the act becomes compulsive, when little material value is placed on the object per se, and an unconscious need is fulfilled in the act of taking or of a particular set of items. In some girls a homosexual component of envy to possess another woman emerges. Objects symbolizing parts of the body, such as the male or female genitals, breasts, body contents such as feces or babies, operates.

Guns and the Adolescent.   With the furor and publicity about possession of guns and the rabid opposition to governmental control over their possession, we are in the midst of a political and constitutional issue. However, there is also the possibility of psychopathological overtones when an adolescent makes this his chosen hobby. No more visible symbolic sign of a sex-role symbol exists for the adolescent boy than the visible possession of a dangerous weapon. Hence, this functions in a sexualized manner to give reassurance in the face of peer demands to prove it and the insecurities attendant upon having to perform. While self-protection is the customary reason given for gun collections (which may be legitimate in certain urban areas where social controls have broken down), for the majority of weapon-toting adolescents, guns secure another goal. When the adolescent male is in a precarious balance with paranoid mentation, the risk of self-protection against projective sexual aggressive attacks from others is increased by virtue of possessing a gun. A way is also opened for parents to act out their phallic needs, coupled with overt aggression, through their sons.

> An angry and disappointed father had moved about the country four times in the preceding five years. His income had been adequate for his wife, son, and daughter, but recognition of his self-sacrifices and dedication, such as working his way through night school, had not been forthcoming. The last move revealed itself as a mistake in a few months after moving a thousand miles, and this new disappointment elicited rage and excessive drinking. The thirteen-year-old son was described as studious, a loner, and inconspicuous in school. He had taken pride in his father's display of various guns kept in a special case with a glass top. No reason could later be given by the boy as to why he had unexpectedly left school one day, returned home, and took one of his father's guns out of the case, and went to a shopping center. There he wandered about and when a woman approached her car in the parking lot, he told her he needed a ride. She observed him standing with a dazed look, holding a gun pointing downward, and told him she would like to make a phone call. He permitted this without comment and she proceeded to call the police. There was no history of drug use in this case—just a confused and angry boy who was sensitively aware of his father's wish to destroy several people.

Arson. Another adolescent behavior which may have a prominent sexual motivation is arson. Many monographs have been written about the subject. An early one was by Stekel.[170] Karpman made a connection between the problem of sex offenses and specifically pyromania and kleptomania.[171] Similar emotional problems were seen in both the latter behaviors. In the earlier clinical literature firesetting was viewed as a particular type of "insanity" characterized by irresistible propensities to light fires. Hence, "pyromania" means fire plus madness. In terms of prevalence, firesetting has been described as the outstanding crime of the adolescent.[172] Several overdetermined factors operate in the act, and by no means can they all be considered indicative of sexual conflict. Most evident are aggressive components which are handled by consuming acts such as burning something up. The act may be an overtly hostile one, but it also fuses the power needs of sexuality and aggressivity in that a puny and insignificant human, with a tiny match, can wreak such damage.

Firesetters are typically, but not exclusively, males. In one study of 1,145 cases, 200 or 14.8 percent, were females.[173] Many fires set by boys relate to revenge or hatred against a female, or rejection of a maternal figure. Some are related to depressive aspects of object loss and sequentially related to menstruation in girls. Although revenge and envy are striking features, the overt wrongs listed are not as one would expect. The act of destruction seems out of proportion to listed grievances.

This betrays unresolved and unconscious hates and the overdetermined nature of the act. While many adolescents are described as impulsive, firesetting occurs episodically. More frequent is the depressed anger and discontent in the juvenile who has chosen such a means of acting out. The syndrome cannot be confined to lighting a match. It includes turning in the alarm, waiting for the firemen and engines to arrive, perhaps watching and assisting in putting out the fire, and establishing a relationship with the firemen as a helper. This recreates a relationship of a junior aid to an older male, and is seen as restitutive.[174] While drive discharge is facilitated by intense sexual excitement and destruction, the behavior additionally signifies the wish for assistance.

Arson requires a thorough assessment. Few of these youths seek out help on their own, and they deny vigorously their behavior when caught in the meshwork of apprehension. The connection to perversion is in the repetitive component if the act has become sexualized. It is at best symbolic and substitutive. However, not all firesetting has these components. It is not naive to say that carelessness operates in the occasional fire. Nor can motives of firesetting for profit be ignored, either directly for insurance or through an adolescent hired to do the dirty work. Some individuals with intellectual and cognitive deficits become entranced by fire much like the boy of four to six years of age. The psychotic juvenile is another type responding to delusional beliefs or even hallucinatory commands to "set the world on fire." Fantasies along the theme of world destruction are evident in their episodes. For the angry adolescent, consumed with rage against authority figures, firesetting falls into the category of setting explosions to shake up or destroy an authority figure or social order. In some cases there are bizarre elements accompanying the firesetting. Since their behavior is logical in other respects, their schizotypal personality organization is often missed with resultant hardship later to all concerned.

> A seventeen year old's firesetting career began ten years earlier when he set fire to a playground building. Over the next few years a typical series of referrals to community clinics and agencies had been done with a melange of diagnoses. A pattern of teasing and provocation from a sadistic father led the boy to chronic absenting from home and school. A series of foster home placements and juvenile court hearings had the theme of his father rescuing him at the last minute. His mother had become an invalid from a vascular accident the year before his firesetting commenced. During his teens, a four-year period was spent in two residential treatment centers with various treatment approaches, depending on the clinician in charge. On one weekend pass home another fire was started. This led to commitment to a state hospital. While there, a fire occurred in a room with a bedridden senile who suffered burns from which he died. The boy was seen leaving the room but since no proof was available that he set the fire, nothing was done. As his eighteenth birthday approached, when he would attain legal majority, a plan was proposed to discharge him with the hope that he would commit a criminal act leading to imprisonment.

Gambling Activities.   Similar to thefts, burglaries, and arson are a host of other antisocial acts which have a conspicuous symbolic element. Gambling may seem like a strictly adult affair rather than something performed by adolescents, yet the term is used to refer to a host of activities which have an element of gaming. Excitement is involved, as well as an all or nothing component. This is seen in such things as games of Russian roulette or drag-racing. Late adolescents express their compulsivity in the form of addiction to cards or games of chance. In fact, large debts may be accumulated in this manner through risking high stakes and marathon card games. To cover losses recourse to thefts and burglaries as well as forgeries and embezzlements may occur.

Developmental components which contribute to gambling have largely been ignored. Such obvious factors as a cognitive readiness to assess alternatives, and make predictions and calculations, are necessary. Built on this is the psychology of risk-taking. Freud saw gambling as similar to masturbation from its operation by use of the hands, a struggle for self-restraint versus indulgence, self-criticism for indulgence, as well as self-punitive trends.[175] Many ego devices come into operation besides the drive component. There is the opportunity to win against superior opponents where the little guy can come through.[176] To win against overwhelming odds restores a temporary feeling of infantile omnipotence. A way to expiate or suffer for transgressions committed in other areas can be facilitated by the high risk of loss. If one does not lose, he has paid the price by laying himself on the line. A feeling of relief is obtained.[177]

A similarity to components of drug usage is conspicuous both for the pleasurable and defensive forms. Outwitting fate or chance when one is an underdog is present. Witness the excitement at sporting events about pulling for the underdog, particularly when long-range chances are taken against the odds to go for broke. Forgeries, swindling, and embezzlements, all operate on the conning principle and touch similar psychological roots. They tell us a good deal about the personality structure of these individuals. What they cannot tell us during adolescence is the relative fixity which can lead to a continuance of the behavior. While adults may resort to sexual substitutes in the form of episodic breakthroughs, the adolescent has the added uncertainty that behaviors may reflect an ego struggling with strong drives rather than a fixed character neurosis. The therapeutic implication is that damage may be done by excessive zeal to cure an adolescent on one hand, or to be punitive on the other.

MISCELLANEOUS EXPRESSIONS OF SEXUALITY

Troilism. Troilistic acts, where three partners jointly participate in sexual activity, are relevant to some aspects of homosexuality. The sharing of partners in terms of the common use of bodies, regression to lack of distinctions between what is mine and yours, raises broad issues. Troilism is not restricted to sexual activities of an overt type. Teenage boys who participate in burglaries with a girl accomplice, or those girls who drive a getaway car, are examples of joint participation in sexualized routines even though coitus is not performed. Girls who participate in these adventures are participants who achieve their gratification as helpers or facilitators. In some cases the role is reversed and a powerful female leader directs a group of boys in a facsimile of a matriarchy.

Bestiality. Bestiality is an act of intercourse between humans and animals, and can involve the vagina, rectum, or mouth. Legally it may be encompassed under sodomy statutes which refer to annoying any person or animal by mouth or anus, or by specific statutes covering activities with animals. The punitive nature of the sanctions against these acts is significant. Punishment of up to twenty years is possible. In England, bestiality is a felony punishable by life imprisonment.[178] The American Law Institute's Model Penal Code recommends the offense be made a misdemeanor.[179] If the acts are performed by a juvenile, he may be handled in the random way characteristic of the handling of juvenile sex offenders. If a particular court or probation officer is personally revulsed by the acts, the juvenile might be waived to an adult criminal court, convicted, and sentenced as a sex offender to a security hospital or commited as mentally ill and dangerous.

These provisions are relevant to adolescents since many relationships with animals have sexual components. What about the adolescent who permits a dog to masturbate on him? Or, taken a step further, the direct masturbation of a dog by an adolescent? Mutual masturbation may occur as well. In some cases the animal organ may be inserted into a human orifice while in other cases the converse appears. As in rape, the degree of penetration appears to satisfy legal criteria. Utilization of animals appears more prevalent in rural areas. As with much sexual behavior in adolescents, the majority of acts are of a transitory or exploratory nature and this should always be considered. Most typically, the acts function as a type of masturbatory equivalent. If seen from this perspective, the severe punishment meted out seems outlandish and tells us more about the anxiety raised in observers and controlling agents than anything else. For some the acts serve as a vicarious homosexual outlet, but again this does not seem to be the preferred object. Except for the hermit, or isolate, about whom diagnostic questions of schizophrenia should arise, the animals rarely function as the continued preference for sexual gratification. A variation is a masochistic exploitation of girls by submitting them to intercourse with animals.

> A humorless youth had spent three years in a teenage marriage attempting to please his wife by way of assisting their dogs to have intercourse with her. He described his wife as 'too wonderful a Christian to be able to engage in sexual relationships with me in the flesh.' However, his wife was the moving party eventually in separating. As an example of devotion to his wife, he seriously described getting rid of their German shepherd dog at one time for a Great Dane which he felt would be more satisfying to his wife. He viewed this as a kind deed. When his wife left him, he was puzzled and sought 'spiritual reasons' for their differences. There was a basis for this since after three years she chanced to read a passage in Leviticus which referred to women not laying down with beasts which led her to resist the acts.

Frottage.   Frottage refers to sexual pleasure obtained by rubbing against bodies. As such, it is often an accompaniment of adolescent petting activities and foreplay. When it occurs by rubbing or touching women in public conveyances and crowds, it is legally classified as a sexual offense. When it takes on a compulsive quality so that the rubbing is the preferred and sought-after activity, we are in the midst of an emerging psychological perversion with all the restrictions stated above about the possible transiency during adolescence. Uninvited rubbing against a woman is actually a mild form of assault, and when a woman is forced to turn and look as well, exhibitionistic features are added.

Coprophilia, Coprophagia, and Undinism.   Coprophilia refers to an obsessive preoccupation with excretory products and processes. Coprophagia is the consumption of bodily secretions or excretions. These are relatively rare among all ages as primary perversions, but their genesis can be observed in the curiosity of children about people going to the bathroom. Cultural shame and secrecy about excretion fosters curiosity, while the interest connected with the genital region provides the nexus. Variations are the desire to excrete on another or be excreted upon.

Such activities occur in the context of homosexual or heterosexual relationships. One boy of sixteen masturbated lying under a glass table while a woman crouched over him on the table defecating. This fulfilled a masturbation fantasy which he had used since attaining puberty. Havlock Ellis mentioned this as one of the services available at Parisian brothels at the turn of the century.[180] Another adolescent boy paid an older woman to let him urinate on her. Self-contempt and contempt for others are manifest. In other cases this is not as clear, and it is the interest in the process itself which is dominant. A thirteen-year-old boy waited and observed cautiously about his home for his mother or sister to urinate. What he sought was hearing the sound of urine splashing against the water in the toilet bowl which excited him and led to masturbation.

This interest in urine and urination is sometimes referred to as undinism. While some theorists attempt explanations of such phenomena as analogous to pica, it seems more complex as well as generically separate. A mixture of biological responses may prompt curiosity in excretions and their fate. These vary from eating at the breast to excretion in infancy. However, a mixture of oral and anal trends have a confluence in coprophilic behaviors. A parallel outcome is seen in coprolalia which has been referred to as a "dilution of coprophagia." While adolescents are known for their use of slang words referring to sexuality and excretion, these utterances need not be part of the peer sexual role. Use of slang words or profanity may become an integral and perhaps necessary, condition for performing sexually. Nor should this be considered as a phenomenon confined to adolescence since for some it continues into adulthood or marriage as an essential for intercourse. Similarly, coprolalia need not be confined to literal sexual situations.

A seventeen-year-old youth was arrested for driving in a crowded section of a large metropolitan city; he became sexually excited when he leaned his head out of the car window and shouted profanities connected with intercourse or defecation. Masturbation would often accompany the yelling. He was arrested after driving his car around one square block several times in succession so that by the sixth trip a police officer was alerted and arrested him.

The varieties or ways language is used are legion. Therefore, these comments are restricted to those most illustrative of sexual psychopathology. The entire realm of primary aggressive discharge by way of words is widely observed. It is interesting to observe in the Gilles de la Tourette syndrome, whose etiology remains obscure, that the verbal expletives used in connections with other tics, are words in the form of sexual or excretory types.

Necrophilia. Necrophilia includes more than "love of dead bodies." Although rare, the connection between this and other developmental anomalies in the sexual sphere can be seen. Groups of adolescents may engage in acts of sadism to corpses (necrosadism), or have intercourse or dismember and mutilate bodies. If parts are eaten, this is called necrophagia, and these acts are all related to the phenomenon of lust murder in which the sexual impulses are gratified by killing a woman. This was noted with rapes and is related to a specific form of sadism required for sexual gratification. A variation is the exhumation of the casket of a loved one as part of a severe adolescent melancholia.

Braid-cutting. Braid-cutting encompasses everything from a playful prank of boys to the performance of a symbolic castration in disguise. There are many equivalents of the act beside the literal cutting off of a pigtail, which gained popularity when little girls used that hairstyle. Most common are a group of latency age boys who engage in teasing and provocative behavior to girls by pulling hair,

or threatening to cut off a piece of hair. Such behavior is tolerated by
adults with humor as the normal behavior of boys. What is sensed is
the anxiety, excitement, and thrill associated with a group of boys
picking on a girl which actually may extend to the point of tears.
Only at that point are the boys warned to stop.

But what about when it is an adolescent who is not just teasing
girls, but acting out such impulses? The behavior is then classified
as a fetishism. Sexual arousal raises the desire and need for
utilization of male sexual organs. If the boy is predisposed by
antecedent experiences to have anxieties about genital use, he is
caught in a dilemma.

Of course, one choice is to avoid sexual activity and exciting
situations of contact with girls. Another choice is to utilize a defense
to reassure the boy against anxiety. The postulated mechanism is
that of identification with the aggressor, whereby the boy feels he
can then obtain control of a situation. He is no longer in danger if he
is the one doing the cutting or mutilating and not being at the mercy
of someone else doing this to him. Yet experiences of play-acting
regarding mock haircutting, as well as situations of literal cutting,
still have the reality-based component that remains cognizant of the
partial nature of such an act. While assertion and control are gained
over one who has been attacked, there is a realization that the hair
will grow back so no real harm has been done. Hence, a counterphobic type of reassurance is given to the boy that he really might not
have to be so fearful of such a reality.

There is the possibility of defects emerging in the body image
when resort to such fetishistic practices are needed for reassurance.[181] When an adolescent literally carries out hairclipping on
unknown girls and women in a compulsively driven manner, while
avoiding them in other respects, we are in the realm of sexually
perverse acts. In some cases, a severed lock of a girl's hair seems to
function as a tangible and visible fetish which will not be destroyed.
As such, it functions to reaffirm the genital integrity of the
adolescent if the behavior is transient, or their future fetishes if this
persists.

A handsome, well-built, athletic looking boy of sixteen was arrested after police
received a report of an assault on a girl. This particular occurrence followed a
pattern of several preceding episodes. On these occasions, he approached a girl
from behind and grabbed her, with one arm around her neck. He brandished a
knife in his extended left arm, held so it was visible to the girl. If the girl fought
or verbally resisted these overtures, the boy usually fled in panic.

Another essential requirement in the sequence was a question he asked each girl. The question was whether she had washed her hair on the preceding day. If she had not, the boy immediately left. If the hair had been washed, he proceeded to the next step of the sequence which was running his hand through her hair for several minutes. The thought of cutting the girl's hair was always present at those times. On occasion, he cut a lock with a knife and left. He had never successfully been able to return home with a lock of hair because he experienced deep shame. Once home, he masturbated with the fantasy of what he had just done. However, at the time of the act the boy was not aware of any sexual impulses nor did he have an erection. He was aware intellectually that 'something sexual' was involved but he had no idea beyond that.

THE TREATMENT SITUATION

Throughout this chapter references have been made to the disposition problems of juveniles involved in sexual behavior viewed as offensive by the community. While complications are added once an official apprehension has been made and the judicial process set in motion, perspectives on management remain desirable whatever approaches are used. The one overriding essential, distinguishing the juvenile situation from adults, is their fluctuating and unpredictable sexual state. This refers to their impulses and desires, as well as controls exercised, and the choices made. For the juveniles who become involved in the judicial machinery, an appraisal of their behavior by a psychiatrist sophisticated in the area of adolescent development and psychopathology is highly important.

In practice this seldom occurs. A major reason is the limited number of juvenile courts or correctional facilities with such experts available. An examination done in an incompetent manner, with haphazard conclusions by an unknowledgable examiner, is better left undone. It lulls everyone into a feeling that something *has* been done. Another reason for inadequate appraisal is the heavy work load of juvenile courts and their need to maintain the flow of a new hearing every ten to fifteen minutes. While many states have statutes requiring a mandatory mental examination prior to sentencing for adult sex offenders, the incongruous fact is that there is no parallel requirement for juveniles. In fact, some statutes even leave a gap between the juvenile jurisdiction and the age for such mandatory examinations. This is seen in requirements which specify that a mandatory examination should be done on convicted sex offenders over twenty-one years of age but which make no reference to those below this age.

The complex problem of many offenses not being perceived as sexual in nature further complicates possibilities for treatment. Part of this is due to efforts at direct concealment by the juvenile. The motivation for offenders of all ages to conceal their behavior in the sexual in nature further complicates possibilities for treatment. Part but just as important are the added legal consequences given such an offense. For the adolescent, there is the perpetual lifetime record of sexual deviancy which remains available despite a pretense of privacy for juvenile court records.[182] This is hardly a situation conducive to accepting help if one does confess his sexual difficulties. Nor does an adolescent find life easier with his peer group if he is remanded to an institution as a sexual delinquent. In practice, he is sent to an institution caring for a heterogeneous mixture of delinquents where the nature of his delinquency—if revealed—opens up opportunities for scapegoating. A further problem case is where the sexual nature of the offense is lost in the context of more blatant charges.

> A fourteen-year-old boy strangled a child several years younger and was then certified to adult criminal court. He stood trial for first-degree murder and was convicted on second-degree charges. No psychiatric evaluation was done at the juvenile level, and prior to trial a simple 'Yes' conclusionary opinion on competency and responsibility questions was rendered by a psychiatrist without elaboration. This occurred despite the fact that the offense was committed while the boy was on leave from a mental hospital. After sentencing arrived, no explanation beyond mentioning the boy's anger had been given. A psychiatric evaluation was later ordered which revealed a past history of pedophilic activity with the victim. The boy was sentenced as a convicted adult criminal to a prison.

In light of recurrent concern about the mental health of children, it is interesting that the Report of the Joint Commission on Mental Health of Children made only one reference to sexual deviation.[183] The reference was in the context of discussing emotional and mental illness problems in pre-school children where reference was made to boys two years of age or younger who may show marked feminine interests along with compulsive patterns of sexual activity.

It appears doubtful that existing mental health approaches will take effective action to implement the needed expertise in diagnostic appraisal and treatment of juveniles with sexually offensive behavior. Issues connected with inadequate assessment and treatments which are often no better, or worse, then doing nothing, should be made clear. This raises contractual questions when a juvenile is sent to an institution for behavior which the state finds offensive and in need of remedy. It does not appear that exposing a juvenile sex offender to the mass approaches offered to juvenile offenders sent to large institutions for delinquents serves many purposes beyond temporary incapacitation. Just as with right to treatment issues being raised for confinement associated with civil commitments, or adult psychopathies, something should presumably be offered to juveniles detected and detained for having committed a sexual offense.[184]

Not to offer a treatment program tailored to the sexual psychopathology of a juvenile makes a sham of the system of justice and a mockery of rehabilitative goals. Better to abandon such goals if the rehabilitative model is not in fact available, and plainly announce to the public, the juvenile, and his family, that he is either being punished or isolated for community protection and that the goal of treatment is largely irrelevant. If nothing else, such an approach has the virtue of honesty.

REFERENCES

1. Group for the Advancement of Psychiatry, *Normal Adolescence: Its Dynamics and Impact* (New York: GAP, 1968).

2. W. H. Masters and V. E. Johnson, *Human Sexual Response* (Boston: Little, Brown, 1966).

3. A. C. Kinsey et al., *Sexual Behavior in the Human Male,* p. 219 (Philadelphia: Saunders, 1948).

4. A. C. Kinsey et al., *Sexual Behavior in the Human Female,* p. 353 (Philadelphia: Saunders, 1953).

5. M. B. Freedman, The sexual behavior of american college women, *Merrill Palmer Quarterly,* 11(1965):33-48.

6. Kinsey, op. cit. 5.

7. S. L. Halleck, Sexual and mental health on the campus, *Journal of the American Medical Association* 200(1967):684-690.

8. I. Reiss, The sexual renaissance: a survey and analysis, *Journal of Sociological Issues* 22(1966):123-137.

9. S. Freud (1912), On the universal tendency to debasement in the sphere of love, *Standard Edition* 11:177-190.

10. G. Legman, *Rationale of the Dirty Joke* (New York: Grove Press, 1968).

11. D. Callahan, *Abortion: Law, Choice and Morality* (New York: Macmillan, 1970).

12. A.M. Seiden, Overview: research on the psychology of women, *American Journal of Psychiatry* 133(1976):995-1007.

13. E. Lewy, Responsibility, free will, and ego psychology, *International Journal of Psycho-Analysis* 42(1961):260-270.
14. L. B. Schwartz, Morals offenses and the model penal code, *Columbia Law Review* 63(1963):669-686.
15. *Davis* v. *Beason,* 133 U.S. 333, 1890.
16. J. Stephen, *History of the Criminal Law,* vol. 2, Chap. 25, 1883.
17. E. P. Powers, *Crime and Punishment in Early Massachusetts* (Boston: Beacon Press, 1966).
18. Psychopathic personality law, *Minnesota Statutes,* Ch. 526.09, 1939.
19. *Huebner* v. *State,* 33 Wis. 2d 503, 147 N.W. 2d 646, 1967.
20. In re psychopathic personality of Benno Dittrich 215, *Minnesota Reports* 234, 1943.
21. *Huebner v. State,* 33 Wis. 2d 505, 147 N.W. 2d 646, 1967.
22. Group for the Advancement of Psychiatry, *Psychiatry and Sex Psychopath Legislation: The 30s to the 80s* (New York: GAP, 1977).
23. A. Ellis and R. Brancale, *The Psychology of Sex Offenders* (Springfield: Charles C Thomas, 1956).
24. B. C. Glueck, Jr., Psychodynamic patterns in the sex offender, *Psychiatric Quarterly* 28(1954):1-21.
25. *Illinois Revised Statutes* Ch. 38, Section 823.a, 1959.
26. Bowman and Engle, op. cit., p. 767.
27. *People* v. *Frontczak,* 286 Mich. 51, 281 N.W. 534, 1938.
28. *State ex rel. Pearson* v. *Probate Court,* 309 U.S. 270, 84L ed. 744, 60 S.Ct. 523, 126 ALR 530, 1940.
29. *Davy v. Sullivan,* 12 Criminal Law Reports 2477 (M.D. Ala. 1973).
30. *Madden* v. *Commonwealth,* 202 Ky. 782, 261 S.W. 273 (1924); *People* v. *Bailey,* 341 Mich. 592, 67 N.W. 2d 785, 1954.
31. N. Ross, The primacy of genitality in the light of ego psychology, *Journal of the American Psychoanalytic Association* 18(1970):267-284.
32. N.Y. Statute on Right to Treatment.
33. *Commonwealth* v. *Page,* 159 N.E. 2d 82, 1959.
34. *In re Maddox,* 351 Mich. 358, 88 N.W. 2d 470, 1958.
35. R. V. Krafft-Ebing, *Psychopathia Sexualis* (New York: Physicians and Surgeons Book Co., 1925).
36. H. Ellis, *Studies in the Psychology of Sex,* 3rd ed. (Philadelphia: F. A. Davis Co., 1930).
37. K. R. Eissler, Notes on problems of technique in the psychoanalytic treatment of adolescents: with some remarks on perversions, *Psychoanalytic Study of the Child* 13(1958):223-254.
38. H. Hartmann, The mutual influences in the development of ego and id, *Psychoanalytic Study of the Child* 7(1952):9-30.
39. E. Jacobson, *The Self and Object World* (New York: International Universities Press, 1964).

40. S. Freud, (1919), A child is being beaten, *Standard Edition* 17:175-204.
41. E. Glover, The relation of perversion formation to the development of reality sense, *International Journal of Psycho-Analysis* 14(1933):486-497.
42. W. H. Gillespie, The psycho-analytic theory of sexual deviation with special reference to fetishism, *The Pathology and Treatment of Sexual Deviations*, ed. by I. Rosen, pp. 123-145. (London: Oxford University Press, 1964).
43. L. Kolb and A. Johnson, Etiology and therapy of overt homosexuality, *Psychoanalytic Quarterly* 24(1955):506-515.
44. A. Freud, *Normality and Pathology in Childhood* (New York: International Universities Press, 1965).
45. C. W. Socarides, *The Overt Homosexual* (New York: Grune and Stratton, 1968).
46. W. J. Gadpaille, Homosexual activity and homosexuality in adolescence, *Science and Psychoanalysis* 15:60-70 (New York: Grune and Stratton, 1969).
47. S. H. Fraiberg, Homosexual conflicts in adolescence, *Adolescents: The Psychoanalytic Approach to Problems in Therapy*, ed. by S. Lorand and H. I. Schneer (New York: Harper, 1962).
48. B. D. Lewin, The body as phallus, *Psychoanalytic Quarterly* 2(1933):24-44.
49. *McKinney's Consolidated Laws of New York (Annotated)* Book 29-A, Judiciary, Part I, Family Court Act, Section 712, 1973.
50. Vernon, *Texas Civil Statutes, Juvenile Court Section*, Criminal Annals Pocket Part, 1970-1971, Article 2338.
51. A. J. Reiss, Sex offenses: the marginal status of the adolescent, *Law and Contemporary Problems* 25(1960):309-333.
52. The pros and cons of conjugal visits in prison institutions, *Journal of Family Law* 9(1970):437-440.
53. A. C. Kinsey, op. cit. p. 224.
54. A. Binet, Le fetichis me dans l'amour, *Revue Philosophique* 24(1887):143.
55. P. H. Gebhard, J. H. Gagnon, W. B. Pomeroy, and C. V. Christenson, *Sex Offenders* (New York: Harper, 1965).
56. R. Bak, Fetishism, *Journal of the American Psychoanalytic Association* 1(1953):285-298.
57. J. Fowles, *The Collector* (Boston: Little, Brown, 1963).
58. M. L. Enelow, Public nuisance offenses: exhibitionism, voyeurism, and transvestism, *Sexual Behavior and the Law*, ed. by R. Slovenko, pp. 478-486. (Springfield: Charles C Thomas, 1965).
59. P. Greenacre, Certain relationships between fetishism and faulty development of the body image, *Psychoanalytic Study of the Child* 8(1953):79-98.
60. H. Benjamin, *The Transsexual Phenomenon* (New York: Julian Press, 1966).
61. R. J. Stoller, A biased view of 'sex transformation' operations, *Journal of Nervous and Mental Diseases* 149(1969):312-317.
62. J. E. Hoopes, N. J. Knorr, and S. R. Wolf, Transsexualism: considerations regarding sexual reassignment, *Journal of Nervous and Mental Diseases* 147(1968):510-516.

63. E. Jacobson, Development of the wish for a child in boys, *Psychoanalytic Study of the Child* 5(1950):139-152.

64. R. Goy, Organizing effects of androgen in the behavior of rhesus monkeys, *Proceedings of the London Conference: Endocrines and Human Behavior* (Oxford: Oxford University Press, 1968).

65. R. M. Oetzel, Selected Bibliography on sex differences, *The Development of Sex Differences in Behavior*, ed. by E. E. Maccoby (Stanford: Stanford University Press, 1966).

66. M. Rabban, Sex-role identification in young children in two diverse social groups, *Genetic Psycholical Monograph* 42(1950):81-158.

67. H. L. Koch, A study of some factors conditioning the social distance between sexes, *Journal of Sociological Psychology* 20(1944):79-107.

68. L. B. Fauls and W. D. Smith, Sex-role learning of five-year-olds, *Journal of Genetic Psychology* 89(1956):105-117.

69. W. Mischel, Sex typing and socialization, *Manual of Child Psychology*, ed. by P. H. Mussen (New York: Wiley, 1970).

70. R. Green, Childhood cross-gender identification, *Journal of Nervous and Mental Diseases* 147(1968):500-509.

71. R. Green and J. Money, Stage-acting, role-taking, and effeminate impersonation during boyhood, *Archives of Genetic Psychiatry* 15(1966):535-538.

72. R. J. Stoller, Male childhood transsexualism, *Journal of the American Academy of Child Psychiatry* 7(1968):193-209.

73. L. E. Newman, Transsexualism in adolescence, *Archives of Genetic Psychiatry* 23(1970):112-121.

74. J. Money and J. G. Brennan, Sexual dimorphism in the psychology of female transsexuals, *Journal of Nervous and Mental Diseases* 147(1968):487-499.

75. E. Revitch and R. G. Weiss, The pedophilic offender, *Diseses of the Nervous System* 23(1962):73-78.

76. Gagnon, Gebhard, Pomeroy, and Christenson, op. cit. p. 71.

77. P. R. Miller, The effeminate passive obligatory homosexual, *Archives of Neurology and Psychiatry* 80(1958):612-618.

78. I. Bieber et al., *Homosexuality: A Psychoanalytic Study* (New York: Basic Books, 1962).

79. L. Z. Freedman, Sexual, aggressive, and acquisitive deviates, *Journal of Nervous and Mental Diseases* 132(1964):44-49.

80. Gagnon, Gebhard, Pomeroy, op. cit., p. 720.

81. B. C. Glueck, Jr., Pedophilia, *Sexual Behavior and the Law*, ed. by R. Slovenko, pp. 539-562 (Springfield: Charles C Thomas, 1965).

82. S. Ferenczi, Confusion of tongues between adults and the child, *Final Contributions to the Problems and Methods of Psycho-Analysis*, pp. 156-167 (London: Hogarth Press, 1955).

83. D. Libai, The protection of the child victim of a sexual offense in the criminal justice system, *Wayne Law Review* 15(1969):977-1032.

84. H. Brunold, Observations after sexual traumata suffered in childhood, *Excerpta Criminologica* 4(1964):5-8.

85. J. Goldstein and J. Katz, Proposed Illinois revised criminal code, *The Family and the Law*, p. 383 (New York: The Free Press, 1965).

86. T. Benedek, Parenthood as a developmental phase: a contribution to libido theory, *Journal of the American Psychoanalytic Association* 7(1959):389-417.

87. S. Freud, Totem and taboo, *Standard Edition* 13.

88. R. Middleton, Brother-sister and father-daughter marriage in ancient Egypt, *American Sociological Review* 27(1962):603-611.

89. Leviticus 18:1-18, *The New English Bible* (New York: Oxford and Cambridge Universities Press, 1970).

90. Genesis, 19:30-38, *The New English Bible* (New York: Oxford and Cambridge Universities Press, 1970).

91. B. Malinowski, Marriage, *Sex, Culture and Myth* (New York: Harcourt, Brace, and World, 1962).

92. T. Parsons, and R. F. Bales, *Family Socialization and Interaction Process* (New York: Free Press, 1955).

93. T. Parsons, The incest taboo in relation to social structure and the socialization of the child, *Social Structure and Personality*, pp. 57-77 (New York: Free Press, 1964).

94. G. Devereux, Why oedipus killed laius, *International Journal of Psycho-Analysis* 34(1953):132-141.

95. Gebhard, Gagnon, Pomeroy, and Christenson, op. cit., p. 207.

96. Kappman, op. cit.

97. Halleck, op. cit.

98. R. E. L. Masters, *Patterns of Incest*, p. 328. (New York: Julian Press, 1963).

99. A. Yoru Koglu and J. P. Kemph, Children not severely damaged by incest with a parent, *Journal of the American Academy of Child Psychiatry* 5(1966):111-124.

100. C. W. Wahl, The psychodynamics of consummated maternal incest, *Archives of Genetic Psychiatry* 3(1960):188-193.

101. P. Sloane and E. Kapinski, Effects of incest on the participants, *American Journal of Orthopsychiatry* 12(1942):666-673.

102. G. E. Williams and A. M. Johnson, Recurrent urinary retention due to emotional factors, *Psychosomatic Medicine* 18(1956):77-80.

103. P. Machotka, F. S. Pittman, and K. Flomenhaft, Incest as a family affair, *Family Process* 6(1967):98-116.

104. I. Kaufman, A. Peck, and C. Tagiuri, The family constellation and overt incestuous relations between father and daughter, *American Journal of Orthopsychiatry* 24(1954):266-277.

105. B. M. Cormier, M. Kennedy, and J. Sangowicz, Psychodynamics of father-daughter incest, *Canadian Psychiatric Association Journal* 7(1962):203-217.

106. M. S. Adams and J. V. Neel, Children of incest, *Pediatrics* 40(1967):55-62.

107. M. Lewis and P. M Sarrel, Some psychological aspects of seduction, incest, and rape in childhood, *Journal of the American Academy of Child Psychiatry* 8(1969):606-619.

108. J. R. Fox, Sibling incest, *British Journal of Sociology* 13(1962):128-150.

109. L. J. Doshay, *The Boy Sex Offender and His Later Career* (New York: Grune and Stratton, 1943).

110. Wahl, op. cit.

111. M. Tramer, The incest problem. Uber das inzest-problem, *Zeitschrift fur Kinderpsychiat.* 22(1955):1-23.

112. G. Vidal, *Myra Breckenridge* (New York: Bantam, 1974).

113. Rape, *American Jurisprudence*, Section 3.

114. Gebhard, et al., *Sex Offenders,* op. cit., p. 178.

115. Crime and its impact—an assessment. *The President's Commission on Law Enforcement and the Administration of Justice* (Washington, D.C.: U.S. Government Printing Office, 1967).

116. Slovenko, *Sexual Behaviors and the Law*, op. cit., p. 52.

117. Gebhard, et al., op. cit., p. 192.

118. M. S. Guttmachen and H. Weihofen, *Psychiatry and the Law* (New York: Norton, 1952).

119. J. M. Reinhart, *Sex Perversions and Sex Crimes* (Springfield: Charles C Thomas, 1957).

120. Gebhard, et al., op. cit., p. 197.

121. G. K. Sturup, Treatment of sexual offenders in Herstedvester Denmark—the rapists, *Acta Psychiatrica Scandinavica Supplement* 204, 1968.

122. G. Legman, *Rationale of the Dirty Joke*, op. cit.

123. W. P. Brown, Police-victim relationship in sex crime investigations, *The Police Chief* January, 1970, pp. 20-24.

124. M. Amir, Forcible rape, *Federal Probation*, 31(1967):51-58.

125. C. Allen, *Sexual Perversions and Abnormalities* (London: Oxford University Press, 1944).

126. A. H. Williams, Rape-murder, *Sexual Behavior and the Law*, op. cit., pp. 563-577.

127. W. H. East and W. H. De B. Hubert, *The Psychological Treatment of Crime* (London: H. M. Stationery Office, 1939).

128. Gebhard, et al., op. cit., p. 397.

129. N. K. Rickles, *Exhibitionism* (Philadelphia: Lippincott, 1950).

130. Karpman, *The Sexual Offender and His Offenses*, op. cit., p. 187.

131. M. Sperling, The analysis of an exhibitionist, *International Journal of Psycho-Analysis* 27(1947):32-45.

132. O. Fenichel, The scoptophilic instinct and identification, *Collected Papers of Otto Fenichel: First Series,* pp. 373-397. (New York: W. W. Norton, 1953).

133. S. Freud, Three essays on sexuality, *Standard Edition* 7:123-245.

134. I. D. Yalom, Aggression and forbiddenness in voyeurism, *Archives of Genetic Psychiatry* 3(1960):305-319.

135. A. K. Gigeroff, J. W. Mohr, and R. E. Turner, Sex offenders on probation: the exhibitionist, *Federal Probation* 32(1968):18-26.

136. Gebhard, et al., op. cit., p. 378.

137. R. P. Nadler, Approach to psychodynamics of obscene telephone calls, *New York State Journal of Medicine* 68(1968):521-526.

138. S. Marcus, *The Other Victorians: A Study of Sexuality and Pornography in Mid-Nineteenth Century England* (New York: Basic Books, 1966).

139. *The Report of the Commission on Obscenity and Pornography* (New York: Bantam Books, 1970).

140. P. Cairns and I. Wishner, Sex censorship: the assumption of anti-obscenity laws and the empirical evidence, *Minnesota Law Review* 46(1962):1009-1065.

141. J. Paul and L. Schwartz, *Federal Censorship: Obscenity in the Mail* (Glencoe: The Free Press, 1961).

142. C. P. Magrath, The obscenity cases: grapes of rath, *The Supreme Court Review* ed. by P. B. Kurlund, pp. 7-77 (Chicago: University of Chicago Press, 1966).

143. *Regina* v. *Hicklin,* 3 Law Reports, 360, Queen's Bench, 1868.

144. *Mishkin* v. *New York,* 383 U.S. 502, 86 Sp. Ct. 958, 1966.

145. R. Dibble, Obscenity—a state quarantine to protect children, *Southern California Law Review* 39(1966):345-359.

146. Gebhard, et al., op. cit., p. 670.

147. Op. cit., p. 675.

148. V. L. Bullough, History of prostitution in the United States, *Medical Aspects of Human Sexuality* 4(1970):64-76.

149. *Minneapolis Vice Commission Report* 1911.

150. *Great Britain Committee on Homosexual Offenses and Prostitution* Report 79, 1957.

151. M. Johnson, Good laws ... good tools, *Journal of Social Hygiene* 38(1952):204-211.

152. R. Shenehon, The prevention and repression of prostitution in North America, *International Review of Criminal Policy* 15(1958):21-23. U.N. Pub. No. 58 IV 4.

153. B. J. George, Jr., Legal, medical and psychiatric considerations in the control of prostitution, *Michigan Law Review* 60(1962):717-760.

154. M. Ploscowe, *Sex and the Law* (New York: Prentice-Hall, 1951).

155. J. H. Bryan, Apprenticeships in prostitution, *Social Problems* 12(1965):287-297.

156. D. Glaser, Criminality theories and behavioral images, *American Journal of Sociology* 61(1956):433-444.

157. S. Shoham and G. Rahav, Social stigma and prostitution, *Ann. Inter. Crim.* 6(1967):479-513.

158. T. C. H. Gibbens, Juvenile prostitution, *British Journal of Delinquency* 8(1957):3-12.

159. E. M. Forster, *A Passage to India* (New York: Grosset and Dunlap, 1924).

160. G. Bychowski, Escapades: a form of dissociation, *Psychoanalytic Quarterly* 31(1962):155-174.

161. H. Deutsch, *Psychology of Women* (New York: Grune and Stratton, 1964).

162. H. Lichtenstein, Identity and sexuality, *Journal of the American Psychoanalytic Association* 9(1961).

163. L. Agoston, Some psychological aspects of prostitution: the pseudo-personality, *International Journal of Psycho-Analysis* 26(1945):62.

164. E. Glover, The psychopathology of prostitution, *The Roots of Crime*, pp. 244-267 (New York: International Universities Press, 1960).

165. P. H. Gebhard, Misconceptions about female prostitutes, *Medical Aspects of Human Sexuality* 3(1969):24-30.

166. J. V. Wallinga, A study of adolescent auto theft, *Journal of the American Academy of Child Psychiatry* 3(1964):126-139.

167. T. C. N. Gibbens, Car thieves, *British Journal of Delinquency* 8(1958):257-265.

168. M. Schmideberg, Delinquent acts as perversions and fetishes, *International Journal of Psycho-Analysis* 37(1956).

169. D. W. Winnicott, Transitional objects and transitional phenomenon, *Collected Papers* (New York: Basic Books, 1958).

170 W. Stekel, *Peculiarities of Behavior Cleptomania and Pyromania* (New York: Boni and Liveright, 1924).

171. B. A. Karpman, The principles and aims of criminal psychopathology, *Journal of Criminal Psychopathology* 1(1940):187-218.

172. N. D. C. Lewis, Pathological finesetting and sexual motivation, *Sexual Behavior and the Law*, ed. by R. Slovenko (Springfield: Charles C Thomas, 1965).

173. N. D. C. Lewis and H. Yarnell, *Pathological Fire-Setting*, Monograph No. 82 (New York: Nervous and Mental Disease Monograph Publishing Co., 1951).

174. L.B.Machl and J.E.Mack, The firesetter syndrome, *Psychiatry* 31(1968):277-288.

175. S. Freud, Dostoevsky and parricide, *Standard Edition* 21:173-196.

176. R. Greenson, On Gambling, *American Imago* 4(1948):61.

177. E. Bergler, *The Psychology of Gambling* (New York: Hill and Wang, 1957).

178. C. Allen, *A Textbook of psychosexual disorders* (London: Oxford University Press, 1969).

179. The American Law Institute, *Model Penal Code,* Proposed Official Draft, 1962.

180. H. Ellis, *Studies in the Psychology of Sex,* 3rd. ed. (Philadelphia: F. A. Davis, 1930).

181. P. Greenacre, Certain relationships between fetishism and the faulty development of the body image, *Psychoanalytic Study of the Child* 8(1953):79-98.

182. C. P. Malmquist, Dilemmas of the juvenile court, *Journal of the American Academy of Child Psychiatry* 6(1967):723-748.

183. Crisis in Child Mental Health—*Report of the Joint Commission on Mental Health of Children* (New York: Harper and Row, 1976).

184. N. M. Kittrie, Can the right to treatment remedy the ills of the juvenile process? *Georgetown Law Journal* 57(1969):848-885.

Chapter Six

The Identity Problem

Aspects connected with sex-role identity are usually discussed as components of a more general problem—that of identity. The terms employed in psychological theory and by clinicians need clarification in this context, for the term *identity* is laden with surplus meaning from its use in fields such as sociology, anthropology, and, more currently, psychohistory. Definitions are rarely provided for such commonly used terms as self, ego, identity, self-representation, self-awareness, and internalization. The concept of identification needs definition in its own right. It applies to identity, and also to a more precise developmental meaning about conflicts in the individual adolescent.

SOCIOLOGICAL ASPECTS

Social Roles and the Psychological Self. Any degree of reflection reveals a sense of self is not a uniform thing, but rather a disjointed sense of *several* selves. Throughout history, poets and dramatists have searched for personal meaning and reality in their relationships with real and imagined people and objects. In one sense this type of working through is similar to the actual and anticipated roles that the adolescent plays out. A recurrent theme deals with the feelings one *has,* as opposed to what he feels he *ought* to have according to a set of norms and values.[1] A realization of different identities, depending on particular situations, becomes manifest. These various identities are like multiple types of realities or, if extreme, multiple personalities.

Some descriptions of adolescence take the position that it is equivalent to a realization that diverse and multiple motives influence human behavior as well as the operation of social institutions. Such limitation of human character is realized by the adolescent in circumstances that are often personally painful. It is not new that parental behavior varies with time and circumstances. Even with children caught up in conflicts predisposing them toward acting out behaviors, the hope persists for idealism in parental behavior. During adolescence, the great awakening enlightens the adolescent not only with respect to parents but the rest of the world as well. Although in part this is a displacement from the disillusionment with parents, it is also a reflection of cognitive enlightenment.

Another group of psychological and social factors contribute to identity problems. These correspond to two opposite types of personality structures: those who exhibit constriction and those who are almost totally at the mercy of their environment. The former show a great deal of rigidity which fulfills inhibitory social needs toward others. In the past they have often been classified as *authoritarian personalities*.[2] Their more tranquil sides give them the potential to fit into a compulsively organized bureaucracy and do a routinized type of work. The limitation is a byproduct of robotized qualities in which identity becomes equivalent to a particular slot where they live a ritualized life of stereotyped organization. The outlets for an adolescent caught in this maze of organizational confines are to experiment in different roles and identities to only a limited degree. There is a simultaneous need to hold on to an early and untested identity, even though it fits into a totalitarian framework and is coupled with impulses to rebel.

The other alternative is a personality configuration so flooded by a plethora of stimuli that the individual is never able to achieve any stable, internalized object representations. (Psychodynamic and developmental components are omitted from the discussion at this point.) These personality configurations have occurred during different historical periods; dilettantes and those in need of living by prominent externalizations are examples. It is much easier in this particular historical period to live by seeking and reacting to external stimulation than to be inner directed.[3] This is even more so now than it was just after World War II. The option seems to perpetuate a diffuse and formless identity, corresponding to an objective world which appears to have its own formlessness.

Portrayals of modern life in literature and art abound in such characterizations. The writings of Kafka, Joyce, Beckett, Sartre, the theater of the absurd, and the depersonalization of sexuality by nudity are common examples. The question of which comes first is an old one between the socio-cultural approach and the psychological-developmental approach. There is evidence for both, and educated opinion argues on both sides. Anthropology has made the distinction between two types of approaches: the structure and functioning of social groups in which the psychology of the individual is not examined, and the study of the relationship between the psychology of the individual, his culture, and the social groups of which he is a member. Although some argue that the former approach suffices in discussions of identity, it appears necessary for any theory of identity with psychiatric implications to include investigations of the individual.

Individual identities are representative of cultural regularities and change, but they are also people whose identity configurations have a psychological history of development within their families. To examine this requires an adequate psychological theory of the individual as well as sufficient cultural theories regarding the processes of cultural standardization of behavior and the interaction necessary for certain types of character structures.

Even for those whose self-identities are not merely porous representations of social institutions, concern arises for the helplessness of the individual in confrontation with these institutions. An antithesis is experienced by the adolescent between subsuming himself to the authority of another or reacting in opposition to individuals or institutional objects. This conflict is strongly influenced by mass media.

Need any more imposing list be compiled for that which confronts the adolescent than the enormous number of advertisers, politicians, and political organizations, as well as the military, industrial, labor groups, and propagandists whose survival may be contingent upon the persuasion of the adolescent generation? The extent of the persuasiveness used by these groups and organizations can be judged when it is realized that their continuance is contingent upon recruitment without abatement of adolescents to their cause. When the persuasiveness utilizes appeals to bodily integrity, narcissism, and family integrity, it becomes extremely difficult to resist, let alone evaluate objectively. Complaints about mass culture and midcult are not new.[4] They have long existed, and at times reach gallows humor. The attempt to joke about one's predicament can be viewed as a rather desperate measure to deny that escape is impossible but to hope for a delay of the full impact of something unpleasant. Defensively, the function may be to give reassurance that an individual is not really helpless since he can joke about it and thus need have no fear. Adolescents epitomize the extremes of gullibility to the system while simultaneously making a last desperate effort to resist it and "lose my identity like my old man."

Vocational and Academic Disappointments. This leads to the problem of vocational and academic disappointments which are sensed by the adolescent not only through his parents but through great numbers of other adult males. Exposure to mass media conveys this theme repeatedly without recourse to intellectual articles or textbooks. Transient appeals of various political causes may lead to contempt for the entire political process, so that short of some radical or anarchic hope, salvation is not seen as residing there.

For most, survival itself requires work. More precisely, to live the way one wishes in an affluent economy requires a sizable income which must be obtained by work. By adolescence this is explicitly clear. More than that, there is a profound investment in work beyond providing monetary support. Academic and vocational success have been noted as male sex-typed traits. What is the impact on the adolescent when numbers of them witness desperate ploys by their fathers to bolster their career failures? At least in the middle classes, the primary problem is not income, despite an ever-increasing need for it. In the lower classes, when families are intact, money needs appear prominent, but the same type of job dissatisfaction operates for many fathers here as well. The adolescent is witness to the frustrated efforts of his elders to affirm one aspect of their identity through the occupational choice which has failed them. The need to justify and confirm oneself in work seems to promise little in the way of achieving a vocational identity over the long run.

Nor does the solution of withdrawal through money-making schemes or social entanglements solve the problem of an identity crisis in the vocational area. More academic aspects have been discussed earlier, but the pervasive effect on the adolescent with respect to his identity is emphasized here. He is witness to career failures in his elders and to that extent has a predisposing void during his adolescence. The over-evaluation of education and work have contributed to this problem because people have been taught that they should spend long years in school and training without asking themselves the value and purpose of this when it is completed. The justification has never seemed to proceed beyond the unexamined level that school is good, without appraising the natural history of the working life of the American male.

Without discussing the psychodynamics of the adolescent student with his frustrations and conflicts, the academic system itself appears to accentuate difficulties. The system cannot be ignored in understanding this predicament. Probably no greater error has occurred in retrospect than the efforts of counselors and therapists to view the individual with school difficulties as the one who by definition needs help in adjusting. Not that several individuals may not need such help, but in the end this contributes to the perpetuation of a format in which institutional practices and myths, in desperate need of change, are not required to do so. So much has been written on the atmosphere of student protest that only a smattering of material as relevant to the problem of identity will be examined.

While the attack on institutions commenced in the universities by students in their late adolescence in the 1960s, the process of questioning was not confined to that group, but progressed downward through the senior and junior high school levels. Some have cautioned the adolescent not to confuse the radical change that society requires with that which universities need.[5] Yet it is exactly such a traditional position of liberals that is challenged by adolescents because it ignores the special representative status quo position that schools of all types represent. One need not see academic facilities and schools as tools of a military-industrial complex to note the necessity of the former for the latter. Education, as the perennial stepping-stone to success as witnessed in their fathers, serves as the fulcrum for the attack. It represents both a false, if not somewhat dishonest, hope that a symbol of the past, which has not been particularly successful in achieving most of its nontechnical goals, can be reformed or eliminated. A historical perspective places student unrest in a pattern of cyclic upheavals which take place when political and social institutions become unstable. A more ultimate explanation has been seen in terms of the "fathers and sons" theme of rebellion.[6]

Whether recapitulation of sons overthrowing fathers is literally correct or not, historical patterns have emerged in terms of romantic movements which appeal to the adolescent. The romantic movements involve a stress on the experiential in contrast to restraint and reason. The stress on experiencing cannot be viewed as an evil by likening it to the German Youth Movement of the Nazi period or the era of Marxist-inspired protest. In a historical context, note the denunciation by Red Guard activists, who are students or young teachers, of senior teachers, and administrative bureaucrats.[7] When the cultural revolution appeared to be getting out of control, Red Guard members were demoted to the status of intellectuals—the essence of a group out of touch with the need for restructuring. Cultivation of feeling over reason has had many historical examples, such as the scene from the 1960s emphasizing drugs and ecstatic ascendance as the route to capture what education did not provide. A new identity was sought by mode of dress, manner, and experience, that appeared outlandish and bizarre to the uninitiated. It was an attempt to replace a previous identity which seemed undesirable. A series of attacks and counterattacks may occur between the challengers and those who feel their own identity threatened by attacks on their myths and institutions.

Adolescents victimize by equating their elders with stagnancy and decay, psychologically equivalent to death. This is not something the elders care to be reminded of, nor from its lack of explicitness is it something with which they can adequately deal. The more stagnant the institutions and their inability to deal with changing demands, the more equivalent to death they are, which is a self-reinforcing process. In turn, the elders strike back and become the victimizers by viewing the criticisms and destructiveness of the young as deadly maneuvers.

In time the process picks up momentum and further separation among divisions occurs. Many sado-masochistic relationships are in evidence. Whether this expresses self-destructive tendencies in terms of a motivational explanation, or represents misguided efforts to change, is open to debate, depending on theoretical preferences. Certainly, the preoccupation with destruction, death, and annihilation permeates many romanticized or revolutionary efforts at change. An error occurs in confusing ideological with empirical aspects, which leads to martyrdom. Death becomes confused, if not equated, with immortality.[8] It is believed derivatively that man will live by his works. If so, is it not worthwhile to die for such a cause? Appeals to the idealism of the adolescent are appeals to live for a cause that is just in contrast to a life which seems unsatisfying in parts and comes to be viewed as not worth living. The influence of group camaraderie reinforces the entire process.

Inherent in the frustrations of attaining an educational and vocational identity is the length of time and the amount of money involved in the preparation for this identity. This holds for the drop out, who gives up along the way, as it does for the remainder who continue student status for varying time periods. For some the preparation extends up to ten or fifteen years of post-high school training to attain a professional identity. While biology creates one kind of destiny, it offers little beyond a baseline for achieving vocational identity.

Social behavior characteristic of the adolescent begins much earlier than the onset of puberty and continues far beyond the attainment of biological stability. One direct consequence of this prolongation of years spent marking time in educational institutions is the perpetuation of adolescent status and expectations. More succinctly, this postpones the assumption of behaviors long since possible by a Pygmalion complex of expectancies that it is normal and right such educational and vocational practices continue.

The perpetuation of adolescence by continuing student status is seen not only in youths of sixteen to twenty-one who remain in school, but also in the professionalization of groups where those established in positions of institutional power continue to demand a multitude of requirements for entrance. Nor are the consequences confined to achieving professional identity by age twenty-five, for in some cases, such as a medical specialist, this period may extend up to age thirty-five before training is completed. Continuance of an individual's identity depends upon a lockstep series by which subservience and dependency remain prominent. One's body never really becomes one's own, but remains subject to infantilization far beyond the time when it is biologically or psychologically necessary. Such identity problems permeate every vocation, from the unskilled laborer to the surgeon or professor. Nor are artistic pursuits an escape, since the perpetuation of right behavior requires one relate to the existent norms or suffer the consequences.

What appears surprising is not the numbers who rebel, but rather the majority who are able to acquiesce in this framework. Data from the 1950s is often cited as indicating that the rebelliousness of youth is actually a myth.[9] Thus, 506 students in four Minnesota rural high schools were asked the question, "Who was the most important reference point in your life—family, school chums, or someone else? When 75 percent indicated parents, this was cited as evidence that rebelliousness was a myth.[10]

Parental influence is cited in these approaches as dominant. Again, the approach is similar in that 3,000 preadolescents and

adolescents were asked to complete a sentence such as, "My father is
———." An overwhelming number give a favorable response, which
is used as evidence for the above conclusion.[11] Another study
involving ten midwestern high schools reported that disapproval by
parents was more difficult to take than disapproval by peers and
teachers, and hence the conclusion that parents are the most
dominant influence on children.[12] Similar findings and methodology are reported in a study of Oklahoma youths.[13]

Another approach cites evidence that voting patterns between
children and parents are similar.[14] In a study of 1,088 students in
thirteen colleges, similarity of religious ideologies between students
and parents was cited.[15] Apart from the usual validity questions
which may be raised about these types of studies and what they tell
us, they convey an attitude that most adolescents remain like their
parents and want to be like them. A subtle fallacy appears related to
the *majority approach bias*. A majority express an opinion and are
then fallaciously viewed as the most influential and significant
members of a group. Radical groups of students, for example,
dedicated to a particular cause, may exert an enormous influence.

Justification for the prolonged educational process is often given
in terms that this length of time is necessary for a student to obtain
the educational qualifications and goals he seeks. Even apart from a
skeptical question whether prolonged education is mainly a device
to deploy adolescents until they can take their place in the ranks of
society, questions should be raised. This type of rationalization can
be seen clearly in the constant appeal to high school students not to
become drop outs with promises that a better job awaits them if they
remain in school. There is little evidence for this for the majority,
who later view it as hypocrisy. However, it does serve to keep
adolescents off the labor market until they are older, similar to the
way military service does.

These double messages contribute to the confusion experienced by
the adolescent when he senses a false basis to formal education. A
concomitant is that the student lacks power to alter such a system,
short of organized demands on those who administer the organizational structure. Yet, administrators and teachers in turn represent
some of the least innovative and most conforming elements in
society to whom the education of the young has been entrusted. They
are constrained by their institutional ties and personal security to
oppose change, and are not equipped to initiate the changes
required. Such dalliance promotes a type of anarchic view which
advocates a complete overhaul and abandonment of the contemporary educational and vocational system.[16]

Relationship to Adult Authority Figures. Since an articulate minority of adolescents continue to feel alienated from the institutional aspects of education, there are few constraints upon their criticisms. What results is a further defensive posture by adult authorities who alternate between citations of the virtues youth possess, such as honesty, duty, and other puritan virtues, and exhortations for adolescents to accept responsibility. Adolescents appear to have shifted back into this identity at present to a much greater degree.

These dilemmas open the way for attack on what education is supposed to provide and what many feel they have not obtained. Many feel that they have been exposed to a process of socialization, so that they can talk in a limited and often superficial manner about what educated people are supposed to say. The problems of attaining high marks and acquiring a superior capacity to pass examinations lend contempt to a process in which the unfortunate consequence is that education becomes condemned. Another result is an overcommitment to discipline and systematic study in the hope of achieving competence.

However, such discipline is rarely acquired and it may lead to disillusionment in the future. A technical proficiency may be obtained by the gifted few, but rarely more. Rather than seeing that they have obtained an exposure to knowledge and a systematic way of thinking, adolescents may turn to things equally trivial. More intense exploration of topics of current interest may take place through group experiences, mystic religious encounters, drugs, rock music, or dabbling in various styles of dress or work. In time, these practices become incorporated within the educational framework, and such things as community participation and involvement, time spent in human-contact work and retreats, may again gain prominence as educational fare, giving a semblance of integrated identity. In the end, this can only give a temporary sense of gratification for performing activities that serve idealistic goals which postpones dealing with the integration required within a personality.

Can anything be more enraging to an adolescent than having criticisms viewed in a patronizing manner by those in authority? A consequence of this attitude is to accentuate more vigorous, if not impulsive, means to attempt to impress those in control that things really are dismal. Limited job opportunities will further contribute to the increasing number of discontents. The failure to gain the support of others, except perhaps a few of their younger followers, may blunt the edge of their message and effectiveness for inducing change.

However, the potential for other discontented groups to join the cause in the hope of resolving some of their own grievances can lead to a state of heightened ambivalence. This frustration can best be encompassed by the idea of the powerlessness which characterizes adolescence in both psychological and social terms.

A feeling of powerlessness has developmental precursors from childhood which can be transformed into re-enacting this state during adolescence or beyond to avoid being regarded as dupes of the system. In this sense parents, teachers, and authority figures meet the criteria. Adolescents have long discovered that educational models may not satisfy their purpose as a means to power. They see other qualities that may lead to real power, such as ruthlessness, ambition, drive, the ability to manipulate smoothly and unobtrusively, and a relatively flexible morality. Books on "how to" gain power reflect this frustration in the population.

Nor do many find their college years an improvement. Alternatives on an undergraduate level provide little beyond scheduled requirements labeled as pre-professional or an assortment of culture courses which do not progress beyond providing a few key principles or terms. The problem is accentuated when college education is as prevalent as high school education and the degree becomes meaningless. However, the potential for discontent may be greater for one who has only graduated from high school and who continues to believe that the lack of education has led to his downfall. When adolescents realize that having a college education does not tap their abilities, and that they may very well end up doing a repetitive and uninspiring type of work, even without physical demands, disillusionment reigns. This may not be the way to social or vocational power, and for many it will not be satisfying either. A college degree for many will only mean some type of secure and slowly expanding income in a technological-industrial society.

Identity conflicts with respect to educational and vocational life have a relationship to what was once viewed historically as a desired goal. For many adolescents the dream of universal education as a coercive demand has ceased to have much meaning, even for those who put their time in for the end result. In view of the lethargy of institutional change, achieving change in the educational and vocational spheres will be difficult. One effort that might help would be to distinguish the cultural function of education as something an individual seeks from the mandatory requirement that an individual be exposed to it. This would restore cultural education to an elective basis for adolescents who wish to absorb it and can utilize it irrespective of social class. Use of education for technical training, or as a system of apprenticeship to fulfill the needs of the economy, should be recognized and acknowledged without confusing it with a system of education that focuses on cultural and humanistic subjects not directly relevant to training people to run industry and government.[17]

Studies demonstrate little or no correlation between the years of education and industrial efficiency—even for highly technical jobs in which most of the technique is learned on the job. Again, the element of fraudulence creeps in from the perspective of youths who spend years training for a certificate whose main role is to permit them to seek a job rather than assist them in doing the technical aspects. Alternatives appear desperately needed. A coercive system of public education is not even serving the needs of the economy except in a pro forma manner. Nor can such a system do more at best than teach the fundamentals of the three R's in the elementary school years. Evidence from college admission tests indicates that even this is not being successfully attained. The need for alternatives to the existing system of formal schooling seems undesirable.

PSYCHOLOGICAL ASPECTS

Role Transition. Psychological approaches to identity tend to view it as part of the phenomenon of role transition. Because of a number of demands in the social milieu, the adolescent is faced with a need to maintain his integrity. This is defined in terms of the obligation to achieve and stabilize his independence, meet certain goals in life, and obtain a sense of inner continuity—all within the social milieu. The need for commitment is present throughout. In one sense, there is the push from within the adolescent for delineating his own future while social institutions and agents simultaneously guide or restrict certain options. George Herbert Mead offered suggestions to bridge the social and psychological.[18] His viewpoint was that the unity of the self reflected the unity and structure of the entire social process. During adolescence a lack of unity is emphasized, with the accompanying disunity and inconsistency contributing to a confused state of identity.

To commit oneself to certain goals and activities means that there is an anticipation of a future of some sort. Even if the future appears hopeless, a commitment to this viewpoint is made and, if honestly believed, will determine some of one's future acts and decisions. How the adolescent perceives the future has implications for personality variables related to a sense of competence, feelings of self-worth, and an appraisal that others will see him in the same light that he sees himself. Uncertainty about his personal worth leaves the adolescent highly vulnerable to the opinions of others.[19] Cognitively, adolescents are equipped for committing themselves to future planning.[20] Planning for the future reverberates upon current behavior.

Competence. Competence is a variable of great importance to the adolescent.[21] Success in manipulating an environment, human or otherwise, contributes immeasurably to a sense of competence. This is related to the feeling of power and assertiveness which has been noted as part of the male sex-role standard and is becoming more so for the female. Experiencing competence can become a powerful motivator which leads to efforts at increasing it further.[22] Competence cannot be viewed as reflecting a general factor of competency, but is related to different tasks. This varies from self-imposed tasks in some areas to the entire interpersonal realm. From what has been said, success or failure in one area will influence the success of the other tasks which are selected. However, the concept of competence can become as elusive as intelligence. A host of personality variables are relevant besides intelligence. These include abilities, aggressiveness, drive level, curiosity, physical stamina, and creativity, to name a few. Beyond these, the environment must be receptive.

Unreceptivity can be related to the type of accomplishment, the fluctuating nature of others to a given performance, and what can be an indifferent response even to an exceptional performance. Examples are those of children with a history of disappointments in school performance who turn elsewhere, such as to delinquent behavior, for their gratifications, or who develop learning problems. Blinders on those from whom rewards are expected is often a crucial variable. Parents who are chronically preoccupied with their own personal difficulties are least likely to respond to the need for competency in their children.[23] A teacher may not see a certain activity or personality trait as desirable, or the cues which she utilizes to make judgments may be different from other norms comprising a standard. In the past this was seen when intelligence tests were being developed and the ratings of teachers were seen as quite inaccurate with respect to test results. It may also be seen in terms of what qualities an individual may have that will give a sense of personal competence.

Related to competency is the belief that an individual has some control over his destiny. This contrasts with a feeling that chance and the whimsy of others determine rewards. The psychoanalytic notion of narcissistic mortification touches this where one feels helpless and maneuvered by some external object.[24] A feeling of personal control and autonomy has developmental relationships from experiences that have been rewarded, if initiated by a child. Experimental studies have indicated that learning is greater when a skill is utilized rather than learned by chance, that attentiveness to cues is greater, past experience given more relevance, and wrong things not learned as often.[25] There is a similar experience when one joins a group which then exerts some type of control over one's future in the direction anticipated prior to joining.[26] This holds for social groups, teams, organizations, or for any self-serving interest.

Research on group participation has indicated greater personal satisfaction in smaller groups in which recognition can be obtained and contributions made according to ability. In terms of the activities which give a feeling of competency in the educational realm, experiences within a large, anonymous school setting, an academic experience which stresses competitiveness, socially and athletically as well as academically, will most likely lead to less competency with its consequent toll on self-identity. Studies on dropouts have indicated long-standing histories of few successes in school and little membership or involvement in group activities, which later give rise to discontent.[27]

Self-esteem and Approval. One component of self-esteem is contingent upon the appraisal given to performances by others. Discrepancies are common between self-appraisal and how others appreciate a performance. Investigation might utilize self-questionnaires, reports of self-rating versus desired ratings, and appraisal by teachers and peers compared to the self. Q-Sort techniques, utilizing self-descriptive items, can be used for self-ratings to compare with an ideal rating, or others could sort another individual.

The way an individual appears to others may be used for illustration. It is significantly associated with peer ratings as a main source of self-esteem. For adolescent girls this has been studied in the same sex and with boys as well. Girls appear to exhibit greater effects on their self-esteem when their physique deviates markedly from the ideal.[28]

The greater the extent of deviation from ideal dimensions, the more negative feelings experienced toward those body parts and their selves. Jourard and Secord studied psychological correlates of deviation from preferred body size in college women.[29] Preferred bust size was larger than the actual size. However, estimated size of hips, waist, height, and weight were smaller than their mean actual size. For the latter, there was a satisfaction with these bodily parts. None of the physical dimensions equaled the desirable in this respect. Such deviations were hypothesized as a source of low self-esteem. Whether this contributes to the greater tendency toward depression in females, which becomes progressive with age, represents an interesting hypothesis.

Peer standards may function to protect adolescents from criticisms by an out-group—specifically critical adults. The more self-esteem possessed, the better one can perform in different roles. This is seen in many endeavors. Conversely, an adolescent with low self-esteem anticipates failure and often gets it. There is a secondary tendency to avoid putting oneself in situations which involve competition and taking a chance on receiving further confirmation of an already deflated self-esteem. Many of the findings related to competency have a bearing on mood lability. Since this involves the subject of cyclothymic personality organization, the question of the genesis and proneness to this type of mood disturbance is germane. The question as to origin is unsettled, such as the extent to which an impaired sense of competency contributes to depressive-proneness, or the extent to which it is a secondary factor reinforcing these tendencies.

Studies of self-esteem in nonclinical populations of adolescents are relevant.[30] A summary of 5,000 eleventh- and twelfth-grade students in ten schools in New York State appraised self-esteem by a ten-item, self-reporting scale. Low self-esteem, depression, anxiety, and low-grade averages were all correlated. Both low- and high-self-esteem adolescents desired occupational success, but those who rated low felt they could not attain success. They prefer an occupation which they believe unattainable, and feel they lack the assets for success. It is apparent that this is not a matter of slight differentials in a few variables, but rather widespread differences which generalize. Those with high self-esteem are more likely to rate themselves high in self-expression, self-confidence, hard work, leadership potential, talent, intelligence, skill, ability to make a good impression, feeling at ease with others, and self-assurance. Those with low self-esteem reveal their incompetencies socially. They tend to provoke others, which leads to further reinforcement of self-depreciation. These self-punitive mechanisms have psychodynamic implications pertaining to masochistic character structure.

How an adolescent perceives the future, then, is related to his self-esteem and sense of competency. A bleak appraisal of the future impairs present performance. The degree and accuracy of self-perceptions, and how they become integrated into the personality structure, are affected. Competency is correlated with a future orientation in which a well-differentiated picture of the future has developed so that what one does is considered important and meaningful.[31] Desire for recognition by others in adolescents cannot be viewed accurately as simply an expression of undesirable narcissism. If developmental processes pertaining to ego integration have been proceeding satisfactorily, there is a need for recognition. The result is to confirm developmental progress and further promote his self-esteem. The path lies open for recognition from activities that may be unacceptable by social mores or legal norms. This is the connection between psychological identity theory and sociological theory in which status within a group enhances the reputation and group identity of the adolescent. It can lead to a confirmation of this identity by the rewards within the group itself and peers outside who view the youth as belonging to a certain group. The process is usually secondarily reinforced by community handling and labeling processes. Learning principles of approach and avoidance operate within peer groups which form the basis for group identity to form similar groups of youths. Since many adolescents perceive adults as hostile, with little understanding or respect for them, they are left with a special vulnerability to form their own oppositional groups.[32]

Incompatibility between adults and adolescents was demonstrated in a study of differences between how a group of adolescents saw themselves compared to how two groups of adults (teachers and other adults) saw them.[33] The youths were from a large, midwestern city and ranged from upper-middle to lower-middle class. Ranking from descriptions of the ideal and actual high school graduate in terms of sixteen orientations was done: religious, economic, political, aesthetic, altruistic, social, hedonistic, physical, ethical, and theoretical (having knowledge of many things and a desire to learn more). The ranking was done by 153 high school teachers, 224 adults from civic and school-related clubs, and by 956 high school students. When a correlation of -0.53 between the real and ideal image of adolescents, who were rated by school teachers, is comprehended, it demonstrates the antagonism present between the groups.

The correlations were 0.15 for other adults, while the adolescents gave themselves a 0.46 correlation. Little difference was present between the three groups of raters in terms of the ideal orientation in contrast to the ratings of actual performance by the adolescent. Educators saw the high school graduate's three highest orientations as making as much money as possible (economic), making friends easily (social), and having as much fun as possible (hedonistic). While the adolescents agreed on the social ranking, they viewed themselves as theoretical and ethical for the other two main orientations. The ethical orientation pertained to being honest and trustworthy. In contrast, teachers and other adults, mainly parents, saw the adolescent as materialistic, personable, and a pursuer of pleasure, and instead wanted him to have moral character and religious interests. When the adolescents committed themselves to what they regarded as these latter attributes, this still did not apparently satisfy the adult group, since it was likely to be a dedication to a moral cause or type of behavior which the adolescents viewed as moral, but the adults did not.

Integrity.   While ego identity in a psychological context is related both to a sense of competency and continuity, it is also related to a sense of distance from the adult group. An ideal result is that of integrity in the sense of a unity of the self which also remains separate from others. Hence the relevance of competency and self-esteem for the adolescents which permits them to maintain separateness without undue dependency on others for integrity.

Other psychological variables contribute to a sense of ego identity. Interactional patterns within a family, including parent-child relations in many spheres, contribute. Identifications have been discussed and will be elaborated in terms of ego development. The adolescent with a strong sense of sex-role identity has a self-concept more congruent with a sex-role standard by which his culture and peer group operate. It would be expected that such an adolescent would have an advantage in establishing a sense of distinctiveness with less conflict and anxiety. Self-perceptions permit them to handle social coercions for certain types of behavior during adolescence with less discomfort. Dealing with heterosexual social encounters as well as sexual impulses is smoother. In contrast to this greater ease of integration of adolescents, note that as youth and young adulthood succeed adolescence, boys with the most secure sex-role identifications retain their masculine behaviors, but their self-perceptions may have suffered.[34]

During adolescence the most masculine were often leaders and self-confident individuals. They were quite accepting of themselves and dominant in groups, but once adolescence was over they declined. A hypothesized answer is that what delineates identity during adolescence may not hold up as such for the male over the long run. The sex-role standard for the adolescent male is often based on overt characteristics which get a higher degree of agreement from those ranking them within an adolescent peer group. When such overt characteristics as physique and dominance no longer define masculinity, it is more difficult to maintain an identity based on stereotypes.

Apart from professional athletes, an identity based on a highly masculine type of work, such as labor or driving a truck, has few accouterments which contribute to identity as an adult male. Even in an overt manner, such things as income, status, and power are not achieved by activities which have succeeded during adolescence. More subtle personality variables give the adult a sense of identity based on the sector of sex-role identity. Vocational roles which combine masculine attributes with feminine ones give greater rewards in terms of personal self-esteem. This is not only because of the social recognition for capabilities which require a fusion of traits, but for the opportunity to be nurturant and sensitive to others, or competitive in ways that utilize intellect, which is barred in blatant forms of adolescent sex-role identity. Heilbrun found that adolescent boys whose fathers were only *moderately* masculine had less difficulty in establishing appropriate sex-role behavior and had fewer discrepancies in their social values than boys whose fathers were at either extreme.[35]

CLINICAL-DEVELOPMENTAL ASPECTS OF IDENTITY

Epigenetic Principle. Overlaps exist between the clinical-developmental approach with the sociological and psychological. The clinical-developmental involves facets of the personality in terms of a structural theory of personality functioning as well as stage-developmental antecedents. There is a sense of sameness and continuity from earlier development, but also an additional need to rework earlier crises for a continuing and new sense of adolescent identity. This is not merely the sum of earlier identifications, but involves experiences at each preceding stage which permit drive endowment to correlate with present opportunities.

A *sense of ego identity* refers to a confidence that one is the same person and has maintained a psychological continuity correspond-ing to the sameness and continuity one has for others. At each earlier developmental crisis more or less self-esteem can eventuate. The epigenetic principle which views things as proceeding from a ground plan, from which parts arise, with special times of ascendancy to form a functioning whole, is the result.[36]

At the time of each ascendancy, a crisis arises from which some type of lasting solution is made. Involved are a progression of psychological forces as well as an encounter with the environment. The phenomena are crises since the individual is then particularly vulnerable. While each stage makes a specific contribution to all that comes after it, as well as certain polarities which follow, there are times of ascendancy which make lasting contributions to components of the personality. During adolescence, identity versus identity diffusion predominates.

Identity in a developmental sense involves a subordination of childhood identifications to a new identification. Sociability and competitiveness with peers are involved which no longer have the playfulness of earlier childhood. Choices and commitments are made which have more finality than previously. Because of this last period of consolidating identity, societies offer a period of psychoso-cial moratoria, during which a pattern of inner identity is scheduled for completion. Lhile latency may be viewed as a period of relative psychosexual moratoria, during adolescence this is no longer possible.

On the other hand, there are no parallels between biological sexual maturity and the capacity for intimacy or parenthood. Instead, role experimentation is carried out to secure a specific niche. If it is found, there is an assured sense of inner continuity and social sameness which reconciles the adolescent's conception and recognition of himself in the community.[37] It is not a mere recognition for achievement that is sought, but a wish to be regarded, in terms of function and status, as having grown. Unless this environmental support is available, development of ego functions specific to adolescence becomes impaired. In broad terms these functions are: (1) to maintain defenses against the increased intensity of impulses accompanying a biological readiness, (2) consolidation of conflict-nree achievements congruent with work opportunities, and (3) resynthesis of childhood identifications in a unique way which accords with the roles available in society. The need for recognition is a mutual one. Those in positions of authority in a community can wreak a terrible vengeance on youths who seem indifferent or rejecting of them in a provocative manner.

Identification and Identity. On reflection, identity is much more than the sum of childhood identifications. All the previously accomplished identifications, whatever their basis, do not add up to a functioning adult personality. Identification can at best be a reaction to the partial attitudes or attributes of individuals, and although these may persist in a desirable or detrimental manner, they do not comprise the sum and substance of a personality. Conversely, the part aspects of another can never be more than a persistent part of someone else.

Identity formation begins where the usefulness of identification ends. Some childhood identifications have been assimilated and others repudiated before a new and individualized identity results. Identity formation is a lifelong and continuous process extending from the beginnings of self-awareness to mutual recognition in the social sphere. A configuration results by a process of successive ego syntheses and resyntheses throughout the developmental years. To the extent that these are successful, the adolescent experiences himself as "being at home in his body," as well as having a distinctive quality to his life accompanied by an inner assuredness of recognition by those who count for him.

Clinical aspects of identification require more detailed examination. The most conspicuous addition to identification usage from a psychodynamic orientation is to view identification as operating not only by conscious and preconscious processes, but by unconscious processes as well. An object that has acquired significance exerts its influence by altering motives and behavior patterns by an accompanying change in self-representation. Several self-representations contribute to a more finalized identification. Object ties are maintained from a variety of sources. There would not only be the biological and ethological aspects of attachment, but a host of developmental processes and conflicts.[38] Not only may many of these transactions initially and subsequently operate unconsciously, but these identifications acquire autonomy from their sources—a type of secondary autonomy operation. Identification is viewed as a sequence of events which are not static and unmodifiable, but continually altered and revised both from environmental encounters as well as from intersystemic and intrasystemic shifts.

A further caveat is needed for those not experienced in the world of childhood identifications. Nonhuman objects, such as pets, animals, monsters, and machines, as well as fictionalized and fantasized characters, who may or may not ever have lived, contribute to identification. Another point is that identification does not take place with a person or object per se, but rather with the representation thereof. Many versions of an object are possible; the conceptions of a particular individual are only one, and perhaps idiosyncratic at that. Questions as to the objective status of external objects open unresolved philosophical issues and psychologically can only be dealt with from a vantage point of whose view and what particular circumstances are present. While some representations correspond to an objective configuration, in the sense of a majority of observers expressing agreement, many factors operate in a particular individual. Developmental factors as well as those referring to the structural status of mental functioning are present, as well as the internal state of a subject at a given time—his drive level, moods, anxiety state, or other distorting factors.

Difficulty is encountered in attempting to determine which parts of objects have been used for identification. Arguments hinge on whether whole or part objects have been used. Again, there may be only one, or several, aspects of an object identified with at one time. If perceptual processes are focused primarily on one component— say the breast or the control one has over another—then that is the whole object. Attempts for an identification with a whole object, meaning the totality of physical and psychological attributes, run into difficulties since this demands a fusion, or a loss of identity. Such attempts are observed in adolescents with their heroes or in states of psychotic regression.

On a more subtle level, a person may be striving to become a certain type, such as an athletic hero, or establish dominance over those with whom he is in contact. This leads to formulations which seem arcane to those not personally acquainted with the workings of the unconscious and primary process thinking. On its surface, a formulation that an individual is identifying with or trying to become a phallus may seem so abstruse or conjectural as to be beyond the realm of science. Yet, considered in the light of identification processes where the power strivings of an external object can be represented in a pars pro toto fashion by a phallic representation with all its detectable consequences, it may not. It is then seen as striving to include the characteristics encompassed within the concept of the phallic character as part of the self.

Cognizance must be given to the irrational and unrealistic aspects of identification, which are based on primary process cognitive operations. To ignore this is to ignore the pre-existing unconscious representations and wishes which determine why a selectivity, as well as generality, operates regarding identification. A simple example: A boy who emulates his father is not just trying to be like him with respect to overt, sex-typed occupational or physical attributes. He is in addition operating by wishes to acquire the masculinity of his father with all the ramifications attached thereto. A more complex example: The identification processes with respect to the development of self-control involve a heterogeneous collection of self-representations, prohibitions, and reorganization of drive aims and objects.

Although approaches to identification which ignore unconscious contributions restrict their usefulness, the opposite type of approach, which gives almost exclusive emphasis to nothing but unconscious formulations, has restrictions of its own. Operationally, we can define conscious determinants as *imitation* while expansion of the concept to use unconscious and preconscious determinants would be *identification*. This is in accord with social learning theory formulations.[39] Imitation would simply be a conscious attempt to be like another person. Imitation implies a high degree of psychological differentiation, in that subjects can recognize themselves as distinct from others so they are capable of deciding which behaviors to copy. Should efforts to be like another person then be regarded as identification processes at all?

It may be in the service of clarification, if not parsimony, to confine the usage of identification to explanatory efforts which include multiple determinants within the personality. Among these determinants the role of fantasy cannot be ignored. Identification operates with respect to overt behaviors as well as fantasies. The result is an alteration in self-representation, which is an essential component of identification. This provides a bridge for understanding how objects with whom an individual is relatively unacquainted can exert strong influences. Some seemingly trivial characteristic may exert great influence because it makes connection with powerful wishes and becomes representative of those wishes. Implicit in such a formulation is the directionality given by early identifications.

While a particular identification of an adolescent may seem crucial, the sine qua non was the previous attachments and identifications that laid the groundwork for a particular one which took in adolescence. This is not to reduce everything to early childhood experiences, but rather to illustrate the developmental process in which whatever the current predicaments, social milieu, or personality state, there are antecedents which contribute to how identification is used. A hierarchy of motives fluctuates and has individual differences.

Even the same identification may serve contradictory purposes. For example, the identification of the oedipal-age boy with his father can be defensive as well as gratifying by taking over many of the activities and locations of his father at times. The wish may be aggressive or sexual, adaptive or not, and progressive or regressive. In terms of the structural aspects of the personality, identification processes may be defined from the ego side as a defensive maneuver, or from the id side as impulse-gratifying. A hierarchical arrangement of motives operates so that it is imprecise to speak in terms of one motive operating.

The Natural History of Identity. Intricacies of identification processes do not account for its ontogenesis. Is there anything in addition to the material discussed as part of sex-role identification that can be added from a clinical vantage point with relevance for identity formation?

1. The inescapable biological variability exerts an influence in its own right. Some children are more active and some passive, some emotive and some constricted, in addition to the entire gamut of constitutional variables which contribute. The biological variables may promote an identification of the parent with the child as much as the converse.[40] An active child finds it easier to identify with aggressive or acting-out parents; the passive child finds identification with a compliant, constricted, or suffering parent easier—other variables being constant. Of course, variables never are constant, which complicates explanations. Yet, it would seem persuasive that constitutional factors of temperament cannot be ignored.

2. The developmental level, in terms of how the child experiences himself and others, is relevant. A host of predisposing elements contributes, such as which drives are in ascendancy, previous types and qualities of object relationships, the developmental level of ego and superego structures, and the fantasy functions attached to drives and their derivatives.

3. A number of wishes are served by any one identification. Schafer refers to these as having "multiple appeal" and acquiring significance by the extent to which they benefit an individual. For example, the oedipal boy's identification with his father gives him a strength in the sense of masculinity, capacity for restraint (resistance to temptation), reassurance against bodily injury, development of less ambivalent and anxious ties to both parents, and preparation for peer relationships.[41] In contrast, a feminine identification is inadequate for the boy by each of these measures.

4. Parental character structures contribute to identity formation. Although a model is distorted by perceptual and projective operations during childhood, an identification with parental styles and the contents of the parents' own fantasies contribute to identification. Especially this is so with respect to parental moral dictates. However, it is not the transmission of moral rules on a cognitive basis that makes the major contribution, but rather the mode of handling moral issues and conflicts which the child witnesses with accompanying affect. Witness the effect on a child whose father handles aggression by identifying with authority figures; counterwise, consider the father whose strategy is to adopt, unconsciously and otherwise, an obsequious manner toward authority.

5. Parental conflict affects identification by polarizing masculinity and femininity for the boy and girl. Particularly does this happen when there is marital conflict. A boy may feel obliged to adopt the most masculine of traits, and the girl the most feminine, or the exact opposite can occur. The reason is the greater difficulty in such situations to integrate successfully masculinity and femininity within one personality. The consequence is an overcompensatory need to demonstrate masculinity or femininity. Conflicted identifications also result from parents whose problems are primarily psychotic, neurotic, or acting-out impulses.[42] [43] [44] Influences on the child are unneutralized consequences which may be overstimulating or too seductive. Other influences operate in the realm of alternating types of deprivation, sadistic, or traumatic experiences.

6. Parental ambivalence about the developing identifications complicate the efforts of children to integrate identifications which are in a transitory state. Both by supporting and opposing identifications, the children sense a confusing split in parents. This can be parental anxiety over sexuality or aggression in the child, or dissatisfaction with themselves in which they hope the child will not be like them. Disillusionment with a marital partner leads to efforts at reinforcing identifications in the child of an opposite type from the spouse. Traumatic influences such as deaths, desertions, separations, abandonments, illnesses, and radical changes in socioeconomic status all exert significant influences on identification processes and identity.

Some identifications have little staying power and exert no lasting influence on the personality. They may involve a temporary regression to identification with a character in a movie or story. This is not to deny predetermining influences as to why such temporary identification takes place, but it illustrates the transiency that is possible. In contrast are identifications which begin early in the context of attachments and object relationships. These make more lasting contributions to personality development.

By shifts and alterations an all-time establishment of identifications for ego and superego functioning is not accomplished once and for all in early childhood, despite the significance of the processes. It is naive to maintain that an adolescent has values and controls which are merely those of a parent or some other type of displaced object. Observation of contradictory adolescent behaviors and goals raises questions, but psychologically by adolescence a degree of autonomy from the experiences which contributed to the original model has been achieved. Rather than demonstrating the pervasive examples of how adolescents rebel against the overt and socially acceptable identifications which their parents represent, consider the opposite. This is seen in cases where the adolescent resists parental efforts to corrupt certain norms which are viewed as more moral. These may be in direct opposition to what was once identified with in the parent.

While the boy may have early identified with his mother for a multitude of reasons, such as to incorporate certain of her traits, to maintain her affection, or to neutralize paternal hostility, these may have little operational influence on how he expresses his maternal feelings during adolescence or adulthood. Other needs and identifications operate so that impulses can be expressed while their overtness may be denied or concealed from the censorious influence of the sex-role standard. Common examples are the helping behaviors of male adolescents toward each other, their maternal behavior toward others—parents themselves, younger siblings, or girl friends. In adulthood their maternal behaviors are manifested toward their children and wife.

A problem is the shifting nature of identifications which occur along with an increasing complexity and psychological growth of the personality related to identifications. If the question is directed toward the individual personality, what changes have occurred within its structure? To appraise personality development solely in terms of external characteristics ignores how it must deal with its impulses, ego development, ideals, and controls. Changes occur within the personality based on identifications with multiple objects. By representations of these objects which persist for an individual, he is able to direct his attachments to these representations and not just their external representations. In fact, the latter may recede or disappear, but the former do not in terms of their influence. By identification with these objects, ego changes occur, as the ego becomes the object toward which id impulses are directed, or an aspect of the self-representation for an object attachment.

Intrapsychic Aspects. Arguments of a theoretical nature have arisen between those who believe that major emphasis should be given to intrapsychic aspects of identification. For those who choose to underemphasize this aspect of the personality as inessential, discussion is beside the point. Early formulations, including those of Freud, viewed the development of "ego-as-id-object" as having quantitative aspects which were inverse from the attachment to external objects. If this process of self-representation occurs at the expense of an external directionality to the personality, questions arise about the relationship to narcissism as well as to self-esteem.[45]

The question of the renunciation of external objects is central to the process of internalization in general, as well as specific types of psychological structures which are perpetuated, such as superego guides. Yet, why does this occur rather than the organism maintaining its behavior subject to environmental inputs or threats? To state it as classic psychoanalytic theory has (in terms of an oedipal renunciation permitting identification to proceed, with an internalized superego structure), does not explain why this has to occur unless one falls back on postulates that the developmental process at that time requires a process of internalization. Personality changes related to a parental identification during the oedipal period take place. An increased capacity for self-love and self-esteem occur, and more defenses become available at that time as well as more realistic self-representations. In addition, the reality testing of the child has been promoted.

Adverse consequences from identification conflicts during the oedipal period result in object representations which are painful or traumatic. Tese representations are associated with low self-esteem, self-destructive tendencies, difficulties in trusting, and affects of helplessness and hopelessness. Personality absorption in such consequences as emerging depressive tendencies, outbursts of rage, sado-masochistic relationships, symptoms and signs associated with repression, withdrawal, reaction formations, and overcompensatory strivings are possible consequences. The result tends toward identifications which stress aims geared toward primitive, yet perhaps precociously developed, activities to protect the individual organism. There may be a hyperalertness, greater sensitivity, and less filtered expressions of impulses, impairing the development of internalized regulation. This is theoretically discussed in terms of an impaired or defective capacity for neutralization.[46]

Objects of identification, which modify and subordinate drive aims to regulatory motives, have an advantage in contrast to those based on a state of semi-emergency. While a type of shrewdness and guardedness develops, the social and psychological handicaps must be questioned. Socially we may question how reliable it would be (if no psychological handicaps were present) to have individual development be in the line of constant alertness for personal threats and attacks or whose needs were self-aggrandizement.

When early identifications have promoted the integration of various motives and drives, a consolidation of identification occurs. If things are progressing satisfactorily, during latency we see models influencing a shift in motives, behavior patterns, and self-representations. A balance may be achieved even earlier between intense involvements with external objects and synthesis of internal representations. Confirmatory observations are behaviors and attitudes such as caring for oneself more independently and in a way which enhances self-approval. Increased initiative and commitment occur with a parallel decrease in expectations that others will take care of the individual. Superego functioning is influenced by identifications in terms of increased moral pride associated with aspirations as well as renunciations. The internalized regulation of self-esteem has come into its own by the capacity for liking or disliking oneself for what one is as well as for what one does.

Manifestations of neutralization of activities are noted in what was once sought in a demanding way. Fewer demands for immediate gratification are made, with an absence of unstable displacements for discharge. Integration of identification objects permits greater interest in activities and objects quite removed from what the original desires were. This can only occur if an internal capacity for satisfaction, delay in gratification, and a belief in emotional comfort are secure. By the ability to gain satisfaction by self-initiated and self-enhancing activities, a further differentiation of self-representations occur with the added feature of further emancipation from others. A qualitative ranking of different representations occurs as well. These changes promote a greater degree of reality confirmation which brings behavior into alignment with perceived reality. Of course, disturbances in development will show up as difficulties in these areas.

IDENTITY DIFFUSION

Definition. Identity difussion as described by Erikson is a syndrome seen in young people who are either incapable of making use of the moratorium which society provides, or incapable of creating and maintaining themselves in their own style. Only a few of the more ingenious can succeed in making their own way.[47] Rather than viewing these adolescents in terms of descriptive nosology or character typologies, they are approached from the point of characteristics representative of the crises from the inability of their egos to establish an identity. In clinics or hospitalized settings, these adolescents are often given diagnoses of schizophrenia, sociopathic personality, or paranoid personality. Careful listening reveals a mixture of depressive and acting-out tendencies with no clear-cut diagnosis, so they are often lumped as *borderlines.*

The period of breakdown into a state of acute identity diffusion is revealing. Typically the breakdown is when an adolescent is exposed to a combination of circumstances which demand simultaneous commitment to physical intimacy, decisive occupational choice, energetic competition, and a psychosocial self-definition. Examples are when the adolescent separates from home, such as entering college or the armed forces. New encounters may involve people from different backgrounds. Friends and enemies are made and physical intimacy (not necessarily involving sex) is attained. Choices are made involving competitive risks which bring to the fore identifications long dormant and which may be in conflict with current identifications. However, the consequences of avoiding such choice and commitment are less appealing. Avoidance leads to an outer isolation and an inner vacuum. Regressive pulls to earlier object ties threaten and a re-emergence of struggles with old introjects takes place.

Signs and Symptoms. Difficulties in establishing intimacies may not be reached during the chronological years associated with adolescence. Pseudo-intimacy may instead be practiced by a series of group participations or happenings which give a spurious reassurance of intimacy. When a serious attempt to become genuinely intimate with one or more individuals of the same or opposite sex occurs, pre-existing weaknesses become manifest. Lacking clear object boundaries, serious contact with others induces a strain due to the threat of interpersonal fusion tantamount to a loss of identity.

Adoption of a facade of reserved coolness, with closeness at a distance is the goal. The threat of intimacy remains, so that ego abandonment or regression becomes forbidden. Since the counterpart of intimacy is distance, there is a readiness to repudiate, ignore, or even destroy, if necessary, those whose existence seems dangerous to the self. Another vulnerability is a tendency to feel that an authority figure can save the adolescent. This need not be an abstract figure, although the attraction therein would seem evident. The old hope for an intimacy at a distance remains. Failing this, a state of ego paralysis may result with a painful awareness of isolation. Inner continuity and sameness are threatened. Feelings of shame accompany an inability to derive a sense of accomplishment and a feeling that life is not being lived but endured. The adolescents remain convinced that they have a psychosocial existence, but it is up to others to prove it given their basic mistrust has to be overcome.

Disturbances in time perspective are another characteristic of identity diffusion. A mild sense of a loss of time as a meaningful component can proceed to a more chronic state in which time seems dissociated. Simultaneous feelings of being childlike exist alongside feelings of being irretrievably old. Adolescent equivalents of what will later be seen as depressive phenomena occur. Once beyond adolescence, complaints take the form of a general dissatisfaction with themselves and the world. Patterns of chronic complaining thinly conceal masochistic provocation. There is a feeling they have never reached their true potential. By that time—in the late twenties—the focus is on vocational and marital dissatisfaction.

Prodromata are seen in adolescent beliefs that they have missed an opportunity to be great at something, be it athletics, artistic pursuits, or attaining academic recognition. Complaints of hanging it up or quitting become typical. Change is wanted, yet feared, which leads to a hesitancy in committing. Slowing down of activities occurs. In more profound cases, the giving up complex associated with depressions is viewed as a desire of the ego to extinguish itself.

Diffusion of industry is related to time diffusion. Concentration difficulties contribute to problems in work, although a skewed preoccupation with one overriding interest may occur. Examples vary from excessive reading to intense absorption in the goals of a particular group. Ego development during preadolescence has been conceptualized as a time when identifications with elders as workers and tradition-bearers succeeds earlier constrictions of elders as sexual or family objects.

If identity diffusion trends predominate, earlier preoccupations recur. In place of industrialization of interests, there is a recurrence of competitiveness and rivalry of earlier years with new anxieties from the changed physical and social milieu. In place of support from work or using one's body physically, fantasies with prominent sexual and aggressive components emerge. Although this is often thought of as more descriptive of boys, it is also seen in girls who alternate between withdrawal into fantasy and aggressive tomboy pursuits. The girl is puzzled as to whether any alternatives are really available.

Choice of a negative identity is a striking feature of the identity diffusion syndrome. It may amount to an abrogation of personal identity. A scornful and snobbish hostility is expressed to roles offered as acceptable or desirable in a community. It can be directed primarily against a particular individual, a role, class, institution, ethnic group, or country. Whatever becomes the object of disdain qualifies. It may take the form of opposition to a sex-role standard of what masculine or feminine attributes are supposed to be. Feminized appearances in male adolescents demonstrate this, as well as attempts to blur or eliminate distinctions between the sexes. Desires to destroy while preserving indicate a high degree of ambivalence.

In most societies there is little difficulty in selecting some object that elicits ambivalence. By viewing themselves as helpless victims, there is denial of their experience as personally weak and helpless individuals. "I am merely the personal victim of an oppressive group. Therefore, it is not I who am weak and helpless since overwhelming and uncontrollable powers decide my fate." This thinking reflects the use of externalization mechanisms.[48] This has analogies to work done on victimology.[49] The resignation to a helpless situation, or protests which entice repressive counterattacks, enable the adolescent to retain or regain a magical position of power since he is, in effect, partially the external aggressor.

Accompanying the negative identity is a self-disparagement. The general dislike and contempt for many things parallels their self-contempt. There are feelings that there is decay and ennui elsewhere while somewhere—true life goes on. Hence, one may feel more comfortable and alive in surroundings and with people quite in contrast to one's background. This may be by living in chosen meager surroundings, engaging in the arts if one has come from a family oriented to social conformity, living with those from a different racial or religious background, or hoping to lose oneself in a peer group who have similarly lost their bearings.

However, these factors do not suffice for a negative identity. For that, a choice is needed based on identifications and roles which have been presented to the individual as undesirable or dangerous, yet real. Different family and developmental antecedents contribute to this choice. Parental conflicts in which one child is selected to replace or repeat patterns from their own past lives, excessively demanding ideals, parental overambitiousness, are a few illustrations. By choosing a negative identity based on a total identification with what one is least supposed to be, reality seems clearer than acquiescing to the powerlessness associated with pursuing socially sanctioned activities.

Family configurations recur in adolescents prone to a diffusion of identity. Mothers have had a prominent awareness of personal status which leads to social climbing. To accept this facade as real is more important than are honest expressions of desires or feelings. When younger, there is often a compliant conformity with this facade by the child. A quality of maternal dominance and omnipresence creates a setting of inescapability to the demands of the mother. In many ways these matters represent an insecure groping for their own identity, which at best has resulted in a use of their families to justify their own existence. There would be little use or place for a paternal figure who could not accommodate. Survival is by compliance and, for a boy, permitting himself to be used as the example of what a boy should not be. In adolescence the boy shies away from his mother as a gesture of survival, but he cannot escape their mutually shared social sensitivity.

The shyness of the boy is seen in the efforts of the father to elude his intrusive wife. Projective complaints are made that the father failed to make a woman of her the way her son has also failed to make her a mother. Girls are more likely to acquiesce into perpetuating this pattern by choosing the kind of life and mate which their mothers want. However, the option of a negative identity to act out their feelings may be chosen. Siblings may be used for projective identification purposes, or fused relationships in which this is one additional route seeking an identity through others. Disappointment on this route induce regressive episodes with psychotic manifestations.

Summing Up.   Identity diffusion is viewed as a particular crisis characteristic of adolescence. Rather than dealing with the diagonal series of psychosocial crises, the focus has been on precursors parallel to the psychosocial crises which are relevant to identity as delineated by Erikson.

During the stage of trust versus mistrust, identity antecedents are conceptualized in terms of "unipolarity versus premature self-differentiation." Success in the realm of trust leads to a dominance of unipolarity, viewed as a sense of goodness prevailing inside and outside oneself. Premature self-differentiation is seen in a diffusion of contradictory introjects and fantasies which coerce the world in an omnipotent manner. Succeeding this is "bipolarity versus autism," in which object representations occur which permit relationships with individuals who have a consistent reality. Autistic preoccupations indicate a continuing search for illusory oneness. The next antecedent deals with play identification versus fantasized identities which lead to work identification, or the negative counterpart of identity foreclosure.

Along a horizontal dimension preceding "identity versus identity diffusion" are achievements of earlier stages as they bear on the particular causes in question. What bearing does an earlier achievement, such as trust, have, in derivative form, on a later stage? Consider the element of time as a derivative of trust. A mistrust of time as such appears in the form of delays being treated as deceit, waits as equivalent to impotence, hope as danger, planning as a catastrophe, and providers as traitors. Resulting from "autonomy versus shame and doubt" can be a self-certainty or a disturbance in identity consciousness. Rather than a certainty about oneself, one may be plagued by doubts as to the desirability of one's visibility (there is something shameful about oneself which should be hidden).

The wish to hide during adolescence does not come only from the supervising adults' presence, but from peers, leaders, and the public at large. Precursors of hidden persecutors who pry into one's privacy are common.

The stage of "initiative versus guilt" has implications for the possible utilization of a negative identity. An overdetermination operates, so that guilt leads to a need to deny ambition while choosing a negative identity is a perverted form of initiative. "Industry versus inferiority" has derivative consequences for identity based on whatever the circumstances are which interfere with a sense that one can achieve. A sense of personal inadequacy about work in its extreme form can lead to a paralysis with all of the connotations this has for later identity diffusion. Many factors contribute—the least of which is usually the lack of identity. There may have been precocious attempts at achievement, an excessively developed ego ideal, or an unfortunate environment which has little room or acceptability for certain talents.

Subsequent to the horizontal and vertical intersections of identity, there are consequents which function as precursors of later psychosocial stages. Sex-role identity makes a definite contribution to the ability for later achievement of intimacy. Heterosexual intimacy may diffuse in two opposite directions, both of which eventually lead to isolation. Such diffusion is a concentration on genital activity per se without intimacy; the other is an absorption in social or intellectual pursuits which minimize genital activity. The progressive importance of social institutions is seen at this stage in that they sanction a psychosocial moratorium.

Socially acceptable alternatives are presented to permit sexual abstinence, such as in religious or social communities. Nor does genital activity require a social commitment, which may be seen in ways which vary from utilization of prostitutes to playing the field. Playing with sexuality becomes an end in itself. Succeeding influences of identity in adulthood and maturity prominently involve social institutions and ideological influences. Difficulties such as diffusion in authority and in ideals portray influences which contribute to self-absorption and later dispair. Absence of ideological influences leads to outcomes where the adverse consequences on identity are accentuated. There are then tendencies to diffusion, in time, appearance, action, personal inhibition, a searching for leaders who can resolve ambivalence by authoritarian solutions, a constant struggle against the world of technology and competition, and a discrepancy between what is viewed as dangerous in one's internal world and the actual dangers of the world.

FEMALE IDENTITY

Are there any particular psychological problems attendant to the attainment of identity by girls? It cannot be assumed that no gender influences operate. The classic psychoanalytic position has been discussed with emphasis on the reactivity of the female to a cognizance of her anatomic lack. Other discussions have dwelt on girls feeling deprived on a cultural basis. To some extent, the girl may be regarded as remaining an adolescen as long as she has not first found her own identity so that she is capable of fusing it in the intimacies of a love relationship. It is not necessary to seek a formulation which abandons in toto the influence of one's body on sex-role identity. In fact, this would fly in the face of overwhelming evidence to the contrary. What is necessary is to give a perspective in the context of multiple influences that are operating.

There is a reality that cannot be denied when a child becomes cognizant of anatomical differences, similar to an opening which many patients, in therapy at least, picture in the form of some type of a wound. The biological function of the wound from which blood issues periodically and its tearing during childbirth support this cognition. There are also dreams, myths, and artistic productions which symbolize the female anatomy as gaping and devouring in a dangerous manner. However, these threatening portrayals do not represent the sum and substance of female identity to the boy or girl. There is the matter of creativity and productivity associated with hollow spaces which can be used for these purposes.[50] Such qualities may give rise to masculine envy.[51] This gives consideration to the contribution of anatomy on a psychological level without abandoning symbolic or somatic influences for a purely social approach.

A theoretical shift is possible from a theory focusing on trauma, which centers on the ramifications of the loss or absence of an appendage, to one centered on a potential which accrues from a given bodily configuration. This is also a shift from a theory based on the idiosyncratic aspects of feminine development, which exist to be sure, but which give a rather fragmented picture of personality functioning. It is then not a matter of superiority or inferiority, or strength or weakness, but of the selective values and potentials which are possible. There is the matter of certain feminine sex-typed qualities, such as compassion, emotional reactivity, sensitivity, and nurturant qualities, which exist in the male as well. These feminine qualities in a male give him some special capacity for artistic or creative ideas and work which allow him to be procreative, and it may result in those who create artistic productions as well as in those who are bent on restructuring society.

Periods of psychosocial moratoria for the adolescent function as stages preceding their commitment to actual functioning as adult females. This serves as a temporary suspension, and in some a denial, of what would be most likely to occur if the girl lives out what her body and sex-typed qualities may utilize. Hence, the moratoria gives her a period of freedom where a variety of identifications can be experimented with. Many of these may have masculine qualities—an extension of the playful peer relationships of the tomboy. The moratoria function in diverse ways by permitting other skills and roles to develop quite apart from childbearing. This is a development in which life has a continuity and meaning apart from sexual procreation, without necessarily abandoning it.

IDENTITY PROBLEMS OF BLACK YOUTHS

Problems of the black adolescent with respect to identity are too complex to discuss in one section of a chapter. They would require consideration of historical aspects pertaining to alternatives of family life during slavery with the attempts to maintain some of the older traditions prior to their slavery status. The status of living as a slave in an agricultural system, which dominated not only the southern half of the United States but extended throughout the Caribbean and Brazil as well, gives an idea of the magnitude of this historical occurrence. Such a background, with the accompanying historical complexities of the last hundred years, gives an origin to the predicament of the black family from which the psychosocial identity of the contemporary black adolescent has originated. In part this is a lower-class socio-economic grouping from which many white adolescents emerge as well. However, it is obvious that cultural backgrounds and identities may be diverse. The black adolescent is part of this lower socio-economic class and affected by it, but not an integrated part of it. This lack of integration has been discussed in terms of an original victimization which was perpetuated by myths of white supremacy, black inferiority, and a system of ghettos and indifference which more recently has emerged as a form of gradualism or violence.[52]

Resulting is an identity in which the process of victimization has been perpetuated. It is equivalent to participation by the stance of the sufferer, or provoking others to remain the victim. To obtain what is believed or felt to be necessary requires that these roles be perpetuated. An overdetermination results from modeling influences and manipulation, as well as a belief in its necessity if certain things are to be obtained at the present time. Note the suffering element in the exploited and minority student or employee, drug user, narcotics peddler, numbers runner, crook, weapon user, con artist, and disloyal marriage partner. Most particularly is the aggression administered within the family unit as well as within their own grouping. It is no accident that law and order are most absent within the ghetto. Paralleling this self-punitive life is the institutional reinforcement which occurs in the form of inadequate schooling, lack of legal rights, and the chaos of inadequate police protection in the decaying central cities where the great majority of blacks live.[53]

In these inner cities of substandard housing live 200,000 to 300,000 black children under fifteen years of age on a poverty level of less than $3,335 per year for a family of four. Housing costs the black family 10 to 15 percent more rent than the whites, which is similar to the higher price of food in ghettos. Part and parcel of this setting is the inadequate medical care given to inner-city ghetto dwellers.

From infancy onward, the pattern is witnessed. Four times as many black mothers die in childbirth compared to white mothers; three times as many black infants die compared to white infants.[54] The medical services blacks receive at public hospitals are largely those run by trainees who are gaining experience in their discipline. It results in a black life-expectancy of 64.1 years compared to seventy-one years for a white.[55] Not even when an occupational or professional skill has been acquired can it be expected to give the benefits and achievements that normally accrue to it. It is often a surprise to learn that suicide among young blacks of both sexes in urban areas, aged twenty to thirty-five, is twice as frequent as among whites in a similar grouping.[56] This would indicate that escape from victimization is not succeeding. Nor do traditional outs, such as song, dance, and folk tales, achieve this now any more than they did in the past.

The matrifocal nature of the black urban family from the lower social classes has been repeatedly discussed. The 1960 United States Census indicated that 47 percent of these families had a female head.[57] When the male leaves, the household is maintained by the mother and they often move in with the maternal grandmother or invite her in. The impact can be discussed in terms of the consequences of the absent father on identity of boys and girls, which will not be further pursued here. A different consequence is postulated in the cognition by family members that their form of family living is different from the remainder of society.

In many ways the family organization, with the myth of a dominant male at its head, evokes envy and ridicule. However, within the black family unit the result is increased tendencies to criticize each other for failing to attain such ideals—without giving cognizance to it as the white man's family structure. The self-critical tendencies influence the ego ideal as well as heighten ambivalence about one's own family. In addition, black adults convey to their children standards of the white, middle-class families, which they themselves do not believe in, and this may lead to many of the same conflicts of duplicity seen in white, middle-class families. Both alternatives contribute to resentment and anger, especially made worse by groups of professionals who intervene in families with their own personal and class biases. These interventions, sanctioned by legal authority, occur at certain key times.

As an example, the lack of division of girls into good and bad by the black adolescent based on sexual activities should be noted.[58] For a woman to be virginal may be viewed as a lack of opportunity or physical immaturity. Hesitation by a girl for intercourse is based more on reality considerations of not being used or getting into trouble with the authorities, than on moral grounds. Willing performance of intercourse by the black adolescent girl may thus be guided more by her spontaneous feelings of genuine affection for a boy than any instrumental function. This is similar to the norms of *situation ethics* which a sizable group of white adolescents have found appealing. It is noted as well in the preparation of a girl for dating by parents who give her contraceptive information in which the implicit norm and standard is that the girl will be having intercourse for which due education should be given. Decisions for or against marriage when pregnancy occurs are made by criteria other than the pregnancy per se, without the compelling sense of urgency that once was attached to this situation. For boys, the attainment of a sex-typed standard based on his reputation as a seducer appears important.[59] He maintains claims on girls within the peer group by virtue of claims which exist independently of marriage possibilities.

Growing up in this type of family configuration contributes to a particular type of identity for the black adolescent. Prior to adolescence, his cognitive and affectional operations are such that the state of other people with whom he relates, and the family itself, are ascribed to his parents. Hence, blames for frustrations tend to be assigned to the family. Threats of disruption to the family integrity, which lurk from within and without, tend to keep the issue of family continuity constantly in question. By a process of victimization and accompanying hostility, challenges to competency are made as part of the hostile attack, in a combination of personal attacks with a tone of demeaning the sexual adequacy of the boy and the overall capabilities of the girl. Further complications arise from difficulties in having external sources of competition and gratification for self-esteem.

By a process of mutual attack and being labeled as no good, by the time adolescence arrives, self-concept and belief about the views of others may have become impaired. The black adolescent, like any other adolescent who gets down on himself, may view himself as having little to offer his environment. Nor does he anticipate that his environment views him in any different light. Negation of this impaired contribution to his identity by a ghettoized existence and caste system persists until quite late in development. It is a factor which contributes to his early and continuing assignment of fault to those within his own family, and which later leads to outbursts of rage against outsiders once there is cognizance that it is not all the fault of his family members. The opposite extreme may be reached so that by projection all fault is assigned outside to negate the contribution of those who have nurtured him.

These factors give a special diathesis to the choice of a negative identity for the black adolescent. Since every child in the course of socialization is exposed to a series of alternatives, both by precept and verbalization, as to what behavior and ideals to emulate, the anlage for negative identities is laid down. This occurs, and is usually justified, by the socializers in terms of the child needing to know what he should not become—be this put in terms of moral evils or unrewarding behaviors. The greater danger exists for the child to select a negative identity when his predisposing personal and family backgrounds have emphasized their respective limitations on offering anything substantive to each other or the family.

There is further reinforcement when a dominant majority holds up their ideals as positive and those of the minority as negative. Even when the elements contributing to identity have been mocking caricatures which could be tolerated by the majority, such as an obstinate meekness, an exaggerated childlikeness, or superficial submissiveness, they indicated a thinly concealed hostility to others as well as themselves by the ridiculed images presented.[61] Yet these same elements, with their corresponding affects, became an integral part of the emerging identity of the black.

One final point needs to be made. A combination of factors can lead to a subtle conviction that one's ways, body, group, or skin color are best. This does not refer to conscious efforts to abandon such stances and convictions, but rather to something in the complex interactions that evoke these feelings in the narcissistic needs and identifications of childhood. It is perpetuated in doctrines that a certain group may be unique because of some particular feature or norm. More abstractly, this is seen in positions about the uniqueness of man himself or a particular subgroup thereof. Phrases and beliefs that one group or species has been specially chosen, or selected, are illustrative of situations that permit one group of homo sapiens to turn on another under a rationalization of morality to justify the imposition of their will. Put in psychological terms, we are dealing with the genesis and maintenance of the need to oppress. A correlative part of this is the need of the oppressor for an oppressee.

More specifically for our discussion of the identity of the black and stimulation, even while a passive participant, may be another way of attaining pseudo-intimacy and pseudo-sexuality. Witness the patterns in dance in which parodies of human relationships take place.[63] Space trips, as well as other kinds of trips, space wars, the preoccupation with speed—meaning velocity and other speed—the preoccupation with cars, car thefts by adolescents and youths, and physical violence, all speak for a motoric culture. This may be the period of the end of ideologies, but it also appears to be an unsuccessful search for one.[64]

Lack of ideology in political or religious institutions leaves a void which contributes to the easy shift of alliances in institutional attachments. Lack of allegiance has a cynicism and distrust, dealt with by putting on so that one never knows whether one is serious. Allegiances are vague and uncertain. In the absence of human relationships which one can accept as sincere, the institutional replacement can at best be only a mockery. However, it cannot be abandoned, but only undermined and replaced as the search goes on to restore counterfeit nurturance.

The Hippie Character. Consider some of the characteristics which were labeled the hippie type in the last decade. Some considered this a personality configuration with specific character-istics.[65] The characteristics were manifested in a new ideology and culture of the dropout. A widespread use of drugs prevailed with a commitment to utopian colonies and communes. In contrast to undertaking types of social action, whose past rationalizations have involved some form of doing good, there was rather a commitment to a tribalism disdainful to many forms of social action. This should be distinguished from passive obstructionism, but was offered as an alternative, free of the tokenism which tends to prolong the tidbit efforts which do not fundamentally change anything. Nor is this conceived in terms of merely a negative identity, although it shares elements with it.

Shifts in the acceptable boundaries of the erotic and pornographic are viewed as part of a more honest ethos. Confused and overdetermined results are seen from the original Free Speech Movement during the student uprising at the University of California at Berkeley, which was succeeded by the Dirty Speech Movement. The latter had not only the facade of a dedication to honesty but was a mockery of its own immediate predecessor which advocated free speech.[66]

Nowhere is it more evident that the same type of characteristics can be conceptualized in different ways than in such formulations as the hippie character. Sociological concepts of "anomie" come to mind with reference to the lack or deficiency of certain values or adaptive conduct. Psychoanalytic theory questions the oral character traits of these youths. Their personality structure exhibits an uneven control over impulse expression. It is not that there is primarily an uncontrolled expression of impulses, but rather that there are alternations and combinations between indulgences and restrictions. A similar situation is present with respect to input. There is both a greater permeability to stimulation, so that less selectivity is exercised, while at the same time there exists a narrowing of perceptive range and withdrawal. Concepts of poorly defined object boundaries and object fusion have been used for explanation. By externalization and attempts to control the self and the environment, a crude attempt to reinstate or gain self and object constancy occurs.

A variety of activities superficially appear contradictory. These vary from drugs, sexual activity, experimentation with different types of religious exercises, types of group experiences which have a pseudo-therapeutic format, and types of self-imposed deprivation. There might be trips to the interior or the pantheistic fusions of Krishna. Any of these can involve relationships. There are oral characteristics, which have been discussed in the context of alienation.[67] Note the following: (1) The predominance of the here and now over the abstract. The physical, visceral, and concrete take precedence over generalizations and the cognitive. (2) Verbalized values are put in terms of immediate experience and the greater the vividness and uninhibitedness, the greater the appeal. (3) Cognitive modes which make for differentiation of self from objects are less emphasized than are such sensory qualities as feelings, texture, touch, and warmth—the ideology of sentience. (4) Visual components are similarly manipulated or fused, with or without psychedelics, so that there is a lack of visual discreteness.

The same personality traits, as noted, can be encompassed by different formulations. By way of contrast, they have been noted in the historical context as the characteristics of the Romantics in the early 19th century.[68] Feelings were trusted over rules, emotion was adolescent, there may be a need for the dominant white majority to maintain the negative identity of the black. Not only does this maintain the superiority of the white, but it permits him to project his own unconscious negative identity onto the black. Such formulations about the social operations of prejudice, and the psychologic mechanisms, are not new. One thing beyond these is new. From educational efforts about the operation of prejudice in the middle classes, two consequences have occurred. One of these has taken the form that since we have now recognized the nature of prejudice, we know what should be done and therefore can undo it. From the above, it is apparent that the social forces, as well as unconscious operants, make it much more complicated. A second consequence has been a hairshirted approach by the white majority, who wish to rectify things by bemoaning the faults and sins of their fathers. The exaggerated nature of these types of confessions alert the clinician to query whether other needs and sources of guilt are being handled in this way.

CONNECTIONS BETWEEN THE SOCIO-PSYCHOLOGICAL
AND CLINICAL-DEVELOPMENTAL IDENTITIES

Protean Man. All formulations stress identity as a process in flux. Although this is also so for such hypothetical constructs as ego and character, it is often lost sight of in construct reification. Identity, as a concept implying a fixed continuity, would be contrary to a structural theory of personality functioning, as well as contrary to a culture whose institutions and symbols themselves are changing and unstable. This contributes to what Lifton has called the creation of protean man.[62] Such a person engages in an interminable series of experiments and explorations—some shallow and some profound—which are easily and readily abandoned for new psychological quests. This is different from the psychopathological connotation attached to identity diffusion syndrome, and is rather viewed as one of the functional patterns of contemporary times. It can be seen in political and sexual behavior or in any area of human experience.

Explanations for this phenomenon have been offered in historical terms. Dislocations, which have separated men from the symbols of their cultural tradition, are offered as one possibility. Unstable symbols representing the family, idea systems, religions, and the life cycle make a special contribution. Another historical tendency is the almost ceaseless bombardment by mass media of vacuous and superficial imagery. This is the McLuhanesque mode of communicating gone mad. One need not resort to clinical examples to illustrate the protean type. Literature abounds with examples. Saul Bellow's *Augie March* and *Herzog,* Jack Kerouac's *On the Road,* J. P. Donleavy's *The Gingerbread Man,* and Philip Roth's *Portnoy* are

American examples. The writings of Sartre and the existentialist group, and German writers represented by Gunter Grass and Jakov Lind, are representatives of a similar type. Examples may be given from the visual and performing arts. Witness action painting and kinetic sculpture—if not the entire abstract expressionist movement in the post-World War II period, culminating in Pop Art and Pop Culture. Another example would be the meaningless movement and cacophony of modern classical music. These examples have been intentionally selected to escape the necessity of using clinical material.

It is no longer clear whether identity diffusion as a meaningful concept referring to deviancy is accurate or whether it is more valid to refer to protean man as in a state of perpetual diffusion as normative, at least in terms of prevalence. In many ways these examples portray almost all aspects of a culture caught up in a caricature of the autonomy of the toddler, mechanized by the adolescent, and extended into all aspects of our culture and age groups. To an extent, there is a conspicuous component of grandiosity and delusion in the feelings and belief that the technologies are for man to control. In reality this may be a denial of the proclivity to control him. The need to experience constant motion good for its own sake, and the exotic and macabre were sought. At times this gave rise to an extravagance in which intensity was sought. This could vary from violence to the inspirational. Forms and rituals were viewed as depleted of value and meaning. Even here, shining through what some might call a lack of standards, was an affirmation of quality in the individual. This was perhaps in reaction to the concept of uniformity in the Enlightenment, which stressed the primacy of reason and the universality of natural law which was to lead to a civility of life and primacy of the group. In contrast, the Romantics appeared contemptuous of the herd by way of affirming the free spontaneity of the individual. Its quality is seen in William Blake's contemptuous reference to exerting self-control. "Those who restrain desire do so because their's is weak enough to be restrained."[69] Glorification of the id over the civilized superego is seen.

Hippies have also been viewed as social types constructed out of variations of role enactment.[70] These social types are a blend between the individual and society. In ways, they can be viewed as folk types in which there is an exaggeration in expected conduct. Settings in which large numbers of individuals occupy undifferentiated positions provide a background for the emergence of stylistic variations. Those who demonstrate some type of variation are designated as types or characters. Some past examples of social types with specific folk-type qualities are groupings within an organizational structure, such as right guys, squares, company men, politicians, or manipulators. A group of adolescents may designate social types as jocks, wheeler-dealers, lady's man, scholar type, or big man. When the need arises for delineating a new social role, which is thought of as possessing certain attributes, individuals to fill these roles are chosen from social types.

Psychological types leads to a consideration of typologies and traits. Theoretical issues pertaining to the nature of bodily or psychological attributes or genotypic characteristics are not utilized. There is rather an emphasis on phenotypic styles in which visible behaviors or value orientations are used for classification. From this, the hippie is viewed as a folk type who is not enacting any social role which would involve complementary roles in a recognized social structure. Hippie status is rather recognized by dress, manner, demeanor, speech patterns, and art preferences. Certain habits may also be involved, such as those pertaining to health, sanitation, or use of drugs.

The hypothesis is that these variations have been selected out as a conspicuous cluster, from their threat to the non-hippie outsiders, that challenges conformity and hence the risk that extreme variation entails. One component of identity involves the confirmation of one's place in the social structure by others reacting in a congruent manner to the valuation of oneself. A belief that status is not congruent with the roles available may result in a dropout from established institutions. Consequently, a lack of social identity results as well. Lacking a search for signs of social meaning, resort is had to the concrete sensory world of raw experience which gives a youth some type of social identity outside of a formal institutional framework. Reassurance that one has a place on some level of existence, even if not in a social order, is then obtained. In fact, a narcissistic gratification may be present in the belief that they are more in the know than others by special avenues to truth, because they have given up the need to place themselves in any particular existing social structure except as onlookers. While names applied to outsiders vary, the character structure which handles affiliation in this manner appears similar over time. What does change historically are the opportunities at any given time for the outsider or the congruence with other sources of stress in a society.

REFERENCES

1. M. R. Stein and A. J. Vidich, Identity and history: an overview, *Identity and Anxiety*, ed. by M. Stein, A. Vidich, and D. M. White, pp. 17-33 (Glencoe: Free Press, 1960).
2. T. W. Adorno, E. Frenkel-Brunswik, D. J. Levinson, and R. N. Sanford, *The Authoritarian Personality* (New York: Harper, 1950).
3. D. Riesman, *Individualism Reconsidered* (Glencoe: Free Press, 1954).
4. B. Rosenberg and D. M White, ed., *Mass Culture: The Popular Arts in America* (Glencoe: Free Press, 1959).
5. S. Spender, *The Year of the Young Rebels* (New York: Vintage, 1969).
6. L. Fuerer, *The Conflict of Generations* (New York: Basic Books, 1969).
7. R. Lifton, *Revolutionary Immortality* (New York: Norton, 1968).
8. R. Lifton, *History and Human Survival* (New York: Random House, 1970).
9. R. C. Bealer, F. K. Willits, and P. R. Maida, The rebellious youth subculture—a myth, *Children* 11(1965):43-48.
10. A. M. Rose, Reference groups of rural high school youth, *Child Development* 27(1956):351-363.
11. D. B. Harris, and S. C. Tseng, Children's attitudes toward peer and parents as revealed by sentence completions, *Child Development* 28(1957):401-411.
12. J. S. Coleman, *The Adolescent Society* (New York: The Free Press of Glencoe, 1961).
13. L. A. Ostlund, Environment-personality relationships, *Rural Sociology*, 1957.
14. S. M. Lipset, *Political Man* (New York: Doubleday, 1960).
15. S. Putney and R. Middleton, Rebellion, conformity, and parental religious ideologies, *Sociometry* 24(1961):125-135.
16. P. Goodman, *Growing Up Absurd: Problems of Youth in the Organized System* (New York: Random House, 1960).
17. A. Toffler, ed., *Learning for Tomorrow* (New York: Vintage, 1974).
18. A. Strauss, ed., *The Social Psychology of George Herbert Mead* (Chicago: University of Chicago Press, 1956).
19. M. Rosenberg, *Society and the Adolescent Self-Image* (Princeton: Princeton University Press, 1965).
20. B. Inhelder and J. Piaget, *The Growth of Logical Thinking* (New York: Basic Books, 1958).
21. R. W. White, Ego and reality in psychoanalytic theory, *Psychological Issues, vol. 3, Monograph II* (New York: International Universities Press, 1963).
22. R. W. White, The experience of efficacy in schizophrenia, *Psychiatry* 28(1965):199-211.
23. D. W. Winnicott, The family affected by depressive illness in one or both parents, *The Family and Individual Development* by D. W. Winnicott (London: Tavistock Publications, 1965).

24. L. Eidelberg, An introduction to the study of the narcissistic mortification, *Psychoanalytic Quarterly* 31(1957):657-668.

25. J. B. Rotter, Generalized expectancies for internal versus external control of reinforcement, *Psychological Monograph, vol. 80* (Entire No. 1 issue), 1966.

26. M. Seeman, Antidote to alienation—learning to belong, *Trans-Action* 3(1966):35-39.

27. S. M. Miller, B. L. Saleem, and H. Bryce, *School Dropouts: A Commentary and Annotated Bibliography* (New York: Syracuse University Press, 1964).

28. E. Douvan and J. Adelson, *The Adolescent Experience* (New York: Wiley, 1966).

29. S. M. Jourard and P. F. Secord, Body-cathexis and the ideal female figure, *Journal of Abnormal Social Psychology* 50(1955):243-246.

30. A. E. Wessman and D. F. Ricks, *Mood and Personality* (New York: Holt, Rinehart, and Winston, 1966).

31. M. B. Smith, Explorations in competence: a study of peace corps teachers in Ghana, *American Psychologist* 21(1966):555-566.

32. R. D. Hess and I. Goldblatt, The status of adolescents in American society: a problem in social identity, *Child Development* 28(1957):459-468.

33. S. Goldman, Profiles of an adolescent, *Journal of Psychology* 54(1962):229-240.

34. P. H. Mussen, Long-term consequents of masculinity of interests in adolescence, *Journal of Consulting Psychology* 26(1962):435-440.

35. H. B. Heilbrun, Jr., Parental model attributes, nurturant reinforcement, and consistency of behavior in adolescents, *Child Development* 35(1964):151-167.

36. E. H. Erikson, Growth and crises of the healthy personality, *Symposium on the Healthy Personality*, ed. by M. J. S. Senn (New York: Josiah Macy, Jr. Foundation, 1950).

37. E. H. Erikson, The problem of ego identity, *Journal of the American Psychoanalytic Association* 4(1956):56-121.

38. J. Bowlby, *Attachment and Loss: Vol. I, Attachment* (New York: Basic Books, 1969).

39. A. Bandura and R. Walters, *Social Learning Personality Development* (New York: Holt, Rinehart, and Winston, 1963).

40. A. Thomas, S. Chess, and H. G. Birch, *Temperament and Behavior Development in Children* (New York: New York University Press, 1968).

41. R. Schafer, *Aspects of Internalization* (New York: International Universities Press, 1968).

42. D. W. Winnicott, The effect of psychosis on family life, *The Family and Individual Development* (London: Tavistock Publications, 1965).

43. E. J. Anthony, A clinical evaluation of children with psychotic parents, *American Journal of Psychiatry* 126(1969):177-184.

44. A. Johnson, and S. A. Szurek, The genesis of antisocial acting out in children and adults, *Psychoanalytic Quarterly* 21(1952):323-343.

45. S. Freud, The economic problem of masochism, *Standard Edition* 19:159-170.

46. H. Hartman, *Ego Psychology and the Problem of Adaptation* (New York: International Universities Press, 1958).
47. Erikson, op. cit.
48. M. W. Brody, Clinical manifestations of ambivalence, *Psychoanalytic Quarterly* 25(1956):505-514.
49. H. Von Hentig, *The Criminal and His Victim* (New Haven: Yale University Press, 1938).
50. E. H. Erikson, Womanhood and the inner space, *Identity-Youth and Crisis* (New York: Norton and Co., 1968).
51. E. Jacobson, Development of the wish for a child in boys, *Psychoanalytic Study of the Child* 5(1950):139-152.
52. S. C. Drake, The social and economic status of the negro in the United States, *Daedalus* 94(1965):772-780.
53. P. M. Hauser, Demographic factors in the integration of the negro, *The Negro American*, ed. by T. Parsons and K. B. Clark (Boston: Houghton Mifflin, 1966).
54. U.S. Dept. of Health, Education, and Welfare, Public Health Service, Vital and Health Statistics. Infant Mentality Trends: U.S. and each State, 1930-1964. Washington, D.C.: Government Printing Office, 1965, Publ. No. 1000, Series 20.
55. J. C. Horman, Medicine in the ghetto, *New England Journal of Medicine* 281(1969):1271-1275.
56. H. Hendin, *Black Suicide* (New York: Basic Books, 1969).
57. U.S. Census: 1960, PC (1) D. U.S. Volume, Table 225; State Volume, Table 140.
58. L. Rainwater, Marital sexuality in four cultures of poverty, *Journal of Marriage and the Family* 26(1964):457-466.
59. I. L. Reiss, Premarital sexual permissiveness among negroes and whites, *American Sociological Review* 29(1964):688-698.
60. L. Rainwater, Crucible of identity: the negro lower-class family, *Daedalus* 95(1966):172-216.
61. E. H. Erikson, The concept of identity in race relations; notes and queries, *Daedalus* 95(1966):145-171.
62. R. J. Lifton, Protean man, *Partisan Review* 25(1968):13-27.
63. L. Roxon, *Rock Encyclopedia* (New York: Grosset and Dunlap, 1969).
64. D. Bell, *The End of Ideology* (Glencoe: The Free Press, 1958).
65. H. Adler, The antinomian personality: the hippie character type, *Psychiatry* 31(1968):325-338.
66. *Confrontation: The Study Rebellion and the Universities*, ed. D. Bell and I. Kristol (New York: Basic Books, 1969).
67. K. Keniston, *The Uncommitted* (New York: Harcourt, Brace and World, 1965).
68. Adler, op. cit., p. 333.
69. W. Blake, The marriage of heaven and hell, *The Poetry and Prose of William Blake* (New York: Doubleday and Co., 1965).
70. T. R. Sarbin, On the distinction between social roles and social types, with special reference to the hippie, *American Journal of Psychiatry* 125(1969):1024-1031.

Chapter Seven

Socialization Aspects of Conscience

MORAL DEVELOPMENT AND CLINICAL CONCERN

The question of whether there are moral stages of development for the human is an intriguing one. In its most conservative form, the developmental approach to moral development espouses a viewpoint analogous to that of a sequential unfolding of physical growth or psychosexual stages. Such a position in its fullest form is rarely held with respect to moral development, due to the socialization processes exhibited in any type of moral transactions. A naive hypothetical example would be to conceive of children living alone on an island developing physically, provided food and water were miraculously present in abundance, and to consider whether moral development would simply unfold sequentially.

Another difficulty concerns which aspects of moral development should be subject to study. Developmental psychologists have largely confined their work to the province of different types of moral judgments which are expressed by children at different developmental stages. This stands in contrast to the area of moral conduct, which varies from observable levels of behavior as conforming to more subtle nuances of interpersonal morality. Some studies have concerned themselves primarily with the verbalization or detection of rules, as expressed by a child, rather than their application. Nor do any of these approaches undertake to evaluate the psychological penalty for violation of certain rules of conduct. Specifically, some studies have considered the emergence of notions such as justice, fairness, or equality. But if moral behavior is being appraised, it must be noted in children themselves, as well as within their family, peer, and cultural setting.

The clinical usage of moral behavior has its own set of criteria involving such poorly defined clinical concepts as those employed with acting out adults. Some of the traits observed in psychopathy may thus be appraised in children, and criteria from the field of adult psychopathology used in studies formulating developmental norms. Confusion has been compounded by clinical contributions to moral development from the utilization of both psychodynamic and psychopathological formulations simultaneously in the developmental realm. These formulations may embody superego functioning with respect to prohibitions as well as idealized norms. Psychoanalytic developmental psychology further considers stages in external conformity as well as the concomitant internalized consequences for transgressions. Questions arise as to when such stirrings commence, what form they take, and the social situations and people to which they are most responsive. Related aspects of psychoanalytic moral development have focused on the forms of self-criticism expressed overtly as well as correlated with harm, self-inflicted or courted from others.

The capacity to observe the self in the sense of critically evaluating both thoughts and acts is often thought of as contingent upon the psychological development of a split into the observing and observed parts of the individual's personality. For this to occur, there is a presupposition that a certain developmental achievement, including the capacity for the reparation of wrongdoing, and to praise and give self-love for resisting wrongdoing or achieving ideals has been attained. Permeating all of this are the interacting contributions of the learning process versus the developmental sequences which are occurring simultaneously. Crucial questions are: (1) To what extent do moral judgments, moral thoughts, and moral conduct occur as an overall concomitant of development versus a byproduct of the socialization processes themselves? (2) What, if any, is the relationship between moral judgments and moral conduct? (3) What is the nature of the evidence that has been presented for different viewpoints on the nature of moral development and socialization with respect to morality?

PIAGETIAN MORAL DEVELOPMENT

Early Concepts. Piaget was meticulous in his study on this subject. In 1932, *The Moral Judgment of the Child* urged caution in interpreting data in terms of stages of moral development. There is the concern for the basis of moral behavior, but which behaviors themselves are to be considered as moral? This is a deceptive problem which philosophers have argued about for centuries, but which behavioral scientists have relatively ignored. Moral behavior is commonly defined as a set of beliefs or values which a social group defines as good or bad. Cognizance is given to cultural variations, as well as moral imperatives found in most cultures. Yet the crux of moral development in a psychological sense hinges on the type of psychological structures which emerge in the individual as he socializes within units, such as the family or culture. Specifically, social intimacies with key individuals are the context in which impulses are handled by the self.

Focusing on the individualized aspects of moral development has two benefits. It permits the appraisal—developmentally and clinically—of how an individual child is progressing or facing arrests or deviations. Second, it permits appraisal of how socialization processes contribute to moral development—without the implication that the sine qua non of moral development for a child is nothing more than a capacity to conform to a set of rules of a culture at a particular time. The danger in equating social conformity with progressing moral development is that of promoting individuals who may be highly developed with respect to the peculiar norms of their own subcultural unit, or merely cognitively gifted in terms of expressing moral judgments. This leads to a *cognitive fallacy*, whereby knowledge of rules becomes equated with moral development with little or no reference to the actual capacity or desire to act on a set of internalized norms.

The methodology of Piaget in his original study was deceptively simple. It consisted of observations on children playing marbles to see if they knew the rules of the game and whether those rules were followed. Another part of the study elicited rules from the child verbally in terms of the nature of the rules themselves, and the attitude of the child toward rules, such as whether rules could be made up, where they came from, and whether they were subject to change. From these observations, Piaget noted stages in how the children used rules. Until about three years of age, there were no detectable rules. The child enjoyed his private playing with the marbles, oblivious of anything but the primitive physical rules which the marbles obeyed themselves. From three to five years of age, processes of imitation began to influence rules as the child followed rules used by other children.

Accompanying imitation, assimilation processes incorporated sensory and motor components from a reflex schemata into what would later be a thought schemata—the basic unit of mental organization in a Piagetian developmental framework. This accounted for the influence of past marble-playing rules and imitations. Yet during the second stage, the operation of private, idiosyncratic schema predominated since the child imposed his own rules when playing, although he continued to believe he was playing by the rules he observed in others.

The discrepancy between cognitive appraisal and behavior is interesting. The rules are verbalized as internal verities not subject to change, yet they continue to be violated ad libitum by the child. Stage three, from seven or eight to eleven or twelve years of age, brings a gradual conformity to rules as part of socialization. Rules could be changed by others, the only requirement being an agreement to abide by the rules since the viewpoint on origin had shifted from an always-existing set of rules to one in which a group of players formulated their own. However, another reversal occurred. Although the rules were viewed as relative, their obedience in practice was viewed as essential, in contrast to the second stage. By age twelve, corresponding to the early adolescent period, rules were understood and utilized routinely with peers. In fact, classifying rules, revising them, and attempting to apply them to new situations took on a positive meaning in its own right. This appears to be the emergence of a legalistic approach in a literal sense, whose fascination for some never ends.

Moral Attitudes. Piaget also conducted experiments dealing with changing moral attitudes. The children were told a number of stories in which an act was to be appraised and an assessment of the relative culpabilities of the actor made. General conclusions were as follows, allowing for individual variations: The younger child viewed an act with the greater objective consequences as more immoral, such as a child breaking a larger number of cups accidentally being most immoral in contrast to one who maliciously broke one cup. Or, a child who stole a loaf of bread to give to the poor was judged as doing a naughtier thing than one who took an object of less monetary worth for his own private use. Not until age nine or ten did the intent behind an act take on significance.

Changing conceptions about clumsiness, stealing, and lying were noted in other investigations. Clumsiness takes on a moral connotation by virtue of the significance given by adults to breaking things, misplacing them, bumping into objects, and preoccupation with tidiness. The anger elicited in response to this gives a moral tone to the clumsy acts, particularly when the notion of carelessness or disobedience is ascribed as the motive. The methodology for this evaluation consisted of presenting contrasting stories in which there were two kinds of clumsiness—one entirely fortuitous or even resulting from a well-intentioned act although considerable damage resulted, and one in which the damage was negligible but resulted from a bad intention. Thus, one boy may push open a door when called to dinner and knock over a chair with fifteen cups on it, which all are broken, in contrast to another boy who is trying to get jam out of a cupboard and knocks over one cup which breaks.

The overall pattern found was that of objective responsibility until about age ten, when the greater amount of damage, as a result of clumsiness, was given a more harsh moral judgment, whatever the motive. Similar results were noted with stealing, in which the amount taken was the guiding index to culpability until about age ten, irrespective of motive. Until age ten, the child did not seem to differentiate between the legal or police aspects of an act from the moral aspects. A larger spot on a coat was naughtier than a small one. They did not ask how and why the spot got there, since the act in itself was wrong. The rules operate as categorical imperatives as though there is a discrepancy between the ability of the child to know the rule and to differentiate the various extraneous factors operating.

Evaluation of lying by the child dealt with such things as definitions of lying to determine whether the child comprehended lying was intentional. Differentiations were made between responsibility as a function of the content of a lie or as a function of its material consequences. First, the youngest children tended to define a lie in terms of language, such as naughty words. This is the example of externalization par excellence, since determination whether a certain word was bad or not was completely a result of linguistic restraint to which the child initially submitted without questioning. In fact, Piaget felt the imposed prohibitions had all the more sanctification to the child because of their inexplicability and the fact that they did not correspond to any of the child's own inner needs. Moral realism is the inevitable outcome of so paradoxical a situation. To lie is to commit a moral fault by means of language, which permits the extension to words or statements that do not conform with fact, apart from any intention.

Note the similarity between uttering an oath and taking one, in which the former consists of using a bad word, and the latter consists of pledging that the child will honestly do something. Only later does the meaning of lying involve the notion of an attempt to deceive. Young children regard a lie as morally wrong if it deviates from the truth, regardless of intent. In fact, a more plausible distortion might be more severely condemned by a child than one in which the untruth is self-evident. The close connection to the emerging appraisal of reality is evident since a subtle distortion promotes greater confusion and uncertainty as to reality. There is also the difficulty of the child in dissociating between ideas of intentionality and those which were not. By age eight, the child can identify mistakes, and lying begins to disappear. Guilt comes to be associated with the motives of lying.

Correspondingly, there are also shifts in which judging a lie by externals is viewed as less deceitful than one which succeeds. Further, it is not mere objective consequences which determine badness; nor does the appraisal of the extent of a lie, as correlated with the degree of punishment. A lie becomes bad if it is punished. Lying to an adult does not continue to be viewed as worse than lying to a peer, since a lie has come to represent a more fundamental deviation from reality, whatever the circumstances. Not lying has come to assume a functional use in terms of securing mutual cooperation on the basis of mutual respect and subjective understanding rather than a unilateral compliance to an absolute command. Three stages are in evidence:

1. A lie is wrong because it is something punished, a type of reverse post hoc, ergo propter hoc fallacy, in which a causal attribution of lying is made once punishment occurs. No punishment, no lie.

2. A lie remains a lie even if there is no punishment.

3. Finally, a lie is wrong because it is in conflict with mutual trust. These are not strictly stages in the sense that they follow each other in a necessary order, but rather broad processes which were distinct from each other in overview, but had some overlap in transition.

Stages of Morality. Piaget used his material to formulate two moralities in childhood along with an intermediate stage. The morality of constraint is based on automatic obedience to rules without reasoning or judgment, and takes place in the context of a unilateral relationship between an adult as superior and omnipotent and the child as inferior and blindly obeying. Rules are moral absolutes which are unquestionable (moral realism). Internal motives are irrelevant to such a morality, nor are the social-interpersonal meanings of an act germane. Other antecedents are not relevant to the moral situation. Only the overt act is assessed as wrong or right, good or bad, by some external appraiser or law-giver, human or divine.

Prior to the emergence of a morality of cooperation (autonomy), an intermediate stage is seen in the internalization of rules by the child without evaluating them or seeking alternative responses to situations. Cooperative morality is based on reciprocity among peers, on a mutual respect rather than unilateral dictates. Comprehension of the role of motives, empathy for other's acts, as well as the social consequences of antisocial behavior, contribute to a beginning cognitive realization of the need for cooperation. This does not lead to practicing this immediately, but it does raise social consequences. For those in whom cooperation emerges, the rules of morality become useful as guidelines for orderly social conduct. They are not arbitrary nor permanent, but subject to revision as the group interest may dictate.

Conceptions of Justice. Integrally related to the moral attitudes of children and types of morality are conceptions of justice. These raise correlative questions as to how transgressions should be dealt with. Three stages in the conceptualization of justice are noted in the course of the moral development of the child: a justice of retribution, immanence, and distribution. Comparison of the similarity of these developmental phenomena with historical and legal notions of dealing with antisocial behavior is striking.

Retributive justice is distinguished by two types of punishments. Expiatory punishment holds that a wrongdoer must suffer in proportion to the gravity of his offense, although the punishment need not be related to the crime in kind. Punishment by reciprocity, on the other hand, does not emphasize the expiatory quality as much. Instead, it directly makes the offender aware a relationship with others has been breached by behavior. Punishment is logically related to the offense. Note that neither of these retributive stages seen in children exhibit retribution in the strict jurisprudential sense in which the talion law exacted measure for measure for no other purpose than a misdeed requiring vengeance. This absence might be explained by the methodology Piaget used of posing hypothetical misdeeds to children and having them choose the best or fairest punishment. Clinicians, with an orientation in sensitivity to primary process thinking, can testify to the abundance of pure vengeance motives and fantasies in the life of the child, as well as the adult. Piaget noted a tendency for younger children to favor expiatory punishments, while older children elected the reciprocal type, indicating that a direct and severe punishment itself, without explanation and discussion, would not be a deterrent.

Immanent justice is the belief that a transgression in itself elicits a punishment even though it may not seem related. The appeal is to nature, God, or some guiding principle that will render justice so no one gets away with anything. It is a view of the physical universe as policeman. This notion is often appealed to in jurisprudential notions that the community needs vengeance, since without apprehension and punishment of a wrongdoer, the sense of law and order in communities suffers. Developmentally, this is contingent on the child believing that punishments emanate from things themselves rather than in a set of contingencies. When a child transgresses, say by stealing, and later falls off his bicycle and is injured, the events are not viewed as independent within the context of an immanent theory of justice. They are viewed in some way as necessarily related. It is the notion seen in certain religions, cultures, and myths wherein members of a sect, tribe, or cult would have to suffer for certain excesses or transgressions of the group, such as the whole earth being flooded as a result of some of its inhabitants being sinful, or famine being visited upon a tribe as a vengeance wrought by the gods. Apart from these expectations, there is the viewpoint that nature is a harmonious whole in which moral accountability operates by principles just like physical laws. If going to bed is always followed by darkness in the cognitive processes of a child, does it not seem just as natural that some type of deviation from parental dictates will be followed by an automatic intervention? By age eight, this type of mentality is progressively disappearing from overt explanations. That it persists in derivative ways throughout subsequent years, as well as in cultural practices, raises interesting psychodynamic and cultural questions, apart from developmental considerations in a strict sense.

Distributive justice refers to the way rewards and punishments are distributed to members of a group. Parallel to the predominant morality of constraint in the first seven or eight years is the acceptance of justice as distributed in an arbitrary manner, depending on whatever an authority figure chooses to dispense. This is referred to, whatever it is, as fair or just by children. Again, caution must be exercised, for Piaget used a series of stories read to children with questions as to the fairness or justice in the story.

Thus, a story was told in which a mother with two girls preferred the more obedient one and gave her the biggest piece of cake. Seventy percent of children aged six to nine approved of this, while only 40 percent of those aged ten to thirteen did so. Both observation and clinical work tell us about the deep hurts children feel in situations in which an authority treats them unfairly or in a discriminatory fashion.

By age seven to twelve years children place stress on the equality of justice, particularly between themselves. All must be treated the same without deviation. An equality justice insists on both getting the same sized piece, or that attempts should be made to have a girl, not treated fairly, become more obedient, but that she should not be given a smaller piece of cake. It is an insistence that no prodigal-son favorites should exist, but that equal justice take place in the here and now. Equality of justice now extends to self-protection and self-defense. If one is hit, it is an act of elementary justice to hit back, while a child of six or seven labels this as "naughty." Although the six-year-old does frequently hit back, he still labels it as wrong. By age twelve, an added emphasis on equity emerges—equal justice tempered by equitable considerations. In the domain of retributive justice, by age twelve, the attenuating circumstances are considered. Distributively, a law comes to be viewed as not identical for all individuals, but needing application to the personal case. Piaget viewed this as a normative end stage which was a product of rational-cognitive processes. He stressed the peer-genesis of the norm, based on the period of reciprocal education children give to each other. This is given emphasis in the evolvement of distributive justice since a morality of constraint operates by duty rather than autonomy in choice, which the development of justice requires.

As the child grows up, the subjection of his conscience to the mind of the adult seems to him less legitimate, and except in cases of arrested moral development, caused either by decisive inner submission (those adults who remain children all their lives), or by sustained revolt, unilateral respect tends of itself to grow into mutual respect and to the state of cooperation which constitutes the normal equilibrium. It is obvious that since in our modern societies the common morality which regulates the relations of adults to each other is that of cooperation, the development of child morality will be accelerated by the examples that surround it. Actually, however, this is more probably a phenomenon of convergence than one simply of social pressure. For if human societies have evolved from heteronomy to autonomy, and from gerontocratic theocracy in all its forms to equalitarian democracy, it may very well be that the phenomena of social condensation so well described by Durkheim have been favorable primarily to the emancipation of one generation from another, and have thus rendered possible in children and adolescents the development we have outlined above.[1]

Piaget in Summary. Before turning to studies stimulated by Piaget's work, there are points of summary on Piagetian moral development that require consideration. The bases of moral judgments are limited by the comprehension of moral rules. When the cognitive processes of a child are not operating on a level beyond that of a realism in which names of objects are viewed as an inherent part of the object, there is a parallel in moral realism in which a child is expected to view announced moral rules as all-time verities. The egocentrism of the child prevents him from having a perspective that someone else may be having different perceptions of the same social setting. Egocentrism also prevents him from being emphatic with the moral behaviors of others.

This cognitive primacy leads to confusions which are not satisfactorily explained. Although there is a pervasive emphasis on moral behavior following the development of cognitive schemas for moral judgments, in his sensitive observations Piaget noted that children often seem to behave morally on a level developmentally more advanced than their formulated moral judgments. Thus, when asked about daily occurrences and failure to assign blame, children will give recognition to the intent of the actor as mitigating. Yet when they are presented with events or stories and asked to evaluate them, they continue to give stereotyped answers based on material consequences for characters in the stories. Although Piaget resorts to the explanation that children will fall back on older and more habitual schemas rather than use the ones in process of formation, since thought lags behind action, it would seem reasonable to question the validity of a methodology of appraising stages in moral development by means of responses to contrived stories.

In other respects, Piaget found that children could verbalize this so-called unchangeable and obligatory rule yet not necessarily follow the rules—an example of cognitive equipment not followed in practice. Piaget accounted for this by explaining that some of the children either lacked the necessary physical and intellectual maturity to put the rules into effect, or were distracted from the task. No contribution of various conflicts or emotional struggles concerning the child's application of a given moral rule was raised. Nor were individual differences in family socialization practices considered, even in their normal parameters, let alone clinically skewed situations. Piaget's preoccupation with determining the modal sequence of moral judgments, and his lack of clinical experience, led him to ignore such variables.

Internalization is a process much referred to in the process of acquiring socialized norms. Piaget uses this term in a manner quite different from psychoanalytic theorists. He wrote that rules become "internalized" through a sequential process in which they are seen as external and imposed, but cannot be questioned, to an acceptance of the rules through reasoning, even though the rule continues to be external. There is a final stage of full interiorization when moral judgments are autonomous. Piaget did not believe this occurred until the mutual social contract basis of society and rule-following was attained at age eleven or twelve. Yet internalization in a psychodynamic sense is a process operating long before the child is ready to participate as an autonomous moral being in a social contract. In fact, internalization in the psychoanalytic sense refers to many processes, some of which have commenced in earliest infancy. Internalization in the latter sense refers not only to processes of incorporation, interjection, identification, and identity, but to such concepts as imitation, self-representation, object representation, external compliance, fantasy development, and parts of the learning process itself.[3]

There is also an interesting emphasis on the notion that justice arises from peer interaction. Piaget extends himself to the point where he holds the sense of justice can be reinforced by the precepts and examples of adults, but it arrives largely independent of these influences. What is necessary is solidarity and mutual respect among children. The authoritarian nature of the "unilateral respect" interferes with the parent promoting a socialization based on mutual respect and cooperation. This is done by other children, especially in the period from seven to twelve, when parental domination is diminishing. Piaget felt that an adult, such as a parent or school teacher, could only contribute to autonomous morality if they were willing to obey the same rules as children and acknowledge the failure of a morality of constraint.

Apart from what may reflect Piaget's entrapment in an older European culture in which strict authority reigned between parent and child, one may question how successful a model of mutual respect and cooperation a group of elementary school-age children really can be. *The Lord of the Flies* is not all a fantasy. The subcultural examples of parents who adapt to childhood mores do not seem to promote autonomous morality, but confusion and uncertainty with respect to norms, in contrast to a cooperative participation of respecting the moral province of others.

SUBSEQUENT WORK ON MORAL DEVELOPMENT

Apart from the Hartshorne and May study on deceit in school children, and Piaget's one work on moral judgment, the field of moral development was dormant for about twenty-five years.[4] Early work inquired into the common-sensical notion that moral character, composed of a set of virtuous traits such as honesty, resistance to temptation, and self-control were part of a set of values to be inculcated into the child. Work took place during the period subsequent to Piaget in terms of social adjustment. Awareness of discrepancies between apparent outward socialization, and tolerance for personal and group asocial and dyssocial acts aroused a renewed interest in internal aspects of moralization.

Subsequent Questions. Questions arose regarding age correlates of certain traits and behaviors taken as reflecting moral character. The implicit developmental question was when these traits and behaviors became detectable. The original work of Hartshorne and May stressed moral conduct as situationally related rather than exemplifying general traits of honesty in the children, although a later factor analysis of the original data indicated a small general factor operating.[5] Wide variation of emergence of factors subsumed under the term *conscience* was found when a developmental perspective was employed. Clarity about definitions and inclusiveness, such as what the defining characteristics of *conscience, moral development,* or *self-control* are, are indispensable for any meaningful discussion on developmental aspects.

Contrasting orientations are used to illustrate purposes about the broad question of the nature of conscience and what is being measured or appraised. Is conscience an internal component of affect, such as guilt, related to an overt transgression? Most clinicians wish to go further and denote painful affective states which may be predominant in response to past, anticipated, or fantasy transgressions as well. They add that if this makes moral development less subject to measurement in terms of correlations, it is more empirical by virtue of dealing with the personality of the child in terms of the way control factors actually operate.

Superego or Habits? The construct superego was decried by some in favor of utilizing common-sense criteria of conscience, such as habits. The assumption was that a good education and family stress on character development should produce good habits, meaning the virtues of the Puritan ethic: honesty, the ability to delay gratification, resistance to temptation, perseverance, and fulfilling obligations and duties. Unfortunately for familes who pinned their hopes on such approaches, as well as the professionals who continued to put their hopes for building and rebuilding a moral society on the inculcation of habits by educational techniques, little evidence supports this position. However, the stress on good habits continues to permeate institutional approaches to deviancy as well as attempts to instill new habits by lectures, exhortations, or group experiences. No positive or consistent relationship has been found between parental practices, such as training and obedience, respect for property, hard work, and honesty, and corresponding measures in the child.[6] Such studies not only illustrate the lack of success by such efforts, but also the complexity of factors involved in a seemingly simple behavior, such as honesty.

Generalizations about the long-range consequences of punitive measures as a technique of instilling moral habits are fraught with dangers. The evidence is confusing and at best illustrates that ad hoc interventions give short-term responses. However, the responses either do not persist or do not generalize to other situations in which moral acts are expected. Undesirable complications also arise from the use of such attempts at moral training. There may be a desire to challenge authority analogous to the conspicuous consumption theory of being willing to risk something that has a high price-tag attached. This is congruent with status achievement in adolescent peer groups achieved by antisocial behavior. Most important, many of the subtle influences operating developmentally and psychodynamically within children and families are ignored.

Another approach, attempting first to delimit conscience development as something between merely acquiring a set of virtues or being cognizant of them on the one hand versus external conformity on the other, has referred moral development to the function of the ego. Caution must be used in evaluating these studies, for the term ego is often used so broadly as to be equivalent to such terms as personality or self. In psychodynamic usage, the ego refers to one hypothetical aspect of the personality in association with id and superego components and its role as an intermediary agency with the external world. In this framework other models of mental functioning may be involved, such as part of ego functioning being unconscious, or the economic aspects of the ego which pertain to narcissism. Keeping these psychodynamic essentials in mind, it can be seen that studies which discuss moral development in children in terms of the ego have predominantly focused not only on conscious ego functioning, but on the part of its functioning which is free from conflict.

As an example, the ability to make choices based on anticipating consequences could be presumed to have some bearing on moral choice. In fact, when crude but typical measures are employed to test this function, such a finding is confirmed. Nondelinquents thus make more use of planning for the future on projective test stories than do delinquents.[7] Delinquents who have supposedly been treated therapeutically with success show a longer time perspective after therapy.[8] Cheaters in an experimental situation choose a small candy bar at the moment in preference to a large one next week.[9] The limiting factor in this type of supporting data is its contrived nature. We simply do not have real responses to stories, time perspective, or wanting a small candy bar, as observed in an experimental setting, compared to what behavior would be like in the complex real world. Nor do we know how reliable such findings about moral development are over the longitudinal perspective to adulthood.

The same general comments pertain to appraising ego strength in terms of volition—a strong-willed youth will supposedly be persistent at tasks, and, therefore, also more resistant to deviance in situations which are tempting. It is somehow overlooked that a strong will may also prove intransigent in whatever activity is undertaken, be it social, asocial, or antisocial. The same type of constriction and isolation effects appear to permeate attempts to equate stable attention-span as an ego variable, with moral strength. Stability of attention correlates with resistance to cheating at levels of r = .68 and .40, but the cheaters possessed more autonomic instability as measured by the Galvanic skin response.[10] This is a result similar to Lykken, who found a primary psychopathic group with a reduced capacity to condition to anxiety and fear.[11] But if these measures are used as indicia of moral development, we are really talking about neurophysiological maturational indicia as related to attention-span.

If we are going to use these physical measures as equivalent to ego strength and part of moral development, we have taken the concept of moral development into a new domain. There are fuzzy lines of demarcation between ego functioning proper and both superego and id activities. To what extent can self-esteem and self-respect be viewed primarily as reflectors of ego strength? There can be little doubt that a feeling of esteem is an ego state, but this is intimately connected with superego sanctioning of such a state. This is similar to the difficulty of distinguishing, in experimental tasks, between the appraisal of a situation as dangerous, and eliciting a warning signal inhibiting an act from an internalized component, such as a feeling of obligation based on superego dictates not to do a certain act. On the other hand, the role of aggression in either a constitutional form with individual differences, or in its complicated interactions with superego and environmental agents, does not permit easy determinations on ego ability to handle aggression as reflecting ego strength and superior moral development. The criterion for moral development is usually given as the ability to control aggressive action. Immediately, one may question if this is a criterion that may validly indicate greater moral development.

Derivative measures may be used as follows: Ratings of the amount of aggressive fantasy in doll play in children have been made which are then correlated with cheating (r = .63). The conclusion is offered by reverse implication that children with smaller degrees of aggressive fantasy exhibit conduct that is moral.[12] It is not surprising that there is no significance when actual aggressive behavior is evaluated. Many other relevant methodological questions permeate this type of research, such as how to measure and detect aggressive fantasies, and how and under what circumstances ego control of aggression should be viewed as a measure of moral development. The problems pertaining to what is "conscience" and "moral development" are obviously conflicting and often not clearly delineated.

Such dilemmas have presented difficulty in determining whether stages of moral development are subject to an age-developmental approach. While there is little ambiguity in noting that ego functions in the non-conflicted child acquire increasing strength as the child ages, the question of which variables most accurately reflect moral development continues to haunt research and theoretical formulations. Even variables included under morally conforming conduct show variation. While resistance to cheating, or stealing remain fairly constant from nursery school to high school, incidents of lying and stealing reported by parents decrease markedly after six to eight years.[13] Yet if conforming conduct remains relatively constant for an individual child throughout development, is it accurate to ascribe this to a unified moral factor?

The young child may be fearful or intimidated, or just plain uninterested enough to transgress. An older child may have a different set of ego and superego factors operating as well as a different set of peer influences.

There is a common theoretical fallacy made by workers who are sophisticated in almost all other respects.[14] This fallacy refers to ego development in terms of a progressive evolvement over time while superego development, in the form of conscience, is viewed as being fixed for all time at a sensitive period of development. Perhaps this viewpoint is due to a misrepresentation of writings on the contribution of the oedipal complex to superego formation. This type of misrepresentation permits the omission of the need to study the variation and complexity of superego functions as developmental phenomena.

Findings on the stability of moral conduct over time are thus sparse and conflicting. The need for sophisticated longitudinal studies in this area is immense. The need is not only to evaluate broad hypotheses of children who are rated morally superior at five years and remain so at ten to fifteen, for example, but to evaluate the components that are believed related to moral knowledge, moral judgment, and, most especially, moral conduct.

MORAL DEVELOPMENT: KOHLBERG

Introduction. Reference to moral stages of development does not imply a necessary sequential unfolding of psychomoral stages, nor does it imply any type of isomorphism with a changing biological organization. The account of moral development by Piaget, as related to the child's conception of the world, had a strong cognitive emphasis on moral development. It stressed the ability of the child to apply logic and notions of justice and obedience to the world. However, the notions were not viewed as unfolding at various age levels but were the result of a cognitive apparatus which permitted the child to reformulate ideas, coupled with relationships which engender feelings, such as sympathy or anger, leading to pragmatic social norms.

A cognitive ability to classify behavior and situations in terms of mutual rights and duties was necessary with a social capacity for empathy. Teaching of values by authority figures would only take if the level of development was such that the child could learn to know the need for certain values in a social order. The emphasis was on attaining a cognitive growth before the child was capable of making variant moral judgments.

Investigation of the types of moral judgments children make was the consequence. Moral judgment was studied in two ways: by rules children use in hypothesized situations, and by the reasons they give for using such rules. Attempts to determine the rightness or wrongness of a rule are bypassed by remaining ethically neutral.

Studying usage and reasons for rules similarly bypasses appraisal of moral knowledge in terms of how much moral knowledge and belief the child has learned, since most investigations reveal that by age six or seven, the basic moral amenities of a culture can be verbalized. They are qualified by socio-economic background, intellectual ability, and idiosyncratic features in a child such as a desire to demonstrate moral prowess or lack of same—which is what the clinician encompasses in assessment.

None of this material has any necessary relevance to moral *behavior*. There is no established correlation between the level of expressed moral judgments or knowledge and moral conduct. Moral conduct does not easily lend itself to a developmental approach after the preschool period in terms of expected sequential behaviors. To investigate this would require knowledge of the superego functioning of a given child as well as appraisals of his interaction within the family and larger social organization. These lead into the realm of psychodynamics rather than stages of moral judgments.

Dimensions. Kohlberg has his own classification of moral judgments.[15] Observations on six dimensions of moral judgment are proposed in terms of increasing regularity with age in western cultures, and regardless of social class, religion, or the particular stories or situations by which the child is questioned. The five other dimensions of Piagetian theory that have not held up are socially derived from the original formulations, while the six that hold up are cognitively derived. The five dimensions found unreliable as indicia of moral judgment are: (1) modification of obedience to rules or authority because of situational demands or human needs; (2) maintenance of peer loyalty over obedience to authority; (3) choosing direct retaliation by a victim rather than punishment by authority; (4) preferring equality of treatment rather than a differential reward for virtue or for conformity to authority, and (5) punishment based on individual rather than collective responsibility.

These measures are viewed as unreliable since they do not tend to increase with age, variation is found between cultural and socio-economic groups, and there is wide variation depending on the particular stories or situations used.[16] The dimensions which hold up illustrate criteria which are taken as evidence of moral stages. They show moral judgments changing over time and do not show unpredictable fluctuations. The judgments are correlated with frequencies in neighboring categories, and demonstrate a greater ease in shifting a child to the adjacent type of judgments than those far distant. Horizontal generalization across situations is present as further evidence of legitimate stage development.

There are six dimensions which meet the criteria for stages of moral judgment. (1) *Intentionality of judgment* is illustrated by older children's appraising the badness of an act in terms of an intent to do harm. (2) Most children achieve *relativity of judgment* by age nine, and are able to recognize that different perspectives on what is right and wrong are possible. (3) *Independence of sanctions*, refer to the shift away from viewing others as bad because they are punished, even when the child has been portrayed as doing a helpful, obedient act. While such moral judgment holds at four years of age, a shift is under way so that in a year, from four to five, some children begin to add that a child who is punished must have done something wrong, even though there has been no reference to it; by age seven, most children are holding that the child was helpful and obedient and not bad just because he was punished. (4) *Naturalistic views of misfortune* are dominated by an immanent theory of justice, so that naturalistic misfortunes cease to be viewed as visitations for misdeeds. (5) *The use of reciprocity* in interaction with others reveals the younger child's reliance on more selfish and concrete components of reciprocity, such as hitting back if hit—an eye for an eye. This predominates until eleven to thirteen years when a shift occurs to an empathic type of reciprocity—putting oneself in place of someone. (6) *The use of punishment as restitution and reform* is seen in young children's advocating painful punishments for misdeeds while older children become more oriented toward giving restitution to victims and reforming culprits.

The last two dimensions do not conform to the actual behavior of children and adults, at least a majority of the time. Again, problems with the use of moral judgments arise. The developmental criterion is the shifting nature of moral judgments which reflect cognitive development and IQ as well. These may have little or nothing to do with behavior. The stages of moral judgment also have low correlation with the intensity of parental disciplinary techniques. The nonintentionality, lack of relativism, and punishment orientations of the young child do not need more than a general type of awareness that some authorities, such as parents, teachers, or police, utilize physical punishment.

From this background and a study of seventy-two boys, aged ten to sixteen, using Piagetian procedures, Kohlberg defined three major levels of moral development and two types in each level:

TABLE 11

Level I. Premoral
    Type 1. Punishment and obedience orientation
    Type 2. Naive instrumental hedonism (conformity to obtain rewards and have favors returned)

Level II. Morality of Conventional Role-Conformity
    Type 3. Good-boy morality of maintaining good relations, approval of others (conformity to avoid disapproval or others disliking one)
    Type 4. Authority maintaining morality (conformity to avoid censure by authorities and resultant guilt)

Level III. Morality of Self-Accepted
Moral Principles (Postconventional)
    Type 5. Morality of contract, of individual rights, and of democratically accepted law (conformity to maintain respect of the individual spectator judged in terms of community welfare)
    Type 6. Morality of individual principles of conscience (conformity to avoid self-condemnation)

With the subject group Kohlberg used, age trends were visible through these stages. The first two types of moral judgment decrease with age, the next two increase until age thirteen and then stabilize, and the last two increase from thirteen to sixteen. In contrast to the interpretation that shifts in moral judgment are primarily due to learning verbal rules of morality within a given culture, in which variation is due to some rules being taught earlier or learned better, moral stage theory holds that stages reflect efforts of the child to organize his thinking about value judgments. Levels of organization would have to be attained before the next level could be reached. Lower stages are displaced when the child is capable of assimilating moral reasoning at a higher stage. The emphasis is on internal patterning of social experiences rather than direct teaching. Hence, the greater correlation of moral judgment with age (greater social exposure) rather than IQ ($r = .59$ to $r = .31$).

Although intellectual development is a necessary condition for development of moral thought, it is not sufficient in and of itself.

Differences in cultural background—such as social class, peer-group participation, and sex—do not vary the sequential stages; the rate of exposure to socialization only accentuates stage attainment. Thus, a popular, middle-class child may express advanced types of judgments earlier. Various social groups, such as family, peers, and the wider society can induce conflict between different value systems, but they can also be a stimulant to the development of a general factor in moral judgments. This general factor can account for much of the co-variance in moral judgments while still permitting individual differences in the *content* of moral judgments.

Yet, this position fails to account for the clinical and sociological findings about individuals who have different rates of attainment in the area of moral judgments, and who appear to remain primitive and unsocialized in some of the basics of moral judgment. There are those who do not attain more than the lowest level of moral judgment, even though they possess normal intelligence. They just do not perceive things the same because of their internal standards. These might be explained by lack of sufficient identification and role-playing to stimulate more advance moral judgments. Instead, their identification might be in terms of parental judgment norms.

This type of theorizing leads to contrasting notions of moral development as viewed from the perspective of moral judgment compared to moral conduct:

1. Moral judgments are viewed as generally stable between individuals, while moral conduct is unstable and more situation-specifc. This is the old Hartshorne-May notion that conduct is situationally determined.

2. Moral judgments are viewed as not becoming moral until early adolescence, while moral conduct develops early. This reflects the opinion of Kohlberg and others that internalization processes do not commence until the second level of moral development where conventional rule-conformity begins. Early conduct is judged as moral in terms of assigning blame and punishment for disobediences.

3. Moral conduct is viewed as development congruent with social class and peer influences whereas moral judgments are viewed, in general, as relatively independent of these influences.

The position that conduct is situationally determined is a thorny problem for those who adhere to sequential stages of moral development. The dilemma resides in the need to avoid tying moral development to the capricious and unpredictable areas of moral conduct, yet to deal simultaneously with the predicament that moral judgment seems unrelated to conduct. There is a necessity to show verbal expression of moral judgments having a relationship to conduct. This is done by attempts to demonstrate that moral judgments and conduct reflect the same developmental processes and are not independent. Experimental studies are cited correlating moral judgment and resistance to cheating or to correlations between moral judgments and teacher's ratings of conscience and fairness to peers (r = .31 and .51 respectively). This attempt to justify an abstract notion of judgment with moral conduct appears unfortunate, for it leads its exponents to fall back on weak evidence to show that cognition and volition are inseparable. How valid a measure of moral conduct resistance to cheating is in a laboratory is highly questionable. Nor can much credence be given to teacher's ratings of conscience in school children. How an individual child will act in the unstructured situations of interpersonal life is the ultimate criterion when conduct is appraised, not expression of moral judgments.

Moral development, as measured by expression of judgments, eventuates in a position of evaluating moral development by idealized Platonic notions of a moral system. In fact, Kohlberg explicitly resorts to philosophy to define what a moral judgment is. He puts it in terms of moral judgments being more mature when they employ such universal criteria as consistency and inclusiveness, and when they are grounded in objective, impersonal, or ideal grounds. These criteria have no reference to moral activity, but are stages of moral development which eventually come closer to philosophical and ethical judgments. Nor are these general criteria related to the rightness or wrongness of an individual moral judgment since these would appeal to personalistic elements, such as aesthetic taste, prudence, or technological or economic preferences. The end result is a fusion of moral judgments in childhood and a philosphic realism. "In this sense we can define a moral judgment as 'moral' without considering its content (the action judged) and without considering whether or not it agrees with our own judgments or standards."[17]

SOCIAL LEARNING CONTRIBUTIONS TO MORAL DEVELOPMENT

General Background. In contrast to cognitive approaches, an emphasis on learned aspects of standards is another alternative. Although some theorists encompass all other approaches under the rubric of learning theories, varying from psychoanalytic models to Skinnerian aversive conditioning, this is a broad category whose impreciseness is confusing. Within developmental psychology the major approach, along with cognitive formulations, has utilized a social learning theory model. Moral behavior is not viewed differently from any learned behavior, subject to principles operating for the genesis of behavior.

Despite differences among learning theorists, such basic concepts as the stimulus-response sequence, reinforcement discrimination, generalization, aversive conditioning, drive, habit strength, and mediation are used. Acquiring moral responses is subject to positive or negative reinforcements. An inherent difficulty is present when some of the responses to be learned do not have their own reinforcement value, such as food, and which may actually involve foregoing immediate pleasure. To sacrifice such inherent pleasures again raises questions about the relative permanence of established controls or their need for periodic external reinforcement by controlling agents.

The concept of internalization is relevant in terms of the ability of an individual to give positive or negative reinforcement to himself. To accomplish this within a social learning theory framework means that self-criticism has to be learned as an internalized prototype which the child replicates in terms of the punishment suffered previously. Rebuking the self physically, verbally, and later symbolically is an observed phenomenon among children (an imitative pattern is noted from adult models). However, there is still a transition before the child adopts self-punitive responses, and there is also a need for resistance to the extinction of self-critical responses.

Although some self-evaluative responses are believed derived from social learning based on reward, some children replicate the punitive and prohibitive functions of socializing agents. The need to explain the persistence and generalization of moral responses which operate outside the stimulus of an immediate transgression has been explained by some on the basis that self-criticism arises because of its anxiety-reducing effect. Originally, evaluative labels were subsumed under or contiguous with external punishment, which permitted anxiety reduction. In effect, a signal theory of self-criticism develops in which the stimulus properties in the critical model operates as a signal for the attenuation of anticipatory anxiety in the child. These processes are held to operate independently of the cognitive substance of responses.[18]

Acquisition of moral behaviors by an extension of imitative practices to modeling and intensification is another theme. There is experimental evidence that behavior can be acquired by observing models without direct reinforcement.[19] The limitation is that the stimulus to the responses produced in the model may be missed or misinterpreted by the child. This may be corrected experimentally by making the cues explicit, but the conflicts and confusion that can arise in a naturalistic setting of child-rearing can be enormous. The cogent effects of mixed messages, such as double-binds or parental acting out, so prevalently noted in clinical acting out situations, can be seen clearly in simplified paradigms of how models influence moral development.

A distinction is made between the *acquisition* of such responses and their *continuance*. Although exposure to mediated violence or television may become a source for acquiring behaviors, to carry out such behaviors a set of reinforcement contingencies are required. Those who control contingencies have the greatest ability to influence which moral acts a child will choose. This has significance in terms of the child performing a certain act in contrast to something happening to him. The distinction amounts to the difference between conditioned *respondents*, which impinge on a child or are done to him, in contrast to actions which appear to originate from within and are *operants*. Further, a child may later employ a respondent to function as an operant, using an internal verbal operant as a stimulus which then elicits a respondent whose external ramifications are noted and reinforced in an operant sense.

Broad questions are relevant about the internal control and purpose of behavior. A child talking to himself in a certain manner ("That was a bad thing to do") or repeating pictorial images of a transgressing act, may elicit positive or negative reinforcements. These originally respondent words and images come to function in a manner that will appear as operant. The behavior that ensues elicits an environmental response. If the responses are positive, the behavior is reinforced. A whole series of respondents may become internalized and act as operants. Unless the reinforcement contingencies change, moral conduct will not change. This inner programming of moral conduct is quite in contrast to cognitive theorists.

How is the question of discrepancies between verbalized moral judgments and moral behavior handled by social learning theory? The degree of correlation between the two is related to the consistency of socialization agents. If there is little generalization of moral conduct from one situation to another, it is presumed that parents use more effective socialization techniques with respect to some behaviors. If there is a strong generalization to many situations, a presumption of great consistency is made. This appears to be a slippery slope argument in some respects. Although there are many gradations in parents as to which behaviors are subject to prohibition, the crucial question of why behaviors generalize remains open. To say that parental consistency is the crucial variable does not tell us why a child may transgress against one individual but not another, or in one situation but not another. Nor does it explain deviations in moral conduct in situations outside of the home, unless one resorts to the simplistic notion that such situations are literally further removed in a physical sense from the original reinforcing agents and are therefore less subject to reinforcement effects. But this is a reversion to the lack of an internalization model in which the presence of big brother socializing agents need to be present. Nor does lack of parental consistency give us more than one variable as to variations between moral judgments and actual conduct.

It is not surprising that results are found such as even a slight negative correlation between parental reports of conscience and measures of resistance to temptation.[20] Similarly, a finding of no correlation between resistance to temptation and guilt over transgression, but rather a correlation between resistance to temptation and parental socialization practices, would appear representative of the types of reinforcement for a specific act by a parent.[21] Artificial situations such as resistance to temptation experiments cannot be expected to have much relationship to internalized variables such as guilt. However, the crucial question is whether resistance to temptation studies have a relationship to the types of control over behavior that are characteristic of a child in his development.

Self-criticism in a child is more related to derogatory comments about transgressions by parents while attempts to repair damage inflicted are more related to the opportunity a child has to administer his own sanctions against himself.[22] These types of studies argue for variation in what may be expected in predicting moral behavior from socialization experiences. They cast doubt not only on formulations adhering to any unitary structure of conscience, but raise questions as to the failure of anxiety generating the basis for acquiring avoidance responses.

The old issue reappears as to the situational nature of many moral responses. Yet if parental modeling and identification, as well as anxiety reduction via anticipating discomfort, are influential for ongoing moral development, how does one account for situational specificity? Answers have raised the issue of the diversity of models available to a child in a pluralistic world which presents gross inconsistencies. This is a resort to a cultural diversity argument to explain the failure of the theory with respect to situational variation and performance.

It is interesting to ponder the recurring psychological debate as to a generalized trait of honesty (a g factor) versus the many factors reflecting situational specificity (an s factor). Since psychology has not yet been able to resolve the question of a general trait even for intelligence, with all the data and research done on this problem, it would seem reasonable to withhold temporarily the need for making a decision regarding morality. A clinician with a focus on developmental psychopathology should point out covert and overt conflicts operating even within one parent as sufficient to explain individual deviations. An aggregation of individual factors operating in the past with respect to behaviors, as well as with the present vulnerability of an individual, would be dispositional.

The Question of Institutional Influences. The presupposition has been that the socializing agents (be they parents, authority figures outside the home, or wider cultural influences), have been relatively homogeneous. The direction was that parents and social institutions both sought the development of a conscience in terms of maximal autonomy, in the sense of exerting controls free from external agents. Another presumption was that commonly accepted goals, as well as some painful affect, such as guilt, were attained in furtherance of the adaptation to adult demands. The investigative methodology presupposes these common goals, as well as the socializing agents being uniform agents administering proper doses of socialization techniques at proper intervals to ensure that these goals be attained. Investigation has focused on the doses, techniques, and intervals between doses, rather than on the variation between agents themselves, such as in parental characteristics or in family differentiation from the wider culture.

Before discussion of parental influences on conscience development, in addition to specific techniques used, institutional influences should be considered. The acquisition of controls in the manner under discussion avoids the issue of decision-making about which values are transmitted. Provision is not then allowed for the impact of changing value systems and the effect this may have on parental disciplinary techniques. Theorists with a sociological bent have noted the lack of evidence to confirm a high correlation between expressed values of parents and their children, although again this points to cognitive differences in relying on expressed values.[23] Changing values have been pointed out intergenerationally, but within a generation, which challenges a position based on accepted values to be transmitted.

As an example, delay of gratification, as a commonly accepted goal or criterion of conscience development, has been increasingly questioned as to its value for inculcation by some techniques. Delay of gratification might be viewed more correctly as a reflection of past morality contingent upon an economy of scarcity in which delay was necessary. The overthrow of delay as a virtue could operate in many sectors, such as sexuality, material possessions, or a generalized hedonistic gratification. Indeed, the commercial and entertainment markets induce individuals to maximize gratification with the shortest delay. In this framework, deviancy would be the individual who develops norms of keeping his nose to the grindstone and feeling a need to work for gratifications. Changes in socio-economic conditions, social institutions and demographic influences produce a flux in moral values. Moral development is felt to be insufficiently explained in terms of internalization or learning of parental norms which give rise to self-control. Rather than values having a fixity due to cognitive-developmental processes or from early learning, the emphasis shifts to the need for continuing reinforcement of standards and controls from social institutions and their caretakers.

There seems to have been a relatively easy transformation for many individuals of values which are presented as normative. Examples have been the ease with which great masses of individuals conform to changing standards of morality, such as in recent German history from the Weimar Republic, the Nazi period, and the post-World War II German government, or the shift in China from the nationalist regime to that of a Communist government. It is not merely the adaptation to different leaders, but rather the ease in carrying out acts, such as acquiescing to concentration camps or genocide. Either there is a lack of a firmly entrenched conscience, or an ease of abandonment to changing authority. Note the ease of acquiescing to an authority in an experimental setting in which the request was made to inflict what appeared to be an injurious amount of electric current on another individual.[24]

It is not that everyone adapts easily, but rather that the majority of a population seem to do so when the external reinforcements change. Those tortured few, guided by the old values, and unable to adapt without internal anguish are viewed as needing psychological refurbishing to help them conform to the new order. Law and order are seen not as absolutes but as relative to the particular demands and power groups setting norms at a particular time. Specific ethical questions are bypassed in this psycho-social presentation, such as competing political ideologies vying with each other on rationalized political grounds of greater freedom, truth, and so on. It is rather that as social norms change, and the agents for enforcing behavior operate with altered norms (courts, schools, churches, police, therapists), the behavior of the majority of a population changes.

Cultural theorists do not wish to say that individuals will conform merely out of fear while in their hearts they know the moral law within. It is rather that the new norms proclaimed become the conscience of the individual which is subject to change under different conditions. Misfits, such as Sir Thomas More, become outcasts.

In wartime, it is thus morally desirable to economize and suffer while in an affluent economy the opposite is true. It is morally desirable to kill in war time, subject to the authority-approving influence of the powers that be. Neither an internalized mental structure, nor the family, are given much significance in mediating or resisting change. Further, parents are viewed as disposed toward accommodating to the new order. The ease with which parents so accommodate is presented as further evidence for the lack of internalization in parents.

What can be said regarding the validity of this type of critique by institutional critics? Is conscience, in the sense of a developmental-learning model, an example of psychological hypostatization for what in reality is a series of adjustments to institutional norms which are reinforced? Apart from semantic differences of words between disciplines, an area of concept clarification is required in this dilemma. The burden should be on someone who defended the beliefs and attitudes of an individual never changing during his lifetime, as well as when value systems are compared in different historical periods. The cognitive position on moral judgments at different developmental periods does not seem directly appropriate beyond the issues referred to above as to whether these are products of acculturation or cognitive development. Nor would a position that attacks the changing nature or accommodation of moral norms seem to demolish the social learning theory regarding certain behaviors unless the social learning theorist is one who is maintaining a position of once learned, always learned, so that further modification would be impossible.

What seems at issue is the matter of personality traits, relevant to moral conduct, and their relative endurability. Psychoanalytic theory does not maintain that the relative balance between id, ego, and superego remains fixed for all time. Clinical evidence is, in fact, directly contrary with respect to changes in the prohibitions and ideals of an individual, and the goals of psychotherapy. Vulnerability to social influences would vary quite widely, and some would argue that adapting to a changing political scene should be viewed as a measure of ego strength rather than being an illustration of individual moral acts reflecting changing edicts in which the individual has little choice or resistance.

Difficulties in the nurturing process seem to result in individual variations in control over conduct. It is extremely difficult to change moral conduct for those individuals, and therapeutic efforts may appear to be hopeless. Although this example is from the realm of conflicted behavior or deviations where adaptation to changing social norms or acquiring new ones is difficult, the corollary is that for the part of an individual which is not conflicted (the conflict-free realm), change would not be expected to be so laborious. It is only in the realm of internalized conflict, reenacted with various individuals or institutions, that change is difficult, and there is resistance as well as repetitive performances based on old values.

Susceptibility of individual children to socialization may lie in their attachment position in which adopting moral norms insures acceptance and survival. The control a powerful adult has over a child, coupled with the intense affect within a family, contribute to the susceptibility for inculcation of norms.[25] A family in which the level of conflict is minimized, particularly with respect to conflicts of the type which lead to acting out solutions, creates an atmosphere in which socialization is facilitated. The problem is not that there is no such thing as learned values which have some autonomous functioning, but that over-socialization induces such a high need for acceptance and affiliation that an individual finds it too anxiety-inducing to resist impositions.

Attention has been given earlier to the assumption that parents have an agreed-upon set of norms which they transmit to their children. The intermediary discussion took up criticisms of this assumption based on the ease of influence to changing norms promulgated by institutions. But how, and in what manner, may parents influence their offspring with respect to the inculcation of moral norms? Within a social learning theory framework the emphasis is placed on such factors as characteristics of parental interaction with children, or more detailed examination of various types of parental disciplinary techniques. From this perspective, the parental techniques, as the independent variable, are viewed as striving toward a homogeneous end result on the child in terms of such criteria as resistance to temptation, or guilt for transgressions.

A preliminary question is related to the nature of the norms which parents attempt to transmit. As discussed, these norms need not and do not remain fixed, but apart from shifts which occur to them, why will a parent socialize a child in a given direction? The physical pain from the personal anxiety which arises from permitting untrammeled aggression, customarily limits aggression in a child. Therefore, consider a more limiting case—the moral norms used by a parent to inculcate cleanliness, which in certain cultures is next to Godliness. The messiness of a child elicits feelings in a parent, dependent upon the degree of mess, the frequency of its occurrence, its accidental versus intentional nature, etc. Parental attempts to control (discipline) such acts weigh the damage done in terms of cost (so much extra money for cleaning up or washing) or the emotional effort needed to teach the child the virtue of cleanliness.

None of these objective measures refer to why a parent wants a child clean, but have presupposed that this is an accepted norm. However, it is precisely at this point that the crucial question can be raised. If a parent merely wants a clean child for the type of reasons given, it should not be too difficult to program a series of habits, much like one does in housebreaking a pet, and for a great many behaviors, which are inculcated in the course of socialization, this appears to be what happens. But, if we say that parents continue to perpetuate such habits because they themselves were so taught, a circular quality is introduced which does not convey the intense personal need of a parent to convert a child to such habits. More is at stake for such moral values from the parental side than merely desiring that a habit be acquired because of economic advantage. To argue that cleanliness is merely a more convenient basis for family living also begs the question. This is not to deny cultural contributions to cleanliness. Simplistically, a culture in which children are led into the bushes for evacuation is one in which we would predict a minimal level of conflict about cleanliness, or one in which there was little social utility in compulsive organization would similarly engender little conflict.

Therefore, certain ecological conditions contribute to socialization practices and are a given.[26] Lack of cleanliness might be much more unpleasant and disruptive to family and communal living in an apartment than in a jungle. But beyond these socio-cultural givens on socialization, the psychological question remains as to variation in parental socialization practices. Social learning theory puts phrases in terms of the reinforcement conditions which sustain a parent with respect to socializing techniques, which would permit explanations and predictions of why and how certain moral norms are conveyed to a child. A psychodynamic model would extend the inquiry into the character structure and personality conflicts of the parental objects and their family interaction.

The Impact of Parental Techniques of Discipline. If one believes parental behavior has something to do with moral conduct in children, investigation becomes a necessity. Two approaches have been used to evaluate the parental contribution. The first is experimental efforts to alter the approach of parents or their surrogates, such as having a parent physically restrain a child from doing something and then waiting until he has attempted it, or rather uttering a verbal request not to do something.[27] Such differences are presumed significant and experimental studies confirm this. However, transmission of laboratory findings to the naturalistic setting of the family or outside world becomes inferential.

A second approach is based on classifying parental disciplinary techniques. A different set of methodological problems arise, such as the reliability of techniques used to observe families and the validity of classifications. Will impressions of parental techniques, based on an interview in terms of, "How do you customarily discipline your child when he disobeys?" have a high reliability between researchers, or on test-retest basis over an interval? If the researcher enters the home as an observer, does he detect the types of parental techniques typically used? The variation contingent upon the astuteness, experience, and theoretical sensitivity of the observer cannot be ignored and is, unfortunately, rarely commented upon. There are also questions regarding whether observation is influenced by some pre-existing theory to which the observer adheres, or whether observation is rather guided by the questions asked, based on a theory. Such difficulties are known but customarily handled by ignoring them on the basis that an experiment can still be validly conducted.

Another approach is to focus rating broad variables, such as degree of parental warmth or hostility. A host of social variables, such as social class, sex of the child, sex of the disciplining parent, age of the child as well as of the parent, are present and often regarded as nuisance variables by psychologists since they do not relate to the theoretical constructs which psychologists are interested in evaluating. Maccoby notes that the problem of intercorrelations among antecedent variables, such as different disciplinary techniques correlated with social class, have been handled in three ways:[28] (1) deliberate selection of samples that are homogenous with respect to the variables whose effect one does not wish to study; (2) efforts to measure the confounding variables so as to hold them constant statistically before the analysis of results; (3) factor analysis of the antecedents so as to reduce large sets of inter-related variables to a smaller number of relatively independent variables.

Other factors are regarded as error variants to be removed, so that the effects of parent practices can be more clearly seen. This has led to studies of both specific techniques as well as to the affective context in which techniques are employed with some holding that these are not independent.

A detailed review of the findings has been done by Becker.[29] Interest in parent disciplinary techniques evolve from many sources. Types of parental disciplines as correlated with various learning theory concepts early interested researchers. There was also the knowledge from clinical observations which were raising questions about parent-child interaction with respect to impulse control. Some studies have tended to use macro concepts, such as parental democratic attitudes, or delinquency as the dependent variable in the child. By 1959, Schaefer had divided parental attitudes and behaviors into two dimensions: love-hostility and control-autonomy. He described a "hypothetical circumplex for maternal behavior."[30] This noted the limitations of attempting to classify parental techniques primarily on the basis of discipline. By factor analysis a minimal number of orthogonal dimensions to account for empirical correlations among variables could be obtained. The dimensions were presented in terms of coordinates.

Becker elaborated this model of parental behavior into three general dimensions by dividing the control-versus-autonomy dimension into "restrictiveness versus permissiveness" and "calm-detachment versus anxious emotional involvement."

The warmth end of the dimension is defined by parental variables such as accepting, affection, approving, child-centered, positive response to dependency, use of explanations, high use of praise and reasons in discipline, low use of physical punishment, and low maternal criticism of husband. The hostility end at its maximum has the polar opposite qualities. The restrictive end is defined in terms of many restrictions and strict enforcement of demands in areas of sex play, modesty behavior, table manners, toilet training, neatness, obedience, orderliness, care of furniture, noise, aggression to siblings and peers and parents, with its opposites at the permissive end. The anxious end, in contrast to the calm end, is characterized by high emotionality in relation to the child, protectiveness, and solicitousness for the welfare of the child.

These dimensions demonstrate that the type of affectional relationship between a parent and child has some correlation with the type of discipline used. Thus, parental variables associated with warmth would more likely use praise and reasoning in discipline, while those tending toward the end of the hostile dimension would be more likely to use physical punishment. The need for considering intersections between the dimensions becomes important, such as the degree of restrictiveness occurring in a warm context. Affectional relationships are not necessarily correlated with one end of the restrictiveness-permissiveness dimension.

Disciplinary techniques have been divided into three types: power-assertive (characterized by physical punishment and material deprivation); non-power-assertive (which is subdivided into love-withdrawal—direct but non-physical expression of disapproval) and induction (parental focusing on the painful consequences of behavior to the parents and others). The non-power types of discipline are sometimes referred to as love-oriented, indirect, or psychological disciplines. Various hypotheses have been proposed to account for differential effects of the initial dichotomy between power-assertive contrasted with non-power-assertive techniques.[31] Some have proposed a difference in the effectiveness of modeling. A child who has a strong attachment to a warm parent with little fear will want to be around such a parent with all of the increased accompaniments for modeling as well as learning.

Experimental work confirms the greater imitation of a nurturant model by a child than a non-nurturant one. Greater contact, coupled with greater modeling of a warm model, provide the groundwork for handling aggression in the manner of the parental model. A model, who discourages ventilation or discharge of anger, in turn has this modeled. However, it would be an unwarranted inference to add that such a child would be one who turns his anger inward since this presumes a hydraulic model where anger has to go somewhere. The variations on what may occur from modeling the non-expression of anger are complicated and would merit a separate section.

A second factor suggested to account for differences between power-assertive and non-power-assertive disciplinary techniques operates with respect to identification. This has been postulated in terms of the self-reassuring effect that internalization of warm parental qualities can have in contrast to power-assertive techniques which lead a child simply to try and avoid a parent as well as his internalization. Withdrawal of love in a warm context may accentuate identification to protect the child against the threat of a loss of such a nurturant object.

A third explanation emphasizes variations in the timing of punishment. The power-assertive parent is more likely to punish at the time of transgression and to end it there, while the non-power-assertive parent tends to expect reparative acts (confession and restitution) which reinforce such acts, since punishment in the form of disapproval or withdrawal continues until such reparation.

Fourth, a power-assertive parent who uses physical punishment dissipates most of the discomfort, such as guilt following a transgression, more readily than one who conveys an expectation of reformed conduct in the future. This means that the child is not off the hook for a prolonged time and is left with greater discomfort than with accompanying motivation to change.

Fifth, some stress a cognitive component to differentiate power-assertive techniques. A parent who delays punishment, and conveys an expectation of reparation, can only have an influence on the child if there is a cognitive ability to grasp the implications of what is expected. Further, cognitive dissonance between the desire to perform an act and not doing so can be reduced by submission to a powerful external authority who forbids, in contrast to a parent who permits the child to abandon his position of wanting to perform an act and thus promotes controls from within.

By way of summary, note the following types of parental disciplinary techniques. Power-assertive techniques utilize a direct power play to control the child. The emphasis is on parental control rather than on cognitively conveying to the child what is expected or relying on affects engendered in the child for control. The techniques may be depriving the child of gratification, physical punishment, or the threat of these.

Love-withdrawal techniques, under non-power-assertive types, either disapprove of the behavior or express anger without accompanying physical punishment. However, the punitive aspects are prominent, such as in the implicit emotional threat of abandonment or not accepting the child after what he has done. The enduring and unpredictable emotional nature of such a withdrawal is another threat, so that the child is unsure whether he is ostracized or not. This type of predicament, where the child is not offered techniques to expiate, is often seen clinically with a host of emotional concomitants and chronic patterns of shame and inferiority.

Induction is the utilization of explanation or persuasion as techniques for inducing behavioral change. The similarity to psychotherapeutic techniques is conspicuous. There is a reliance on pointing out to a child the reasonable thing to do or the harmful possibilities in a certain type of behavior as well as to others. Appeals to norms that already exist within the child ("Don't pick on him since he's smaller") to certain sensitive components in the personality such as pride, autonomy, or maturity ("Don't quit now") or to empathic appeals may be used ("How would you like some of your property taken?"). Another approach is to explain the needs or motives of others ("Don't tell on him, he was hungry and needed the money"). This technique relies on appeals to the ego-ideal of the child for control of conduct, and seeks to bolster norms which have been inculcated in a normative context.

Power-assertive techniques are used more by hostile parents. The result is seen in the promotion of aggression in young children accompanied by their use of power-assertive techniques with others. The control is in terms of an external authority who will punish, and there is attendant resistance to authority as well. The consistent use of power-assertive techniques over time may lead to an inhibition of overt aggressiveness, where hostility is handled by projection, prosocial aggression, or self-aggression. In contrast, non-power-assertive techniques promote acceptance of internalized responses to transgression in the form of self-responsibility and guilt, if the technique is working at its optimum.

Effects of the control-versus-autonomy dimension are vaguer. Their effects vary by the predominance of an accompanying warm or hostile context. High degree of control exerted in a warm parental context tend to produce children who are conforming, obedient, polite, and neat, but not creative or independent. Baumrind's work on authoritative parental control showed that authoritative techniques, coupled with warmth, have a maximization of qualities such as competence and friendliness, with an absence of anxious-withdrawal or impulsive, disruptive types of behaviors.[32]

Semantics enter the situation if autonomy is defined in terms of parental permissiveness. Permissiveness per se in the face of disturbing conduct does not simply prevent autonomy, but may interfere with assuming personal responsibility or leadership. Some use control as equivalent to parental consistency, and in that sense the parent may go beyond reasoned explanations to ensure that a type of behavior occurs. Yet, there are perplexing findings such as the expectation that warm disciplinary techniques would induce a more socialized child in terms of controls, who should need minimal control by parents. However, such children seem to have parents who use high control techniques. Questions of antecedents and consequences, causal relationships, as well as weightings to be given to various variables, are still in need of clarification.

DELAYED GRATIFICATION

The capacity to delay gratification is seen by many as the sine qua non of internalized conscience functioning. Without the capacity to delay, neither reflective choice nor taking heed of painful affective signals are operationally functional. Some would reverse the formulation: delay of gratification may not be possible if the cognitive or affective systems are not performing adequately. However, delay can be viewed as an essential index of moral development. Nor is this position vitiated by arguments that since delays might be self-serving, there is something impure about delay as an index. Such an argument could be used with every criteria held to function as internalized guides in contrast to a plain fear of external punishment. If temptation is resisted apart from an external agency, it would be from some internal self-serving, just as heeding internal anxiety signals is. One series confronted children with choices between an immediate, but less valued, object, and a delayed choice for a more valued object.[33] Findings indicated an increase in delay with age, but also the ability to increase delay by lowering the waiting interval or strengthening the probability that the chosen delayed object would be forthcoming. Conflicting questions are raised on research methodology.

Consider a study in which two groups of children, in the fourth and fifth grades, were given a choice of fourteen paired items in which each pair had a less valued item available immediately or its mate available in one to four weeks.[34] Several weeks later the two groups of children, divided into low and high-delay groups, were exposed to models who not only demonstrated the opposite choice, but verbally expounded their rationale. The test was readministered a third time four and five weeks after the modeling exposure for reliability. While the high-delay children showed a marked preference toward immediate rewards, the low-delay group did not. The question arises as to whether the delay group is composed of children who may have been cognitively and intellectually superior to begin with, which may have aided delay.

An explanation solely in terms of modeling does not suffice although it is certainly relevant. Predisposing factors for influence on the part of authority figures, differential susceptibilities to persuasion, varying abilities to grasp verbal statements, and such factors as individual acquisitiveness or drive level, have been raised as possibilities. It is significant that a control group which did not witness the model shifted in a retest trial. It might be that peer interaction in seeing more valued objects other children received after a delay became relevant. Plaguing possibilities as to the desire for variety in choices, or responses to other unmeasured variables in the children or their environment remain unanswered.

Experiments in the modeling effects of promoting delayed expression of impulses suffer from such ambiguous implications. Although there is evidence that experimental exposure to a model who deviates can induce behavior temporarily, there is not sufficient evidence to substantiate that such an effect would hold up over time. When an effort is made to establish pre-existing base rates for children, the rates are usually relatively fixed once the experiment is over. This would argue for an ad hoc type of situation that is structured in such experiments. It appears that a child with usual controls can be induced to lower his inhibitions with respect to certain types of experimental deviations, but a child who is having difficulty with impulse control is relatively little influenced by a conforming model. However, the reverse question can be raised in terms of the influence of models in a naturalistic setting not being known, so that it would not be warranted to infer that conforming models in the natural setting of the child or a therapeutic center are without influence.

Apart from believers one way or another, coupled with individual (clinical) examples, we just do not know the impact of modeling in the complex life of a child outside of laboratories. The evidence is confusing on parental modeling due to the prolonged and intensive exposure to parents. There are studies that parents and children express similar moral judgments, but again questions arise in the cognitive realm regarding the expressions of judgment or testing hypothetical possibilities, such as in story completions. Even being able to appraise the moral modeling of a parent in terms of overt conduct is fraught with difficulties in making inferences as to the expectation that a child will so model.

Clinicians see cases in which model parents have children with massive acting out and antisocial tendencies. This leads to genetic and psychodynamic explanatory models. Identification in terms of overt attributes is rarely sufficient. One study dealt with conscious efforts of children to be like their parents in terms of moral indices (internal moral guilt, confession, and consideration for others). Identification did not seem related to moral development, although boys identified with fathers gave more internal reasons for their moral judgments.[35] Individuals with difficulty in the realm of impulse control appear far too complicated for intervention to affect by simply telling a parent to act in a certain way or say a certain thing so their child will change. The same limitation is unfortunately present in attempts to appraise experimentally the effect of an indulgent model versus one who denies.

Although it can be demonstrated that an object who models taking a candy will have children emulate him when the laboratory situation is one based on gain, extension is difficult. When experiments become more complicated, and hence more naturalistic, the results are complicated. Such factors as who the model is in terms of age, sex, degree of competence, all become relevant, as are the prior experiences and needs of the child to tolerate disappointments. Nor can we assume that the behavior of a child in a group is a group performance or that who the model may be is insignificant. In one thorough study which employed multivariate design, six different and independent tests were used and it was noted that those whose performance did not reach that of the model while initially not rewarding themselves were found on later tests to become more indulgent than those in control groups who had no model.[36] This could be conceptualized in terms of the cumulative frustration effect of not equaling the performance of a model which then induces acting out. The clinical model is that of the parent with exceedingly perfectionistic standards which the child cannot attain.

Determination of the variables in deferring gratification is extremely complex. External conditions, such as the influence of a model, parent, or other authority, have been investigated to delineate their specific contributions to those of the motives of the child. The vulnerability of individuals to external authority has been noted in the discussion on institutional influences. Psychodynamic formulations are relevant to exerting choice and resisting impulse expression. Experimental work on resistance to temptation has attempted to develop some type of objective external measure.

Temptation studies go back to the original Hartshorne and May work and that of MacKinnon.[37] School children were studied with respect to resistance to cheating. Variations on this methodology have requested children to complete a story in which a hero is tempted to transgress.

Another approach has been to devise a tempting situation in which to place a child. Although the child believes he is not being observed, and may have even been told so, he is in fact being observed in some manner by the experimenter, such as through a one-way mirror. The independent variable which is being studied is a situation such as the taking of a toy or candy, going where he is forbidden, or a test of increasing difficulty which the experimenter knows the child will fail. Some type of incentive beyond conformity is needed to fulfill the criterion of a tempting situation. However, note the following types of limitations. There is usually a baseline on intellectual or cognitive components which have some bearing on making choices in general as well as specifically in a situation of temptation. Nor do we know about antecedents in the individual child or his family which contribute to variability due to such factors as a high or low need to achieve or for praise. The lack of standardization of tasks used should also be noted. The need to cheat for a candy bar in a simulated situation might be more relevant as a discriminating variable for some type of developmental deviation in a child than as a measure of morality. Broader social variables are relevant as well, such as social class backgrounds of the children and their correlative attitudes about cheating and differentials connected with gender.

Consider the following paradigmatic experimental design for appraising resistance to temptation as an index of conscience functioning in a child. Only the most carefully designed features of such experiments will be included. The hypothesis is to determine how subject to an external model a child is with respect to moral behavior, such as a tempting situation or an altruistic act. Therefore, although there is some presupposition that a child has a desire for a tempting object, the manipulated variables are external to the child (the independent variable is the model and his various behaviors). In its most stringent formulation, no reference to identification processes is believed necessary since imitation is all that is required. Hence, references to earlier attachment behaviors, motives, or the requirement of identification before similar responses would occur in the absence of the model, are all viewed as unnecessary and undesirable. There is merely the development of matching behaviors between the child and the model. In its most sophisticated form, this is ascribed to temporal stimulus sequences in the model.[38] These sequences elicit perceptual responses that are later retrievable as images which guide the appropriate modeling behavior. There are accompanying verbal representations which can activate the image, given the right environmental cue. Reinforcers, which determine whether an act will occur, are based on external events, self-administration, or those vicariously experienced from any number of models.

Continuing the paradigm, does the presence of a model who yields to a situation of temptation, or resists it, have an effect on the observing child? The situation may have an activity carried out or something the child wants presented, presumably on the basis of previous conditioning. The tempting situation might be some toy or candy which is available but verbally forbidden for use or consumption. In some cases the inculcation of certain morals may be used, such as sharing or demonstrating helping behaviors.

In one experiment, fourth-grade boys were placed in a room while a movie was shown outside their range of vision.[39] Their job was to perform a boring task by pushing a button when a light came on. Models were then introduced for two groups of children, before being placed in the room, based on a "yielding" or "resisting" model in terms of motor behavior and verbal comments. A control group employed no model. The boys exposed to a yielding model were found to show less inhibition in getting up to see the movie than the resistor group. However, this disinhibition by a model was matched by the finding of no difference between the resistor group and the group with no model. The conclusion is that observing a resisting model does not contribute to resistance to temptation. However, there is nothing in modeling theory which says that only a model who promotes acting on one's desires should be imitated and not one who restrains activities.

A variation is peer models for vicarious reinforcement where the peers are witnessed receiving punishment directly or on a screen. The punishment is viewed as a cue for the prohibited nature of an act, and it is assumed that the emotional response in the observer will be analogous to that of the punished child.[40] The situation may involve a forbidden act with punishment for the deviator and no punishment, or actually a reward for the other group; it is difficult to assess whether a model who ignores a prohibited transgression is rewarding or neutral. Again, a control group with no exposure of the consequences to a child from the model by deviating is used.

In one experiment, six-year-old boys were forbidden to touch toys, and then exposed to a film with three endings. The first part of the film showed a small boy being forbidden to play with toys by a mother figure, but after she left, he played with the toys for two minutes. Ending number one showed the mother returning to play with the boy in an affectionate manner; ending number two showed the mother returning, snatching the toy and shaking the boy; ending number three was terminated at the point where the mother left and did not return; a fourth control group were boys who did not see the film at all.

Again, it is of interest that the subjects who observed the model punished deviated less with respect to touching toys in the experiment, but they deviated more than the group who did not see the film, and the group who saw neither the punishment or rewarded ends of the film had as much deviation as the reward group. Resort is made to auxiliary explanations, such as the influence of differences in social classes, where punishment may be more effective in the lower classes for inhibition.

The problem with auxiliaries is that there is no limit to such possibilities. They are used to retain a theory when findings are not convergent with implications, or to ignore inconsistent findings. Is it the punishment of the peer model which inhibits the act, or does a rewarded model have no influence in comparison to a "no exposure" group? Questions concerning the salience of the situations used to test moral behavior become relevant. Are they merely eliciting a baseline of behavior in children of a certain sex, age, and socio-economic class? Some argue that children put in a new laboratory and beginning to play with toys have a low prior probability and that, therefore, this is not de facto testing inhibition of acts to begin with. General inhibition in such situations seems operative, not necessarily countered by observing a structured model on a screen or in a laboratory setting. It would be difficult to say that observing punishment in a laboratory model for violation can be taken as sufficient evidence compared to a situation of an absent model or rewarded model who inhibits forbidden acts.

These experimental paradigms have not been discussed from the perspective of how valid they are portraying moral conduct of children in natural settings. The variables become complicated and unwieldy and, unfortunately, laboratory findings of moral conduct are not easily generalized. Even within an experimental setting such factors as intelligence are acknowledged but rarely viewed as primary determiners of moral conduct. Reference is frequently made to such factors as the children being bright, coming from academically oriented families, or citing the socio-economic situation of their school. This conflation of social class references and intelligence is frequently made.

When one is measuring something as irrelevant or monotonous as a task of button-pressing, for example, intelligence might ordinarily be a crucial variable in how to outwit or beat the monotony. Nor would reference to achievement tests or group intelligence test data suffice. There is the distinction between expressed moral judgments which correlate with resistance to temptation in which both are influenced by intelligence, social class, and status within a peer group.[41] The salience of the experimental situation for the child is another significant variable for how well he may do in performing a task—namely not responding to a certain temptation. The more intelligent and the more the child is attuned to interpersonal nuances, the better he will comprehend the nature of the experiment. As two six-year-olds put it so cogently after a resistance-to-temptation situation, "They wanted to catch me cheating," while a more bodacious one displayed his creative divergency by commenting, "I thought I'd see what would happen if I tried it."

The question of what really is being measured in such experiments cannot be answered. Should the situations described be referred to as measuring moral conduct? They are psychological behaviors operating, but whether they are in the realm of the cognitive or psychomotor realm is the question. In many situations it appears that it is the activity level of the child, or his reactivity-impulsivity level, that is in question. This holds apart from any pre-existing emotional conflict in the child or family psychopathology for which there is rarely any baseline or data given. These variables are either ignored by presuming they are irrelevant to moral conduct, or the children are considered as free of psychopathology. Even excluding these emotional components, it appears that cognitive functioning is what is being measured, such as the ability to direct attention to a task, the ability to tolerate boredom on a task without deviating or engaging in distracting motor activities or daydreams, competency at certain activities, or the capacity to occupy oneself in a position of boredom.

A cogent study offers support in this direction in which both first- and sixth-graders were appraised in terms of two independent studies which used the same subjects.[42] One study was concerned with tension, while the second examined the inter-relationships between psychomotor performance, psycho-physiological recordings, teachers' ratings of moral behavior, and cheating on tests adapted from the Hartshorne and May type of test. Persuasive evidence was presented that high correlations between experimental measures of morality and measures of attention reflect tension as the causal variable. In this type of situation, a distracting and supposedly interesting stimulus situation is created in which there is an unusual opportunity to short-cut a task. Cheating was defined as incidence of short-cutting a monotonous task or attending to illicit novel and interesting cues in the task. Experimental morality amounted to the greatest ability to stick to a boring task (possessing lower distractibility), while experimental cheating amounted to utilizing novel ways of doing a task.

The authors of the study refer to findings that adolescents high in measures of distractibility and cheating are those high in measures of divergent thinking and associating in terms of the novel and unusual. This raises possibilities for the relationship between immoral behavior and creativity. It would seem that what experimental tasks measure may be a cognitive attentional function as a variable relating to performing a task in a certain manner. Generalizations about moral behavior, apart from the discreet situation, seem hazardous.

THE ROLE OF AFFECTS IN REGULATING BEHAVIOR

The role of painful affects as a signal to cease and desist certain tendencies, or as a consequence of a deviant act, has long held a prominent place in discussions regarding moral conduct. Although guilt is the most commonly thought of affect, it is unjustified to restrict discussions to guilt while ignoring shame, rage, and disgust as painful or emergency emotions. There is also the role of welfare emotions such as joy, happiness, pride, or self-respect. The classification of the presence or absence of one affect is an oversimplification.

Focusing on guilt in experimental studies may be related to its seeming relationship to transgressions as well as lack of acquaintance with the psychological ramifications of other affects. Detection and measurement of affects raise problems for clinicians and non-clinicians alike. Similar methodological problems confront experimental attempts to confirm or deny guilt. Judging guilt solely by externals is fraught with invalidity, nor is it much help to ask, "Are you feeling guilty?" Most typically this is approached by administering projective tests or obtaining free-floating projective responses if a child, a peer, or model has deviated. A variant is having the child complete a story or give completion responses to transgressive themes.

With younger children a structured doll or puppet play theme may be used to detect guilt by permitting them to provide their own ending or describe the feelings the doll or puppet has. Such an extra step is needed even if there are indications of guilt to delineate meaningful connections to factors such as resistance to temptation, level of moral judgment, or actual deviant behavior. There are theoretical issues of cognitive precedence as discussed. If a structural framework is used, superego components must be differentiated from ego processes which have been approached experimentally, such as attention, task-conformity, and low distractibility in contrast to a superego directionality forbidding behaviors.

There is a fundamental problem. No one denies children have feelings. Yet how and to what extent are these affects involved with moral behavior and controls? Discussion in this chapter will limit itself to experimental and developmental work and keep to a minimum psychodynamic formulations which utilize affects. Only a few comments will be made to point out the difficulty in appraising the presence, degree thereof, and behavioral relevance of guilt, to illustrate how far removed many of the experimental procedures are from the role which psychodynamic formulations ascribe. This does not mean that the laboratory measures are irrelevant, but that they are analogous to resistance-to-temptation measures; they may not be dealing with moral behavior in more than a tangential sense, and hardly at all with guilt in a psychodynamic sense.

If we consider one of the necessary assumptions of guilt measurements, the discrepancy becomes more apparent. Although the story of a child who transgresses may evoke interest and feeling in a listener, it is always subject to a screening process whereby the situation itself is unreal. Unless the reality appraisal of the child is so impaired that distinguishing a fantasy production from an actual occurrence cannot take place, artificiality is present.

Philosophical considerations aside concerning arguments about realism, the child beyond infancy is making a progressively sophisticated differentiation of objects in his inner and outer life. The differentiation is aided by virtue of experimental stories being presented in terms of a child who has transgressed and not been detected, but the child is to give a pretended ending regarding the feelings of the hero. The child who actually experiences some affect, such as guilt, in this type of a situation prompts a clinical question regarding his conflicts about some aspect of his life rather than being viewed as a subject with an excessive degree of guilt as an index of his conscience functioning from the story. Rather than having an independent appraisal of the function of guilt from the story, it would be presumed that this type of child is predisposed toward the response from aspects of his past and present life. But then we are not measuring guilt with respect to a given transgression in a concocted story but the guilt of a particular child at the time of the examination.

Another type of predicament arises if a list of external criteria of guilt are used, such as overt expressions of fear. This usually amounts to summarizing expressed themes of punishment when someone in a story transgresses, which are taken as manifestations of guilt. Again, such a correlation need not hold. An expression that the subject in the story is to be punished may be an intellectual-cognitive operation without any particular affective correlates in a given subject. Some of the most blatant sociopathic individuals can invent stories in which the actors say and do the proper thing. The crux of these comments is that these measures may not be dealing with guilt or guilt-sensitivity, and they cannot be expected to be reliable as predictors of guilt, even for overt transgressions.

Many developmental questions remain unresolved concerning guilt in children and its role in controlling behavior (apart from the clinical and psychodynamic material). The age at which verbalized self-criticism emerges might be one index of guilt functioning; this is rare in young children, but common by preadolescence.[43] A study with institutionalized delinquent boys noted a correlation between degree of guilt based on content analysis, a global clinical rating subsequent to interviews, a guilt scale, and the level or moral development utilizing Kohlberg's scales.[44]

The role of punishment with respect to guilt induction in a child is also confusing. Low correlations between physically punitive parents and degrees of guilt in children remind us that punitive parents are not the main variable in guilty children. Nor is the key relationship the quantity of punishment. While children have a low but significant positive correlation between physical punishment and punishment fantasies as a consequence of transgressing, there is not such a correlation with types of transgression reactions more representative of guilt. Children who have never been physically punished may be filled with themes of punishment in their stories, which dovetails with clinical observations on guilt-ridden and impulse-ridden character problems. Hence, the vulnerability of a child toward guilt-proneness for deviating must remain elsewhere.

Another source examined is the type of parental discipline. While love-withdrawal seems a natural for guilt induction, and some findings do indicate this for measures such as confession, the results are not confirmed for self-criticism. The use of reasoning, when a child is capable of making self-critical judgments, is rather what is found necessary.

We are back to the question of why some children cannot merely ignore disturbing inner feelings subsequent to a transgression, but over a developmental period continue to experience painful affect if they transgress or are tempted to. The resort is to theories of identification to explain the greater acceptance of moral standards in a child in which there is a strong identification with adults who hold certain norms. Yet the old problems remain. Greater acceptance of parental norms, where a child strongly identifies with a warm parent, does not lead to greater moral action in terms of those norms. Even a theory of identification-based guilt with parental warmth and dependency ties has one necessary variable, as questioned from Kibbutzim data, in which the parents as affectional objects are distinct from the main source of socialization demands.[45] Bear in mind that these comments are made without taking into consideration clinical and psychodynamic formulations.

MODELING CONTROL OF AGGRESSION

The topic of delaying impulse expression cannot be discussed without reference to withholding the expression of aggression. Is this control exerted by some type of concomitant or succeeding affective warning signal, or is it due to modeling influences? Again, developmental psychology resorts to modeling influences, such as using film-mediated aggressive models.[46] Their methodology consists of exposing experimental and control groups of nursery school children to different portrayals of aggression. In one situation, an adult model appropriates the possessions of another adult and is rewarded for doing so; in another the model is punished. Two control groups are used as well, in which children observe models in vigorous but non-aggressive play, and one in which no modeling exposure occurs. The children are subsequently observed in a free-play situation and rated on their aggression.

In this case, the children who witnessed the movie where the model was punished exhibited less aggressive play than the children who saw the model rewarded, but the punishment group did not show less aggression than the control groups. A similar approach and result was obtained in which an adult model behaved aggressively toward an inflated rubber doll, Bobo. If the model was punished, the exposed children were rated as showing less aggressive behavior than children exposed to a model who received no punishment consequences for hitting Bobo, or another group who observed the model rewarded.[47]

Comments about the validity and generalizability of these experimental findings are similar to those made regarding the influence of modeling on delay or resistance. Although in the latter situation the modeling was based on something usually forbidden socially, and with aggression the modeling was of asocial behavior, the format of the experiment is not different. Within the confines of these experiments questions arise, such as the meaning of the amount of aggression in the children who see the model punished still being no less than children without any model. The question is how to interpret such data? Is the appropriate control group a group of children who see the model neither punished nor rewarded (*no consequences*), or rather one has no exposure to the model? If the no consequences group is used, it is found they demonstrate approximately the same amount of aggression as a group which sees the model rewarded; the interpretation may be given that in these cases there is a sanctioning of the aggression either by the permissiveness for it or by a reward.

Therefore, if either of these two groups are used as controls, we would expect an inordinate amount of aggressions to be present since a disinhibiting effect has been operating. The tendency would be to exaggerate the differences operating between groups. The appropriate control group would be a group not exposed to a model. When this is done, the model-punished group shows no less aggression than the amount in a no-model exposure group, while compared to a no-consequences group, a differential would be found and a conclusion offered regarding inhibition. But to explain this, auxiliary hypotheses are introduced at the low level of aggression in a group not exposed to a model, which vitiates conclusions regarding the inhibiting effect of a punished model. May this have been due to other socialization experiences the children have had in the past?

Resort to outside hypotheses, exclusive of the experimental situation, permits hypotheses regarding the effects of punishing a model to stand. But how much significance these findings have in the world of peers, social groups, multiple authority objects, and mass media, which all impinge on children in their natural habitat, is unknown.

REFERENCES

1. J. Piaget, *The World Judgment of the Child* (New York: The Free Press, 1965.).
2. *Ibid.* p. 324.
3. R. Schafer, *Aspects of Internalization* (New York: International Universities Press, 1968).
4. H. Hartshorne and M. A. May, *Studies in the Nature of Character* vols. 1-3 (New York: Macmillan, (1929-1936).
5. R. V. Burton, The generality of honesty reconsidered, *Psychological Review*, 70(1963):481-500.
6. A. Bandura and R. Walters, *Adolescent Aggression* (New York: Ronald Press, 1959).
7. R. Barndt and D. Johnson, Time orientation in delinquents, *Journal of Abnormal Social Psychology*, 51(1955):343-347.
8. D. Ricks and C. Umbarger, A measure of increased temporal perspective, Paper presented at the Eastern Psychological Association, April, 1963.
9. W. Mischel, Delay of gratification and deviant behavior, Paper presented at the Society for Research in Child Development, Berkeley, California, April, 1963.
10. L. Kohlberg, Development of moral character and moral ideology, *Review of Child Development Research*, 1:391. (New York: Russell Sage Foundation, 1964).
11. D. Lykken, A study of anxiety in the sociopathic personality, *Journal of Abnormal Social Psychology*, 55(1957):6-10.
12. Conscience, ed. by R. Sears, L. Raw and R. Alpert, *Identification and Child-Rearing* (Stanford: University Press, 1965).
13. Kohlberg, op. cit., p. 392.
14. R. Sears, E. Maccoby and H. Levin, *Patterns of Child Rearing* (Evanston: Row, Peterson, and Co., 1957).

15. L. Kohlberg, The development of children's quantitives toward a moral order. I: sequence in the development of moral thought, *Vita Humana* 6(1963):11-33.

16. L. Kohlberg, Moral development and identification, *Child Psychology, 62nd Yearbook of the National Society for the Study of Education*, ed. H. Stevenson (Chicago: University of Chicago Press, 1963).

17. L. Kohlberg, op. cit., p. 405.

18. J. Aronfreed, The origin of self-criticism, *Psychological Review* 71(1964):193-218.

19. A. Bandura and R. H. Walters, *Social Learning and Personality Development* (New York: Holt, Rinehart and Winston, 1963).

20. R. V. Burton, E. E. Maccoby, and W. Allinsmith, Antecedents of resistence to temptation in four-year-old children, *Child Development* 32(1961):689-710.

21. R. Sears, L. Rau, and R. Alpert, *Identification and Child Rearing* (Stanford: Stanford University Press, 1965).

22. J. Aronfreed, The effects of experimental socialization paradigms upon two moral responses to transgression, *Journal of Abnormal Social Psychology* 66(1963:437-448.

23. A. J. Reiss, Social organization and socialization: variations on a theme about generations, Paper 1, Center for Research on Social Organization (Ann Arbor: University of Michigan, 1965).

24. S. Milgram, *Obedience to Authority: An Experimental View* (New York: Harper and Row, 1974).

25. O. G. Brim, Jr. and S. Wheeler, *Socialization After Childhood.* (New York: John Wiley and Sons, 1966).

26. J. W. M. Whiting, et al., The learning of values, in *People of Rimrock*, ed. E. Z. Vogt, and E. M. Albert (Cambridge: Harvard University Press, 1966).

27. R. H. Walters and L. DemKow, Timing of punishment as a determinant of response, *Child Development* 34(1963):207-214.

28. E. E. Maccoby, The development of moral values and behavior in childhood, *Socialization and Society*, ed. J. A. Clausen (Boston: Little, Brown and Co., 1968).

29. W. C. Becker, Consequences of different kinds of parental discipline, *Review of Child Development Research vol. 1.* pp.169-208 (New York: Russell Sage Foundation, 1964).

30. E. S. Schaefer, Converging conceptual models for maternal behavior and for child behavior, *Parental Attitudes and Child Behavior*, ed. J. C. Glidewell (Springfield: Charles C Thomas, 1961).

31. M. J. Hoffman, Childrearing practices and moral development: generalizations from emperical research, *Child Development* 34(1963):295-318.

32. D. Baumrind, Effects of authoritative parental control on child behavior, *Child Development* 37(1966):887-907.

33. W. Mischel, Theory and research on the antecendents of self-imposed delay of reward, *Progress in Experimental Personality Research*, ed. B. A. Maher, vol. 2 (New York: Academic Press, 1965).

34. A. Bandura and W. Mischel, Modification and self-imposed delay of reward through exposure to live and symbolic models, *Journal of Personality and Social Psychology* 2(1965):698-705.
35. M. L. Hoffman and H. D. Saltzstein, Parent discipline and the child's moral development, *Journal of Personality and Social Psychology* 5(1967):45-57.
36. A. Bandura and C. Whalen, The influence of antecedent reinforcement and divergent modeling cues on patterns of self-reward, *Journal of Personality and Social Psychology* 3(1966):373-382.
37. D. W. Mackinnon, Violation of prohibitions, *Exploration in Personality*, ed. H. W. Murray, pp. 491-501 (New York: Oxford University Press, 1938).
38. A. Bandura, Social-learning theory of identity processes, *Handbook of Socialization Theory and Research*, ed. D. A. Goslin (Chicago: Rand McNally, 1968).
39. A. H. Stein, Imitation of resistance to temptation, *Child Development* 38(1967):157-169.
40. R. H. Walters and R. D. Parke, Emotional arousal, isolation, and discrimination learning in children, *Journal of Experimental Child Psychology* 1(1964):163-173.
41. Kohlberg, op. cit., p. 409.
42. P. F. Grim, L. Kohlberg, and S. H. White, Some relationships between conscience and attentional processes, *Journal of Personality and Social Psychology* 8(1968):239-252.
43. J. Aronfreed, The nature, variety, and social patterning of moral responses to transgression, *Journal of Abnormal Psychology* 63(1961):223-241.
44. E. H. Ruma and D. L. Mosher, Relationship between moral judgement and guilt in delinquent boys, *Journal of Abnormal Psychology* 72(1967):122-127.
45. A. I. Rabin, *Growing Up in the Kibbutz* (New York: Springer Publishing, 1965).
46. A. Bandura, D. Ross and S. Ross, Vicarious reinforcement and imitative learning, *Journal of Abnormal Psychology* 67(1963):601-607.
47. A. Bandura, Influences of models reinforcement contingencies in the acquisition of imitative responses, *Journal of Personality and Social Psychology* 1(1965):589-595.

Chapter Eight

Self-Control as a Power Game

Past decades have witnessed the expansion and clarification of concepts related to an emerging ego psychology. In turn, presently we see a growing preoccupation with problems related to a superego psychology. Although the shaft may not be dramatic, it does lead to the necessity for a clarification of systems. Interactions between different psychological structures, and a general re-evaluation of the development of a functional superego system, need examination. The functions ascribed to the construct *superego*, examined in the context of clinical experience, illustrate how and why psychopathological deviations originate.

The manifestations of self-control in the child until approximately six years of age represent an anlage that is given freer rein in adolescence. Focus is on the developmental fluctuations of conscience in the young child. Emphasis is placed upon the susceptibility to experiential influences which affect the manner in which the child achieves discharge, mastery, and control over his impulse life. The perfection of such a mental structure occurs from two main sources: (1) inhibition of certain desires, (2) idealizations which emerge and the nature of the early narcissistic injuries which lead to lifelong reparative efforts.

The early moral activities of the child are seen as amoral.page 3 Behavior initially is controlled by fundamental biological strivings for pleasure-seeking or pain-avoidance. Tendencies to re-live and cope with experiences by repetition are not necessarily congruent with the avoidance of pain. Fundamental questions are implicit: How is it that guilt and subsequent needs for penance arise? What are the psychological processes which propel such affective development? In a broader sense, how does a child become socialized and acquire a control system? Is it all just a matter of drives seeking gratification and defenses arising?

DEVELOPMENTAL ISSUES

The first humans with whom an infant is intimate can inculcate in him feelings of trust and confidence—basic feeling states responsible for how the world comes to be viewed by the child. Work done in the area of maternal deprivation makes apparent that the infant can sustain multiple and critical injuries which predispose toward later emotional disturbances. The debatable issue is whether techniques can be found to predict which type of specific psychopathology might develop from these unfortunate experiences occurring at vulnerable developmental stages. With respect to a control system the question is: What disturbances of later superego functioning result from influences operating at particular ages, or what were once described as "critical periods" of development?

Infantile Narcissism. Infantile narcissism as a developmental stage is relevant to the development of a system of controls. It is believed that narcissistic disturbances originate from conflicts in this early phase, and struggles with narcissism are of great significance for a conscience template. Unfortunately, the concept of narcissism has been plagued by theoretical confusion. It has been used to refer to: type of libido or its object in the psychoanalytic literature; a stage of development, a type or mode of object choice; an attitude (sold on oneself); psychological structures or personality types. To complicate matters further, some of these refer to normal development and some to pathological.[1]

Primary narcissism is used as a hypothetical construct referring to a state of psychological equilibrium in a person analogous to an idealized nirvana state. Since conditions of perfect bliss are unattainable, except briefly, objects are perceived as existing primarily to gratify oneself so a relative narcissistic balance is maintained. Empirically, the earliest interactions with objects for receiving and taking as well as loving and being loved are put into operation. Infantile omnipotence is compromised repeatedly by the gradual realization that others must be depended upon for satisfaction. The antithesis of narcissism is not an independent existence of another object, but rather a quality and feeling state of love for an object. Such qualitative relationships allow an infant to experience a narcissistic equilibrium rather than merely a profusion of random object contacts. Early narcissistic injuries contribute toward many later clinical phenomena, such as proneness to depression, acting out, and schizoid withdrawal. Each of these has its own developmental deviation for conscience functioning, but the feeling of helplessness before another power appears basic.

From the External to the Internal. Transmitting and absorbing external objects, and their multiple representations and associated feelings, into the mental life of a child remains a psychological problem with many unanswered questions. The answers are relevant to the topic of how humans socialize and interpersonally affect one another. Clinical discussions of the development of progressive controls over feelings and impulses presuppose some type of differentiation process which occurs within a mental structure.

Ego psychology assumes that the infant possesses inhibitory apparatuses even before a set of ego processes has emerged from an undifferentiated matrix.[2] This type of theorizing receives its greatest criticism from behaviorally oriented psychologists for whom such terms as conscience or superego carry too much surplus meaning. References to "inner controls" are viewed as reifications. Only descriptions of "self-control," defined in terms of self-generated stimuli which observably control certain responses, are permitted. "If any of the critical responses or response-produced stimuli are not observable, then no application of the concept of self-control can justifiably be made."[3] Inhibition of acts without an accompanying verbal indicator of the response-produced stimulation would be considered an unwarranted inference. Such parsimonious theorizing cannot be quarreled with if the limits to which it is applicable are clearly stated. It would even hold for very discrete situations in which a child is willing to oblige with observable stimulus and response patterns which the experimenter considers necessary for a description of functional relationships. There is acknowledgment of difficulties with physiological processes in this regard, but behaviorally oriented workers continue to hope that more of such processes will become observable, even though the physiological processes themselves are intraorganismic.

A clinician is greatly restricted in attempting to confine data to nothing but observables as defined above. Though the rigorously empiricist part of the clinician may resonate to the neatness of the approach, its constrictiveness restricts working operations. Clinical data are not neat, nor are they often directly observable. On the contrary, they are usually quite complex and multi-determined. Particularly is this so when efforts are made not merely to describe phenomena, such as the choices a child has made, but to account for and make predictions as to why the child has made particular choices. The development and execution of judgments are directly relevant to the types of controls which begin to be exercised. At present there does not appear to be a valid philosophical criticism to utilizing concepts with surplus meanings which many other scientific theories employ. If critics object to such theories, it becomes a matter of empirically demonstrating the usefulness, or lack of usefulness, of employing specific hypothetical constructs which allow for cognitive referents beyond observable data.

Internalization is a concept derived from empirical data. Children beginning to imitate parental behavior verbally and nonverbally is an example. Children also directly observe incorporative acts when objects are ingested, such as in eating. Internalization also extends to psychological processes referred to as "introjection," where mental representations occur apart from external and observable data. This permits data from fantasies to be treated as significant and usable. If a critic argues that such data are not observable and therefore not scientific, another can maintain that the construct is useful since it permits further empirical propositions to be derived which are connectable to observables. Moreover, the derivations are subject to scientific criteria such as testability, preciseness, predictability, generality, coherence, and consistency. Internalization is a principle operating with imitation, introjection, and identification in two ways: defensive and developmental. Development of a control system by virtue of these processes allow for the gradual replacement of controls based solely on the presence of external supports.[4] In place of, or in preference to, a dependency on the outside world or stimuli for regulation by societal threats or coercion, an autonomy or gradual independence of control is gained as a progressive developmental landmark. Whether this is an ideal that can be entirely attained is another debatable issue.

Empirical Data. Empirical evidence indicates a primitive struggle in infants for control over impulses. In the context of their frustration, they are led to attempts at taking it out on oneself. A common example is the physiological need to bite, appearing at approximately six months and which is not only pain-relieving to tender gums but pleasurable in its own right. Yet the response of the mother sets sharp limits to these activities which are punished. Erikson feels that, "This point in the individual's early history can be the origin of an evil dividedness, where anger against gnawing teeth, and anger against the withdrawing mother, and anger with one's impotent anger all lead to a forceful experience of sadistic and masochistic confusion, leaving the general impression that once upon a time one destroyed one's unity with a maternal matrix. This earliest catastrophe in the individual's relation to himself and to the world is probably the ontogenetic contribution to the Biblical stage of paradise, where the first people on earth forfeited forever the right to pluck without effort what had been put at their disposal; they bit into the forbidden apple, and made God angry. . . . A drastic loss of accustomed mother love without proper substitution at this time can lead (under otherwise aggravating conditions) to acute infantile depression or to a mild but chronic state of mourning which may give a depressive undertone to the whole remainder of life."[5]

Does this fatalistically predispose each individual to a potential feeling of badness and depression based on infantile impulses to bite? The nurturer must be viewed as a source of both gratification and deprivation, depending on whether the situation is one of pleasure or of inflicting pain in some manner (as an enemy might). Such potentials might be actualized in varying degrees, depending upon the intensity of infantile losses and deprivations, but they would also seem to be contingent upon many subsequent experiences.

Somewhere in the period between nine and twelve months infants begin to shake their heads from side to side as though communicating a no by gesture. The shaking is associated with behavior of the parenting condemning in the form of a verbal *no-no*. The head shaking is based on a biological pattern which earlier led the infant to rotate his head sideways toward the nipple, and by six months to rotate his head away from the breast when satiated as an expression of withdrawal. Spitz viewed the no-no as the first semantic symbol to function on an abstract level, in contrast to such global expressions as "ma-ma," which have innumerable meanings. That a process of internalization going beyond the initial imitative efforts has begun, is evident when the child is observed to shake his head as he approaches a forbidden object. Thus, a ten-month-old child who has knocked over a lamp and been punished by a slap may subsequently be observed standing near the tempting object shaking his head, or a fourteen-month-old who has turned on the burner of a stove and been similarly reprimanded may be seen standing in front of the stove saying no-no verbally and physically.

Efforts to conceptualize these behaviors purely as a change from a social positive reinforcement of receiving parental attention to a social negative reinforcement based on discriminating punishment do not seem adequate even at this early age, nor do they serve as a sufficient explanatory premise for the meaning of the no-no. Rather, they are descriptions of what is immediately observable. Even with such operational theorizing, the situation is more comparable to a conflict situation where the infant must choose between alternatives, such as to touch or not to touch, but parental attention is also sustained—along with a negative reinforcement—so that the child is not confronted merely with a mutually exclusive choice. Such maintenance of parental attention is believed conducive to internalization.

Attempts to conceal or escape also emerge in infancy which acquire subtlety. A child of one year who has been caught doing something prohibited may seek to run away from the parent, or hide a hand behind their back when they have touched a forbidden object. Struggles to control impulses and evade external control now appear. A twelve-month-old infant may be forbidden to touch an object. However, the infant is observed repeatedly pushing an object closer and closer to the forbidden object and gingerly reaching out toward it. When the parent does not watch, the child is observed to smile and perhaps touch the object. One of the earliest power games has been won.

Another facet of the early phase of these struggles for internalization is self-punitive behavior. During the first year, motor disturbances occur in the form of head banging, head rolling, and self hitting, which are rather frequent occurrences. These may progress to bruises and other injuries which are viewed as maladaptive patterns in handling aggression. (Cases in which such patterns are due to organic factors, such as headaches or otitis media are not considered here.) Originally, such behavior was believed a response to frustrating conditions or stimuli, a miscarried attempt to express hostility toward others or against external objects. It was hypothesized that the hostility was being retroflexed against the initiator.

These self-punitive mechanisms for coping with anger are one prototype for a type of depression associated with defective internal regulation of affect. However, the model of retroflexed aggression, when external expression is blocked, does not generalize to many cases. Such behavior can simply be discharge-oriented, irrespective of the recipient, or it can be a response to the need for stimulation as a counterirritant to offset other psychological or physiological states.[7] As an external object is introjected, retroflection of an impulse may refer to aggression directed against this internalized psychic representation, or to defensive identification with an external object. In some cases, autoaggression also functions as an aid to delineate body boundaries, or to project blame from one part of the body to another. An eighteen-month-old child who has touched a forbidden object is observed hiding his hand as though saying, "My hand (not I) did it." When caught for such a misdeed, some children actually slap the guilty hand with the innocent one.

Theorists differ as to whether such turning of aggression against the self can occur before, or only after, the existence of a functioning superego. Observational and developmental evidence indicates it occurs much before that time. Psychophysiological skin disorders illustrate a similar mechanism. Some infants compulsively scratch themselves when angry, or push their fists into their eyes. Undoubtedly, blending of equipmental sensitivities and situational factors subtly occurs in the individual who focuses on the skin as a place to express feelings.

More dramatic are instances of self biting, to the point of bleeding. Such phenomena have too frequently been passed off as extreme degrees of psychopathology confined to retarded, brain-damaged, or psychotic children. However, many sporadic instances of similar behavior can be observed among infants and children taken from normative investigations without such malignant diagnoses. Whatever varied and individually determined motivation such autoaggressive activity has, the self-aggressive element is overtly evident. Although it may be theoretically impossible to direct aggression against the *self* (ego), before a distinct concept of the self and its boundaries exists, aggression may be directed against the *body* from the earliest period of life. Attacks upon the psychological structure of the ego necessitate a higher degree of psychological structuralization and understanding of masochism.

THE QUEST FOR CONTROL

Increasing Ego Capacity. The entire period from the second to the fourth year is crucial for the template of future superego functioning. Not only the battle of the pot, but general increases in motor, language, and perceptual activites occur. The very act of walking allows for a broader field in which conflict or forbidden behavior can be expressed. Emergence of communicative language allows verbal opposition, or the capacity to comply verbally but not in deed as another power game. Language development permits the utilization of a mode other than motor discharge for handling feelings. It may allow for a confirmation of feelings by those with whom the child is intimate, and make a contribution to the ability of the child to accept such feelings as an inner reality.

In contrast to primitive societies where older children lead the young into the bushes without the complicated paraphernalia of modern bathrooms, the setting for toilet training is further complicated by the cultural impact of the need for cleanliness. The child now has sphincter control as a potent weapon in coercive, defiant, or manipulative attempts. Control over feeding is a relatively mutual process between mother and infant, but sphincter control tips the balance in favor of the child. Anxieties related to lack or loss of body control become equated with lack of sphincter control and concern that things might remain so. Parental behavior can convey shame and disgust, and by use of techniques such as cajolery, bribery, and begging convey models for exercising control over others and for dealing with oneself.

The Feeling of Uncontrollability. Literal sensations of having an uncontrollable monster within are related to fantasies in the two-three year old. Feelings of alienation result from attempts to isolate oneself from the foreign presence. Struggles over impulse mastery may persist into adolescence, with secret fantasies that when one is threatened by the possibility of impulse expression, an animal takes over. In some severely conflicted adolescents the fantasy may be experienced in a concrete manner and be associated with a pictorial image of a specific animal or a specific name. A boy with an overt obsessional neurosis revealed a secret fear of suspecting a dead animal, probably a rat, had remained in his bowel for years. He believed that when he was three an animal had crawled into his anus from the toilet bowl, which accounted for the smell associated with bowel movements. Intellectually he realized that this was not so, but the feeling state persisted in isolation and undiminished intensity for years.

Abstract world systems and communal practices of purifying a contaminated body before acceptance or redemption may have genetic psychological connections with efforts to get rid of the enemy within. Such children develop a distorted body image and feel compelled to wage a constant war against an evil which is part of them. Self-hatred generated in this manner may induce a child to seek punishment or project hate onto others so he feels external objects hate him—one origin of persecutors. Nor can the transactional element be ignored with respect to feeling one is hated. The hate is generated not only in attempts to control forbidden strivings, but is also sensed in the feelings of those on whom one is dependent. A chronically hostile, conflicted parent induces self-hate in a child. By four years of age, a child may candidly tell a parent, "Daddy, you don't like me and then I don't like myself." Such reciprocal exchanges of affect between parent and child begin in the earliest imitations, and continue in multiple ways throughout subsequent developmental periods.

During this period, a rudimentary system of self-regulation arises which Ferenczi designated as "sphincter morality."[8] This refers to the child's self-esteem being contingent upon complying with the toilet-training requests of the parent. "I am good only if I have a bowel movement in such and such a place, and bad if I do it in my pants." In a context of mutual trust and respect, rather than hatred and rage, the child's control over his body progresses with decreasing remnants of oppositional behavior. A preponderance of negative emotions such as hate, rage, or jealousy are later perpetuated via overt defiance and sneaky behavior. The association of such characterological traits with resistance to socialization and later antisocial behavior is apparent. The stage is set for acting out feelings of rage associated with conflicts of whether to give in or not. Emotional paralysis associated with helplessness promotes behavior leading to its alleviation. Feelings of gross injustice or a need to get even are derivatives of such struggles, and they can break through a deficient control system at adolescence.

Encopresis is a paradigmatic symptom of unresolved conflicts of this stage. In such expressions parents and children play morality games of hiding soiled underwear or throwing it away. Usually sadistic elements are involved. The parent may force the child to wash the soiled underclothing with bare hands, or demand that the clothing be exhibited to neighbors or visitors under the guise of teaching morals.

One eleven-year-old encopretic girl, without signs of organicity or mental deficiency, would crawl under her porch steps and defecate crouching and barking like a dog. A large collection of soiled underclothing was collected in her hideaway. An adolescent boy, when angry at teachers, would leave a stool lying on the washroom floor to convey his hate and contempt. Fecal calling cards may be left at the scene of crimes—especially burglary and thefts—to convey similar feelings. Soldiers abandoning an area to the enemy may leave feces scattered about as an expression of their feelings. The discomfort and humiliation attendant upon conflicts about obedience and authority are one source of a lasting resentment and persistent desire for vengeance.

Negativisim. Strivings for autonomy are discernible in the changed manner in which the two- or three-year-old uses the word no. Attempts to master the impulse to negate appear in the form of games which children play. At bedtime children three years of age state repetitiously, "No, no, no, no"; or they may indulge in games of reversal, such as looking in a mirror and calling the image a copycat or a not me as part of the struggle to differentiate themselves. Cognitive and affective splits occur in the ego preparatory to observing and evaluating oneself as later superego functions. Depersonalization is developmentally connected with these experiences.

About 50 percent of American children learn no as their first word, an interesting cultural observation in its own right. Developmentally, it reflects strivings for autonomy. A child may be flexing his controls in an effort to test whether he can make a decision. For example, a child may refuse to accept something which he really desires. This may indicate a struggle to master his own impulses in a learning situation with other people. It is the beginning of his ability to say no to his impulses.

A similar principle is witnessed in three-year-olds who constantly change their minds. Behavior which an adult interprets as antagonistic may in reality function as a self-testing device. A child who repeatedly asks for permission to go outside finally gets an adult to agree, but often the child responds with a no after receiving the desired permission. If the adult accepts this at face value, he may be chagrined to find the child protesting and reiterating, "I want to." One alternative is to quash and ridicule such strivings for autonomy. From the standpoint of superego formation, the use of *shame* as an educational technique results in an affective state of nakedness and humiliation about one's impulses and the self from which they originate. Feelings of worthlessness and hatefulness toward oneself arise rather than condemnation of certain acts. Such a device for controlling behavior says, "You as a person are worthless and shameful." Feelings of social ostracism and alienation become the norm. Another result may be a repetitious seeking to get away with things, since detection brings such painful humiliation. Brooding about ways to get even against the rule givers may begin.

The Precocious Conscience. A more specific danger for conscience structure is the precocious or overmanipulative one. "Denied the gradual and well-guided experience of the autonomy of free choice, or weakened by an initial loss of trust, the sensitive child may turn against himself all his urge to discriminate and to manipulate. Repetitiveness becomes an end for its own defensive sake rather than serving any productive purposes."[9] This is often an accompaniment of a control system based on repetition and perfectionism. These qualities are used to manipulate authorities who are viewed as arbitrary and unjust. When there is a desire to deceive, even the wish may lead to attempts at negation, to convince oneself that controls will not falter. The child alternates between a pseudohumility and feelings of shame. An apologetic manner is coupled with fears of exposure punctuated by precipitous attempts to achieve a defiant autonomy.

Obsessional devices are observed developmentally as a control measure. Magic words and rituals counter talion fears. Elements of caricature taper as well as ridicule external authority's demand for conformity and cleanliness. Early obsessional behavior can thus be a mimicry to taper the standards being placed upon the child prior to their defensive use: "I will not only clean my hands but wash them five times before every meal."

This parody of a moral system once led Freud to describe the obsessional neuroses as a private religion.[10] Such behavior is related to the ego function of observing oneself in action as well as on reflection. Multiple levels of discharge and control operate when a five-year-old demands her mother participate in her hand-washing rituals, with angry outbursts if the mother does not comply. The raw, red hands of the child also effect a self-punitive regulatory mechanism for transggression and a punishment for the mother who cannot avoid seeing damage.

A good deal of civilized behavior is based on the fear and avoidance of being caught. Since an external agency is still the prime regulator of behavior, one cannot yet speak of a functioning superego, conceived of as an internal agency. Moreover, for the preoedipal child, feelings and impulses often have greater reality than do external objective criteria. It takes until the fourth year for the child cognitively to become aware of what truth is in the sense of differentiating external reality from inner experiences, desires, fancies, and aspirations. The straightforward factual contradictions which a child denies are examples.

At times, drive strength coupled with a weak ego determines deviations even when externalized control is present. Hence, the phrase that the pleasure was worth the price. By age seven the child has become almost obsessively preoccupied with the problem of lying and cheating, but by eight years he can again comfortably lie, boast, or put on since he knows himself what external reality is and is not. Behavioral regulation based primarily on not getting caught suffers from several unfortunate consequences from the standpoint of the individual who does not progress beyond it and for society.

Parental prohibitions are often greatly exaggerated, so that the child fears horrible punishment for transgressions which have overtones of oral or anal destruction, such as being eaten or blown apart. A six-year-old psychotic boy whose behavior fluctuated between autistic withdrawal and devious ward behavior repetitively expressed fears in therapy of being "bombed by shit." He had panic episodes in which he lay crouching in a corner or under a table. Minor reprimands led to smearing feces on himself.

External authority may be evaded, but the danger of detection by some type of magnified and distorted inner authority is an ever-present reality. Various guises develop to appease authority which contribute to sneaky qualities. Traits of becoming a stickler, or pretending to feel sorry while no such feelings are experienced portray this. As Ferenczi stated, "And out of this lie morality came into existence."[11] Such feignings of regret must be distinguished from the emerging capacity for genuine *empathy* as a forerunner of an ego capacity, in contrast to a superego defect permitting such pretending.[12] The child is capable of identifying with another person and sensing that person's painful feelings. He then indicates he is sorry. Such concern is viewed as a step leading to an ability to console oneself when needed (the loving aspects of the superego) by "identification with the comforter." To ensure the continuance of gratifications from pleasure-giving objects in the environment, there is a continuous introjection in fantasy. The threat of separation from these objects engenders anxiety (which may be one factor contributing to the nucleus for later propensities to act out).

The presence of conscious fantasies of merging with love objects is part of normal development up to three years of age. Beyond that age transitory fusions between the self and external objects occur which contribute to an individual's empathic capacity to relate. The tendency toward fusion always remains, and under stressful conditions (catastrophies, dominating authority figures) may be seen in efforts to merge with each other or with their persecutors. This explains some cases of false confession as well as group regressions in moral standards.[13]

At this developmental level of conscience categorical judgments begin. People and objects are either good or bad and compromises tolerated poorly (if at all). A child feels he is bad, regardless of whether the behavior was motivated by an attempt to control bad impulses or was actually a forbidden bad activity. Unsophisticated and blatant attempts to manipulate adults in the environment make their appearance. A four-year-old unabashedly tells an adult how much he loves him shortly after having performed a prohibited act, or prior to carrying out forbidden behavior. Such behavior is the beginning of bribery, first directed toward external objects and later toward agencies of the superego. The goal is to obtain permission from a poorly integrated authority—external or internal—to perform or think prohibited acts or thoughts. A similar defect is the corruptibility of the superego in which a first act leads to a second act of atonement which is then used as permission for further transgressions in a vicious cycle.

Such a pattern is observed in acts of sexual perversity as well, in which unresolved problems of shame are present. This may have components of bribing the superego: the child performs a meritorious act but punishes himself to purchase the pleasure he is seeking. A comparable attitude is seen in storing up little acts of denial as the price for future indulgences. Exaggerated kindness before or following transgressions indicate similar types of efforts to manipulate one's control system.

Role of Defenses. As the defensive capacities of the ego develop, certain defenses are used to consolidate the superego and alleviate the discomfort attendant upon wishes or acts which have been prohibited. These are defenses directed against guilt which is the sina qua non of superego functioning. These defenses make their appearance at about three years of age, when projection of blame is common. "You shouldn't have left the cookie jar out for me to take one," implying that the mother is responsible for the child eating the cookie. The same mechanism is seen in adults who are struggling to control behavior, as a woman who carries on an affair when her husband is out of town blames him for putting her in such a tempting situation.

Displacement and externalization are seen in efforts to hypostasize an external control system which will stop one from misbehaving. Hence, the games and associated fears of being detected by bogeymen or policemen. Externalization is employed to portray the conflict emerging between impulses and their prohibition. Theories of the good guys versus the bad guys are repetitively re-enacted, with the forces of evil often represented by some thief, monster, or beast over which smaller, but more virtuous individuals (perhaps toy soldiers or cowboys) triumph in the end. Pervasiveness of such dichotomies in society indicate they are not resolved easily. Once it is realized that in the psychic life of the child, actually committed acts, wishes, fantasies, and words are equated, and have the same economic-dynamic function, the universality of such mechanisms becomes clearer.

Themes of guilt and atonement attain prominence and are observed in dreams and play activities of children at this transitional stage of superego formation. Devices like Pinocchio's Jiminy Cricket may help an immature conscience decide what to do and admonish it when a control system falters. Questions pertaining to power and submission become frequent when the child's psychological structure is solidifying—a process reinforced by religio-cultural norms. A five-year-old asks, "Who is more powerful than God?" Or, he comes up with unanswerable philosophical questions as, "Who punishes God when He is naughty?" or, "Why is swearing bad?"

Another phenomenon seen in immature or defective consciences is superego isolation. Isolation allows prohibitions to be experienced at one time but not at another. By temporarily vacating controls, the child acts out impulses he would not otherwise be capable of acting upon. In some, such periods of selective license remain as a consolidated structure within the personality. The behavior of suffering first as permission for later indulgence, or the need to expiate after having experienced pleasure, are analogous. Some use therapy as a justification for indulgence outside therapy hours. Another example of maladaptive patterns is compulsive hard work, either preceding or following indulgence in pleasure. These measures are reinforced by cultural practices such as holidays of indulgence, or by cultural myths such as hard work being rewarded or success not be achievable by other means. When their fallacies are revealed, anger and a need for revenge on authorities who perpetuate such myths is seen. Explosive forms of acting out aggression by fighting, sending threatening letters, or planting explosives. are not uncommon. The disillusioned terrorist shares many of these characteristics.

Carrying out condemned acts with equanimity under certain conditions is similarly based on dissociation of certain superego functions. In such cases, the child's identification figures are unsatisfactory or defective, so that a license to carry out behavior varies with the situation the child is in. For this reason a consistent degree of internalized controls does not progress. Instead, a hybrid set of standards give the character structure a quality of unpredictability. Amazement is registered when a nine-year-old boy who is a model and an outstanding student is caught hanging cats, or when a girl, known only for her assiduous hard work and shyness, is found to enjoy experiments of burning live animals.

Many of these behaviors reveal reaction formations. There is a breakthrough of impulses that were not renounced and toward which adequate defenses were never accomplished. Consider the sixteen-year-old honor student with a lifetime of laudatory reports who suddenly takes a rifle and kills several pedestrians before committing suicide. These are extreme examples of the struggle that occurs in all children, though most of them achieve greater synthesis.

There is the famous case of Charles Whitman who killed fourteen people and wounded thirty-one by a rifle with a telescope sight from a tower at the University of Texas. The night before Whitman had killed his mother and wife and meticulously arranged deatils for what he knew would be called an atrocity.[14] However, it should be noted that the most civilized nations also reward their citizens for carrying out antisocial acts under the banner of national defense. The ease of vacating internalized standards varies widely among people. At one end of the scale are those who reveal they were never able to pull a trigger or who shot over the enemy's head; at the other end are men who idealize manifestations of their aggression by referring to them as noble causes or serving a higher purpose.

CULTURAL ASPECTS

A culmination of superego precursors occurs during the oedipal period. The attempt of Freud to establish an ultimate phylogenetic basis of all guilt is rarely accepted today without qualifications and questions.[15] He speculated that the claims of religious and moral codes which gave them cogency were based on a primeval act of parricide which permitted the appropriation of the women who belonged to the father. An everlasting guilt and need for repentance was established in mankind.

One obvious difficulty in this explanation lies in its failure to account for guilt in women. Freud did not hypothesize that the females of the tribe practiced matricide. In a variation of this theme, Margaret Mead hypothesized, on the basis of recent paleological and ethological work, that an actual deed of parricide may have occurred, although not in the time perspective of our species, but possibly at an earlier time when no physiological latency occurred. The young prehuman may have repeated parricidal acts for hundreds of thousands of years.

A standard psychoanalytic view holds that the establishment of a moral system is related to attempts at resolution of the oedipal struggle, so that at the beginning of the Oedipus situation one cannot yet speak of a superego. Superego development is contingent upon the subsequent utilization of the hatred felt at that time for rivals within the family matrix. The two specific components of the oedipal conflict—incestuous wishes toward the parent of the opposite sex, and death wishes toward the parent of the same sex— are believed crucial for internalization and the perpetuation of a superego structure. Fears of retaliatory punishment exist, as well as fears of losing parental love and support. The resultant ambivalence is the driving force that impels the finalization of a mental structure which is a conglomerate of functions in the service of self-control and self-esteem. Psychoanalytic theory assumes that introjection of parental standards is continuously and progressively solidified by an identification with the oedipal introjection. Castration anxiety in the boy, and its analogue in the girl, is posited to be phase specific fear that provides the motivational impetus to renounce oedipal strivings.

In theoretical terms, it is a shift of instinctual cathexes from the original objects to their identification models within the ego. These later become part of the superego, which is the heir of and substitute for oedipal relationships. Further ongoing identifications crystallize the superego and give it the strength for control of behavior. Drive neutralization and the enlargement of conflict-free ego functions are promoted. The ego behaves toward the superego as an internal and irrevocable—although not unmodifiable—educator. Maturation of ego functions such as reality testing, synthesis, memory, conceptual capacity, and the experiencing of affect also contribute to a stabilized conscience. In this way superego development cannot actually be discussed apart from ego development. A level of ego maturation for conceptualization is needed for effective superego functioning.

Introjected are largely the values, conflicts and conscience defects of parental figures. The process contributes a stabilizing, conservative element in the sense that similar values are perpetuated. However, the potential for a disorganizing effect exists if adult educators transmit their conflicts to the child. Moreover, there is an element of inevitability: if the parents express tenderness and affection, children do not appear capable of escaping some degree of socialization and at least a rudimentary conscience structure. Closely related is the question of the universality of the oedipal situation. The wide ramifications of this issue will only be noted by reference to problems of conscience development in different cultures.

If conflict about oedipal obejcts plays a crucial role in the solidification of conscience, different conflicts in various cultures determine which processes pertain to conscience formation. Several of these issues were debated over fifty years ago between Ernest Jones and the anthropologist Bronislaw Malinowski. They remain confused.[16] The issue is not solely a matter of semantics but partially a matter of how data should be interpreted, as well as a controversy about the nature of oedipal objects. One of the issues pertains to the question of whether the oedipal struggle takes place only with parents and whether it is necessary to explain variations as denials or displacements from this one relationship.

With the increasing work on the relationship between personality and culture and the expansion of ego psychology, a wider framework has evolved. However, even with an instinctual approach, a greater latitude was possible. Instincts were viewed in terms of having a source, aim, or object (external or internal representation), which could be displaced. A great number of variations in different societies with different family and social patterns could take place. Clinical and sociological investigations show that a number of objects, not just parents, are the focus of oedipal strivings. The developing personality is based on multiple identifications with different aspects of people. Such a perspective does not sacrifice instinctual strivings and infantile sexuality for a purely culturalist position. Cultural absolutism oversimplifies the situation by viewing personality as strictly determined by social situations. Contrawise, the concept of a mental apparatus which is constructed to control drives and operate within a social framework does justice to the drive vicissitudes as well as to the multiple objects which significantly influence a child's development.

ASPECTS OF DEVELOPMENTAL PSYCHOLOGY

We have presented the works from the fields of learning and developmental psychology about moral development. Most typically, controls are viewed as a form of learned behavior as a result of reward and punishment, as well as of secondary and vicarious reinforcement. Superego development is ascribed to the desire for parental approval, and, conversely, anxiety in response to parental rejection and criticism. Elaborate empirical and laboratory data have been amassed by utilizing social learning theory in an effort to describe the acquisition and maintenance of self-control as well as transgressions.[17]

One of the difficulties in the concept of identification is the different referents to which it is applied. In the above discussion of the development of an internalized control system, identification has been used as a process by which external models in their complexity become part of the psychological structure of the child. This is an anaclitic type of identifcation which serves a developmental function: the child thinks, feels, and behaves as though the characteristics of another person, or group of people, belong to him. He patterns his behavior, consciously and unconsciously, after such a model.[18] Other usages have become known since delineation of the defensive process as observed in depressions. These other usages have mainly seen service in nonclinical areas. Some think of identification as behaving like another person or imitation while others have extended the concept to have motivational implications such as the need to be like another person. The concept has been used as the belief of a child that the attributes of a model belong to the child himself.[19]

It may be that resort to a biological theory such as imprinting and its derivatives is needed. An element of circularity is inherent in much of the theory of anaclitic identification. Thus, "I want to be like my parents and therefore I identify, and I identify because I want to be like them." It is not much better to say that children behave in the way parents do because that is the way to get approval and avoid disapproval. Apart from overt situations such as those obtaining in classical conditioning or instrumental learning, the *how* and *why* of the manifold variations seen in the development of control systems are not given a sufficient explanation. Explanations to account for pathological phenomena which are believed to be related to identification problems also seem insufficient if the explanations restrict themselves to acquiring the attributes of another. This is not to deny that adaptive and defensive identifications occur in learning situations, but a theory with additional explanatory power is necessary.

Identification with the aggressor as a defensive maneuver usually begins during the second year of life, and is believed significant for crystallization of the superego. It builds on the attachment the child has earlier made to a parent, and is almost always described in the oedipal context of the boy fearing castration from his father as retaliation for his sensual wishes toward his mother. The wish to eliminate the rival is repressed and gives rise to guilt. The coexisting affectionate tie permits the child to identify with the threatening parent as well as with the mother who is loved by both child and father. The establishment of this defense by the ego is viewed as necessary but not sufficient for the development of internalized controls.

This method of handling anxiety by adopting the behavior of the person who is feared offers an explanation of how a child can identify with an adult with whom he has had unpleasant experiences. A common example is playing doctor, which allows children to change from a helpless, passive state to active mastery. They repetitively re-enact on playmates the unpleasant experiences and anxiety which they have experienced. They put themselves in the role of an aggressor and do to others what adults have done to them.

Such processes originate in the infant's helplessness and are primitive attempts to master a situation by becoming the protective or frustrating adult. A change from passivity to activity allows aggression to be discharged against external objects, but also against the self. The defense, initially directed against a feared object, is now available to the child's own psychological self as a restrictive mechanism. In economic terms, energy is withdrawn (decathected) from the external objects by a process of desexualization and deaggressivization. This energy becomes available to the superego for its primitive aggressive and loving activities.[20] Guilt is not experienced until this level of development is reached, when the ego can direct against itself some of its functions. A separate group of functions are then developed under the control of the superego, such as self-evaluation and self-punishment, a need to expiate for transgression of standards, the bestowing of self-esteem for virtuous thoughts, acts, and wishes, and the withholding of self-esteem for their contraries. Intersystemic conflicts now supersede intrasystemic ones.[21]

The loss of the object during the oedipal period has elements in common with the mourning processes accompanying loss of an object. The renunciation of a loved object is facilitated by becoming like that object. This is seen in persons who take on the qualities, or symptoms, of those they mourn. In theoretical terms, the loss of oedipal objects entails an instinctual defusion which liberates the child from aggressive attachment to parental figures. The fate of the liberated aggression and the precise mechanism utilized by the individual child in attempts to neutralize it are of significance. One result is an intra-punitive superego which wars against its introjects. A control structure which does not permit sufficient discharge of aggression use the aggression against part of the self. Harshness of educators, premature attempts to develop inner controls, anger generated by repeatedly inconsistent or disappointing parents, use of shaming techniques, masochistic adaptations to authorities, and parental conflicts with respect to handling their own impulses, are some factors contributing to the quality of conscience established.

Attempts to examine conscience formation from the external aspects of conformity have delayed a conjoint consideration of the complex psychological processes involved in the emergence of controls—the aspect with which the clinician is more familiar. As we have discussed in the preceding chapter, studies subsequent to Hartshorne and May viewed "moral character" as overt conformity, (adherence to rules and not cheating on school tests, resistance to temptation).[22] Clinicians are interested in such behavior, but are more curious about the meaning of such outward conformity. They are aware of the fact that such external rule-following can be present in children, yet be accompanied by severe conscience deficits, as witnessed repeatedly in therapeutic work. In fact, conformity to moral rules seems to have little correlation with the strength of verbalized beliefs in rules or the intensity of guilt feelings following transgressions. Judgments and verbalizations about what a moral act is are of little value in predicting whether the individual child or adult will actually act in such a manner. Rather, knowledge of morality is simply indicative of the child's cognitive and cultural background and the desire to make a good impression.[23]

If moral character actually refers to a *knowledge* of moral acts, clinicians are interested in knowing the age norms when children can verbalize certain standards. If moral character refers to the *performance* of acts that are judged virtuous (moral conduct), the clinician is interested in which acts a given culture considers so, and in sociological data about which classes of children behave in such ways. Yet he is still left with the feeling that the problem of superego functioning has merely been skimmed.

Some have attempted a synthesis by viewing moral character as part of the developing ego strength of the child. Moral behavior, or the effectiveness of a control system, is then an ego rather than the superego function. This is consistent with the theory that emphasizes a cognitive rather than an affect-motivated system of controls. The primary basis of behavior of all types is seen in the decision-making processes of the ego. On that basis, the stronger one's ego, the more moral will be the child's behavior insofar as that behavior is subject to the controls and the sanctions of society. A mature superego is contingent upon the organization of the ego which has achieved a level of development that corresponds to the psychosexual stage of development and is adequate to the task of handling impulses and external pressures.

A degree of conceptual capacity is needed before an operational conscience can exist. Many of the functions indicating some type of control system are precursors of a conscience system. The viewpoint of developmental stages is still crucial, since the superego is a structural part of mental functioning which evolves in the early years of life. Ego functions, such as reality testing, memory, and judgment, are necessary for the elaboration of conscience, but to say that these are equivalent to conscience gives a totally different perspective on a mental agency that functions in the realm of personal values, ideals and social controls. Furthermore, it is not an agency concerned merely with conformity as judged by external criteria (such as being detected cheating on school tests), but refers specifically to part of an interpsychic system that develops by interaction with the social environment from contact with the inner world of wishes and strivings. Moreover, at a certain point in development, this psychological structure survives in its own right, independent of specific social and environmental pressures.

THE ROLE OF AFFECTS

Superego Precursors. In the young child diverse manifestations of controls exist prior to a functioning superego. As noted, some inhibition of direct impulse expression is observed in children during infancy. Originally based on imitation and fear, it later expands to the stage of an inner danger. Since warning functions are attributable to the ego, impulse-controlled behavior or conformity does not by itself signify superego activity or restriction. It is rather that ego development is a precursor of superego development. Outward social conformity may thus be a protective device of the ego and not be influenced by the superego.

Similarly, the existence of defenses does not imply a superego since they too are ego functions. What does occur is that the superego lends a more skilled and specific direction to ego activities. The presence of a superego is detected by a different kind of warning signal experienced by the ego—the affect of guilt—in contrast to other affects experienced. Defenses, moreoever, are not always initiated by or in the service of the superego. They can be employed by the ego when the latter is in conflict with the environment. Reaction formation may thus result in cleanliness to counter the expression of anal impulses when these are prohibited by a strict environment and need not be the result of a harsh superego. It may be very difficult to distinguish whether a behavior is due to the influence of the superego or that of a defensive ego function. To make such an evaluation we need to know whether other superego functions pertaining to ideals or controls, such as self-evaluation, prohibitions, injunctions, social feelings, and the necessary sense of guilt are present. Only these will give us a clue to the developmental level attained.

The morality of the preoedipal child, and those who remain on this level of moral functioning, implies an absolutism that can be not only uncomfortable but actually portray a lack of personal controls and values. Lack of stabilized identification processes contributes in part. Disturbances become manifest when a separate identity fails to develop. Subsequent developmental periods, particularly adolescence, are of great importance. Unless the child can progress beyond a level of object relationships based solely on identification, autonomous moral functioning is not possible and environmental models continue to exert inordinate influence. Such children may be considered to have "preceptual superegos" which constantly plead for external percepts to guide their behavior.[24]

A striking feature of such immature morality systems is not only harshness, as noted in studies of obsessionals, but the indecisiveness inherent in such a conscience. There is confusion as to how one should behave and an inability to decide which are not just cognitive defects. Such children vacillate between groping for and rejecting the opinions of others, and never really achieve any consistent synthesis throughout their lives. Relationships to others involve not only ambivalent submission, but envy of those who possess greater freedom in their lives.

Role of Guilt. If a sense of guilt is the hallmark of an internalized conscience and value system, as well as one of the most important problems in a civilized person, its development may be one of the most important problems of child development. Guilt has been viewed in an ultimate sense as serving the biological survival of men who must live together with restrictions on their behavior. Some have gone beyond by holding that the price of civilization is a heightening of the sense of guilt. Such broad questions are beyond the scope of this chapter which is focused on the development of guilt as a regulator and power moves to evade it.

Psychologically, guilt is an affective state which denotes equilibrium between ego and superego, or a feeling of anxiety in the ego with respect to the superego. There may be a conscious awareness of guilt, or derivatives of unconscious guilt that manifest themselves in inferiority feelings, self-depreciation, self-punishment, or depressive states. Guilt as an affective state is also related to the ego ideal. While the ego ideal is a substitute for the lost narcissism of childhood, in which the child takes himself as his own ideal, disturbances in the narcissistic problem give rise to diverse power moves on the self and others.

Evidence of conscience development, which proceeds simultaneously with other developmental processes, can be observed in the three- to six-year-old child. A child who has transgressed may look guilty, or he may be led to communicate his deed in a manner that contains the seed for future subtle deceptions about his behavior. For example, when a child of four who has taken an object not belonging to him comes to his mother hiding it behind his back asking, "What will happen to so-and-so (a friend) if he takes my gun?" the child seems to be groping for some help and direction with respect to control of impulses. A child may transgress and then verbalize in a choked voice, and a tear or two, how he feels bad. If one asks what this is like, he may answer, "It's like I feel lonesome when mommy is gone," illustrating his fears of abandonment because of a misdeed.

If a child in this age group is punished, hostile feelings lead to expressions of dislike. Such anger serves as a defense against a fear of losing the loved object and expresses the child's hope that the parent will seek reconciliation. It is as though his anger initially denied the possibility of such a loss. When the child has not been accepted back into a close relationship for some time, he may be unable to separate. Unresolved sleep disturbances may be associated with parents who utilize such situations to prolong the discomfort of the child and do not allow him to get close for some time. Such parents are often identified with this bad part in the child and punish themselves for their own unresolved infantile conflicts and transgressions. When sleep will not come, the child may, in time, swallow his anger and repeatedly come out of his bedroom until things are good again, or he may provoke punishment which soothes his conscience. Children use all of these devices to restore themselves to the good graces of the people who nurture them and to their own needs for such reconciliation.

The Need to Feel Good. What gives the need for restoring a good relationship with dependency objects so prominent a place in the motivational structure of the child? If such behavior is conceptualized as fear of losing love, are we helped in understanding it? It could be argued that since survival is ultimately the key to all behavior, maintenance of a dependecy relationship is necessary for existence. This would be a variation of the earlier ego-instincts approach.

However, such an abstraction lacks the vitality of the actual feeling states which accompany observed behavior. This has led to a concept of guilt as a feeling state so painful and threatening to the ego that failure to resolve it produces feelings of annihilation and emptiness akin to death. The association of guilt feelings with gastrointestinal complains was noted by clinicians early in their work with depressed patients. It was also found in the "masked depressions" of children who often present recurrent abdominal pains for which organic pathology is not demonstrable. Such children have been labeled little bellyachers by some clinicians.

Guilt over a transgression is initially related to a state of starvation on an emotional level. It is as though the child were saying, "Unless you are restored to your parents' good graces you will starve. You will be empty and isolated." The concept relied on as explaining this is loss of self-esteem, which regulates the intrapsychic hunger for a feeling of well-being. Guilt or lack of self-esteem are anticipated by signal affects which also lead to an elaboration of defenses against affect. A bad conscience is equivalent to a feeling of emotional hunger. To relieve it, the child seeks to be restored to a loving relationship in which he will be fed, physically and emotionally, so that he can again think and feel well about himself.

With the appearance at four to six years of superego anxiety (guilt), in contrast to the fear of an external authority, a major landmark has been achieved. The brief period in the life of the child before an internalized, automatized conscience is present is analogous to the problem that existed with prehistoric man. As the first social codes to guide behavior evolved in the fourth millennium B.C., there were no words such as right and wrong. Rather, such phrases as, "He who does that is *loved*," and "He who does that is *hated*," were used to approve or disapprove of behavior. These were transitional periods on the way toward an internalization of individual standards. It would appear that the group conscience and the standards of society since then can be as inconsistent and riddled with conflicts as the conscience of the individual. The events and feelings that each child experiences in the course of his development are reflected and result in some type of internalized mechanism for guiding behavior in both a prohibitory and a striving manner. That defects exist does not seem as surprising as the fact that such processes and structures result.

A byproduct of successful internalization is that the child now sins in thought, word, and deed as institutionalized religions emphasize in their prayers. Not only actual transgressions but fantasied ones induce feelings of discomfort which serve multiple functions. They may serve as a warning against the deed and thought, or they may represent a concomitant punishment via displeasure for even having the thought. In the developmental anomaly of an overdeveloped conscience, we can see persons in a state of dysphoria, lacking satisfaction, and feeling a chronic need to do something like fulfilling an obligation. "It also expresses itself in an exaggerated helpfulness and an exaggerated generosity, and in spending money. Some patients have the feeling that they must give their innermost souls to free themselves from the unbearable tension. The aim of all these strivings is reconciliation. The feeling of guilt appears in a variety of forms, in forebodings of disaster, humility, suffering, striving for punishment, repentance, self-sacrifice, compulsion for purification, etc."[26] When guilty feelings become manifest, a discordance between ego and superego can be discerned. The mechanisms to achieve reconciliation often betray an urgency. Moreover, by five to six years, the ways in which the child handles conscious and unconscious misdeeds give us clues as to how he is consolidating character traits. Regressive phenomena such as merging with protective authorities, delusional systems with magical overtones, the beginning use of formalized religious devices, and sublimatory activity now achieve prominence. Awareness of loneliness and fear of social ostracism are cognitively and affectively present. The need of the child to belong and to be accepted in a group has then acquired deeper significance. At the same time it brings with it the propensity for many pathological neurotic disturbances.

Not only a hated authority, but also a loved one has been internalized. In the young child the *ego* is loved by the id as one has earlier loved the external and actual parents.[27] Similarly, the ego is loved by the superego as one wished to be loved by parents. The hostile aspects of the superego have object hate transformed into self-hate. The benign aspects of the superego have object love transformed into an aspect of self-love or narcissism, felt as pride and security in relation to society and destiny as well as one's own conscience and ideas. The superego builds and upholds as well as splits and tears down, just as the ego. A great many psychopathological and clinical conditions result if the hating aspects of the superego take precedence.

In young children the need to suffer may result in psychophysiological or neurotic illnesses, manifested in behaviors such as the constant courting of punishment or humiliation, or accident proneness. Future delinquent behaviors are foreshadowed by defects in the emerging superego. Some are related to faulty object relations which hamper the development of a structurally intact superego. Internalization of defective parental models is another possibility. An overriding sense of guilt may lead to compulsive criminality. An ego-ideal system which tends toward high aspirations gives a vulnerability to acting out when these disillusionments occur.

IN CONCLUSION

In this chapter the processes of acquiring an internalized set of controls has been explored as a developmental phenomena with concomitant needs to escape from the controls. The emphasis has been on developmental observations and clinical material of children up to the age of six, although implications for later normal and pathological functioning have been pointed out. The diversity of data from these early years has led to the development of theories from different branches of psychology. The approach utilized in this book emphasizes the emergence of structuralized mental agencies, but takes into account the significant contributions made by learning theory and experimental investigations of moral development. Current theoretical issues such as the cognitive or affect-based theory of controls have been elaborated. There is a need to understand the vicissitudes of normal conscience development from infancy onward in order to comprehend the diverse clinical syndromes that are possible with conscience defects. The emergence of guilt as a phenomenon of conscience has been viewed as indicating the establishment of a delineated and functioning superego structure with idealized and prohibitory aspects.

REFERENCES

1. B. E. Moore, Toward a clarification of the concept of narcissism *Psychoanalytic Study of the Child* 30(1975):243-265.
2. H. Hartmann, *Ego Psychology and the Problem of Adaptation* (New York: International University Press, 1958).
3. S. E. Bijou and D. M. Baer, *Child Development—A Systematic and Empirical Theory* (New York: Appleton-Century-Crofts, 1961).
4. H. Hartmann and R. M. Loewenstein, Notes on the superego, *Psychoanalytic Study of the Child* 17(1962):42-81.
5. E. Erikson, Growth and crises of the healthy personality, *Identity and the Life Cycle* (Psychological Issues, Monograph 1) (New York: International Universities Press, 1950).
6. R. Spitz, *No and Yes: On the Genesis of Human Communication* (New York: International Universities Press, 1957).
7. A. C. Cain, The presuperego turning-inward of aggression, *Psychoanalytic Quarterly* 30(1961):171-208.
8. S. Ferenczi, Psychoanalysis of sexual habits, *Further Contributions to the Therapy and Technique of Psycho-Analysis* (London: Hogarth Press, 1926).
9. Erikson, op. cit., p. 70.
10. S. Freud, Obsessive action and religious practices, *Standard Edition* 9:115-127.
11. O. Fenichel, *The Psychoanalytic Theory of Neurosis* (New York: W.W. Norton and Co.,1945).
12. A. B. Szalita, Some thoughts on empathy, *Psychiatry* 39(1976):142-152.
13. E. Jacobson, *The Self and the Obejct World* (New York: International Universities Press, 1964).
14. B. Porter, The many faces of murder, *Playboy* 17(1970):218-219.
15. S. Freud, Totem and taboo, *Standard Edition* 13:1-161.
16. E. Jones, Mother-right and the sexual ignorance of savages, *Essays in Applied Psycho-Analysis* 2:145-173. (New York: International Universities Press, 1964).
17. A. Bandura and R. H. Walters, *Social Learning and Personality Development* (New York: Holt, Rinehart and Winston, 1913).
18. U. Bronfenbrenner, Freudian theories of identification and their derivatives, *Child Development* 31(1960):15-40.
19. J. Kagan, The concept of identification, *Psychological Review* 15(1958):296-305.
20. S. Hammerman, Conceptions of superego development, *Journal of the American Psychoanalytic Association* 13(1965):332-355.

21. D. Beres, Vicissitudes of superego functions, *Psychoanalytic Study of the Child* 13(1958):324-351.
22. J. Hartshorne and M. A. May, *Studies in the Nature of Character*, 3 vol. (New York: Macmillan, 1928-1930).
23. L. Kohlberg, *Moral Development* (New York: Holt, Rinehart and Winston, 1970).
24. D. Beres, op. cit.
25. J. H. Breastad, *The Dawn of Conscience* (New York: Charles Scribners, 1947).
26. H. Nunberg, The feeling of guilt, *Practice and Theory of Psychoanalysis* (New York: International Universities Press, 1948).
27. R. Schafer, The loving and beloved superego in Freud's structural theory, *Psychoanalytic Study of the Child* 15(1960):163-188.

Chapter Nine

Antisocial Behavior: Sociogenic Aspects

Various perspectives on antisocial behavior can be taken. Unfortunately, in practice only passing reference is usually given by one approach to the others. Adolescents are caught up in a matrix of possibilities, yet only a few pages in texts on adolescence are allotted to contrasting viewpoints, and books often take a condescending tone toward the diverse fields. It is appropriate to state directly that no one approach provides sufficient answers as to what encourages antisocial behavior. Nor is it desirable to assume that one causal theory does justice to the multiple factors which contribute to such behavior. Expecting to find a single causal etiologic agent reflects an outdated model which stems from the 19th-century viewpoint on bacterial agents, long ago seen as too simplistic for infectious diseases.

This chapter reviews two approaches to delinquent behavior: the sociological and psychometric. In succeeding chapters psychiatric (from the biological to the descriptive) and psychodynamic models are discussed. Comparative evaluation and extraction of what seems valuable in the different approaches is emphasized, as is adequate appraisal of different behaviors for an individual in a particular culture with a given set of personality traits and conflicts.

An assumption cannot be made that a high correlation exists between a given professional background and a particular attitude toward delinquency. Some psychiatrists lean toward a social explanation to account for antisocial behavior, and occasionally one meets a sociologist who stresses an ultimate explanation in the context of personality theory. It is not so much a matter of choosing one theory or another, but rather that in practice everyone is predisposed toward a particular viewpoint. These predispositions lead to the advocacy of certain practices in diagnosis, treatment, and rehabilitation for juveniles or adults whose behavior exhibits a repetitive pattern of deviancy from personal controls or social norms. Contact with law enforcement agencies may or may not eventuate. Clinicians are not solely interested in those who are caught, since they are aware of a great deal of undetected psychopathological behavior in individuals and families with whom they deal. These hidden figures on crime call attention to the selectivity in detection and apprehension.

SOCIOLOGICAL VIEWPOINTS

Common Terms. Some commonly used technical terms are employed when groupings of antisocial adolescents are made. It is desirable to keep these in mind to avoid overlapping and confusion. No definition of delinquency by itself is given, since the usages of this term depend upon how a given source is using it.

Juvenile Population. This usually refers to all children below a stated age, such as sixteen or eighteen. It is customarily defined by statute in the laws of different states.

Juvenile Deviants. These are children exhibiting deviant or odd behavior, whether antisocial in a legal sense or not. Hence, this term may be used to encompass the bizarre behavior in adolescent schizophrenia on the one hand, to varieties of drug usage on the other.

Legal Delinquents. This group encompasses all deviants committing antisocial acts as specified by law. This is not equivalent to criminal acts since by definition the forbidden acts may not transgress the legal rules which make the behavior criminal for an adult. Still the juvenile is handled through the civil procedures of the juvenile court unless his case is waived to a criminal court. There are many behaviors considered delinquent for a minor which are not so for an adult, such as truancy or incorrigibility.

Detected Delinquents. These are the juveniles under a stated age who are apprehended for antisocial behavior. They represent a small number of the total juvenile group who are deviants, and the even smaller number who are apprehended.

Agency Delinquents. These are delinquents who are detected and then reach an agency or community facility.

Alleged Delinquents. This is a subgroup of antisocial deviants who are apprehended and brought into court.

Adjudicated Delinquents. These represent the antisocial delinquents who are found guilty at a juvenile court hearing.

Committed Delinquents. The adjudicated delinquents who are committed to some type of correctional institution or program.

Juvenile Criminals. Those within the state definition of a minor who are waived to an adult criminal court and, therefore, removed from the juvenile population. They are found guilty or not guilty of committing a criminal offense by the procedures of adult criminal courts, and their subsequent disposition of such cases is determined accordingly.

Antisocial behavior. A phrase mainly used by clinicians to refer to a variety of personality disorders which may give rise to acts directed against others to relieve conflict, in contrast to other diagnostic groupings, such as neuroses or psychoses. They are usually ascribed to developmental lags or defects which result in personality trends which utilize or permit behavior which can be contrary to the social standards of a community, but more specifically reflects difficulties in the ego and superego development in a given individual.

Acting Out. Acting out is a phrase with multiple and confusing meanings. Its use has spread from its original meaning, within the context of intensive psychotherapy, to a broad usage which has made it almost parallel to the behavior of any subgroup of juvenile or adult deviants. Its original usage involved the painful remembering which occurred during the course of psychoanalytic therapy. Rather than dealing with the return of painful memories and affects, there was a compelling urge to repeat the forgotten past within the context of a therapy setting by reliving certain repressed emotional experiences. These were transferred onto the therapist as well as onto other aspects of the current life situation.

In time the meaning of the concept shifted to refer to repetitions of unresolved past conflicts outside the therapeutic setting to avoid dealing with them in therapy. The original concept had in mind an individual with a sufficiently strong ego so that a forgotten past did not ordinarily express itself in action except under intense conditions, such as the involvement in therapy.

When many other types of behavior problems were dealt with in psychoanalysis and other forms of psychotherapy, the term acting out was used. However, it now applied to repetitions occurring

outside the treatment situation and to individuals whose control
over their impulses was precarious. Such individuals were seen to
spend a good deal of their life in efforts to change the external world
or manipulate their human contacts. The term has thus changed
from a special type of remembering to an action instead of a
recollection. The reference was to a type of alloplastic rather than
autoplastic action, in which the change is something outside the
self. In some cases it is equivalent to antisocial acts which are part of
a pattern or style of living. In terms of ego functioning, the acting out
may serve as a defense against the recognition of impulses in which
a wish or fantasy is instead lived out impulsively in behavior.

The Sociological Approach as Epidemiology.   There is no one
sociological theory to encompass antisocial behavior. Rather, there
is an interlacing context of factors assessed as causal. These usually
include cultural, socio-economic, political, and religious factors with
varying degrees of emphasis. Although past historical factors
within the individual may be noted, there is an emphasis on socio-
cultural and ideological factors which have contributed to the
development of the child. In this sense it is an epidemiological
theory, since the interest is in the incidence and prevalence of
certain behaviors within a population. This is similar to a public
health approach to disease than that of the clinician faced with
specific pathology within an individual patient or family.

By analogy variations in the incidence of the disease (delinquent
behavior), are ascribed to variables such as economic barriers,
ethnic groupings, social class, situational crises, geographical
location, or other demographic data. More specific explanations
within this framework attribute. variables for high rates of
delinquency to factors such as the lapses attendant upon perpetual
unresolved international tensions, the lowering of acting out
thresholds in an atmosphere of permissiveness, tendencies toward
the abandonment of law and order, or the increased academic and
social stresses at progressively lower ages. The emphasis is on how a
certain number of children or adolescents in a population, at a given
time in history, react to such conditions by delinquent behavior.

In contrast are explanations of how a specific individual behaves
and the configurations within his personality and family. For the
former, individual variations are acknowledged but deemed
insignificant. The analogy is taking a global interest in the state of
the economy compared to studying the reasons some individual
firms go into bankruptcy.

Religious Orientation. Perhaps the oldest, and still most widely held, cultural viewpoint on delinquent behavior is taken from a religious perspective. Historically, this has greatly influenced legal thinking. It is the epitome of the common-sense belief of the man on the street since its seeming rationality coalesces with the childhood teachings of parents and substitutes. Many confluent trends have operated from the influence of the Old and New Testaments which give a heavy stress to concepts such as personal responsibility, free choice, blameworthy behavior, punishment for wrongdoing, guilt, and expiation.

Wrongdoing is felt to demand vengeance to restore or to maintain order in a community. A retributive view of transgressions gives an emphasis to the act. Of course, there were always those considered doli incapax for some reason, such as childhood or intellectual immaturity, but these were the exceptions to the general rule. Implicit in this approach is that continued wrongdoing reflects either insufficient punishment, or the continued operation of a guilty mind in an individual so that expiation has not occurred.

A moral approach cannot be discounted as simply the archaic residue of an outdated theology perpetuated by anti-intellectuals. Kant, for example, as representative of a great philosphical tradition, argued that it appeared self-evident that the dessert of crime is punishment, and that justice demanded that a man who had willed an unjust act be penalized in a strictly proportional manner.[1] Kant anticipated a modern therapeutic position for dealing with acting out behavior in his position that a society which fails to punish one who violates the norms in effect sanctions his principles and thereby becomes particeps criminis. Hence the therapist passively sanctions antisocial behavior by failing to deal with it in treatment.

In contrast is a position utilizing individual punishment to serve more general ends, such as deterring others from similar types of behavior. Since one of Kant's basic ethical tenets was his stricture against any man using another as a means to a desired end, there would be no justification for the use of one transgressor as an example to deter others. This is not dissimilar from contemporary writers on youth who stress that among the many resentments of the youth and underprivileged, including delinquent and criminal groups who are mainly under twenty-five, is the unfair distribution of punishment. While they bear the brunt of punishment, many of the more skilled, powerful, and affluent go unpunished or are allowed to plea bargain for minor punishments. Rage and hatred are kindled.

The individual responsibility position on deviant behavior has been elaborated to illustrate one of the most historically influential theories. It holds that a deviant act requires punishment in its own right. This position was modified by innumerable theorists, from Plato, Aristotle, Aquinas, Hobbes, and Beccaria, to the 19th-century utilitarians, such as Mill and Bentham. These thinkers felt that the only justification for inflicting punishment is an ultimate goal of greater welfare to the members of a community. The welfare could be through future deterrence of such behavior in the transgressor or in others who weigh the circumstances and then decide to forego a transgression. "The general object which all laws have, or ought to have, in common is to augment the total happiness of the community; and, therefore, in the first place to exclude, as far as may be, everything that tends to subtract from that happiness, in other words to exclude mischief.... But all punishment is mischief; all punishment in itself is evil. Upon the principal of utility, if it ought at all to be admitted, it ought only to be admitted inasmuch as it promises to exclude some greater evil."[2]

In a contemporary form this has been incorporated within certain learning theories of delinquency which emphasize the need for reinforcers to strengthen less deviant responses, or the use of punishment to extinguish rewarding antisocial acts. Mowrer once viewed antisocial behavior as due to inadequate teaching of moral standards.[3] In a similar vein Menninger asks, "Whatever became of sin?"[4]

INCIDENCE AND PREVALENCE PROBLEMS

Attention should be called to the problems of incidence of delinquent behavior prior to elaboration of the sociological contributions to its genesis. From the various definitional meanings given to delinquency, there is an immediate problem as to how a delinquent population should be constituted in attempts to measure the overall incidence of delinqunecy and delinquency rates. There are not only different statutory definitions of delinquent acts in the fifty states, but enforcement of the statutes varies at different times. The sources of data on crime and delinquency in the United States are primarily based on the records available from two Federal agencies: the Children's Bureau of the Department of Health, Education, and Welfare, and the Federal Bureau of Investigation's annual *Uniform Crime Reports* (UCR).

The Children's Bureau relies on a representative sampling of various courts throughout the countrs for figures on the annual number of juveniles officially adjudicated delinquent and the type of offense. The most widely used source of data for the incidence of various types of frequencies of criminal behavior is the UCR. These data are compiled from 8,000 towns and cities in the United States with a population of over 2,500 which gives a Crime Index based on seven major offenses known to the police. These offenses are chosen since they are most likely to be reported to the police (see Table 12).

Other sources of data are the Federal Bureau of Prisons in the United States Department of Justice, which records the individuals incarcerated in prisons each year, and the National Office of Vital Statistics, which collects information on homicide through records from coroners' offices.

TABLE 12

National Index of Serious Crimes, 1975

OFFENSES	NUMBER KNOWN TO POLICE
A. *Violent*	
1. Murder and Non-negligent Manslaughter (Criminal homicide)	20,570
2. Forcible Rape	56,090
3. Robbery	464,970
4. Aggravated Assault	484,710
B. *Property Crimes:*	
5. Burglary	3,252,100
6. Larceny—Theft	5,977,700
7. Motor Vehicle Theft	1,500,000

Total Violent Crimes Against the Person: 828,150
Total Property Crimes: 5,063,800

Source: *Uniform Crime Reports*, Wash., D.C., U.S. Dept. of Justice, 1975, p. 11.

These sources of statistics have come under increasing criticism in recent years. A standard criticism involves the differential enforcement involving social class and racial factors. A more updated version adds the intellectual differential, whereby the less intelligent and cognitively creative are the most likely to be apprehended. It has long been known that the availability of community referral sources and clinicians in private practice in any given community influence the number of adolescents who become listed as adjudicated delinquents. Most cogent of these statistical records of crime is the criticism of their failure to distinguish law violation from rates of apprehension. These are not distinguished by police records but require field surveys and skilled data collection from outside the realm of police arrests. There is also the yet smaller sample who are finally institutionalized. The incidence of unofficial delinquency as judged by non-reported and non-detected acts is undoubtedly very high. Some surveys indicate it is the rare (deviant?) adolescent who has never committed an act that could not be called delinquent.[5]

Unless discussing serious crimes, such data should raise serious questions about what delinquent behaviors are. Another problem is that of duplication.[6] This refers to juveniles who have committed multiple offenses, such as absenting and incorrigibility, which are lumped into delinquency figures involving many acts which are not simply acts for which only minors are charged.

Despite these initial caveats, some of the types of statistical records evident in the *Uniform Crime Reports* will be used for illustration with particular application to adolescents and youths. Selective tables will be used for drawing implications for these populations.[7] In Table 13 the arrests and rate by size of population groups illustrates the different potentialities for various offenses per 100,000 inhabitants, based on the size of the community. The six basic divisions by population size include suburban and rural areas. Among many inferences from such data is the notation that the rate for serious crimes in rural areas is not necessarily the lowest. While the rate may be low for robbery and burglary, for murder and non-negligent manslaughter, as well as rape, rural areas are in the middle. For negligent manslaughter, the rural areas actually have the highest per-capita rate of all.

However, the types of offenses must also be distinguished, since there is evidence that rural boys do not exhibit the characteristics (such as having as early an onset of delinquent behavior) of adolescents in larger metropolitan areas. Earlier onset leads to many antisocial techniques, accompanied by a self-concept of being a delinquent and future criminal.

It should be noted that this argument can be used in support of the delinquent subculture theory as a necessary spawning group for development of future delinquency. This may be true for some offenses, such as criminal homicides, robberies, auto thefts, prostitution, narcotics violations, and gambling. Less significant differences may be present between sizes of communities for offenses involving financial trust (forgery, fraud, and embezzlement) and offenses against the family and children.

Another set of revealing data pertain to the distribution of arrests for youths by different age groupings, such as under fifteen, eighteen, twenty-one, and twenty-five (see Table 14).

Although this is not strictly a juvenile population in the sense of cases confined to the juvenile court system, it does illustrate the frequencies of some of the major offenses in the late juvenile and youth groups. The total arrests in these city populations show that 53 percent of these arrests involve those under twenty-five years of age—the basic adolescent and youth group populations. Those under eighteen, who make up a bulk of the juvenile court adjudication process, account for about 25 percent of all arrests. Fifty percent of property crimes and about 25 percent of violent crimes against people are committed by juveniles. Specifically, more juveniles under eighteen are arrested than are adults for burglary, larceny, arson, auto thefts, and vandalism. Even conceding the methodological flaws in assuming that these data are equivalent to an incidence of actual law violations, such figures as 83.8 percent of auto theft arrests, 83.0 percent of burglaries, 76.2 percent of robberies, and 62.8 percent of forcible rapes, composed of individuals under age twenty-five, are highly impressive.

SOCIOLOGICAL EXPLANATIONS OF ANTISOCIAL BEHAVIOR: SOCIAL CLASS ROLE AND ECOLOGY

Traditionally there are four approaches emphasizing social components as contributory to antisocial behavior: (1) social class, role, and ecology; (2) group delinquency or what has sometimes been called gang delinquency; (3) institutional influences on delinquency, such as the mass media and schools; (4) family configurational patterns. The first is discussed in this section and the others in succeeding sections, but they are all seen as a set of complementary sociogenic hypotheses about certain types of antisocial behavior.

Early Work. Some of the early work on the contribution of social class factors and delinquency in the United States came from Chicago in the second and third decades of this century. These early approaches attempted to set up distributions for special demographic areas of the city to study a variety of social problems. An early approach was an effort to plot the residences of children coming into the juvenile court over a ten-year period.[8] In fact, these were early

TABLE 13

Arrests. Number and Rate, 1975, by Population Groups

(rate per 100,000; 1975 estimated population)

	Cities			
Offense charged	Total (8,051 agencies; total population 179,191,219)	Total city arrest (6,237 cities; population 130,409,771)	Group I (55 cities over 250,000; population 41,193,011)	Group II (105 cities 100,000 to 250,000; population 15,072,581)
TOTAL	**7,984,547**	**6,392,792**	**2,166,143**	**797,969**
Rate per 100,000 inhabitants	**4,455.9**	**4,902.1**	**5,258.5**	**5,294.2**
Criminal homicide:				
(a) Murder and nonnegligent manslaughter	16,485	12,692	7,335	1,485
Rate per 100,000	9.2	9.7	17.8	9.9
(b) Manslaughter by negligence	3,041	1,797	664	221
Rate per 100,000	1.7	1.4	1.6	1.5
Forcible rape	21,963	16,860	8,738	2,202
Rate per 100,000	12.3	12.9	21.2	14.6
Robbery	129,788	114,596	67,171	13,302
Rate per 100,000	72.4	87.9	163.1	88.3
Aggravated assault	202,217	156,398	67,150	18,969
Rate per 100,000	112.8	119.9	163.0	125.9
Burglary—breaking or entering	449,155	348,233	123,291	46,219
Rate per 100,000	250.7	267.0	299.3	306.6
Larceny—theft	958,938	821,451	242,876	113,755
Rate per 100,000	535.1	629.9	589.6	754.7
Motor vehicle theft	120,224	97,069	41,034	11,986
Rate per 100,000	67.1	74.4	99.6	79.5
Violent crime[2]	370,453	300,546	150,394	35,958
Rate per 100,000	206.7	230.5	365.1	238.6
Property crime[3]	1,528,317	1,266,753	407,201	171,960
Rate per 100,000	852.9	971.4	988.5	1,140.9
Subtotal for above offenses	1,901,811	1,569,096	558,259	208,139
Rate per 100,000	1,061.3	1,203.2	1,355.2	1,380.9
Other assaults	352,648	292,113	95,944	44,571
Rate per 100,000	196.8	224.0	232.9	295.7
Arson	14,589	10,941	3,648	1,254
Rate per 100,000	8.1	8.4	8.9	8.3
Forgery and counterfeiting	57,803	43,790	13,727	6,511
Rate per 100,000	32.3	33.6	33.3	43.2
Fraud	146,253	92,311	23,061	19,889
Rate per 100,000	81.6	70.8	56.0	132.0
Embezzlement	9,302	7,457	1,309	2,939
Rate per 100,000	5.2	5.7	3.2	19.5
Stolen property; buying, receiving, possessing	100,903	81,881	29,875	9,655
Rate per 100,000	56.3	62.8	72.5	64.1

Source: UNIFORM CRIME REPORTS, 1975, p. 180

				Other areas	
Group III (259 cities 50,000 to 100,000; population 17,931,065)	Group IV (556 cities 25,000 50,000; population 19,327,825)	Group V (1,317 cities 10,000 to 25,000; population 20,717,252)	Group VI (3,945 cities under 10,000; population 16,168,037)	Suburban area,[1] (3,733 agencies; population 64,765,536)	Rural area (1,373 agencies; population 21,200,683)
835,669	**867,690**	**918,076**	**807,245**	**2,426,821**	**675,625**
4,660.5	**4,489.3**	**4,431.5**	**4,992.8**	**3,747.1**	**3,186.8**
1,366	1,094	855	557	3,566	1,735
7.6	5.7	4.1	3.4	5.5	8.2
251	234	232	195	1,108	605
1.4	1.2	.1.1	1.2	1.7	2.9
1,922	1,614	1,381	1,003	5,682	2,092
10.7	8.4	6.7	6.2	8.8	9.9
13,177	10,174	7,083	3,689	26,082	4,506
73.5	52.6	34.2	22.8	40.3	21.3
19,965	17,639	17,857	14,818	56,736	19,662
111.3	91.3	86.2	91.6	87.6	92.7
52,187	48,174	44,979	33,383	145,552	39,220
291.0	249.2	217.1	206.5	224.7	185.0
124,328	136,738	124,947	78,807	311,124	43,368
693.4	707.5	603.1	487.4	480.4	204.6
13,235	11,876	10,715	8,223	34,857	8,651
73.8	61.4	51.7	50.9	53.8	40.8
36,430	30,521	27,176	20,067	92,066	27,995
203.2	157.9	131.2	124.1	142.2	132.0
189,750	196,788	180,641	120,413	491,533	91,239
1,058.2	1,018.2	871.9	744.8	758.9	430.4
226,431	227,543	208,049	140,675	584,707	119,839
1,262.8	1,177.3	1,004.2	870.1	902.8	565.3
38,695	40,957	42,061	29,885	105,593	25,637
215.8	211.9	203.0	184.8	163.0	120.9
1,481	1,632	1,586	1,340	5,450	1,393
8.3	8.4	7.7	8.3	8.4	6.6
6,471	6,381	6,518	4,182	17,300	6,177
36.1	33.0	31.5	25.9	26.8	29.1
11,071	14,318	15,513	8,459	45,617	28,582
61.7	74.1	74.9	52.3	70.4	134.8
1,710	672	471	356	2,012	803
9.5	3.5	2.3	2.2	3.1	3.8
11,806	11,784	11,387	7,374	34,715	6,329
65.8	61.0	55.0	45.6	53.6	29.9

TABLE 14

City Arrest of Persons under Twenty-Five Years of Age, 1975

Offense charged	Grand total all ages	Number of persons	
		Under 15	Under 18
TOTAL	**8,013,645**	**716,206**	**2,078,459**
Criminal homicide:			
(a) Murder and nonnegligent manslaughter	**16,485**	184	1,573
(b) Manslaughter by negligence	**3,041**	80	368
Forcible rape	**21,963**	867	3,863
Robbery	**129,788**	12,515	44,470
Aggravated assault	**202,217**	10,600	35,512
Burglary—breaking or entering	**449,155**	90,189	236,192
Larceny—theft...............................	**958,938**	192,495	432,019
Motor vehicle theft.........................	**120,224**	17,290	65,564
Violent crime[1]	**370,453**	24,166	85,418
Property crime[2]	**1,528,317**	299,974	733,775
Subtotal for above offenses.................	**1,901,811**	324,220	819,561
Other assaults	**352,648**	26,280	69,965
Arson	**14,589**	4,904	7,727
Forgery and counterfeiting	**57,803**	1,215	7,320
Fraud	**146,253**	851	4,665
Embezzlement	**9,302**	157	679
Stolen property; buying, receiving, possessing....	**100,903**	9,445	32,891
Vandalism	**175,865**	66,663	115,046
Weapons; carring, possessing, etc	**130,933**	5,127	21,365
Prostitution and commercialized vice	**50,229**	177	2,362
Sex offenses (except forcible rape and prostitution)............................	**50,837**	3,928	10,876
Narcotic drug laws	**508,189**	16,229	122,857
Gambling...................................	**49,469**	263	1,763
Offenses against family and children...........	**53,332**	2,884	6,271
Driving under the influence	**908,680**	289	17,020
Liquor laws	**267,057**	9,429	105,813
Drunkenness	**1,176,121**	4,243	41,457
Disorderly conduct.........................	**632,561**	34,989	120,278
Vagrancy	**59,277**	1,296	5,323
All other offenses (except traffic)..............	**1,037,754**	95,020	265,568
Suspicion	**29,098**	2,365	7,718
Curfew and loitering law violations.............	**112,117**	29,974	112,117
Runaways...................................	**188,817**	76,258	188,817

[1] Violent crime is offenses of murder, forcible rape, robbery and aggravated assault.

[2] Property crime is offenses of burglary, larceny—theft and motor vehicle theft.

[3] Less than one-tenth of 1 percent.

Source: UNIFORM CRIME REPORTS, 1975, p. 190.

arrested		Percentage			
Under 21	Under 25	Under 15	Under 18	Under 21	Under 25
3,360,830	**4,560,693**	**8.9**	**25.9**	**41.9**	**56.9**
4,149	7,396	1.1	9.5	25.2	44.9
974	1,539	2.6	12.1	32.0	50.6
8,137	12,743	3.9	17.6	37.0	58.0
74,903	99,953	9.6	34.3	57.7	77.0
65,316	100,282	5.2	17.6	32.3	49.6
325,970	382,708	20.1	52.6	72.6	85.2
602,132	723,451	20.1	45.1	62.8	75.4
87,843	101,707	14.4	54.5	73.1	84.6
152,505	220,374	6.5	23.1	41.2	59.5
1,015,945	1,207,866	19.6	48.0	66.5	79.0
1,169,424	1,429,779	17.0	43.1	61.5	75.2
121,179	183,161	7.5	19.8	34.4	51.9
9,530	10,898	33.6	53.0	65.3	74.7
18,797	32,695	2.1	12.7	32.5	56.6
20,735	52,292	.6	3.2	14.2	35.8
1,703	3,683	1.7	7.3	18.3	39.6
54,999	72,367	9.4	32.6	54.5	71.7
136,879	515,233	37.9	65.4	77.8	86.0
43,129	67,021	3.9	16.3	32.9	51.2
16,115	33,080	.4	4.7	32.1	65.9
17,790	25,844	7.7	21.4	35.0	50.8
270,824	391,394	3.2	24.2	53.3	77.0
4,718	9,367	.5	3.6	9.5	18.9
13,391	22,348	5.4	11.8	25.1	41.9
110,349	246,623	(³)	1.9	12.1	27.1
192,963	215,668	3.5	39.6	72.3	80.8
147,263	280,758	.4	3.5	12.5	23.9
239,504	362,824	5.5	19.0	37.9	57.4
12,392	19,657	2.2	9.0	20.9	33.2
443,180	628,360	9.2	24.7	42.7	60.5
15,032	20,707	8.1	26.5	51.7	71.2
112,117	112,117	26.7	100.0	100.0	100.0
118,817	118,817	40.4	100.0	100.0	100.0

attempts to plot areas with a high incidence of delinquency. The leading figure in extending this type of research was Clifford R. Shaw.[9] In a series of studies, he employed three measures to investigate delinquency petitions: (a) *Area Rates* for a square mileage area based on census tracts, (b) *Zone Rates* extending outward from the center of the city by mile-wide concentric circles, and (c) *Radical Rates*, which extended via main thoroughfares from the center of the city to the outskirts.

Some of the early findings were a higher incidence of delinquency near the center of the city and in areas characterized by physical deterioration and declining population. Distribution of delinquency paralleled the distribution of poverty, vice, broken homes, and other evidence of socio-economic deterioration—a conclusion that has subsequently been assumed as causal for the remainder of the century. Delinquency rates remained high in these areas even when the ethnic composition of the population shifted. It was emphasized that delinquents from the high-incidence areas were also those most likely to become future recidivists and the tendency for the behaviors of younger delinquents increasingly to become part of a group activity was noted.

This pioneering effort resulted in a host of debates about the conclusions which have continued on a more sophisticated level to the present day. The original study of Shaw was attacked on statistical grounds that his delinquency rates included cases later dismissed as well as tests of statistical significance which did not bear out. Another criticism was that the differential distribution of police as well as community agencies in the areas studied was ignored, and that use of concentric residence zones was inappropriate.[10] A pragmatic result was to stimulate debate and promote area-wide research. Many of the ecological approaches currently employed are in need of reformulations due to the rapidly changing patterns of urban living. The geographical mobility of the American population shows that it is a rare occurrence for a child to spend his developmental years all in one locality. In addition, urban development has destroyed many older areas of cities, which has been accompanied by a burgeoning of high-rise apartments and suburban living, together with a breakup of the old ethnic communities.

Role. This early focusing on slums as a source of delinquency expanded by use of such traditional sociological concepts as *role* and *class* as playing contributory parts. As with most concepts in the social sciences these have been employed in a number of ways. Role is used as a social position characterized by a set of personal qualities and activities, such as those possessed by a parent or child in a family. Some sociologists add a further distinction between role and status. If this distinction is used, status is viewed as a collection of rights and duties (obligations), and role is then the pattern of behavior in a group corresponding to a given system of obligations. Status can come from age, sex, race, and class, or it may result by way of certain achievements.

Role has assertive qualities which accrue to status; it involves putting rights and duties into effect. The distinction is between recognized social rules of behavior and their application. Some have extended the meaning of role to include role-playing in which a pattern of learned acts are performed by a person in an interactional situation. This is related to how people present themselves to one another or what they expect of each other. In both of these usages, role has an intermediate position between the individual and the larger society in the manner of individual behavior becoming social conduct. The implications from this are that when social roles are clearly defined, there is less tendency for conflict between individual and collective goals. To the extent that there is social flux, due to any number of factors, such as shifting geographical boundaries or breakdowns in racial barriers, one may expect difficulty in defining how an individual shall behave.

As an illustration of some earlier work dealing with delinquency and roles, one study distinguished stealing done by boys and girls in terms of boys' acts being predominantly role-expressive.[11] The act of stealing is oriented to its social context, which is described as an enhancement of maleness. A girl who steals is role-supportive, in that she is seeking certain objects, such as jewelry, which enhance her femaleness. Mention is made of the possibilities of stealing being symptomatic, or defined as a substitute gratification, but this is not viewed as significant.

Differences in role and status in members of a group are components of social organization which have some effect on how individuals relate and communicate with each other. This is crucial with respect to social class distinctions in which one group of society receives less deference, or some other indicia of status, than another group. Criteria for class inclusion in the United States have become increasingly vague, with subtle criteria utilized. Occupation, income, education, or residence location are typical criteria utilized. Past efforts at defining social class by occupation when there was a correlation with income demonstrate how difficult it is to peg someone. This is not a defense of the position that social class distinctions are desirable, but rather that such distinctions are made by groups who also have accompanying personal correlates, such as people who rank themselves in a higher social class than others rank them, and the ever-present wish to succeed which is present in most classes to some extent. Such upgrading is true for that large figment called the middle class, which was once described by Weber as being guided by the "Protestant ethic" of hard work, frugality, cleanliness (a white collar), self-advancement, deference to authority, and postponement of pleasures for the long-run (including the hereafter?).[12]

The Theory of Walter Miller. One widely cited approach utilizing social class as a determining factor in delinquency is that of the anthropoligist Walter B. Miller. The source for much of his theory was from work with lower-class black youths in the Boston area. His thesis was that delinquent behavior in the lower classes was not a reaction to the frustrations in meeting the middle-class ethic. Rather, it was ascribed to an independent set of behaviors derived from their lower-class culture.[13] In contrast to the middle-class norms, Miller saw the lower classes as utilizing four norms in particular: toughness, avoidance of trouble, outsmarting others, and excitement.

Toughness stressed physical strength and endurance, which became equated with masculinity. The reason suggested for such development was the matriarchal family, which in turn was due to the high frequency of illigitimacy, divorce, and abandonment in such families. The absent father has been widely discussed in the literature as a generator of delinquent norms.

Even when the father is physically present in a home, he tends to be involved in only a haphazard manner. Serial monogamy is a frequent phenomenon in which there is a succession of temporary mating partners who come and go over the procreative period of the mother. Lack of a cohesive family structure enhances peer-standards as a guiding role in the adolescent male even more than in a two-sex household. The female-based household has a primary role in forming a one-sex peer unit which becomes the main socializer of the boy—or so the theory goes. Other studies confirm that a delinquent group may have a higher incidence of paternal deprivation which is age-related. Yet, other studies point more to a disturbance in father-child relationships as the predisposing factor for future delinquency rather than absence per se.[14] An absent father at a particular age, such as four to seven, is a more specific hypothesis.[15]

Socialization and internalization of controls in the male appear to be the concomitant psychological variables affected by familial-cultural situations in which toughness is a reaction-formation to a controlling female in the house. Stress has been placed on the matrifocalness of families due to the occupational instability of the male which has historically been true from the educational and occupational deficits they present. This is true not only for economically deprived blacks but for any group suffering from male occupational instability. The result for the male is devastating in terms of self-image and aspiration. It leads to an exaggerated need for toughness and to survive by outmaneuvering. The pattern is perpetuated generationally since family life is not a pattern which has had much positive reinforcement, nor does the type of family life offered have much appeal.

Avoidance of trouble is listed as a second normative standard by Miller for lower-class youths. These youths are seen as reacting to trouble with a double meaning, since trouble refers to both law-abiding and law-violating behavior. Trouble is defined not primarily by wrongness but by getting involved in predicaments. It is not wrong to steal, fight, skip school, or get drunk, but it is wrong to get caught and have to deal with all of the blundering paraphernalia of community agencies and courts. A youth who is not caught may attain definite individual benefits and group status. In fact, this may happen even if he is caught. Threat of exclusion from a peer group may compel law-violating behavior.

Outsmarting others is a third norm viewed as a skill in duplicity and conning others in contrast to academic achievement. The theory does not satisfactorily explain the exceptions who somehow do assimilate the norms of academic achievement except to view them as deviants since they do not conform to the patterns and expectations of their group. Little status is conferred for acts of penitence to an authority when caught, but there is for beating the rap. In fact, the more intelligent and perceptive of these youths learn that the smart approach is not to play the tough guy when apprehended, but to feign contriteness and cooperation with the authorities—bartering for time by a withering away of the authorities' need to do something, much like what adolescents witness with adults in the white-collar crime area. The question left unresolved is who the subgroup are who learn to con intelligently.

Excitement is a fourth norm, but it is not a search for thrills and stimulation, but rather an effort to avoid the dull monotony and barrenness of the home environment coupled with the stultifying educational experiences most of these youths have had. Forms of this are drugs, drinking, gambling, stealing, car theft, joy-riding, or destruction of public property. There is a high stress on luck, which accounts for the risks and daring in these adventures. Similarly note the emphasis on mobility and autonomy: "No one is going to confine me," "I'm my own boss," which reveal both striving and the end, where the youth is ultimately deprived of his liberty through incarceration. A clinician assesses depressive components both symptomatically, and as a defensive effort, to deal with depressive affect.[16]

The stable lower classes are those who adapt by eventually performing in unskilled or semi-skilled jobs. They may or may not finish high school. Those who are the achievers from this group, the aspiring but conflicted, are the ones who are most intelligent but perpetuate their antisocial behavior from the frustrations necessary to surmount their backgrounds. The result is a self-perpetuating system of lack of opportunity integrally related to their lack of exposure to adequate educational and social institutions. There is a doubly reinforcing effect of lack of opportunities dampening aspirations, and without adequate aspirations the opportunities promoted by social planners are not utilized. Some feel there is good evidence to show that educational aspirations are actually quite high in lower-class communities, but a variety of factors erode this as the children are socialized into the self-perpetuating lower-class culture. Social reformers advocated educational opportunities so the aspirations would not be evaded as frequently.[17] Needless to say, the multiple factors operating beyond educational opportunity per se are often enough to cloud adequate evaluation.

Theories Emphasizing Lower-Class Etiology. Cultural blindness in theorists from various disciplines has at times proceeded to the extent that some view delinquency as normative behavior in the lower classes. This represents the ultimate in sociolocial determinism. Criteria for lower-class membership are taken as either being a member of a group with its own identifiying features, such as Miller proposed, or being a member of the lower class by standing in opposition to the standards of the middle class—an equally unpleasant position to be in. Thrown in with this argument are such positions, voluminously written about, as the *differential association* theory (which holds that delinquent and criminal behavior are basically learned by association with antisocial elements[18]). "The statistics on ordinary crime so consistently show an overrepresentation of lower-class persons that it is reasonable to assume that there is a real difference between the behavior of the social classes, so far as criminality is concerned."[19]

Cloward and Ohlin pointed out that delinquents are easily recruited into adult criminal activity, but this is no longer viable due to the progressive isolation of youths from adults in all social class groups.[20] The autonomy of many youths has itself provided a breakdown in the direct continuity into adult criminality. A subgroup is posited who are failures in terms of any conventional norms. These are seen as most likely to resort to consistent use of whatever narcotics are predominant at a particular time or alcoholic problems.

This is probably too sweeping a generalization and would certainly not be valid based on the large number of adolescents who have periodically resorted to drugs or alcohol from all social classes. Cloward and Ohlin actually struck a variation on the differential distribution theory. While acknowledging that such a differential exists in their thinking, they went on to argue that the delinquent subculture actually is more important among the lower classes because of the greater social problems in terms of differential costs, commitments, and consequences.

The concept of anomie has also been used in descriptions of dysfunction between culturally prescribed goals and socially organized access to such goals.[21] Anomie was used in the sense of certain groups having only relative accessability to the means for achievement which induces a state of normlessness in their group. These sociological descriptions are parallel to the affective states of helplessness and hopelessness, induced in individuals exposed to the types of disparities which are prominent affective states in depressed people. All of these trends could be encompassed by the *opportunity theory* of delinquency, based on the lack of opportunities which contribute to delinquency.

The value of these theories to the clinician is to stress how behavior cannot be viewed in isolation from the milieu in which it occurs. None of them compel an abandonment of the psychodynamic model of explanation since they focus on a different dimension and level of explanation. Plaguing questions remain: why do some individuals not take advantage of opportunities to advance themselves when they are offered? Why do some join borderline illegal groups while others do not? Is there in fact a differential use of drugs and alcohol among different social classes of youths? What differences in goals, values, and ideals of individuals and family units expressed in a particular social setting are relevant to delinquent acts? There is the pervasive problem of evaluation in all theories dealing with delinquency. It is not that advocates of theories do not believe that evidence confirms their theories, but that ways to subject them to tests where they can be disconfirmed are again lacking. Since this cannon of a scientific theory is not met, theories continue to abound.

Practical differences take the issue out of academic pedagogy. Some of this is due to the pressures by citizens and professionals in communities that something must be done. The result is that every proposed theory of delinquency is seized upon as offering the latest in intervention techniques so that an adequate evaluation is never achieved. What does occur is that theories are recycled without ever being laid to rest.

GROUP DELINQUENCY

Another approach to the origins of delinquent behavior focuses on a subgroup of those engaged in delinquency. Early studies considered the nature of gangs in terms of age, intelligence, ethnic grouping, and descriptive characteristics. There are descriptions of Irish and German gangs in New York City at the turn of the century which have more recently been supplanted by descriptions of black, Puerto Rican, and Cuban gangs. Thrasher, working in Chicago at the same time as Shaw, used case histories and statistical techniques in his book, *The Gang.* He pointed out the functions served by belonging to a group: lessening intrafamilial ties, different opportunities for excitement not available to a lone individual, opportunities for heterosexual contacts, and a vehicle for action. According to Thrasher, "Each gang as a whole, and other types of social groups as well, may be conceived of as possessing an action pattern. Every person in the group performs his characteristic function with reference to others. . . . Lacking the group, personality in the sense used here would not exist." Since then a plethora of community experiences and writings on the nature of gangs has occurred.

What Constitutes a Gang? Glueck and Whelan differentiated four types of gangs: street-corner gangs, clubs, conflict gangs, and pathologically delinquent gangs.[23]

The needs satisfied by gang membership are:

1. The need to convince one's self that he is a person of worth
2. The need for acceptance, belonging, and recognition
3. The need for new experiences, shared interests, and ideals

4. The need for common support on a peer level in a subculture of society toward which tremendous punitiveness, hostility, and conflict is directed
5. The need to possess, own, and control
6. The need for status in the neighborhood and community in which one lives
7. The need to identify with something in the subculture which symbolizes culture, authority, and prestige
8. The need to have an impersonal medium through which to rebel against the environment, both physically and socially; to deal with and express fears, anxieties, and insecurities, as well as feelings of hostility, aggression, and anger
9. The need for protection from real or fantasized threat
10. The need for opportunity for sublimating and expressing basic drives
11. The need for peer group-evolved concepts of equality, justice, and control
12. The teenage need for symbolic group ceremonies and activities

More recent work has centered on the criteria for membership in a gang in terms of how cohesive its boundaries must be. Some have extended the concept to make it closer to the theory of collective behavior or a social movement. Gangs are seen as varying from peer groupings as a phenomenon of adolescence, which are not under consideration here, to social gangs which predominantly engage in mild delinquency, on to highly formalized conflict groups dedicated to reform with or without the use of violence. Yablonsky refers to a *near-group* for one in the middle of a continuum between amorphous mobs on one end and organizations with definite measurement criteria at the other end.[24] In some there is only a small core of active organizers who persistently identify with the gang, but in times of stress or excitement the size of a group may be multiplied manyfold.

The relationship between individual psychopathology and group funtioning is illustrated in the thesis that core membership of violent gangs may be composed of paranoid psychopaths, analogous to what is described as being in the delusional world of a paranoid pseudo-community with huge membership myths available at the beck and call of a leader.[25] The interlacing of these processes is in need of depth explanations to delineate the personal and family characteristics of the leaders as well as members.

The Role of the Gang Leader. The effectiveness of small numbers of self-proclaimed leaders with an evangelistic fervor is striking.

These leaders often govern by fiat, or veto any proposal which might threaten them. Investigations are even more desirable when the forces of adolescent group activity appear on the way from strictly illegal acts against property (such as theft or gang fights over turf) to a shift to bigger things which border on terrorism. The appeal for youths of politicized revolutionary groups, committed to radical solutions and acts to the point of sacrificing life, has long been an intriguing puzzle. Ascribing such commitments to group influence alone does not suffice for it appears to involve personal components such as a sense of betrayal of disillusionment with ideals once cherished. The relevance to questions of the political criminal are evident.[26] Nor is this just a contemporary problem, as witnessed by Dostoyevsky's portayal of young revolutionaries in *The Possessed.*[27]

One investigation of adolescent gang leaders in New York City found them to be suffering from severe personal psychopathology.[28] Their extreme violence and readiness to fight give them qualities which attract followers. These findings stand in stark contrast to the viewpoint that such delinquent gang leaders are psychologically intact adolescents rebelling against an unjust environment. The thrust is not to ignore contibutory social pathology but rather to reinstate a personal component in the equation which involves a question for understanding rather than just opposition. The frequent use of narcotics among some gang leaders, a finding which is also in opposition to the beliefs of many others, is viewed as the instigator to other members of the gang. The resultant narcotizing effect has been seen as one of the main pacifying instruments which can lead to a tapering of some gang delinquency over the years in some major metropolitan areas.

> A case example is that of a twenty-year-old who was the leader of the most feared street gang in his community at age fifteen. He achieved this position as a result of the admiration and awe which his intrepid and extravagant outbursts of violence elicited. He fought often, used all types of weapons, and was known as a 'sneaky' and 'dirty' fighter who could attack viciously without provocation or warning. He was arrested for one homicide and probably committed one more. He began using drugs at the age of fifteen and immediately became less violent. Many of his followers also began using drugs as a result of indoctrination and emulation, and the gang changed from a fighting group to a coterie of drug addicts which soon split into groups of two and three. A few tries at communal living with mixed sexes seeking 'love' were unsuccessful.

He never worked and maintained himself by armed robbery, burglary, selling drugs, and 'scheming' on his family, friends, and street associates. In addition to the murder, he was arrested in connection with assault, robbery, larceny, and narcotics, serving some prison time.

His father became concerned about the boy's fighting only when he was apprehended by the police. As a child he performed sadistic acts on animals and engaged in petty thefts. He did not get along well with other children, and began to have sexual intercourse at the age of thirteen, associating sexual desire with evil and dirt. In later years he suffered from impotence and premature ejaculations.

In recent years he has had feelings of desperation, tantrums, crying fits, and uncontrollable violent outbursts which frightened him. He expected to die young. During his last incarceration he got into many fights and was isolated as a security risk. Thereafter he became grandiosely delusional, believing his wild exaggerations were true, and planning litigious actions against prison personnel. He began to fear for his sanity and developed a pseudohomosexual panic. After his last release from prison he went through a period of agitation which he 'treated' by resorting to drugs.

He has chronic and pervasive fears and explosive, unpredictable rages which endanger his life and freedom. Drugs have provided a partial way out of his dilemma as well as an escape from sex, work, and competition, for all of which he is incapacitated. There is minimal capacity for empathic resonance with people except in terms of violence, heroic doings, vengeance, and a desire for power and effortlessly gained money.

Delinquency as part of a subculture opposed to the middle-class norms raises preliminary definitional problems. The term subculture, like acting out, has been subject to a variety of meanings. The sub prefix has reference to a sector of the larger culture. This is not the place to expand upon the 160 definitions of culture which have been critically reviewed.[29] From these various usages it is felt that the essential core of a culture is the traditional patterns and ideas to which values attach and which are selectively and historically transmitted. These are involved in promoting action as well as being the product of action.

Kroeber and Parsons advocated a distinction between *culture* as the content and pattern of values and ideas which are transmitted and help shape human behavior, and *society* as the social system which designates the relations between individuals and collectivities.[30] The meaning of subculture has varied from the original conceptions which viewed it as part of the larger culture, while still possessing a unity of its own based on class, ethnicity, residence, and religion. The emphasis shifted to the value system espoused by this subset, acknowledging that in any culture there is a distribution of a norm, very much like a standard deviation, which varies from extreme affirmation to negation. Such variants are what give cogency to a subcultural group.

The Theory of Albert Cohen. This was expanded in a contemporary fashion with reference to delinquent boys by Albert Cohen. He noted that subcultural norms are shared among the actors in a group who stand to profit by these norms and find a sympathetic moral climate with each other where the norms can be realized.[31] The subcultural group has value judgments and a social value system which are both part of, but also apart from, the larger or central value system. This subvalue system is perpetuated as long as it continues to serve the needs of those who follow the original group. The subcultural values may retain some of the elements of the central value system of the broader culture while partially accepting others and also adopting contradictory values as needed.

The amalgamation separates the subculture and prevents total integration within a culture. The degree of separateness is derived in part by the response of the larger cultural group to the subset, and in part by their mutual interactions. However, the result is an ethos of shared values which are learned, reinforced, and used and which differ from those of the general culture. The concept of the subculture is not confined merely to an ethnic group or geographical area, but is used with reference to deviants of any type, so that such groupings may be composed of groups of chronically ill medical patients, the mentally ill, enlisted men, drug users, prison inmates, or delinquents.

Cohen has explicitly raised a question as to the subculture of the delinquent in terms of the values, beliefs, and practices which encourage delinquent behavior and delineate relationships to those who are outside the group. Whether this subculture is a negative reaction to the larger culture, or rather a positive outgrowth from it, Cohen depicts it as a reaction formation as opposed to the pious legalities of middle-class life. The future delinquent is seen as emerging from an initial state of indecisiveness and ambivalence to repudiate the set of middle-class values with a substitute set of his own. A set of norms evolves which is primarily opposed to the larger culture. If a boy is to accept these alternative norms, he has to reject two alternatives: striving for upward mobility via aspirations to make it by following middle-class rules, or to temporize in an intermediate position of a corner boy whose activities are of a borderline delinquency nature.

To reject these solutions is to participate in the creation and maintenance of a new culture—a delinquent subculture—which has six main characteristics:

1. *Non-utilitarianism* is seen in social acts, such as stealing, not being performed from need or some community or group need, but rather for the hell of it. In this setting stolen objects are rarely converted to money, which is also a distinction from adult criminal groups.

2. *Maliciousness* flouts or challenges the conventional middle-class norms rather than trying to evade the norms. Dirty tricks may be done for fun. However, Cohen does not ignore the internalization of middle-class norms which the lower-class boy cannot totally escape. His internalization of middle-class standards, coupled with limited access to the goals of the middle-class, contribute to status anxiety. It is the lack of clear channels for attaining such goals that gives the lower-class boy a feeling of being at an unfair disadvantage.[32] This added source of frustration is handled by a reaction formation against heightened hostilities. The end result is an irrational and unaccountable hostility which makes impulse control more difficult toward externalized targets for aggression who represent hated objects. The mechanism is applicable to the situation of any deprived group with legitimate grievances who direct their hostility against the representative of the oppressors. Racial and religious groups easily mobilize such feelings in their members over a cause that touches old hurts and sensitivities.

3. *Negativism* is a characteristic in the sense of subcultural norms being in opposition to those of the middle class. Opposition takes root from resistance to evaluating themselves by middle-class measuring rods which are applied at school and work. A state of personal anxiety and alienation is induced from the larger group which makes any proffered solution with status overtones seem appealing.

4. *Versatility* is represented by a degree of non-specialization to perform delinquent acts, so that adaptability to antisocial behavior is present. There is no one particular technique that is exclusively employed in antisocial behavior.

5. *Group autonomy* is represented by a low tolerance for externally imposed restraints. It is coupled with a feeling that decisions should be self-imposed in contrast to being imposed by an outside authority.

6. *Hedonistic activities* are noted by the short-run gratifications and impulsivity present in many of the activities. Application to academic pursuits becomes frustrating and progressively unrewarding. It also contributes to status anxiety in which feelings of

inferiority are attached. These have been described as follows:[33]

> That lower-class youth (mainly the sons of dependent families or of low-income laborers and service workers) are disadvantaged in the struggle for 'success' is certain. Two decades of solid research have reminded us that schools and churches, courts and social agencies uphold middle-nlass values and virtues, and peg the working-class child at the bottom. His opportunities to acquire the vocabulary, health, personal characteristics, social skills, and manners approved in these places are few. At home, the occupational models he encounters among his older brothers, friends, relatives, father, and father's friends are generally of low status; the sustained pressure for school performance is lacking. At school, he experiences consequent discomfort. The testing and grading system puts a premium on information and abilities developed in middle- and upper-class homes. Discipline will be unequally administered by middle-class teachers—to his disadvantage. The conduct thought proper and rewarded by the school—stay on the job, learn your lessons, budget your time, obey authority, develop the ambition, initiative, self-control, good character, and sociability to get ahead—this ideal conduct which supports the home and neighborhood training of the middle-class child, contradicts that of the slum child.

Status is cultivated by a set of standards opposed to the middle class. This is done by attacking authority objects, expressions of aggressivity, and the use of gang membership to participate in the rewards by a new set of standards. The gang need not take one specific form of opposition, such as fighting rival groups, but it can be organized around an activity such as theft, vandalism, escapades, sexual liberties, or drug usage, as a few examples. In much of their value system, one can sense overt opposition to the middle-class ethic and what the lower classes view as a mockery of the more honest values which they aggressively espouse. Three examples illustrate this.

1. The middle-class ethic of individual responsibility as a moral imperative is viewed as a rationalization for exploitation. The proverb that "the poor help the poor" contrasts to the paternalistic help via philanthropic enterprises which the middle classes use to protect their own interests from a discontent lower class.

2. The doctrine of honesty is used by the middle-class in a legalistic manner to refer to meeting one's obligations on time, such as rent, while the subcultural opposition thinks of honesty as personal integrity to the group. The perversion of honesty by those in power manipulating their own power-ridden needs is seen as a mockery.

3. The emphasis on appearances, or selling one's self as part of the middle-class stress on achievement, is seen as the false front of advertising. Being able to sell oneself is quite close to conning others.

Opposition to these middle-class attributes has widened to adolescents in almost all social classes. It is manifest in ways warying from a deliberately ostentatious caricature of physical appearance (old or contrasting clothing), to middle-class college youth revolting against the regimented education imposed upon them to take their place in the rat race. The ultimate in defeat is seen in the collapse of youth movements when their members rejoin the rat race, with a quiet resolution to abandon personal ethics and to be as cleverly corrupt as current models in power.

Extension of The Theory and Critique. The original model of a subcultural gang presented by Cohen has been expanded. The expansion recognizes groups with different attributes and goals. In addition to the model of a male, subcultural, delinquent group, a *conflict-oriented subcultural* group has been elaborated, composed primarily of large gangs with a formal organization who engage in overt physical aggression.

A drug-addict or withdrawn subculture might be present which is non-violent and utilitarian. This takes the form of active participation in an addict subculture, or merely withdrawing into a group that stands in opposition to the goals of middle-class life.

A semi-professional thief group is a transition from petty offenses to organized crime. Although most of the juveniles drop out by age sixteen or seventeen, a few take up this lifestyle which becomes part of an adult criminal subculture. The gangs can be elaborated into highly organized criminal activities involving car thefts, store robberies, apartment burglaries and eventually, once into the youth period, some drift into the rackets. [34]

A subculture of violence is possible, in which a cluster of values laden toward violence are present in the lifestyle, socialization processes, and interpersonal relationships of a group living in similar conditions. [35] The behavior ranges from assault to homicide. Those considered psychotic or legally insane who engage in such activities are excluded. Since only about 5 percent of homicidal acts are premeditated, intentional killings, the bulk of such acts are often an inherent part of a pattern of explosive violence and mutual provocation.

A middle-class delinquent subculture is a variation which needs a satisfactory explanation. Such a variation is challenging to the subcultural theory of delinquency since if the same type of delinquent behavior can flourish outside the lower classes, it challenges the presupposition that there is something about the lower classes which is endemic to the development of delinquency. Theorizing from the subcultural delinquency school becomes must elusive at this junction. Thus, an explanation for middle-class delinquency says it is not purely economic criteria which are determiners, but the aspects of family arrangements and methods of child-rearing. Yet to accept this slips away from a cultural explanation per se, and puts the focus on intrafamilial factors.

Although Cohen adheres to a theoretical position that subcultural delinquency in different social classes is qualitatively a different response to qualitatively different problems occurring in varying contexts of interaction, this presumes what is to be proven. At times Cohen is biased in favor of not letting us forget how delinquency is disproportionately concentrated in the lower classes. If we acknowledge that data on overall incidence and types of delinquency are grossly deficient, even for the lower classes, are we not further pressed in holding to a position that middle-class delinquency is qualitatively distinct? Even with respect to juvenile groups, the question is whether the groups are responding more to the psychological and social problems which they are facing than to differences based primarily on social class level, defined non-economically.

Resort must be had to a fused psychological-sociological model in the form of masculine-protest in the middle-class boy, linked to a motif in the family and the occupational system. The emphasis is on modern society, where the father is relatively unknown to the boy due to preoccupation and absence for the sake of his work. The mother is the example of morality, discipline, and an object for identification to separate himself from since she is the symbol of goodness. The middle-class boy then engages in bad behavior to prove his masculinity. Yet this hypothesis adds too much of the wrong thing. At one point it not only holds that one significant variable is the relatively absent father, but, conversely, the lower-class boy has a clearer delineation of the male and female sex roles. However, when it is realized that for much of the lower-class the male model is either physically absent or inadequate when present, the subcultural theory falls back on the greater mobility hypothesis. This hypothesis holds that the lower-class boy has wider access to different male models than the middle-class boy which is at least questionable if not fallacious.

Explanations of female delinquency within the subcultural theory are also vague and unsatisfying. From the framework of a girl being exposed to the presence of her middle-class mother, even the hypothesis raised concerning the middle-class boy is not available. If we rely on the argument that girls of all classes may have conflicts within their families, we do not have a theory of subcultural delinquency. One variation offers an explanation based on the rejection of legitimate status goals, in which a girl seeks status by attracting male attention through sexual activity rather than through other attributes. Such activity, can hardly be described as a class-linked problem. Female delinquent subcultures are much in need of explanation from the viewpoint of how class-associated they in fact are. There are psychosocial factors operating with girls who deviate from the social norm in their behavior. Sex-role confusion would be only one variable.

General criticisms have been raised about subcultural theories of delinquency. The emphasis on groups has impressed some as an example of a culture-bound theory, at best applicable only to some of the large metropolitan areas of the United States with high-density population and urban slums—and then at variable times. From another vantage point, the nature of adolescent group action in gangs is in constant flux. Descriptions of a gang subculture may not fit overtime. Some hold the descriptions did not even fit gangs at the time Cohen published. The theory that gang activity is non-utilitarian has been much criticized, as it holds that organized delinquent activity with a rational goal was not carried out. There were too many overtones that gang behavior represented the angry outburst of lower-class juveniles against a different social class rather than angry expressions from feelings of apprehension based on multiple factors.

Some early formulations held that subcultural delinquents did not comply with society's norms simply because they did not know what the norms were. This position, basically that of a cognitive deficit, is usually not put so directly but is concealed as part of theoretical jargon. Excluding those with intellectual malfunction on some basis, this is a weak theory. A cogent criticism is that the subcultural delinquent group operates by many of the same standards as those in broader society. As noted, partial adherence to middle-class norms is not contrary to subcultural groups, yet many of the same motives and affects operate in these individuals as they do with those in other classes. Needs for status, not available by conventional channels, promote deviant ways to obtain it. A clinican phrases this as deficiencies in self-esteem, leading people into pathways to bolster it. Nor can anyone, believe self-esteem problems are confined particularly to one social class. Feelings of guilt and shame for transgressions or shortcomings as a common psychological core do not seem to restrict much of this behavior. If such a critique is tentatively accepted, an explanation for the intermittent violation of middle-class rules may be offered based on the technique of neutralization.

Neutralization Theory. Delinquents rarely violate norms without some excuse. Except for certain extreme groups, a pretense of justification is usually offered.[36] This is not different from justifications being offered for types of killings in wars, self-defense, coercion, duress, or undue provocation. Justifications permit a neutralization of the inhibitions against certain anti-social acts which are supposed to operate.

There are various techniques of neutralization which have a good deal of overlap with certain psychodynamic formulations:

1. Denial of responsibility operates by assigning the responsibility for one's acts to someone or something else. The assignment may be to parents as unloving, living in a slum, or having bad friends. Unfortunately, these are the very reasons often seized upon by public media or conscious community groups to account for delinquency. It provides a convenient rationale for a delinquent to continue his behavior until others shape up.

2. Denial of injury is an attempt to negate wrongdoing. "The guy wasn't hurt just because I took his car and drove it, was he?" Such borrowing is distorted into being a purely private affair.

3. Attempts to assign blame to the injured party involve projection. This may be by attacking an outsider, such as a member of a minority group, cops, homosexuals, drunks. It can be more removed, as in the form of property offenses: "Corporations don't feel it."

4. Condemnation of the condemners is another device to shift the focus of being blamed for transgressions. It is a red-herring, operating by pointing out that the rules of society are unjust, cops are stupid, shrinks are crazy, and teachers have favorites—all in the service of deflecting negative sanctions from themselves.

5. Appeals to higher loyalties, such as dedication to the gang or old friendships, take precedence over the demands laid down by the rules of the larger society. Indeed, higher loyalty argues that a lower-class boy is not really so sensitive of his exclusion by the middle class since his gang dedication would be paramount. What would have to be added would be psychological explanations such as reaction formation, so that the lower-class boy really could aspire for middle-class status.

Explanations on a level which could confirm or deny such defensive operations would be required. Hence, the motivational dynamics for the emergence of the delinquent subculture ultimately reside in offering psychological hypotheses, although maintenance of the subculture may occur independently once it is functioning.[37] Neutralization techniques could be equally well conceptualized from the vantage point of ego defenses. Again, the techniques need not be restricted to a single social class, but seem applicable to antisocial behavior in many situations with a particular twist where the social class differential operates.

INSTITUTIONAL INFLUENCES

Schools. Three other major social approaches to delinquency remain for discussion: institutional influences, the role of communication media, and family configurations.

There is no area more laden with feelings and fewer facts than the relationship between the practices employed by educational institutions and juvenile delinquency. Perhaps the respective difficulties in evaluation in each of the spheres is responsible: educating the child, and treating his nonconformity. The result is a series of antagonisms and accusations which the public occasionally joins. Confusion about the functions of courts and schools is noted in positions that one of the major causes of delinquency lies in the failure of the schools. Since the schools, along with churches and families, are one of the basic institutions influencing the socialization of children, causal factors in socialization do not result but are rather ascribed to these institutions.

Although there has lately been a temporary rejuvenation of the argument that schools are soft on discipline and thus responsible for delinquency and moral decay in American youth, this does not focus on many relevant issues which merit discussion. One can detect, when the juvenile court is used as an agency for dealing with school problems, an underlying belief that a child having problems in school needs some special type of schooling. The need might be because of an intellectual deficit or special physical handicap, but if it is associated with problems of attendance or behavior disorders, a special type of schooling is needed.

The types of schools suggested vary as much as the viewpoint of a special relationship between schooling and delinquency espoused. For some, special types of disciplinary schools are seen as necessary, including reform schools with military-type settings (be they private schools or work camps). Some see a special need for substitute family settings, with substitute parents who can help the children learn. Others feel more freedom and openness, in contrast to structure, allows curiosity to flourish and learning to take place, in institutions like Summerhill or open schools.

A specific issue is the reading disabilities seen in antisocial youths. Deficits in reading level in delinquents are well known to those working in courts and correctional facilities. In some cases the disability is profound.

Has the school system failed because it is their responsibility to teach reading? We expect a child with a major learning handicap to have a disadvantage in adjusting to community demands, yet there is really no such thing as a reading problem, but rather a series of biological-psychological-social problems which may all operate in a child not reading well. Further details will not be repeated here, except to question whether the schools should be able to provide diagnostic remedial, and treatment measures as soon as possible. The burden is then properly placed on the school to explain why such large numbers of children receive inadequate evaluations and management. It does not suffice to point out that some children have predisposing family and cultural problems before they come to school, since that merely extends the question.

The use of uniform teaching methods for all children may be a major detrimental influence on the child who performs poorly and progressively becomes less motivated. Problems with authority and hostile rejection of the rejectors is reinforced. It is not any more reasonable to expect every child to learn in the same manner than to expect any one psychotherapeutic approach to suffice. Rather than place blame on the schools, courts, or families, we must face two basic problems in the area of learning disability and potential asociability. The first is the limitation on how much can actually be done for children with certain kinds of limitations. The second raises fundamental questions about the deficits in the tangled web of community resources involving school personnel, clinics, diverse agencies, hospitals, professionals, and paraprofessionals.

Does truancy contribute to delinquency? Is truancy the first step in delinquency as one so often hears? Does the willful missing of school constitute a causal factor toward antisocial behavior? Perhaps such accusations make school authorities eager to resort to the courts to solve their problems. A cross-cultural comparison is relevant since most European delinquency codes do not contain truancy. Permitting children to leave school earlier, coupled with screening out those not deemed competent for further academic training, accounts in part for the difference. More fundamental is something for everyone in contrast to seeing it as something for a more restricted group who can meet high criteria with commitment. In the United States college education is considered almost as a right. Conflict is inherent, for the right is given on one level even when it cannot be exercised as a viable option on another.

The only equitable solution would be to eliminate the judicial dumping approach by schools and communities and place instead the emphasis on early detection of problems in schools when they begin to emerge. Delinquency in a community may or may not be altered. If any sense is to be made of the diversion of youngsters from the juvenile justice system, it means that what is needed will have to be supplied somewhere other than by court authority. At most court intake could function in an assessment and referral manner, but this is just one more step in what could presumably have been handled before that by the school if problems in performance or attendance were involved.[38] It is questionable whether the coercive sanction of the courts is capable of inculcating the desire to learn which is basic to any educational venture. Of course, the elimination of slum schools, unqualified personnel, and an improvement in the quality and quantity of teachers and auxiliary personnel as once recommended by the President's Commission on Law Enforcement and Administration of Justice would be needed.[39]

The Media. How much impact do movies and television have on the incidence of delinquency as well as specific acts of violence? What influence do comic books and pornographic literature have on promoting delinquent behavior? Does some of the literature for children exert an influence toward acting out? Is there clinical evidence of adverse consequences from such influences in promoting delinquency or in enhancing conflict?

The figures seem startling. One television survey indicated the average American child between five and fifteen will see 13,000 violent deaths in ten years, usually in some detail, and frequently with sadistic and sexual overtones. A survey of one week of evening television, plus the Saturday morning children's cartoons, revealed eighty-four killings and 372 other acts of violence.[40] The Mass Media Task Force of the National Commission on the Causes and Prevention of Violence concluded, after reviewing research, that a general reduction in the level of televised violence was needed— especially an elimination of the violence in children's cartoon programming.[41]

What can be made of data which reveal 6,500 murders by gun annually in the United States compared to thirty-seven in Japan, sixty-eight in West Germany, thirty in England and ninety-nine in Canada, where the combined populations are equal to ours? Or the realization that since 1900 more than 500,000 Americans have died from lethal weapons, mainly guns, which are more deaths than in all our wars put together. Untangling the myriad variables resulting in these figures is unbelievably complicated, and raises questions of a historical and political nature. However, it is legitimate to wonder whether there is evidence that the mass media to which children and adolescents are exposed has any delineated consequences in delinquent behavior. Many behavioral scientists are skeptical about the evidence. A typical approach is to cite a few experimental situations, which seem constricted compared to the broad questions being asked, and say that no definitive evidence is available, or that the problem might not even be researchable because it is so complex. Yet, it would be inconsistent to say that the themes and emotions portrayed on television are not a source of learning, and that they have no specific impacts on violence.

Many insights about television and movies have been based on clinical work with selected groups of children. Evaluations have often been made in retrospect. It is not surprising that movies and television, like any other compelling emotional contact, have a significant impact on a person. Why some individuals accept aspects of a potentially traumatic situation, but do not react to others which are even more traumatic, lies within the confines of the individual's life history. If one is asked for experimental studies outside the therapeutic situation, data is scanty. Another major deficit is that the type of experimental situation is often quite contrived, focusing on the dependent variable of attempting to assess changes in aggression—which is different from subsequent development of antisocial or criminal behavior. However, some studies have noted what they believe is a consistent and reliable relationship between preferences for viewing violent television programs and engaging in aggressive or delinquent acts.[42] [43]

One study was carried out in Sweden by exposing 160 children, aged eleven to eighteen, to a series of movies which previously had been banned for children by a government board of censors.[44] Scenes in the movies contained rapes, mob killings, sadistic beatings, and sexual orgies. Evaluation of the children was done by direct observation during the showings, obtaining the opinions of the subjects about the reaction after the showing, as well as their own estimates of the emotional response of the film characters, and finally psychiatric interviews. The investigators were unable to find any perceptible reactions after the showing in 80 percent, and in the remaining 20 percent only transitory minor symptoms of anxiety, depression, or poor sleep patterns occurred. On a nine-month follow-up, no further adverse consequences were noted, nor did any differences appear when one of the movies was shown to a group of delinquent boys. Only one thirteen-year-old girl with obsessive traits showed a prolonged depressive reaction (which could be taken as an indication of an altered response in a girl with predisposing conflicts).

In contrast to the ad hoc exposure given to a violent movie, what is the effect on children from chronic exposure to a deluge of cartoons on television? The cartoons are heavily loaded with violence and killing, and may have sadistic themes. The closer to real life, the more upsetting films appear to be as judged by public protest. This may account for the controversy over films stressing male chauvinism, sadism, machismo, and territorial imperatives. Many of these deal with the deficits of internalized controls when dependency conflicts and rage are kindled.[45] The nightly impact of killings from war newsreels as witnessed for years until the end of the Vietnam War may be even more detrimental. The fear is that violence is seen as an acceptable norm for settling disputes. Shootouts between police and those committing crimes seen routinely on news shows may play a similar role. There is also the impact of massive conditioning processes, with resultant habituation to the use of violence and tolerance for such behavior when used by groups for whatever purposes.

The model for studying the impact of an aggressive model can be seen in an experiment which utilized a film-mediated model to exhibit three novel aggressive responses accompanied by verbalization.[46] In one situation the model was punished, in a second the model was rewarded with approval and food reinforcers, while in a third no response-consequences occurred. During the acquisition period the children neither performed any overt responses nor received direct reinforcement, so that learning was purely observational or vicarious. Children in the model-punished condition were noted to perform fewer imitative responses than those in the other two groups. Boys showed more imitative responses than girls, especially in the model-punished condition.

The study was then extended. Children in all three groups were given positive incentives to reproduce the responses of the model.

The result was to wipe out any previously observed performance differences which indicated that motivational factors or anticipation of positive or negative reinforcement could augment or decrease the probability of certain responses. A reward or punishment may follow closely upon an act, or there may be knowledge of how the behavior is later rewarded, such as by prestige or power. But does a child who spends several hours weekly watching the violence of professional football on television become more predisposed to the use of physical violence since he is aware of the enormous adulation given to the players? Such a question may have more significance than the impact of the caricatures in cartoons.

One study exposed young children to a situation where an aggressive model was rewarded or punished. One control group had no exposure to the models, while a second group had highly expressive but non-aggressive models.[47] The models were filmed adult males who employed considerable physical and verbal aggression in taking the possessions of another adult. In one situation the behavior resulted in the adult being severely punished. Children who witnessed the aggressive model rewarded showed more imitative physical and verbal aggression than the children who saw the model punished. The latter were no different from the control groups. Further, a general disinhibiting effect on aggressive responses was noted in the group exposed to rewarded aggression, so that new aggressive responses were added. This occurred even though the children were able to voice disapproval of the model's behavior, so that the values which had been taught were still transgressed. Understanding of portrayed motives and consequences has little impact on postviewing aggressive behavior.[48]

While the material presented has sought to deal with the psychosocial evidence and arguments about the impact of violence on television and in movies, the issues are not confined to that sphere. One argument for delinquency due to the mass media has used the moral argument. Communication media of all types are seen as cogent inculcators of attitudes and standards in the young, particularly in view of the massive amount of exposure—and hence modeling influence—coupled with the decline of family influence. A movie which not only employs a great deal of violence, but portrays individuals as amoral—people who degrade others by using them as vehicles for some goal, conquest, or sexual gratification—presents this as an acceptable norm to the child. Advertising illustrates the impact made through the mass media to induce certain behaviors, and that similar inducements should operate from whatever else is being shown, particularly since many desires are stimulated.

The argument is that there is at least a tempting offer to give a try by emulation, if not more extensively. Most significant is a longitudinal study designed to follow the development of aggressive behavior in boys and girls from ages eight to eighteen.[49] Originally, several measures of each child's aggressive behavior were made and related to their preference for violent television programs. At age eighteen, when the subjects were out of high school, similar measures of program preferences and aggressive behavior were obtained. The results indicated that preferences for violent programs at age eight were significantly related to aggressive and delinquent behavior at age eighteen; for girls the relationship was in the same direction, but less strong.

Many questions dealing with the impact of television and violence are left unanswered in any definitive sense. Yet, the impact of the mass media is too important to be ignored either in a prosocial or antisocial sense. There might be a difference in impact depending on the ages of the children in question, as well as the quantity of television exposure. Besides modeling and identification effects, there is the promotion of acting on impulses without the benefit of ego mediation or delay. There are also the diverse ways people are portrayed as relating to one another, such as expressing affection, solving conflicts, relating to children, parents, peers or authority figures. The number of programs portraying police officers, detectives or government officials as dishonest is striking. While this may portray the world as it is, it also functions as a norm-giver to the young viewer. It is striking when we realize that the power of the media industry, including producers and writers, is only minimally governed by anyone. No citizen group has a significant impact in influencing television programming, nor in appraising the competence of writers, performers or the script.[50]

Movies, whether shown on television or theatres, raise similar issues regarding the impact of violence. Restricting their showing raises constitutional questions. The endless debate that the wrong kind of movie will promote juvenile lawlessness has been raised in terms of film censorship for over fifty years. In the United States there have been widely varying standards, as well as ridiculous pronouncements, since movie censorship is largely a matter for local and state government regulation. It has only been since a 1952 Supreme Court decision that movies have been considered to fall within the First Amendment protections of speech and press, which overrules an earlier 1915 case that had paved the way for restrictive legislation.[51] Most of the cases have dealt with dirty movies and not with the question of limiting crime and violence in movies.

Limiting the exposure to film media on the basis of their alleged inducement to crime and violence is discussed under three headings:

1. Restrictions under the First Amendment
2. Crime and violence should be treated like obscenity where it has been established that the state does have regulatory powers
3. Portray of crime and violence must be regulated to prevent antisocial behavior

The analogy to obscenity regulations enters a legal and verbal maze of phrases which have behavioral implications. Obscenity statutes may merely codify that antisocial behavior is prevented or that the goal is to prevent exposure. Obscene material may be regarded as something which "excites impure thoughts," or which has a "tendency to excite lustful thoughts."[52] If so, would not regulations of films based on that which excites thoughts of violence, and which have a tendency to be acted upon, be considered in order? Such reasoning has not been accepted by the courts.

That the primary criterion for regulation of obscenity is not to view it as speech, but rather to give arguments based on reasons of history and public policy as to why obscenity regulation is valid. However, these reasons are not applicable to themes of crime and violence. Nor does it appear defensible to uphold a position that it might be all right to let adults choose which exposures to crime and violence they want, except for those under a stated age, such as sixteen.

Not only is there a problem of lack of confirmatory evidence, but it would lead to a restrictive type of social exposure for children which allows them to hear and see only what a group of government officials or local citizen's groups deem desirable. There is little hope that permitting individuals of such boards to control the media has any merit, and the long-range consequences for the psychological development of a child and society from such imposed conformity could be quite detrimental. There are many reasons for cautiousness in attempts to restrict portrayal of films with violent themes. While there has been little study of the psychology of the censor, security officer, and investigator, it appears that those attracted to these positions have personality structures which are more than ordinarily influenced by the fear, prejudices, and emotions which furnish the driving force for suppression. Daily administrative work is controlled by persons in the lower echelons of a bureaucracy. Their narrow adherence to rules, fear of superiors, and sensitivity to pressures carry the application of restrictions to an extreme limit.[53]

If movies or television are to be censored because they contribute to antisocial conduct, it would be necessary to demonstrate significant evidence. Even free speech is not an absolute, depending on the circumstances of its use. The burden is on the regulators, such as some state authority, to demonstrate an impending social harm, such as delinquent behavior, if certain movies are to come within a standard. Of course, the causal issue is exactly what is in question: Would removing certain movies or films serve to lessen antisocial behavior? The evidence we have for the genesis of antisocial behavior does not appear to be based on exposure to films. The exception would be the idiosyncratic case where a combination of predisposing factors in a current crisis situation are combined with the eliciting influence of the right film which leads to an eruption of violence. This latter type of situation is unpredictable.

In the above discussion, a fusion of movie films and television programs has been made. This type of generalization may not be valid for a particular case, but the approach seems warranted when the topic is the theme of crime and violence associated with such media. When the discussion is broadened, it is not necessarily warranted to use conclusions offered from studies about reasoning in one medium with another. Research about motion pictures may be valid for television, but what about the impact of photographs, painting, sculpture, radio, books, or comic strips? Comic books were the subject of Congressional Hearings as a response to parents and legislators who believed that crime comic books were behind delinquency.[54] Yet the President's Commission on Law Enforcement and the Administration of Justice did not even mention comic books, pictures, or movies in its survey of the causes of crime.[55] At one time Wertham was one of the leading advocates of danger in comic books. He felt the greatest impact of the comics was on normal children, since children were exposed to glorifications of murder, rape, obscenity, and crimes of violence. In his opinion such portrayals enticed children into experimenting with such behavior.[56]

A host of statutes continue to forbid sales of comic books to juveniles where deeds of bloodshed, violence and crime are the main themes. In fact, some statutes do not specify any age limit, but prosecute such book sales on the basis of portraying brutality and violence, or sadistic and masochistic themes.[57] While this type of media is subjected to control under obscenity regulations, there are almost nonexistent restrictions on movie themes which deal with crime and violence. This should not be interpreted as a plea to censor movies, but rather to illustrate how publicity and conflicting expert opinions result in measures aimed at controlling delinquency which have little basis in fact and are inconsistent.

Under the rationale of obscenity, many works of major writers would have been restricted. A list would have included Salinger, Hemmingway, Moravia, Joyce, Maugham, Dumas, Voltaire, DeMaupassant, Tolstoy, Zola and Freud. These writings would have been deemed unfit for adults let alone children. When the welfare and development of the child are at stake, all varieties of lay and professional opinion are mustered to regulate exposure to visual materials. One approach is not to permit the publication and distribution of what some censor or group thinks is obscene. Another is to bowdlerize many of the classic myths and fairy tales or eliminate the sensual along with the blood and guts. Others maintain that the old fairy stories are not only safe but helpful to children as a way of coping with their emotions such as love, hate, courage, fidelity and a sense of justice.[58] However, this might not apply to such modern-day myths as the comic book. Children whose conflicts give them a vulnerability to retreat into excessive fantasy, which have accompanying themes of violence, are most likely do so with whatever material coalesces with their needs at a particular stage. The source for such retreating might vary from childhood versions of Greek gods destroying each other to Batman.

A personally unsatisfaying or frustrating environment, coupled with unsatisfied needs, is what should be given primacy as determiners rather than ad hoc exposures. In this connection fairy tales can be viewed as cautionary tales to children who are struggling to renounce early gratifications, such as the primary process world dominated by the pleasure principle, for the world of delay, postponement, and work.

Comic books are an integral part of today's literature for children, and their reading fulfillls an important psychic function in the inner life of those latency and preadolescent children whom they attract. In both form and content they seem to appeal to a transitional phase of development, making the shift from a predominantly infantile pleasure-principle-dominated level to a more reality-principle level of functioning; and like the myth and fairy tale, they facilitate the working-through process. They do so in part by externalizing the conflict, enabling the child to identify and come to grips with some of the conflicts and reflect on a variety of potential resolutions, facilitated in this by the opportunity for catharsis, abreaction, identification, etc. It has been suggested that myths must originally have served an ego need; to explain existing phenomena, albeit in a prelogical fashion. . . Superman readers regress to that prelogical state in order to relax for a while and become all the more logical thereafter.[59]

FAMILY CONFIGURATIONAL PATTERNS

Family contributions to delinquency require clarification. Almost everyone at times joins in the chorus that families are responsible for delinquency. However, when specifics are requested, it becomes apparent that some theorists are referring to sociological characteristics such as deviations in descriptive characteristics of the family unit (the impact of broken homes, inadequate incomes to meet certain basic living needs, or the significance of a working mother). It quickly becomes apparent that once these broad approaches and the relationship to delinquency are examined, the borderline between the psychological and sociological becomes blurred. Pursuing the variables that affect not only the family constellation, but the interactions within a family, one is soon involved with questions about whether a parent is absent or neglectful, and with details about the impact on a given child as well as intrafamilial interactions. The extension to psychosocial processes such as identity, identification, self-concept, and the development of self-control has then taken place.

In the past broad-based social factors have held sway. Broken homes as a significant variable was thought to be one of the main determinants of delinquency. It soon became evident that studies did not employ control groups so that variables such as age, sex, ethnicity, social class, and neighborhood were controlled before a higher incidence of broken homes could be said to have been established as the antecedent for a delinquent population to develop. The impact of psychological variables could not be ignored, so that the generic phrase broken home became almost meaningless.

Parental death is different from abandonment, which is different from divorce. The age of the child at the time of such an occurrence is also significant. A group with an older set of parents would be more likely to sustain some kind of parental loss or family alteration. Subtle influences operate within intact families which are not amenable to observation on a macroscopic level. These only become visible when the clinician is involved with one or more members of a family and is alerted to the forms of psychopathology that may be contributing to delinquent behavior.

Similar complexities reside in hypotheses on delinquency regarding the contribution of a mother who is employed and hence absent as a child-rearer. The fallacy in many of these hypotheses is due to isolation of one factor and making unwarranted inferences from it. There are multiple reasons why some mothers work and some do not. The emphasis would not be merely on a certain number of mothers working in a delinquent group compared to a delinquent population for statistical significance, but on greater specificity in determining what the characteristics of the mother and family are when a mother does work. Investigating present interactional variables, such as the attitude of both parents toward the working mother, arrangements made for the child, and the rearrangements necessary within a family would be required.[60] The subtleties of family psychodynamics do not allow causal significance to be assigned to a sole descriptive factor.

The following are some of the family influences which have affected development adversely with respect to delinquency. It is evident that they are in reality psychosocial factors:

1. Inconsistent or extreme discipline is noted where an ignoring of antisocial acts occurs at one time while at another time there has been severe punishment. Control is then achieved by external force, which established this as a pattern to be reacted to or challenged during adolescence. A variant is a permissive pattern. Permissiveness may be by virtue of other time-consuming demands on the parents so that discipline is lax, although it can be associated with parental exposure to popular publications advocating greater autonomy for children, or to more complex personal conflicts about using authority with children. The result is a child who resents the demands of authority figures or the need to conform. Processes of internalizing these demands have remained underdeveloped.

2. Family structure as related to delinquency can have an effect on the child in terms of a reduction in parental control. When there is parental absence or marital conflict, the child is exposed to inconsistent and less parental control. The factors alluded to above are relevant, such as the impact of a missing father, parental age, size of family, and the ordinal position of a child.

3. More significant may be the quality of parental functioning, such as the sporadic presence of the father, the physical and emotional demands of coping with a family too large for a given couple, the unpredictable use of authority such as when a parent is intoxicated, and parental disharmony with its multiple consequences. The latter situation has an effect of dethroning authority when it is witnessed in a parental context of disagreement.

4. Rather than dealing with lack of discipline, another series of studies has emphasized the parental deprivation theme in terms of a

lack of affection. This hypothesis has become more sophisticated than earlier studies which considered parental physical absence. Glueck and Glueck, and others following them, felt that the failure of boys to win the affection of their fathers is an important factor contributing to delinquency.[61] Deficits in meeting the early dependency needs of a child have also been held relevant to the predisposition to aggressive delinquency.[62] The extensive work on attachment and loss with the anger when faced with separation or the threat of separation are relevant.[63]

5. The traditional emphasis on the status of a family cannot be ignored. A family whose members feel integrated within a community in terms of various institutions such as schools, churches, and neighboring families, has a model of social identification and conformity provided for its members. There are also the fringe benefits of providing reinforcement for identification of children with parents in types of participations which have status within the rules of a society. Asocial patterns present in certain subcultural groups foster group solidarity and identification with norms that are contrary to those of the larger community. These groups tend to be diagnosed by psychiatrists as being dyssocial, which is an effort to dissociate these groups from others manifesting a psychiatraic disorder in the narrower sense.

PROBLEMS OF SAMPLING AND PREDICTION

Prediction is considered one of the essential criteria for the viability of a scientific enterprise. It is not an absolute in all sciences, such as in geology or paleontology, which are retrospective in nature. However, with human behavior one of the requisite efforts is to make forecasts so that there is not only a feedback on various hypotheses, but in addition a criterion of falsifiability to discount or taper some hypotheses.

As noted elsewhere, definitions of subgroups, populations, and characteristics must be clearly delineated before efforts attain significance. In studies this is rarely achieved. Part of the difficulty is due to the lack of viewing delinquency from the perspective of an individual's behavior as the only dependent variable. Factors of variability in quantity and quality of law enforcement, changes in social and legal policies, influences from those interacting with a potential delinquent from his family as well as victims, simultaneously operate and interfere with predictive efforts. The difficulty in getting theorists to agree on what behavior should be considered delinquent, as well as to substantiate predictions which are not merely truisms, is no small task. As an example, conclusions about slum families in a culture with a high incidence of antisocial behavior as the most likely to have delinquent children continue to be cited and replicated. The questions at present extend far beyond, into the realm of selectivity of data when social class is a variable.

If part of the problem of prediction is related to the validity of which groups are designated delinquent to begin with, the types of distortions in definitions, theories, and statistics are not irrelevant. If the statistics regarding crimes cover only a part of the actual incidence, subsequent efforts at prediction based on these minimized figures would either be inaccurate or irelevant. In actuality the error is even greater, since the figures are not only erroneous in terms of the true incidence of offenses, but also with respect to offenders.

Since the clearance rate itself (cases of reported offenses for which there was an arrest—not a conviction), varies widely, it is doubly significant when it is realized that the underestimation of offenses is quite high. The clearance rate for forcible rapes is estimated at 57 percent, robberies at 30 percent, and auto theft at 17 percent, but not until we deal with offenses against the person such as murder, negligent mansalughter, and aggravated assault, do we get clearance rates up to 82, 92, and 66 percent respectively.[64] However, statistics on offenders are compiled from records of convicted offenders, and obviously represent a small proportion of actual offenders. A caveat is raised about studies of offenders based on convicted offenders who seem clustered in the lower social strata. A similar stricture holds for research conclusions drawn from probation records. Any assumptions about equal representation from different social classes are entirely unwarranted.

There is also the problem of the uneven and unrepresentative nature of crime reporting. Even excluding crimes of violence against the person, crimes against property such as robbery, burglary, and larceny, are reported to the police much more frequently than are respectable crimes such as fraud, forgery, embezzlement, shoplifting, tax evasion, and corporate crimes. Even if the clearance rates were equalized a bias would exist, since fewer respectable offenses are reported to the police.[65] Of course, this makes the figures on adolescent and youth age groups weighted against them, since few of them as yet are in a position to commit respectable crimes.

For property offenses, the two main sources of searching for suspects do not come from the general population but rather from that euphemism called typical criminal neighborhoods and youth populations. These groups contribute excessively to official categories of criminals and delinquents. Besides lower class areas being located where investigations are directed, there are differences between adolescents in different social classes. The middle-class youth learns to play the game of contriteness—much as he will later when engaged in respectable business offenses. Surely, passive-aggressive behavior in a juvenile elicits arrests. One study indicated that nearly 67 percent of adolescents who misbehaved when encountered by police were arrested in contrast to only 11 percent of the adolescents who were well-behaved.[66]

While one might be tempted from such a critique to come to the opposite conclusion—that the class-related hypothesis has been refuted—this is unwarranted. The only valid conclusion is that the issue of the relationship between law violations and social class is not resolved.[67] The closest one can come to disproving the class-related hypothesis actually involves self-reports of delinquent acts committed by adolescents. The limitations are that other variables possibly related to delinquency are not controlled, such as the size of the communities in which the assessments are being made. Some studies are restricted to school populations, thus omitting drop outs. Others only study drop outs. Some lump together as delinquent acts not only those which legally qualify as crimes but the usual acts, such as truancy, which can bring an adolescent into the juvenile court. However, some go further and include a miscellany of aggressive acts and misbehaviors so that what is being measured remains unclear.

Gold's study is one of the best which tried to obviate these difficulties.[68] Both in and out of school adolescents were included, and interviews were conducted so that an authority did not have to be pleased on questionaires or surveys. They did not leave the behaviors in question vague, such as whether the behavior was simply unruly or nonconforming versus actually delinquent. By initial screening alone, half of the acts of property destruction, one-fourth of the confidence games, and one-fifth of the assaults were eliminated as chargeable offenses. Informers were used to check the truthfulness of respondents, although cases of exaggerators or loners could not be so evaluated. From these multiple checks they were able to determine that five times more lowest than highest status boys appear in the official records, and that unselected records would have a ratio closer to 1.5 to 1.0. The correlation between social class and delinquency utilizing the two highest delinquency groups was only 0.12 which accounted for only 4 percent of the variance.

Studies combining environmental factors make it possible to delineate groups of individuals in which statements are offered that 50-80 percent will engage in future delinquent behavior.[69] Yet, as discussed, multiple complex issues are involved in this type of seemingly simple probability statement. Despite the continued outpouring of reports on delinquency prediction, a persistent realization of the limitation of such methods is needed despite this more skeptical conclusion being at variance with popular opinion and much theorizing. The entire problem of prediction is treated elsewhere.[70] [71] Here it is important simply to summarize some of the problems, with a few of the major studies so often cited, as to why the criteria of reliability and validity in such studies are so difficult of attainment.

A frequent problem is the lack of adequate discrimination between group studies to which later predictions are made. Hence, a predictor item found useful with one group, or in one geographical area, is not necessarily applicable elsewhere. A prediction item for drug usage among adolescents in Harlem may have little generalizability. There is often a lack of cross-validation studies where a predictive device is confined to usage with the groups from which it was originally developed and not tried elsewhere. Results become spuriously high and contribute to erroneous predictions and judgments about other groups. Beyond systematic sampling bias, such as the type of study mentioned which uses samples from a high-delinquency area, the hypotheses are regarded as established without testing in other populations. Nor is the superior accuracy of a predictive device established by a favorable comparison with a different group rather than within a group. Predicting a higher incidence of delinquency in a Class V socio-economic area compared to Class I, does not lend validity to a device when the question is the rate within each class, and how to distinguish the incidence of delinquency within a social group.

There is a need to appraise items considered as predictors of delinquency independently. Heterogenous sources of data are now used: self-reports of subjects, raters whose experience and theoretical orientations vary widely, use of selective historical data for an individual or his family, preselected environmental factors, personal interviews which vary from those performed by workers in correctional settings and with little other professional training to those by mental health workers who have had experience clinically but perhaps little with delinquents, and in many cases by volunteers (paid or unpaid) or students working part-time as assistants. A host of different psychological measures are used, which include not only objective or projective personality tests, but measures of interests, attitudes, and vocational aptitudes. From this diverse batch of approaches, forecasting behaviors labelled delinquent takes place.

Prediction studies are also handicapped since unless the criterion problem of classifying delinquency has been met, vagueness and uncertainty persist as to how valid and reliable delinquency predictions are. Certainly a criterion of delinquency based on the whims of a social agency lacks confidence, but to some extent the criteria employed by various juvenile court jurisdictions suffers from the same handicap although it is disguised under official designations. A common example is the criteria in prediction studies utilizing confined delinquents which ignores not only the varying bases for confinement, but assumes the confined population have been validly convicted while the nonconfined group have in turn been validly excluded. Whether this limitation can be remedied, is questionable in itself. Unless it is, substantial doubt is cast on the predictive enterprise since efforts are geared toward an elusive criteria which has low reliability itself. Random variation is introduced, which decreases the strength of relations between any items used as predictors and what is supposed to be predicted— namely, delinquency.

Base-rate determination is another factor which stands as a challenge to predictive devices. It refers to the proportion of individuals in a population who fall into the designated category one wishes to predict. It refers to the number of delinquents in a population which would occur simply on the basis of experience or an actuarial table. In many situations base rates have not been determined, so that devices claimed as predictors really do not have the first criterion for a comparison established. Until one knows what the occurrence of a class of events would be by experience, there is no basis for the claim that superior measures of prediction are available. When the event being predicted is rare, the number of valid predictive guides is smaller and the results more untrustworthy. Unless a prediction method can beat the base-rate alone, i.e., provide more and better information, its validity is negated since past experience is at least as good a guide (and much more economical). If 20 percent of the adolescents in a given population are expected to become delinquent, a predictive device which cannot improve upon this by predicting better than 20 percent has little value.

The point is significant but overlooked in many studies. It leads to the fallacy of prediction studies being based on equal number of delinquents and non-delinquents, a factor not comparable to the distribution of delinquency in the general population. The result is a spurious overestimation of the effectiveness of predictive criteria or instruments. This error is present in one of the most widely cited series of prediction studies on juvenile delinquency, by Glueck and Glueck.[72] Prediction tables were devised, and one called *Social Factors* was subjected to long-term evaluation. The tables were based on a comparison of 500 delinquents and 500 non-delinquents. Over ten years a two- and three-factor scale was retained based on family cohesiveness, supervision of the boy by his mother, and supervision of the boy by his father.

Conclusions were offered that the Three-Factor Table yielded a 70 percent accuracy in predicting delinquents and an 85 percent accuracy in predicting non-delinquents.[73] The base-rate criticism of the study is germane in that when the base-rate is set more accurately, rather than at 50 percent, the prediction tables are far less discriminating. Sampling criticisms have also pointed out the non-representative character of the high delinquency area of New York City used in the study. It has also been noted that extrapolations made after the boys had been institutionalized are quite different from studying them in childhood anterespectively.[74]

Nor can the group and personal consequences of erroneous predictions of delinquency be treated casually. Group consequences represent erroneous decisions and policies which may not only be a waste of resources, but actually have the adverse effect of promoting delinquency. Individual repercussions may be in terms of the self-fulfilling prophecy, in which individuals designated as potentially or pre-delinquent develop expectations regarding themselves. It could also be added that others similarly develop expectations about youths. The error is two-fold; some will be predicted for delinquency which does not materialize, and some will not be predicted who do materialize. With the low predictive value for most current devices, does society wish to stigmatize certain individuals as potential delinquents? Even if such predictive devices were to achieve greater accuracy, are there treatment and rehabilitative devices which can be employed with confidence? If not, we have arrived at a social policy using sanctions against large numbers based on uncertain predictions which employ even more uncertain cures.

There have been other efforts at developing predictive measures which are amply discussed elsewhere.[75] The Bristol Social Adjustment Guide, developed in England, is based on the incidence of symptoms of non-delinquent behavior disturbances in those on probation versus a control group. Kvaraceus originally attempted to develop a rating scale of delinquency-proneness based on multiple-choice items. The revision was the "Non-Verbal KD Proneness Scale" with sixty-two pictorially presented items based on concepts concerning reported differences between delinquents and non-delinquents. He reported his most significant result as teacher nominations, based on pupil behavior, being equal to the test as predictors of future delinquency.

Approaches of combining predictor items to improve predictive ability have also been tried. Some have been utilized without a waiting system, others have employed a number of predictive characteristics with a waiting system, such as those in the Glueck's studies while others have employed elaborate statistical models utilizing multiple linear regression and linear discriminant function. Association analysis to subdivide a heterogenous population into subgroups in combination with regression methods has been suggested, but despite the methods proposed for combining predictors, empirical comparisons of predictive power are as rare as are validated tools.

PERSONALITY FACTORS AND DELINQUENCY

Personality theories and delinquency are often discussed in broad generic terms to encompass almost every perspective short of the sociological. In fact, some would consider the last section on prediction as a discussion of personality theory and delinquency. In this last section data from the realm of personality studies are examined, but with the explicit qualification that this does not include clinical theory from those who work with juveniles and their families in treatment. The failure to make this distinction is prevalent, so that "personality theories and delinquency" in many textbooks become limited to psychometric studies.

Comments on studies utilizing the Minnesota Multiphasic Personality Inventory (MMPI) in relationship to delinquency have been reserved until now. This psychometric device has been utilized in delinquency prediction, and was initially used in such a study with 87 percent of the entire ninth-grade population of Minneapolis who had a periodic follow-up. Two and four years later the files of the Hennepin County Probation Office and the Juvenile Division of the Minneapolis Police Department were checked for records indicating contact with the subject. A second sample was obtained six years later, based on ninety-two schools and eighty-six communities and the test was administered to 11,329 additional ninth-graders.

Included were 28 percent of all the ninth-grade population in Minnesota. Similar checks with court and police files were made as well as microfilms of school records, personal data sheets, and teacher-administered ratings and predictions on the students most likely to have legal and emotional difficulties.

In terms of delinquency prediction, code types based on the first two high-point scales on the MMPI were compared for delinquent and non-delinquent groups; the base-rate was the percent distribution for the overall population. Deviancy from the base rate in certain codes was then detected such as the "4-9" classification, where the delinquency rate was 38 percent while with a "2-7" profile the delinquency rate was lower than that of the general population. Attempts to develop an independent scale to predict juvenile delinquency were unsuccessful since it was noted that code patterns with a high delinquency rate were more accurate than if a single scale was used. Perhaps this was due to the multiple factors which contribute to delinquency.

Teachers' estimates revealed a social class bias in predicting delinquency more for the lower socio-economic groups. A marked influence on their judgments from intelligence and school achievement existed. Elaborations have employed a successive hurdles approach of first screening those boys with excitor scale codes of 4, 8, 9, and then further screening for illness within the family. This subpopulation was twice as dense with predelinquent cases as the general population.[77] Further, taking the boys with delinquency-prone personality profiles, when the family was known to some social agency by records, the delinquency rate was 42 percent, in contrast to that of 23 percent when the family was not so known.

Apart from MMPI studies, approaches have sought out identifiable personality variables that might be related to delinquent tendencies. Although past reviews have concluded there was no support for the hypothesis that criminal tendencies and personality elements were associated, there has been more refined work since then utilizing the Rorschach, Guilford-Martin, and Porteus Mazes in addition to the MMPI. Unfortunately, many of these studies have merely been confirmatory, such as tests demonstrating time concepts in delinquents more oriented toward the present. Concern with the present and impulsivity are diagnostic features of psychopathy, and hence not independent findings. Similar are findings of inferior performance on the Bender-Gestalt when groups are matched for age, intelligence, and absence of motor defects, believed related to the same factors of impulsivity and lack of control as are exhibited in a poor qualitative performance on the Porteus test.

With the expansion of cognitive psychology, more sophisticated explanations for delinquency have been proposed. As we have noted, cognitive approaches in the early part of this century had assumptions that knowledge of moral rules was significantly related to moral behavior. Various pencil-and-paper assessment devices were developed with the goal of differentiating adolescents with delinquent tendencies. Fernald developed a battery of perceptual motor and paper-and-pencil tests in 1912, designed to identify defective delinquents.[78] Unfortunately, the inability to dissociate knowledge of norms and a preoccupation with conventional notions of morality has continued in efforts at developing measurement devices to evaluate personality factors such as self-control. The test instruments developed continue to be either irrelevant or devoted to an approach which has little correlation with delinquent behavior. By contrast, a role-theoretical approach to psychopathy, utilizing a socialization scale, demonstrated an ability to predict certain types of moral behavior in individuals without reference to conventional moral standards.[79] The irrelevancy of knowledge of moral standards and moral behavior, unless one is dealing with a questionable case of intellectual deficit, was demonstrated.

Some cognitive approaches have employed a developmental model in which a lag in the perceptual-cognitive spheres is hypothesized. An earlier form of this stated that psychopaths "don't learn from experience," manifested in their repeated transgressions, but also in traits of poor judgment and impulsivity. An immediate difficulty is to establish whether such a cognitive deficit is the primary deficiency which accounts for given behavioral traits, or whether behaviors like impulsivity rather give rise to perceptual-cognitive distortions. Are general disturbances in ego functioning involved with perceptual-cognitive areas one of several impairments?

Experimental approaches have tested such hypotheses but answers to these more basic questions are not forthcoming. One approach presented partially complete drawings of familiar objects to an experimental group of incarcerated adolescents who had been convicted of at least three serious offenses. Compared to a controlled sample of males, significantly few delinquents arrived at a solution.[80]

Cognitive defects have also been postulated as one basis for why socialization processes have gone awry in the delinquent. While a

child without cognitive defects may respond to praise and punishment in predicted directions, the child with difficulty in discrimination either fails to generalize or responds in the opposite manner,
such as to praise as though being blamed. It is difficult for the
clinician to accept such misinterpretations as due solely to cognitive
influences. However, past oversight of cognitive contributions has
been evident. No valid reason exists why cognitive disturbances in
thinking are cited, but omitted in acting out problems. The
implications for socialization processes from a defective discriminatory ability are enormous.

In one study 750 adolescent males and 160 adolescent delinquents
were given a series of story situations to choose between an
interpretation indicating a positive or negative self-evaluation. The
delinquents less frequently interpreted positive events as self-
positive, and they also interpreted positive events more self-
negative.[81] Of course, such deficits do not necessitate a developmental deficit in the realm of cognition. The interaction with peer groups
and especially the continuing influence of parents is highly
significant. An adolescent who perceives parental concern is more
likely to have a higher self-evaluation.

The ramifications from the psychological to the socio-cultural are
wide. Adolescents with low self-esteem are not only adversely
affected in school achievement and occupational expectation, but
interpersonally are more withdrawn, sensitive, and suspicious.[82]
Such findings are from interpersonal or self-descriptive ratings and
have not even involved intrapsychic components. Data from
interviewing techniques and story-completion studies indicate
delinquents from both lower and middle-class backgrounds exhibit
fewer self-critical guilt responses.[83] An entire complex of family and
social factors are operating, so that the moral arrest of the
delinquent seems more related to living in a milieu which
corresponds to the early developmental stages of moral thought in a
child. A child of eight to twelve years begins to discriminate self-
serving behavior in himself and others. If he perceives most of the
models and authority figures operating primarily from selfish or
power motives, despite what is verbalized, an amoral world view is
developed.[84] Once antisocial acts are undertaken, there is a tendency
to appraise them as worthy or desirable, which tends to lower
cognitive inconsistencies between the acts and normative standards.[85]

Another personality approach has applied trait and typology
theory to delinquents, seeking clusters. An early study by Hewitt

and Jenkins applied ninety-four descriptive phrases about behavior to 500 children with behavior problems referred to a child guidance clinic.[86] Forty-five items were retained and a cluster of internalized traits were derived. The criterion for a cluster was a group of traits with an intercorrelation of 0.30 and logically consistent with clinical judgment. On this basis, three syndromes were separated: (1) *unsocialized aggressive* (assaultive, fights, cruel, defiant of authority, malicious mischief, and inadequate guilt), (2) *socialized delinquent* (various types of cooperative or furtive stealing, truancy, absenting, late hours, bad companions), and (3) *overinhibited* (seclusive, shy, apathetic, sensitive, submissive, and worrying).

These three classifications easily correspond to what clinicians describe as sociopathic, neurotic delinquent, and neurotic disturbances. Methodological criticisms have been made, such as 97 percent of the cases being white, the unrepresentative nature of the population in which legally delinquent children were under-represented, and the reliance on child guidance records which are notably unreliable. A partial remedy was effected in a study involving a group of 300 adjudicated delinquents.[87] Two-thirds of the sample was found classifiable in one of the three categories. The approach gave rise to subsequent factor analytic studies whose aim was to separate traits which hung together. Such efforts may be viewed as an effort to gain increased diagnostic accuracy within the group of delinquent or acting out individuals. In this sense it is part of a descriptive psychiatry and hopefully may lessen the diagnostic confusion prevalent when such behavior gains prominence.

Attention has been called to the distinction between a typology and a cluster of traits. While factor analysis, or clinical description, might group certain signs, symptoms, or traits together, there need not be a given type who possesses only the traits clustered. Such diagnostic purity is never attainable. In fact, there have been failures experimentally to confirm the groups of delinquents by trait systems.[88] This has led some to advocate that the various traits observed in certain delinquents be viewed as different dimensions of personality rather than seeking a typology. This would be more in accord with psychodynamic formulations, which stress functions of the personality which perform at different levels of efficiency or regression, interacting with each other and environmental precipitants.

REFERENCES

1. I. Kant, *Foundations of the Metaphysics of Morals*, translated by L.W. Beck (New York: The Liberal Arts Division of the Bobbs–Merrill Co., 1959).
2. J. Bentham, *Principles of Morals and Legislation* (Oxford: 1879).
3. O. H. Mowrer, *The Crisis in Psychiatry and Religion* (Princeton: Van Nostrand, 1961).
4. K. A. Menninger, *Whatever Happened to Sin?* (New York: Hawthorn Books, 1973).
5. W. B. Miller, The impact of a 'total community' delinquency control project, *Social Problems* 10(1962):168-191.
6. T. Sellin and M. E. Wolfgang, *The Measurement of Delinquency* (New York: John Wiley and Sons, Inc., 1964).
7. *Uniform Crime Reports* (Washington., D.C.: Department of Justice, 1975.
8. S. P. Breckenridge and E. Abbott, *The Delinquent Child and the Home* (New York: Russell Sage Foundation, 1912).
9. C. R. Shaw, *Delinquency Areas* (Chicago: University of Chicago Press, 1929).
10. S. M. Robison, *Can Delinquency Be Measured?* (New York: Columbia University Press, 1936).
11. S. M. Robison, *Juvenile Delinquency—Its Nature and Control*, pp. 101-102 (New York: Holt, Rinehart, and Winston, 1960).
12. M. Weber, *The Protestant Ethic and the Spirit of Capitalism* (London: George Allen and Unwin, 1930).
13. W. B. Miller, Lower class culture as a generating milieu of gang delinquency, *Jounal of Social Issues* 14(1958):5-19.
14. R. G. Andry, *Delinquency and Parental Pathology* (London: Methuen, 1960).
15. R. E. Anderson, Where's dad? *Archives of Genetic Psychiatry.* 18(1968):641-649.
16. C.P. Malmquist, Psychiatric perspectives on the socially disadvantaged child *Comprehensive Psychiatry* 6(1964):176-183.
17. H. I. Gans, Urban poverty and social planning, *The Uses of Sociology*, ed. by P. F. Lazarsfeld, M. H. Sewell, and H. L. Wilensky, pp. 437-476 (New York: Basic Books, 1967).
18. E. H. Sutherland and D. R. Cressy, *Criminology*, 9th ed. (Philadelphia: J. B. Lippincott, 1974).
19. D. R. Cressy, *Delinquency, Crime and Differential Association*, p. 500. (Amersterdam: Martinus Nijhoff, 1964).
20. R. A. Cloward and L. E. Ohlin, *Delinquency and Opportunity: A Theory of Delinquent Gangs* (Glencoe: The Free Press, 1960).
21. R. K. Merton, Social theory and social structure pp. 125-149. *Social Structure and Anomie* (Glencoe: The Free Press, 1949).
22. F. M. Thrasher, *The Gang* (Chicago: University of Chicago Press, 1927).
23. S. Glueck and R. W. Whelan, *Reaching the Fighting Gang*, p. 18 (New York: New York City Youth Board, 1960).

24. L. Yablonsky, The delinquent gang as a near-group, *Social Problems* 7(1954)108-117.
25. L. Yablonsky, *The Violent Gang* (New York: Macmillan, 1962).
26. S. Schafer, *The Political Criminal* (New York: The Free Press, Macmillan, 1974).
27. F. Dostoyevsky, *The Possessed*, trans. by C. Garnett (New York: The Modern Library, 1936).
28. H. Davidman and E. Preble, Schizophrenia among adolescent street gang leaders, *Psychopathology of Schizophrenia*, pp. 372-387. ed. by P. Hoch and J. Zubin (New York: Grune and Stratton, 1966).
29. A. L. Kroeber and C. Kluckhohn, Critical review of concepts and definitions, *Papers of the Peabody Museum of American Archealogy and Ethnology* vol. 47, no. 1, 1952.
30. A. L. Kroeber and R. Parsons, The concepts of culture and social system *American Sociological Review* 29(1964):633-669.
31. A. K. Cohen, *Delinquent Boys: The Culture of the Gang* (Glencoe: The Free Press, 1955).
32. H. L. Wilensky and C. G. Lebeaux, *Industrial Society and Social Welfare* (New York: Russell Sage Foundation, 1958).
33. W. L. Warner, R. T. Havighurst, and M. B. Loeb, Who shall be educated? *Industrial Society and Social Welfare*, pp. 191-192 (New York: Russell Sage Foundation, 1958).
34. I. Spergel, *Racketville, Slamtown and Haulberg* (Chicago: University of Chicago Press, 1964).
35. M. E. Wolfgang and F. Ferracuti, pp. 1-387. *The Subculture of Violence* (London: Tavistock Publications, 1967).
36. G. Sykes and D. Matza, Techniques of neutralization: a theory of delinquency, *American Sociological Review* 22(1957):664-670.
37. T. I. Kituse and D. Dietrick, Delinquent boys: a critique, *American Sociological Review* 24(1959):208-215.
38. National Advisory Commission on Criminal Justice Standards and Goals, *Corrections* (Washington D. C.: U. S. Government Printing Office, 1973).
39. The President's Commission on Law Enforcement and Administration of Justice *The Challenge of Crime in a Free Society*, (Washington, D. C.: U. S. Government Printing Office, 1967), pp. 69-73.
40. S. Blum, De-Escalating the violence on tv, *New York Times Sunday Magazine*, Dec. 8, 1968, p. 129.
41. R. K. Baker and S. J. Ball, *Mass Media and Violence: A Staff Report to the National Commission on the Causes and Prevention of Violence* (Washington, D. C.: U. S. Government Printing Office, 1969).
42. J. McIntyre and J. Teevan, Television and deviant behavior, *Television and Social Behavior*, vol. 3, *Television and Adolescent Aggressiveness*, ed. by G. A. Comstock, and E. A. Rubenstein (Washington, D. C.: U. S. Government Printing Office, 1972).

43. J. McLeod, C. Atkin, and S. Chaffee, Adolescents, parents, and television use: self-report and other-report measures from the Wisconsin sample, *Television and Social Behavior*, vol. 3, *Television and Adolescent Aggressiveness* (Washington, D. C.: U. S. Government Printing Office, 1973).

44. Children unaffected by violent films, *Psychiatric News*, July, 1968.

45. F. Hagenauer and J. W. Hamilton, 'Straw dogs': aggression and violence in modern film, *American Image* 30(1973):221-249.

46. A. Bandura and R. H. Walters, *Imitation of film-mediated aggressive models, Journal of Abnormal Social Psychology* 66(1963):3-11.

48. A. D. Liefer and D. F. Roberts, Children's responses to television violence, *Television and Social Behavior*, vol. 2, *Television and Social Learning*, ed. by J. P. Murray and E. H. Rubenstein (Washington, D. C.: U. S. Government Printing Office, 1972).

49. M. Lefkowitz, et al. Television violence and child aggression: a follow up study, *Television and Social Behavior*, vol. 3, *Television and Adolescent Aggressiveness* (Washington, D. C.: U. S. Government Printing Office, 1972).

50. R. M. Liebert, J. M. Neale, and E. S. Davidson, *The Early Window: Effects of Television on Children and Youth* (New York: Pergamon, 1973).

51. *Joseph Burstgn, Inc. v. Wilson*, 343 U. S. 495, 1952.

52. *Roth v. United States*, 354 U. S. 476, 1957.

53. T. Emerson, *The System of Freedom of Expression* (New York: Random House, 1970).

54. Hearings on Juvenile Delinquency (Comic Books) *Subcommittee to Investigate Juvenile Delinquency of the Senate Committee on Indecency*, 83rd Congress, 2nd Session, 1954.

55. *The Challenge of Crime in a Free Society*, op. cit., pp. 55-90.

56. F. Wertham, *Seduction of the Innocent* (New York: Rinehart, 1954).

57. Exclusion of children from violent worries, *Columbia Law Review* 67(1967):1148-1168.

58. B. Bettelheim, *The Uses of Enchantment* (New York: A. Knopf, 1976).

59. E. Caruth, Hercules and superman: the modern-day mythology of the comic book: some clinical applications *Journal of the American Academy of Child Psychiatry* 7(1968):1-12.

60. E. Herzog and C. E. Sudia, Fatherless homes: a review of research, *Children* 15(1968):177-182).

61. S. Glueck and E. Glueck, *Unraveling Juvenile Delinquency* (New York: Commonwealth Funds, 1950).

62. A. Bandura and R. W. Walters, *Adolescent Aggression* (New York: Ronald Press, 1959).

63. J. Bowlby, Separation: Anxiety and Anger, vol. 2 *Attachment and Loss* (New York: Basic Books, 1973).

64. *Uniform Crime Reports*, 1975, op. cit., pp. 1-30.

65. E. O. Smigel and H. J. Ross, *Crimes Against Bureaucracy* (New York: Van Nostrand Reinhold Co., 1970).
66. I. Piliavin and S. Briar, Police encounters with juveniles, *American Journal of Sociology.* 70(1964):206-214.
67. S. Box and J. Ford, The facts don't fit: on the relationship between social class and criminal behavior, *The Sociological Review* 19(1971):31-52.
68. M. Gold, Undetected delinquent behavior, *Journal of Research of Crime and Delinquency.* 3(1966):27-46.
69. P. F. Burggs, R. D. Went, and R. Johnson, An application of prediction tables to the study of delinquency, *Journal of Consulting Psychology.* 25(1961):46-50.
70. P. E. Meehl, *Clincal Versus Statistical Prediction* (Minneapolis: University of Minnesota Press, 1954).
71. H. Gough, Clinical *versus* statistical prediction, *Psychology in the Making,* ed. by L. Postman, p. 526 (New York: A. Knopf, 1962).
72. Glueck and Glueck, op. cit.
73. M. M. Craig and S. J. Glick, Ten years experience with the Glueck social prediction table, *Crime and Delinquency,* July, 1963, pp. 249-261.
74. W. C. Kvaraceus, Programs of early identification and prevention of delinquency, *Social Deviancy Among Youth,* 65th Yearbook of the NSSF (Chicago: National Society for the Study of Education, 1966), pp. 189-220.
75. D. M. Gottfredson, Assessment and prediction methods in crime and delinquency, *Task Force Report: Juvenile Delinquency and Youth Crime* (Washington, D. C.: U. S. Government Printing Office, 1967).
76. Kvaraceus, op. cit. p. 193.
77. P. F. Briggs and R. D. Wirt, Prediction, *Juvenile Delinquency,* ed. by H. C. Quay (Princeton: Van Nostrand, 1965).
78. S. M. Pittel and G. A. Mendelsohn, Measurement of moral values: a review and critique, *Psychology Bulletin.* 66(1966):22-35.
79. G. G. Gough, Theory and measurement of socialization, *Journal of consulting Psychology.* 24(1960):23-30.
80. D.D. Jones, N.H. Livson, and T.R. Sarbia, Perceptual completion behavior in juvenile delinquents, *Perceptual and Motion Skills* 5(1955):141-146.
81. J. McDavid and H.M. Schroeder, he interpretation of approval and disapproval by delinquent and non-delinquent adolescents, *Journal of Personality* 25(1957):539-549.
82. M. Rosenberg, *Society and the Adolescent Self-Image* (Princeton: Princeton University Press, 1965).
83. W. McCord and T. McCord, *Psychopathy and Delinquency* (New York: Grune and Stratton, 1956).
84. L. Kohldreg, Development of moral character and moral ideology *Review Of Child Development Research.* 1(1964):383-431.(New York: Russell Sage Foundation).

85. L. Festinger, *A Theory of Cognitive Dissonance* (Evanston: Row and Peterson, 1957).

86. L. E. Hewitt and R. L. Jenkins, *Fundamental Patterns of Maladjustment: The Dynamics of Their Origin* (Springfield: State of Illinois, 1946).

87. R. L. Jenkins and S. Glickman, Patterns of personality organization among delinquents, *Nervous Child.* 6(1957):329-339.

88. T. L. Tiffany, D. R. Peterson, and H. C. Quay, Types and traits in the study of juvenile delinquency, *Journal of Clinical Psychology.* 17(1961):19-24.

Chapter Ten

Antisocial Behavior: Psychiatric Aspects

THE CONCEPT OF CHARACTER

Temperament and The Emergence of Character.   Character has a variety of ambiguous meanings. Clinicians use it one way, personality theorists another, and moralists yet another. Courts rely on all of these and add in jurisprudential notions as well. Before resorting to clinical material involving antisocial conduct, the validity and relevance of character concepts will be reviewed.

It is difficult to purge the concept of character of moral overtones. In everyday usage people are spoken of as having a good or a bad character, which is equivalent to saying they are good or bad people. Ancient classifications of personality, such as that employed by Hippocrates, held to a humoral basis for personality development. Combinations and balances of humors were seen as determining personality traits. Four classic types of temperaments were sorted out: melancholic, choleric, phlegmatic, and sanguine. Although lacking knowledge of modern endocrinology, Hippocratic theory was a forerunner of later propositions about endocrine influences on personality development. It illustrates the ever-present search to classify personalities into types.

In recent centuries, this emphasis evolved into theories emphasizing the somatic or hereditary determination of temperament. A major problem with the temperamental hypothesis is the difficulty of separating genetic factors from multiple biological influences. These occur in utero, as well as from direct influences on processes of

chromosomal division (assuming these influences are not hereditary). A second difficulty is the complexity of specifying which
attributes should be ascribed to temperament. A third unresolved
problem is the lack of a bimodal distribution of personality traits.
What we have instead is a normal distribution, which makes it
difficult to distinguish distinct mechanisms or populations. Sufficient details to explain the transmission and manifestation of
personality traits to temperaments are not available. Nor do we
know the mechanisms of how temperament becomes established
and continues to persist throughout life with what seems to be a good
deal of consistency. A final predicament involves the vagueness in
specifications as to what the essential characteristics of temperament are. Unless specified, references are made to any number of
variables. The most common are: body constitution, brain size or
weight, psychomotor characteristics (coordination, posture, kinesthetic performance), drive manifestations (activity level, degree of
aggressivity, plasticity of sexuality), differences in physiological
functioning, and types of socialization patterns which reflect
temperament.

Theories on temperament from the 19th century emphasized
physique. Such theories paralleled the preoccupation in psychiatry,
particularly in France, with splitting-out innumerable psychiatric
types. Thinking about   bodily constitutions gave rise to
Kretschmer's famous four types: athletic, leptosomic, pyknic and
dysplastic.[1] He believed these constitutions not only led to certain
personality types, but also toward predispositions to mental illness.
However, Kretschmer was unable to demonstrate this to a degree
sufficient for general acceptance. A modernized version was seen in
the postulates of Sheldon and Stevens regarding their three
somatotypes:[2] (1) endomorphs (abdominal prominence, large,
round body cavities and contours); (2) mesomorphs (prominence of
bone and muscle), and (3) ectomorphs (thin, with a prominence of
skin and neural tissue).

A correlative relationship was postulated between the somatotypes and temperaments: viscerotonia (hedonistic, Dionysian
qualities of joy in eating and joviality); somatotonia (joy in
competitiveness, energetic movement, high drive level, and aggressiveness); and cerebretonia (hypersensitivity, shyness, cogitation,
and apprehensiveness). Each type had a rating of one to seven in a
given person in an effort to establish correlational clusters with
psychological temperaments. The visceratonic and cerebretonic
types corresponded in a crude way to what Jung later hypothesized
as extrovert-introvert dichotomy.[3]

A different but fascinating evolvement was the attempt to use temperament as a basis for explaining criminal tendencies. Phrenology, although later associated with charlatans, had its origins in the work of a Viennese physician, Franz Gall, who performed post-mortem examinations on criminals in an effort to establish clues to criminal propensities.[4] In 1809, Gall hypothesized that the lobes of the brain, as represented in skull protuberances, permitted the mental faculties of an individual to be determined. This was judged by the size of his bumps. The larger a bump, the more influential the underlying brain lobe was considered. Traits of combativeness, secretiveness, and acquisitiveness were believed associated with criminality and supposedly identified.

An early leader of American psychiatry, Dr. Amariah Brigham, believed in phrenology and used it as an explanatory model for criminal behavior. Such behavior was ascribed to a preponderance of the "lower propensities" without the counterbalancing effect of "higher faculties."[5] The theory blossomed under the advocacy of Cesare Lombroso and the school of classical criminology.[6] Lombroso and his group held criminal tendencies were inborn and detectable in the physical characteristics of the skull and skeleton, such as prominent ears, frontal sinuses, thin upper lips, and a voluminous jaw and zygoma bone. Biological determinism in extremis reigned in such a theory. Phenotypic manifestations were seen in violent passions, tattooing, strong insistence on obtaining vengeance, wild courage, and a lack of foresight. Lombroso later attempted to correlate moral imbecility, epilepsy, and the born criminal as an atavistic grouping.

Another model formulated during the 19th century viewed criminal temperament as reflecting a degenerative central nervous system. Hereditary theories, along with Darwinian evolutionary theory, were simultaneously emerging. It was an era which sought to identify the criminal man, moral degenerate, the mentally deficient, and the emotionally disturbed through stigmata. The theory was used both ways: signs of stigmata meant a criminal type and a criminal was taken to have stigmatic signs. Existence of a criminal temperament was indicative of degeneration—either an atavistic throwback to primitive man, or as a form of neuropathy much like the explanation given for varieties of psychopathological behaviors.

Benedict August Morel (1809-1873) taught that the mentally ill were degenerative deviates. Little distinction was made between hereditary factors and temperament in most of these theories—let alone an attempt to segregate environmental and social multivariate correlations. An interesting by-product was the psychiatic diagnosis of "moral insanity" advocated by such leading physicians of the time as Prichert, Isaac Ray, and Esquirol from 1820 to 1870. This influence extended to the sexual psychopathies, as illustrated in the writings of Kraft-Ebing (1840-1902) who ascribed sexual deviation to neuropathological degeneration. The assumption was that the central nervous system had developed differently for those who exhibited sexual deviation. The modernized form of these temperamental determinants of antisocial tendencies is seen in the "Constitutional Psychopathic Inferior" diagnosis used by Adolph Meyer who otherwise was quite environmentally oriented.[7] Contemporary theorizers now hold to subtle polygenic influences, biochemical or endocrinological abnormalities, or neurophysiological derivatives, as the temperamental loadings toward deviant antisocial behavior.

Alternative approaches try to establish a relationship between temperament and character. Research in the area of cognition is one example. The delineation of cognitive styles, and ways of exercising moral judgment, are approaches which utilize developmental differences. They may also be used to illustrate constitutional differences which manifest themselves in different cognitive approaches and predispose toward antisocial behavior. Differences in autonomic functioning and regulation, such as dominance of the sympathetic over cholinergic functioning, may also contribute to characterological differences. Prenatal influences contribute to biological variability and require consideration for the range of disparate characteristics that can result.

The problem of the relationship between groupings of uniqueness in psychological attributes or functions, is relevant to temperamental differences. What has been labelled *constitutional differences* in the past is now studied as part of the spectrum of individual differences which begin on a genetic basis. These are seen in discreet areas such as motility, perceptual responses, sleeping and feeding patterns, drive endowment, quality and intensity of emotionality, sensory threshold, social responsiveness, biochemical or enzymatic individuality, and neurophysiological functioning. All of these temperamental factors contribute to the development of character by themselves as well as by interaction with each other. In turn they elicit responses from parents and other socializing agents. Such a viewpoint goes beyond the implicit assumption in studies such as that of Sheldon where temperament was viewed as a direct consequence of physical traits. Instead a flexibility is permitted for differential environmental responses which certain physiques elicit. Each of the variations can function in this manner and lead to a different set of behavioral consequences.

One group of investigators attempted to assess individuality and behavioral functioning in children by means of a longitudinal investigation beginning in infancy.[89] Ratings on nine behavioral characteristics were utilized: activity level, rhythmicity, approach or withdrawal, adaptability, intensity of reaction, threshold of responsiveness, quality of mood, distractibility, and persistence. This is a more contemporary version of temperament based on empirical observations within a developmental framework.

Character, Traits, and Dispositions. Clinicians are accustomed to thinking of *character* either as related to temperament, or as part of a descriptive nosology related to a psychopathological framework. A clinician thinks of customary diagnoses which use phrases such as "passive-aggressive" or "compulsive character." There is a domain of psychology which is also interested in the problem of traits as related to dispositions as well as to a conceptual analysis of traits. The theoretical problem has relevance not only to the area of types of character problems but to tendencies of a dispositional sort toward antisocial behavior.

Distinctions between phenotypic and genotypic traits are relevant. The former deal with observable data conceived of in behavioral or descriptive terms. Critics feel the phenotype deals with superficial aspects of the personality since the data are so observable. In contrast, genotypic traits refer to theoretical, source or depth manifestaions. Of course, to maintain an either-or dichotomy is fallacious since there is overlap. At the extremes, delineations can be made by statements such as, "*X* had an inclination to hit *Y*," as a piece of descriptive-behavioral data, versus, "*X* felt guilty after he hit *Y* because of his punitive superego." Distinctions between intervening variables and hypothetical constructs are relevant.

Developmental implications are present in studying traits. The association of psychological uniqueness or style with the idea of character is related to studies in temperament. While most clinicians and personality theorists think of character as equaling a cluster of personality traits, they rarely bother to explain their notions about the origin of the concept of *traits* itself. At best, traits are thought of as a cluster of behaviors which remain stable over time. In actuality, this employs a crude categorization of phenotypic traits without further analysis. As examples, a clinician may point to the penuriousness of an individual, or use a phrase such as, "Smith is up to his old type of manipulative behavior." The consistency of these behaviors over time is noted as an index of reliability with predictive implications.

In addition to consistency, variability is inherent in the trait concept when differentiating clusters. A behavior with only minimal variability would not suffice from its lack of distinctiveness in spite of stability in other respects. In these general terms, a man speaking with a Midwestern accent would not indicate a trait distinction, but a pattern of wearing the latest fashions in a conspicuous manner would. In the clinical realm, a psychoanalytic framework is interested in the uniqueness of motives, defenses, and displays of affect. Social learning theorists share an interest in observables, but place an emphasis on observational settings where traits can be listed, such as in modeling behaviors or identification processes.

Factor-analytic or psychometric approaches, such as the Minnesota Multiphasic Personality Inventory, have been used to link certain broad traits, such as psychopathy, neuroticism, depression, or extroversion-introversion. A cognitive perspective on traits is seen in the way an individual categorizes familiar and unfamiliar stimuli, performance on complex perceptual discrimination tasks, or the speed of decision-making in problem situations. There is overlapping material from the cognitive and affective realms when an individual is categorized as having "impulsive traits" which then lead him into behavioral difficulties.

Further clarification is needed when it is realized that not all traits are perceived as having the same level of meaning or explanatory power. Explication requires some knowledge of theory formation. Despite the oft-repeated phrase that science studies observables and then defines them in terms of incidents supposedly directly registered by sense impressions, such as the eyes and ears, a brief examination reveals this as only partly true. Such dustbowl empiricism fails to give more than a series of finite measurements, $X_1, X_2 \text{----} X_n$— even apart from the problem of lack of precision in measurements. Going beyond this requires processes of inference or exercising inductive logic so that an extension can be made beyond the level of summation, resulting in an interesting series of inferring dispositions and powers to certain individuals.

Conceiving of character as a group of personality traits which remain consistent as a developmental phenomenon refers to a consistency of dispostions to behave in a phenotypic manner. Character involves enduring qualities or capacities to react in a certain way under a given set of conditions. Dispositions are viewed in terms of conferring hierarchical tendencies or powers.[10] These dispositions are not isolated sets of responses but rather potential states which have an extended duration. Orders of dispositionality can be delineated:

A first-order disposition with respect to characterology involves observable traits. These vary, depending on different personality theories. A tendency to react under stress with acting out behaviors as a rather consistent trait of an individual is an example of a disposition of the first order.

The tendency to possess these traits, or more precisely the conferring on an individual of a capacity to react in such a manner under certain conditions, is a disposition of the second order. While no one, including the most latent psychopath, exists in a state of constant acting out, under suitable external and internal circumstances, the behavior can be elicited or produced in a manner not possible in another individual who does not possess such powers. The more an acting out disposition is present, the greater the tendency for its actualization.

A combination of factors account for a given predisposition to a trait. If the primary disposition in the example used is the tendency to behave in such a manner, the tertiary disposition is the factor responsible for an individual possessing the tendencies (or power) which give him an acting out capacity at all. Dispositions of the third order are factors such as biochemical propensities, genetic loadings, etc. For illustrative purposes, the analogy of solving a mathematical problem will be used. One may have the capacity to solve a mathematics problem which can be utilized at a particular time and place. This power is used selectively in response to a combination of environmental and inner needs. The mathematical disposition of a first order of actually solving a math problem is conferred by a disposition of the second order which gives such a capacity. However, the power to confer would be lacking if a certain baseline of genetic loadings were not present in terms of a disposition of the third order to permit the potential for solving mathematics to be present (secondary) which in turn allows the actual solution to be achieved when necessary (primary).

Conceptual clarity demands that a distinction be made between normative happenings and dispositions. Methodologically it is a continuum.[11] These vary from the level of highest theoretical formulation to empirical, discreet events as follows: (a) hypothetical constructs, (b) traits of varying complexity and generality, (c) atomic dispositions, and (d) episodes which are single, dated occurrences; concrete happenings in time.

Atomic dispostions are indicators of evidence for a trait. Episodes are consequently bits of behavior which occur at a certain time and place. *Atomic dispositions* are slightly more theoretical formulations than are singular episodes. Their distinguishing properties are: temporal restriction, physically describable, and maximal covariance. The temporal restriction merely exemplifies the time period of the episodes, which restrict them to a brief period, such as seconds or minutes. This is the reason for the atomic—to distinguish these dispositions from those which are more enduring.

There are other types of dispositions characteristic of the life-style or ideals of an individual, illustrated by statements such as, "He has never been an ardent revolutionary all his life," or, "Being a manipulator is a way of life with him." The property of *physically describable* creates problems for those with a social or developmental perspective since it means that episodes exemplifying atomic dispositions must be topographically identifiable in time and space. Again, this is in distinction to some usages of disposition in psychology which refer to it in terms of manipulation-consequences, social stimuli, or attainments or achievements. *Maximal covariation*, or equivalence, refers to the continued lawfulness of atomic dispositions even when subdivided. There is no improvement in the curve smoothness or predictability of continuing to make finer subdivisions in either a quantitative or qualitative sense. On a simple level, this is illustrated by saying that the social disposition to utter four-letter words by an adolescent, which is noted by observing a series of such episodes, may have a difference if the profanity occurs when the boy is dressed in jeans or a suit, if a mixed, heterosexual group is present or not, and so on. The question that emerges from a series of collected episodes is whether they constitute an atomic disposition to swear, and whether it makes a difference in the response emitted if the boy was in jeans, or in a heterosexual group or not. The point is that the covariation would remain lawful.

Critics of a trait approach say that *trait-talk* is like discussions involving the number of angels on the head of a pin. The ontological status of traits is put in question. Distinctions which have overtones of old philosophical arguments between realism and nominalism are maintained on the contemporary scene in the elucidation of traits. If an alleged trait is viewed as a composite of a disposition-family, the basis for clustering relies on behavioral data or language. If behavioral data are used, the correlation based on empirical covariation must be demonstrated. A trait based on language should demonstrate a shared content based on logic and psychological material. If all that can be demonstrated is the semantic grouping of data, which seems logical but has no consistent set of empirical groupings which are conjunctively present, it can be maintained that a psychological reality has not been demonstrated.

This is the theoretical background with respect to moral character, from the early work of Hartshorne and May on lying, to the present day in which an alleged trait of honesty cannot be demonstrated to have an empirical covariation.[12] One becomes aware clinically and experimentally of the nontrasferability from one situation to another of what logically is classified as behavior exemplifying honesty. Empirically, low correlations exist between measures of honesty, such as resistance to temptation, honesty in test performance, type of parental discipline, or degrees of guilt ratings. When a trait has both empirical and semantic covariation, the reality situation is one where a phenotypic trait exists. If only the empirical condition is met, the trait may be viewed as genotypic. It is in the latter case where theoretical entities fully come into play in the form of hypothetical constructs. If the semanto-logical basis is lacking, we are dealing with a theoretical construct in the form of a source trait. This is an inferred entity-type trait rather than a descriptive trait with dispositional tendencies.

CLINICAL BACKGROUND
OF PSYCHOPATHOLOGICAL DELINQUENCY

Delinquency as a Product of Conflict. Clinical contributions to delinquency and acting out have a varied and confusing history. Part of this is due to the diversity of professional and lay groups involved with attempts to rescue wayward children.[13] Research and theoretical formulations have emerged from different professional disciplines and approaches. With these factors in mind, selective milestones will be discussed to illustrate the complexities in understanding delinquency, in psychopathological terms. The presentation of the types of problems utilizing a descriptive nosology is followed by one relying on psychodynamic formulations which involve characterology and family interaction in the genesis and maintenance of such behavior.

Some of the earliest clinical approaches to antisocial conduct were reactions against rigid classificatory schemes. They attempted to replace static categories, such as *moral imbecility*, with their attendant notions of irremediable deterioration, with alternatives involving environmental components. Most striking was the emphasis given decades ago to factors which continue to receive attention as though they are now original. Healy's 1915 classic, *The Individual Delinquent*, listed factors such as broken homes, poor parental control, bad companions, and unhealthy mental interests as antecedents of delinquency.[14] In Healy's list was the role of mental conflicts with accompanying repressions. In the same year, Healy applied his approach specifically to problems of lying and swindling.[15] The seeming purposelessness of much deviant behavior raised questions about its source, such as having a basis in conflict. Maintenance of a strict legal dichotomy between delinquency and criminality was seen as redundant. Many insights about behavior found by those working with adults were seen applicable to juveniles, and in turn a developmental perspective was present in seeing the relevancy of childhood antecedents.

Contributions by the famous psychiatrist William Allanson White illustrated these changes. As superintendent of a mental hospital, Dr. White dealt primarily with adults. A considerable number had previously been adjudicated criminally insane. In several landmark cases he was able not only to expand the viewpoint that criminal acts were unconsciously determined, but to use the courtroom as a place where a psychiatrist could raise questions about criminal responsibility and punishment.[16] Although many of his efforts were legal failures, in the sense that the cases were lost, White introduced the model of a competent psychiatrist who offered explanations for behavior beyond mere legal categorizations.

Two cases are illustrative. In the Schmidt case, a priest killed a girl parishioner in a bizarre murder. Although the prosecution was successful in having him electrocuted, White offered an explanation for the behavior in terms of a longstanding schizophrenic process in which the murder was a symbolic sacrifice and atonement. White's testimony in the Leopold and Loeb case again raised an alternative explanation for their behavior. Although Clarence Darrow, the defender of Leopold and Loeb, offered similar conclusions, he stressed the criminal as a product of a sick society—an argument not dissimilar from current explanations which stress the helplessness of an individual caught up in a corrupt social milieu.[17] Darrow's favorite saying—"I may hate the sin, but never the sinner"—is reminiscent of the adage of those treating institutionalized patients or inmates who condemn the act but not the actor. Working with White at St. Elizabeth's Hospital was Dr. Bernard Glueck, Sr. In a 1918 study of the inmates of Sing Sing Prison, he concluded that more than half the inmates were mentally ill.[18] What was present before confinement, and what was induced by institutional confinement was not known, but it did offer a commentary on the status of prisoners. Almost a half a century later, the estimate was still placed at almost the same number with half the prisoner population diagnosed as psychotic.[19]

By the third decade of the 20th century some studies dealing with adolescence were being included in discussions of delinquent behavior. As discussed earlier, the work had a sociological focus emphasizing the impact of slums and the concomitant gang culture with the failure of urban planning. It is striking to note the similarity of hypotheses offered decades ago and to see how little has changed in professional and popular writings on the problems. Richmond called attention to the frequency of antisocial acts in adolescent girls seen as a difficulty in adapting to a world of adults.[20] Discrimination in enforcement of delinquency provisions against girls was noted in the large number of their offenses involving sexual acting out which then, as now, are relatively ignored in boys.

In most cases, the antisocial tendencies phase out over the course of adolescence. Where this does not occur, attempts at reformation and punishment have had little effect. The point was emphasized by Judge Lindsey and Evans, who stressed the danger when punishment fails since dangerousness and criminality are accentuated.[21] During the third decade applications of psychoanalytic hypotheses to delinquent behavior emerged. Stekel's interest in the sexual symbolization of acting out behaviors led him to view kleptomania and pyromania as substitute sexual gratifications.[22]

In *Wayward Youth*, Aichhorn discussed the application of psychoanalytic principles to delinquent adolescents living in a group setting.[23] Symptom removal by directing activities toward other goals rather than repressing impulses was advocated for those burdened with neurotic character disturbances. While recognizing the role of guilt and aggressiveness, the family matrix of inadequate affection was stressed as a background in delinquent boys. Despite a treatment setting of a shack with a dozen incorrigible delinquent boys, Aichhorn believed he was able to achieve a transference relationship. He was not beyond thinking that manipulative structuring was legitimate and necessary, and that it provided the sine qua non for therapeutic success.

An extension was provided by Clark during the same period, who illustrated some types of pilfering were related to a desire for revenge upon fathers.[24] The egocentric child was viewed as having selfish demands acted out against the limit-setting of the parents who have power and possessions. A simple model of identification was proposed, such as children trying on parental clothing having their appetites stimulated. While parental discipline was viewed as a restraining influence, the child coveted parental possessions. What was lacking was a sufficient explanation of how socialization processes actually occur in children—a subject still in need of further explanation. This was a period when delinquent acts, such as pilfering, truancy, and assault, were being minimized as inefficient.[25]

The vitality of the approach at that time could not anticipate the subsequent disillusionment forty years later from misguided and poorly conceived therapeutic efforts. Still present were explanations which stressed delinquency as a failure of the will. Burt's *The Young Delinquent* was an example.[26] The intellectual viability of these explanations should not be discounted merely because they appealed to the masses from their notion of an ethical life as propagated by institutional representatives, such as families, schools, and churches.

Criminality As A Result of Guilt. Awareness of the ramifications of guilt in neurotic symptom formation led theorists to delineate types of delinquent acts based on efforts to alleviate it. As with so many theories, it was quickly seized upon by many as the explanation for criminality. What resulted was a predictable cycle whereby the popularity of the explanation gave rise to its being discredited. No clearer example of the need for competent diagnostic appraisal can be given than in this area. It is not that guilt does not contribute to criminality, but that its ramifications need to be demonstrated by clinical and empirical appraisal to determine its role in a particular case. The difference is between begging the question by assuming excessive guilt as causal versus demonstrating clinically how it operates.

In 1916 Freud discussed three character types he had encountered.[27] All three have relevance for the potentiality of antisocial behavior. By "the exceptions," he referred to those who expect to be treated as special, in which their personality is dominated by irrational desires for impulse gratification. Their life is dominated by a belief that they have once been unjustly wronged and consequently are entitled to obtain special privileges thereafter. Such an attitude contributes to difficulties in social adjustment. Overtones from several convergent areas of knowledge converge, particularly contemporary work on narcissistic personality disorders.[28] In terms of descriptive psychiatry, these traits are relevant to passive-agressive personalities whose resentment, pouty insubordination, passive obstructionism, procrastination, and stubbornness predominate. Given these dispositional tendencies—all related to aggressiveness—it is not surprising that acts periodically reach antisocial proportions.

A second character type mentioned by Freud was individuals who are ruined by success. Achievement leads to activation of a need to undo the gain due to the influence of guilt. To pay for their successes or neutralize them, they unconsciously maneuver into such painful predicaments by provoking others to dethrone them or squandering the results of their accomplishments. Borderline illegal activities, such as gambling or promiscuity in adulthood, or all manner of risk-taking and daredevil activities are possibilities. This is not proposed as a sole explanation for such behaviors, but rather stressed as on operational model. More commonly these potentials are manifested in the disposition toward *success phobias*, referring to the avoidance of success or ambitious goals, because they fear others may not like them as well, or that those not so successful may retaliate against them. The result is avoidance of competition and chronic patterns of academic and vocational underachievement. Some learning problems are encompassed within this grouping. More malignant trends operate when paranoid tendencies emerge from fear of one's competitors.[29]

After observing that Nietzsche discoursed on "pale criminals" whose deeds rationalized their guilt, Freud referred to a third type of character. Individuals, respected in their communities, continue to talk about earlier transgressions. They find it easier to call attention to some misdeed, or to commit such a deed, than to deal with the unconscious wishes which stimulate guilt. Observations of "naughty children" who provoke punishment and then feel relieved were cited in support of this theory, which proposed that a strict conscience externalizes a situation so that an overt pronouncement of guilt could occur rather than face internalized judges. Punishment is not only sought but carries a moral surplus, since it is received for unexpressed desires as well. Simultaneously, a feeling of relief is experienced for not needing to become aware of what the impulses promoting guilt really are. Unfortunately, the relief in such situations is temporary and leads to repetitions. Given sufficient strength of the desires which induce guilt, they continue their influence and may lead to illegal acts performed repetitively. The requirements are that the desired punishment be obtained as well as that the impulse be expressed in some derivative and concealed manner.

From these fomulations based on drive manifestations, a shift of interest to ego functioning occurred. Explanation shifted from the myriad expression of impulses to the conscious and unconscious responses elicited by an individual. Paradoxical behavior, which seemingly led to punishment and suffering, aroused interest. It appeared to go beyond, if not directly be opposed to, the maximization of pleasure in an individual.[30] Changing theories with respect to the nature of masochism are relevant.

Early work gave rise to ideas about the neurotic character—a mixture of neuroses and character disturbance. While Freud raised the hypothesis of a death instinct for self-destructive behavior, other possibilties were possible. Ernest Jones and Reich tied self-destructive tendencies to aggression turned against the self already seen to operate in some depressions.[31] [32] Those with neurotic character disorders, in contrast to neuroses, were seen as leading an active and eventful life. As children and adolescents, they were not ambivalent ruminators but rather driven toward high achievements. There is a greater living out of their impulse life than with the neurotic.[33] While the neurotic builds fantasized castles, and the psychotic lives in them, the neurotic character actually builds in a way that is sure to bring disaster. The distinction is clearer if a contrast is made with obsessional behavior which is closely related developmentally. In both cases there is a semblance of rational acts which have a sensical and nonsensical component. Obsessional development is sensical, since it permits temporary alleviation of guilt coupled with impulse gratification in the act itself; the nonsensical component is the purposeless and wasteful quality of the act. A neurotic character may be caught up in similar irrationality. Kleptomanic behavior, where the object taken is often worthless and frequently discarded, has a significant subjective and symbolic meaning for a given person. Yet, these are not antisocial personalities in the sense of sociopathy or psychopathy in which there is a rather unified directionality to impulse life.

The neurotic character is most accurately described as someone whose asocial impulses are ego dystonic since they are not integrated within the personality, nor are they under any adequate control. By way of an ego-splitting device one part of the personality restrains and punishes another for some of its acting out of impulses, or better yet—for some of its desires to transgress. Therapeutic work began to appreciate that approaches based on admonitions or punishments rarely had any lasting effect. Nor did self-resolves to mend their ways usually achieve desired results unless some other factors had influenced the personality. Formulations about the neurotic character were applied to children described as *neurotic delinquents*. They expressed their aggressiveness in unconscious ways which sought punishment and disapproval by external authorities. While these adolescents temporarily adjusted in institutional settings, the same factors which stirred their delinquency in the community stirred them to act out aggressively in institutions or to run. Bender and Schilder described types of childhood suicide as escapes from an unbearable situation by directing aggression against those who denied them affection and security. With sufficient guilt, the aggressive tendencies were turned against the self.[34]

The need for dramatic action is suggestive of the theatrics of the hysteric, yet in place of alloplastic symptom formation acting out of neurotic impulses occurs. However, the environment definitely becomes implicated in acting out patterns not only by way of their possible illegal nature, but because their lives are filled with action. Running through their acts is a theme common to many adolescents—the need to demonstrate the absurdity of adult authority by eliciting an unjustifiable punishment. Acting as though guilty is seen in young children who put on by way of intimation that they have done something wrong. When the punishment is forthcoming, they feel a self-satisfied sense of having tricked the authority into a wrongful outrage. An adolescent engages in these games by acting guilty when passing near the police, which often elicits an interrogation.

Elements of mockery can also lead to guises of the imposter.[35] One type is the *Munchausen Syndrome*. These individuals demonstrate their prowess in fooling doctors into falsely believing they have an illness so that medical procedures are carried out.[36] All varieties of impersonations may be seen from forgers to those who simulate success or failure. In one case an adolescent boy, who had moved from one part of the country to another, succeeded in changing his school records prior to moving. He succeeded in playing the dummy with his IQ of 138 for two years in a class with retarded children before revealing himself.

Strong needs to dethrone authority have been connected with frustrated idealism in some cases. Pursuit of unattainable goals can lead to Don Juanism.[37] Dichotomizing between tender sensuality and a series of impersonal conquests is a component of adolescent sexuality and permits an isolation between sensuality and tenderness. Continued as a rationalized way of life, the same incessant demands for conquests which become harder to attain continues. Decades ago David Levy attempted to fuse the sociological with the psychodynamic by holding that the breeding potential for delinquent behavior was based on loadings from delinquency-fostering milieus (high-delinquency neighborhoods, criminal fathers, alcoholic mothers, etc.) and unsocialized aggression in the boy.[38] Antisocial acts represented disguised techniques for bringing disgrace on a family, such as by making it hot for them. Neurotic delinquency arose from unsuccessful attempts to prevent impulse expression with irrational explanations offered. Rather than the cultural setting creating these trends for the neurotic delinquent, the patient creates delinquency in the environment as an attempted solution.

In the neurotic character infantile expectations continue with little insight and are played out in erotic relationships, vocational quests or other spheres of life. The near-panic when these individuals are required to give up their pursuits, or subordinate them to an authority, can hardly be overemphasized. Since they are only comfortable in the role of dominance or exploitation of others, anxiety mounts when control is vitiated or challenged. When pushed, paranoid symptomatology emerges in some. Yet, a self-injurious component is present which tempers goal-attainment. The character of Cassanova is an illustrative example.[39] Alexander and Staub gave a masterful description of Cassanova which is still applicable to contemporary neurotic characters.[40] Cassanova never gave up anything. He was a fighter for the freedom of the individual's instinctual wishes, boldly challenging the monotonously gray ideals of the community. He even succeeded in bringing a note of ethical protest into his battles. He appears to us as the heroic apologist of free thought who protests against the tyrannical spirit of the Inquisition and superstition. Yet, even these catchwords, by means of which he justified his acts, did not allay his unconscious need for punishment. He would bring about his arrest as an atonement for his protest against those in authority—a protest which, unconsciously and symbolically, he continued to fight in terms of early and internalized representations of authority.

POWER-STRIVINGS AND DELINQUENT BEHAVIOR

Introduction. Strivings for power have had a varied background as an explanation for certain forms of delinquency or ruthlessness. The closeness of these strivings to what can easily lead to the accoutrements of social and political success is striking.[41] Theories about primary or secondary aggressive drives, or compensatory responses to feelings of inferiority, have been used as baselines for psychological conflict. Yet there is not sufficient specificity in such formulations. We are left with the injunction that power corrupts, but we do not know where to go from there.

There are distinctions between the use of power in overt acts, in contrast to role definitions (who is in charge?). In a clinical sense power is significant in an experimental manner since a person feels limited, hindered, or oppressed, by someone or something which has the force to incapacitate him. When a person comes to see the future as hopeless and without promise, the potential to challenge authorities increases immensely. Again, it is a small step to see himself hemmed in and threatened from without so that paranoid mentation enters the picture. Rather than facing the feeling of lacking power, a person may act out his aggression.

Power definciencies which contribute to delinquency-proneness are not a new theme. Winifred Richmond, in 1933, stressed the desire of the adolescent to feel important, be successful, and sell himself to others.[42] No psychological sophistication is required to observe this in people, but to provide an adequate explanation is more complicated. An explanation must include a consideration of attaining biological maturity, sex-role identity, and a culture in which power and success at any price are stressed as ideals. Consider the sports fantacism associated with the philosophy of winning at any price.[43] To cop out in seeking power can lead to varying psychological consequences. It can be seen in a lowering of self-esteem or in passive obstructionism, which is an effort to control others. Myriad combinations of power exert their influence on the individual.

Berle listed five laws of power:[44]

1. It fills vacuums in known organizations
2. It is based on a system of ideas or a philosophy
3. It is exercised through institutions on which it is dependent
4. It confronts with and acts in the presence of a field of responsibility
5. It is invariably personal

The last point is crucial to psychological explanations of power since ultimately the individual is confronted with threats to narcissism and self-esteem which are basic to a motivational system.

Responses to Powerlessness.   In response to states of powerlessness, the adolescent experiences a feeling of oppression. It is related to states of narcissistic mortification in which he feels at the mercy of another—be it a person or institution. This is the ultimate in negation of individual autonomy but, in contrast to the giving up complex seen in depressions, it is a loss of autonomy by external coercion toward which the individual feels helpless. The key phrase with respect to oppression appears to be "helplessness imposed from without." There may be a feeling of muted anger and rage, overt at times, but not necessarily having internalized responses of anxiety.

Alternatives are available for the classification of oppression. The oppression may be biological, psychological, socio-economic, or political. Another approach involves the degree of awareness an individual has regarding his oppressed state, since some oppressions can be subtle and indirect. Common examples are the oppressed feelings of a minority group, but the same feelings arise in a subcultural group in which one is an outsider. Oppressions are possible within family matrices beyond such commonplaces as the proverbial second-child syndrome. There is also the sensitized child who reacts to minor slights with suspiciousness or feelings of being intruded upon. His oppressive coefficient is quite high from many contributing factors. Halleck offers the following classification of oppression:[45]

TABLE 15

A. Objectively Measurable Oppression

1. Social and interpersonal stresses which are real, direct, and recognized
2. Social and interpersonal stresses which are real, but indirect and totally or partially unrecognized

B. Oppression which is perceived but which does not have an apparent source in the observable environment

1. Misunderstood oppression
2. Internal oppression (superego pressures)
3. Projected oppression

From this classification, the situations most likely to give rise to oppression are more apparent. What remains elusive is the problem of specificity which plagues all classifications of psychopathology. We do not know why an experiential state of oppression, as a developmental phenomenon, leads a person toward an antisocial solution while another develops overcompensatory ambitions to achieve. Yet another may accentuate neurotic conflicts while others have bodily changes induced by way of psychophysiological processes. Yet others react by periodic psychotic episodes.

All of these have varying combinations of intrapunitive efforts as well as extractive efforts aimed at the environment. We also lack genetic information which would allow us to account for dispositions in these directions. Clinical reconstruction allows ideas as to what happened to a particular individual with a set of personality traits in a given psychosocial milieu, but prior prediction is extremely difficult. Apart from outcome, the particular behavior selected is a result of multiple influences which have been operating and either give a supposed gain, or are the results of massive conditioning so that cognitive operations without affective signals lead to chronic behavioral patterns.

Discussions of power abuse usually select an extreme example for illustration. It is more efficacious to consider a less dramatic but more pervasive situation illustrating the genesis of hopelessness. Instead of considering an individual with a terminal illness, or someone confined in a prison or maximum security hospital, the predicament of an adolescent caught up in alternatives which seem equally unappealing illustrates several points. The alternatives are unappealing because they induce little self-esteem related to what the adolescent does or intitiates. The solution, proposed by sociological theorists is to join a gang or some other deviant group with its concomitant values of excitement and cohesiveness. From the vantage point of the adolescent a commitment is made to an identity which gives the ego a feeling of carrying out acts for which he is a responsible agent.

Rather than engaging in linguistic and legal subterfuges of denying intent or cognitive awareness of acts, the commitment appears to be just the opposite. There is pride in carrying out acts which he personally intends. While this may not be the epitome of individual responsibility, it does achieve a direct result. It exerts a counterforce on the environment stronger than almost any other type of activity—barring the bizarre outbreak of violence at the peak of a psychotic episode. Witness the absence of a personally unfavorable stigma to adolescents who are designated delinquents versus mentally ill. The latter phrase, with its associated framework of community approaches by a sundry group of helpers, has almost passed the stage of adverse stigma to one associated with laughter if not derision.

A dichotomy between activism associated with delinquency—in contrast to the conformity and passivity of being mentally ill— operates. Neuroses are seen by most as something not under one's personal control, and this dichotomy is accepted by juvenile and adult criminal courts. To throw oneself at the mercy of authorities and the institutions which are viewed as unjust or corrupt holds little promise as a way of regaining self-esteem.

Additional values are present in actively seeking out those identified as oppressive agents. Externalization of conflict is more easily facilitated. A child, previously conforming and self-critical during the latency period, may emerge as a different person during adolescence. Previous self-effacing trends, which led to blame for minor transgressions without insight, are not overthrown by mobilizing an attack against something concrete and external. In addition, a discharge of aggression is permitted precluding guilt. Identification of external sources heightens the burden and functions by displacement as well. It is more comfortable to have sources of oppression supposedly identified than to experience them as unknown, and there is less need to torment oneself when the cause is seen elsewhere. Individuals and institutions are singled out and called weak, ambilvalent, and indecisive thus becoming a focus for grievances. Hence, an adolescent might seek out relatively ineffectual and incompetent teachers to confront (rather than the strong and truly oppressive). No matter that bureaucratic agents are themselves caught up in self-hate and feelings of oppression—for they have remained in the system and are vulnerable targets. Projection appears by blaming intellectual or academic inadequacy on the system—a part-truth which increases its cogency.

Cogency of Power-strivings. What gives power strivings such driving force? To go beyond an explanation which states that the narcissism of childhood continuously seeks to regain an initial state of fantasized omnipotence requires appraisal of the dynamics of power strivings and their compromise. Developmental antecedents are presented as power strivings being a defensive maneuver in response to the anxiety of helplessness before an actual or fantasized powerful being.

Work with older children, and reconstructive work with adult patients, permits the use of a construct that children attempt to participate in the power of figures. Fantasies of devouring powerful objects or fusing with them are common. Participation can take place by sharing in the possessions of a great one or having a relic or object. Witness the mania to touch or see athletes, or movie stars, rub against them, or tear off parts of their clothing in a fetishistic manner. To take from someone in this way becomes a source of self-esteem, and it is analogous to one form of kleptomania. To possess something from the powerful in a magical way permits participation in their power. The sign or talisman confer power, protection and omnipotence. Implicit is a set of cognitive operations which regard power as having reified qualities. "If I do not get or take the power, someone else will." Taking from another—by hook or by crook—has a close connection to acts of piety. Beseeching a powerful creature for mercy has a similar motivational basis and goal, as does preserving mementos of departed ones. Appropriating parts of them brings protection or good luck (hence, customs such as athletic trophies, letter-sweaters or jackets with athletic insignias, special gold awards to hang from belts or watch chains, pictures of old teams, offices with pictures of famous men or senior colleagues, and stuffed animals). All of these let the individual retain a feeling of power from old victories, or share in the power of someone who was once great.

Derivative forms of fusions with greatness are seen in exuberant patriotism ("My country, right or wrong") or religious zealotry in the form of merging with a superior being on a cognitive and affective level. Varieties of submitting to a powerful or authoritarian figure have a similar goal. These vary from the commonplace submission to authority of a legally constituted type to a blind submission carrying out the will of a leader. Harlotized young women devote themselves to their owners in a dehumanized manner of carrying out their desires for a homicide.[46] Drug-induced experiences, with a loss of ego boundaries, are another phenomenon of expanding beyond oneself.

Feelings of powerlessness induce strong conflict in an individual. On one hand there are desires to share the power of some object or institution; on the other hand there are desires to seize or aggressively take power beyond what is perhaps willfully ceded. Those who adopt the former solution are predisposed to identify with existing powers and perhaps occupy a frustrated role in an institutional framework. Those who go beyond and challenge the system for a niche of their own making occasionally attain historical significance, but they most often pursue a path of opposition to authority figures.

We will not pursue the devices which various societies have instituted with respect to substitute satisfactions to alleviate power strivings. These vary from aggressive contests and spectacles to substitutes for power, such as exposure to television, which is filled with ersatz possibilities to indulge fantasies. Such illusory participation in power reconciles people to the impotency of their situations by the self-delusion that they are participants. Given that actual showing and utilization of power are very difficult in most forms of society, the person must look for some means of acquiring power.

Gaining self-esteem through academic or athletic prowess is available only to those with special talents, even if equal opportunity to excel is provided. Even more oppressive is the realization of how short-lived these gratifications are, as well as the failure to resolve the recurrent need for power. A youth learns that good behaviors do not beat the system as readily as more devious ways do. Our discussion about the formation of delinquent gangs where power and status can be achieved is relevant. The capacity to seize power, or to one day share in it, is seen with depressive variations as life progresses.[47]

For a dwindling few, the hope of an ultimate sharing of power in the hereafter suffices. During adolescence the hope and striving to attain power persists as part of the ego-ideal. Achievement expectations maintain a degree of hope mixed with unrealism. Projections of blame onto the system work as an ameliorating device to forestall disillusionment. Every experience (and every projection of blame) serves as a reinforcement that one can ultimately share in power.

A realization that one may not be succeeding mobilizes rage and anger, which are acted out. However, the very need to conquer and to be assertive can come close to antisocial conduct—one reason for the high incidence of delinquent tendencies during adolescence. Overcoming a fear of authority figures is tried by taking or borrowing from them. This raises objective possibilities for retaliation. In addition there are introjected psychological controls. These formulations can be seen in terms of a goal being needed to attain power or its equivalent in the form of a trophy.[48]

Primitive mechanisms of oral incorporation or introjection are the forerunners, but adolescents later generalize to many kinds of needing to defeat others or take from them. The experience is one of triumph. However, the process is an ambivalent one—not only due to fear and anxiety but from love for those who possess power. There are also feelings of remorse after deeds of seizure. Failure to give at least token representation of trophies to adolescents kindles their feeling of estrangement and a need to take in their own way. Alternatively, tokens of external rewards from power figures permit the adolescent to identify with the group and conform. The problem is not only adolescent rebellion, but why authority objects resist sharing so vigorously. Witness the resistance to lowering the voting age to eighteen when most adults, as seen in the small percent voting, regard this as a meaningless exercise of power.

PSYCHOPATHY

Diagnostic Confusion. The concept of the psychopath has had a long and confusing history. No one is ever sure of what the term psychopath means. Nor has the validity of the label in the past or present been accepted by many. The following terms in some combination have all been applied to the group under discussion: constitutional psychopath, constitutional inferior, psychopathic personality, moral insanity, moral imbecility, moral idiocy, melancholia sans delire, manie sans delire, defective delinquent, emotionally unstable, and sociopath. Various diagnostic schemas are proposed from time to time in an effort to categorize symptoms. The American Psychiatric Association's *Diagnostic and Statistical Manual of Mental Disorders* utilizes a descriptive approach which lists the diagnosis of *antisocial personality* as one category of personality disorders.[49]

The latter are defined as deeply ingrained, maladaptive patterns of behavior perceptibly different from psychotic or neurotic behaviors. It is specified that these behaviors should be recognizable by adolescence or even earlier. The antisocial types are viewed as unsocialized beings whose behavior brings them into conflict with society. The customary descriptive symptoms are : lack of loyalty to others, low frustration-tolerance, blaming others for their difficulties, selfishness, callousness, impulsivity, irresponsibility, lack of guilt, and an inability to learn from experience or from punishment. Such a cluster if taken literally, would hardly describe someone able to operate and survive with the cleverness and cunning which such individuals manifest.

The difficulties in diagnosing psychopathy in the adolescent group are even more complicated than with adults. The term *psychopath* implies a fixity of behavior and a prognostic accuracy which does not exist. There is the further problem of applying the term in a loose and vague manner to those who deviate from the predominant mores of the group. Some classifications, such as the one from the American Psychiatric Association, also provide for a *dyssocial reaction* for those whose norms conform to a deviant social subgroup within society. But this does not account for the situation where the values of the child or family differ from those of the clinician who is doing the evaluation. In the past, what resulted were behavior problems being diagnosed as psychopathy once schizophrenia or manic-depressive psychoses had been ruled out. As an example of a classification of psychopathy gone amuck, Kahn's 1931 book, *Psychopathic Personalities*, is a classic. He listed anxious psychopaths, compulsive psychopaths, depressive psychopaths, etc.[50]

Another difficulty with the concept of psychopathy is attendant on diagnoses made on the basis of delinquent acts. These diagnoses are fraught with unreliability, since delinquent conduct can occur in a multitude of situations and under diverse environmental stresses. Nor can the response to psychotherapy, or any type of therapy, be adequate criteria for the diagnosis of psychopathy. Difficulty in diagnosis is complicated by the presence of childhood histories of deprivation which some studies take as a significant antecedent for antisocial development. Statistical studies indicate some loading from deprivation when populations are compared. However, not all psychopathic individuals come from deprived backgrounds, nor does a deprived background mean one is destined for psychopathy. These limitations reveal difficulties with the concept and why some believe the diagnosis can never amount to more than a subjective impression that a person has less emotional attachment in relating to others. Furthermore, all kinds and degrees of difficulty in relating to others may be present, depending on the situation, to whom one is relating, and the internal variations.

Part of the difficulty is associated with the multiple causes believed present in the development of psychopathy. Some hold to a special psychological vulnerability which permits the exertion of familial and cultural influences. Heterogenous factors are lumped under personality disorders. Multiple etiology results in a confusion of etiology with psychodymanic explanations, further compounded by confusing moral and legal issues of responsibility for behavior with psychological explanations. Reasons given for behavior are then treated as equivalent to causation and both are confused with exculpability.

By adolescence behavioral traits or symptoms are emerging in the potential antisocial individual. Noshpitz stresses three antecedents in their childhood background:[51]

1. A situation of overstimulation which can occur in a variety of ways. For example this may have been manifested in sleeping with a parent of the opposite sex until an advanced age, or excessive bodily concern accentuated by stimulation, tickling, or whippings. The result can be adverse in terms of anticipation that this level of high stimulation will continue.

2. Overgratification from inadequate limit-setting by parental or authority figures.

3. Overdeprivation in the senses mentioned previously where there has been an inadequate meeting of basic needs for development to progress satisfactorily.

Certain early life experiences leave a proneness to delinquency.[52] (1) lack of opportunity to form attachments to maternal figures in the first three years of live; (2) emotional deprivation for a limited period of at least more than three months prior to age three or four, and (3) changing of maternal objects during the same period.

By adolescence, only a semblance of superficial relationships may have developed with no deep attachments. By then such individuals may be inaccessible to the kinds of help or assistance available. The result is exasperation, since cooperation or a change in behavior occurs more on the changing needs of the moment than anything more enduring. Further puzzlement and exasperation result from deceitful or evasive behaviors which appear pointless. When most of their wishes are being met—such as during preadolescence—little may be noticed as deviant, although careful histories reveal episodes of acting out and earlier impulsivity. Temper outbursts and oppositional behavior appear as background factors. This behavior should be distinguished from a strong tolerance for pain, or taking calculated risks in the line of duty. Those with budding psychopathic traits take risks more for the hell of it, and for no apparent purpose beyond seeking excitement. If an injury is sustained, their pain tolerance is not particularly high.

Historical Points. Before more specific and contemporary formulations of psychopathy are discussed, the historical development of the concept lends a perspective. It illustrates how a particular idea about behavior begins and evolves with varying cultural influences. There is a groping to assimilate diverse observations about personalities who deviate. Whether the concept has relevance and validity at the present time, or it has become outdated, is another problem. Initial observations are credited to a German, Ettmuller, who called it *melancholie sans delire* (melancholia without delusions) in the latter part of the 18th century. Pinel (1745-1826), the father of modern psychiatry, working at the Bicetre in Paris viewed psychopathy as connected with mania. He called it *manie sans delire* (mania without delusions).[53]

Two things in these early formulations remain prominent: (a) cognitive exclusion by which delusions were ruled out, and (b) references to mood disturbance so that the cross-reliability of diagnoses between different clinicains is low from contamination of psychopathic traits with mood disturbances.

The consideration about whether there was as a pure culture of psychopathy began to enter the picture. By 1837, Prichard in Bristol, England, was dividing insanity into two types: moral and intellectual.[54] Moral insanity was a morbid perversion of feelings, affections, inclinations, temper, habits, and moral dispositions. No defect of intelligence or cognition was held to be present, especially not hallucinations or perceptual abberations such as illusions. Prichard gave a prominent place to states of gloom and sorrow alternating with excitement. The role of object loss was acknowledged by Prichard in references to personality changes whereby a reverse of fortune or loss of a beloved relative deeply affected a person. All kinds of diagnostic conditions were subsumed under this category—apart from those with overt disturbances in thinking.

For the remainder of the 19th century arguments waxed and waned about the presence of intellectual defects in moral insanity. Rather than carefully delineating a syndrome and symptoms, the controversy centered on whether such an entity as moral insanity existed. By such phraseology the confirmation or disconfirmation of this idea as a concept having existential validity was actually precluded. The argument about cognitive defect in moral insanity was not an empty one in terms of its social and legal implications. The famous McNaughten rules for legal insanity formulated in 1843 in England, were phrased in terms of cognitive responsibility as the criterion for criminal responsibility. If someone with a mental illness did not know the difference between right and wrong, or the nature and quality of an act, he was not criminally responsible.

Hence, establishment of cognitive impairment was not a moot point. It was rather that during that century, a methodology was not available to demonstrate cognitive impairment, if it was alleged, so the argument did not progress beyond semantic and moralistic levels. Even with modern insights into the nature of mental functioning, we are still unsure about the type of cognitive disturbance present in psychopathy. With or without cognitive disturbance, the moral and legal responsibility of the psychopath continues as a debatable point.

Innumerable articles dealing with the psychopath appeared in the literature of medicine, psychiatry, law, and lay journals during the 19th century. It would be fascinating in its own right for a social historian to study the preoccupation with these nosological and moral questions. In 1879 Bonfigli, a leading Italian forensic psychiatrist, reviewed over a hundred authorities of the day who took adamant pro or con positions on the cognitive-defect question in "moral imbecility."[55] A beginning effort to set down the characteristics of moral insanity was made by Gouster in 1878.[56] Childhood antecedents were put in terms of characteristics becoming "perverted in infancy." Children who were potential psychopaths were described as headstrong, malicious, disobedient, irrascible, liars, neglectful, and at times violent. As childhood progressed, they were seen as delighting in intrigue and mischief, given to excess, excitable, and later passing themselves off as heroes or martyrs.

The issue running throughout the commentaries was the debate about whether such behavior was a concomitant part of a disease—moral insanity—or whether it was really a cloak for vice. Was the recalcitrant and unruly child reacting to a disease process or was he using this explanation as a cover for mischieviousness? Similarities of the behaviors, in the absence of any agreed-upon criteria for a disease, prevented closure then as it does today. The appeal of organic deficits to explain the phenomenon became apparent. If organic deficits were significant, such individuals could legitimately be viewed as diseased and suffering from a constitutional defect—genetic or acquired. Professional groups, families, institutions, and relatives would then have a sanction to view them as such.

Failure of the moral sense to develop could be congenital or destroyed by disease. Examples given for the latter are general paralysis or congenital syphilis. The implicit assumption then, as now, is that organicity negates responsibility. If the explanation for psychopathy were to reside primarily in an interlacing series of environmental events, everyone could dredge up adversities, yet it would still be no excuse for antisocial behavior. Explanations which would satisfy exculpability required defects in the central nervous system. In the United States during the 19th century the issue of moral insanity received a thorough airing at the trial of Guiteau, the assassin of President Garfield.[57] As before, contrasting viewpoints were presented by leading forensic psychiatrists of the day without further clarification, similar to the present. The current version of the debate is being played out with respect to the XYY chromosome, despite inconclusive evidence for its role in psychopathic or violent behavior.

Tuke, the great English psychiatrist, in 1885 supported the idea of moral insanity based on a weakening of the higher centers of the brain which permitted excessive emotionality and paralyzed the will.[58] Perhaps this was due to the influence of Darwinian evolutionary theory in which the higher levels of evaluation were viewed as underdeveloped or diseased. Moral insanity was viewed by some as an atavistic manifestation of anomalous development where the moral sense could not develop. Theorizing about atavism was close to the anthropological theories of Lombroso which we have cited.[59]

Lombroso did not maintain that the born criminal theory explained all criminality. All children were viewed as born delinquents in need to be exposed to education. Failure of education produced delinquent types, but they did not become as deviant as born criminals. Degeneration into criminality as a type was allowed—similar to developing a seizure condition. Hence, both a congenital and acquired moral insanity was permitted. Not every born criminal engaged in criminal acts. Education and favorable circumstances could delay or conceal it, but the disposition was much greater. Over his lifetime Lombroso reduced his born criminal type from approximately 100 percent to 40 percent.

By the end of the 19th century subvarieties of opinion existed about moral insanity. The main supporters of the diagnoses were certain that some organic deficit on neurological or anthropological grounds was crucial. Old arguments about the need to establish a diseased intellect persisted, as did arguments about the origins and location of the moral sense. Opponents of the doctrine were either those who were not persuaded a disease was detectable, or those who saw such a doctrine having a pernicious influence on holding people not responsible for their behavior.

At the commencement of the 20th century the standoff between the two orientations resulted in efforts to fuse the most acceptable parts. German psychiatrists spoke of "psychopathic inferiors." The inferiority in question referred to the defects that prevented an individual from adjusting in his environment—be they predisposition, defect, or degeneration. In America, Adolph Meyer introduced the term "constitutional inferiority," and originally excluded the term "psychopathic," which was taken as synonomous with insanity. A fusion into "constitutional psychopathic inferior" soon resulted.

Renewed interest in the diagnostic problem came from different sources. One was the realization that varieties of organicity, from seizure patterns to infectious diseases of the central nervous system, might be relevant to behaviors encompassed under psychopathy. A second influence was the beginning delineation of what would constitute the mentally subnormal, then called moral imbeciles, and for whom an incapacity to acquire the moral sense was seen. A further subdistinction was realized betweeen those who could not (the subnormal), and those not given adequate training in moral development. A further contribution was from work involving dementia praecox, which could present with psychopathic behaviors (now more commonly seen as varieties of "pseudopsychopathic schizophrenias.") Episodic confusional and psychotic states with impairment of intellect were observed in these individuals, who on occasion were clumped with the morally insane.

An important contribution was made by Karl Birnbaum in 1914.[61] The introduction of psychometric testing made possible the confirmation that no intellectual defect existed in most psychopaths. The old argument about the pros and cons of intellectual deficit in psychopathic individuals was then resolved. Psychopathy was viewed as a pathological affectivity by Birnbaum, whose views were strikingly advanced for the time. Unfortunately, they were ignored for decades. He stressed that the subnormal could have psychopathic traits but a superior intelligence might permit the neutralization of antisocial tendencies. The psychopath, as a diagnostic type, was distinguished from the criminal—a confusion which had permeated the 19th century. Lack of evidence for degenerative processes was cited (if a physical impairment was present and contributing to antisocial behavior, it was viewed as separate from the psychopathic element. The argument continued with a host of articles referring to nervous instability, poor emotional balance, and bad moral standards as characteristic. However, a transition occurred when these were considered as personality traits of the individual. A later shift would view them as responses of an adaptive or maladaptive type.

Froukel pointed out in 1920 that the concept of the psychopath lacked objectivity and hence required diagnostic criteria.[62] He felt that interpretations based on degeneracy had lacked explanatory power, and that diagnosis was only possible on a retrospective basis after certain patterns of behavior had occurred and a history compiled. Further, the notion of relativity was introduced, in that psychopathy was viewed as a composite. Froukel listed as examples of psychopathy all of the following:

1. Imbeciles
2. Those leading unstable lives, (pathological swindlers and liars)
3. Lack of balance as seen in a sense of superiority in which individuals were striving for unattainable goals
4. Lack of normal inhibitions and restraints
5. Neurasthenic features of hypochondriacal complaints and vasomotor instability
6. Sensitivity which showed itself in seclusiveness, few friends, anxiety dreams, alcohol intolerance, and timidity with women
7. Cyclothymic tendencies which revealed the persistence of early notions involving affectivity.

The grouping corresponded with Kraepelin's list of seven kinds of psychopaths: antisocial, eccentric, excitable, impulsive, liars and swindlers, quarrelsome, and unstable.[63] The condition was ascribed to heredity, but did not provide anything close to the clarifying value which his classification of schizophrenics did.

The symptomatic approach was further used in attempts to obtain a descriptive picture of the psychopath. Weakness and inhibitions were attributed to motivations being based on the desire to obtain pleasure at the moment. Johnson ascribed this to a deficiency in socialization processes which left a weak moral impressionability.[64] The recognition gave rise to the realization that similar behaviors could be observed in the oversocialized who were excessively morally impressionable. Ben Karpman at St. Elizabeth's Hospital began his extensive writings on this problem in the 1920s which continued for the next forty years. One of his early contributions stressed the "psychotic-like" schizoid or cycloid manifestations in some of the psychopathic group. He stressed they should be regarded as "larval psychotics."[65] Another group showed a manifest grossness and crudeness in their affective life which gave them a primitive quality and led them into constant conflict with others. These were viewed as warranting the diagnosis of constitutional psychopaths. Their impulsivity and lack of resilience prevented them from acquiring stable habits. The end of permitting themselves indulgences justified any means to achieve a goal. No defect in sexual performance was noted, in contrast to opinions of earlier writers, but they did show deficiencies in functioning in roles of husbands or fathers. Their selfish and narcissistic attitudes toward others prevented them from responding with the loyalties required for a commitment to family life. On deeper exploration, some revealed sado-masochistic sexual trends.

Wittels felt the "oversexed" promiscuous person was the primal representation of the psychopath.[66] In contrast to fears of bisexuality in the neurotic psychopath, the plain psychopath enjoyed bisexual indulgences and was the epitome of the phallic narcissist. The "sexual psychopath" showed florid bisexuality when opportunity presented itself. Connection with other miscellaneous impulsive misdemeanors occurred by the inability of the psychopath to deal with sexual impulses when they were aroused but incapable of being fulfilled.

Cleckley's Syndrome. Descriptive attempts to establish diagnostic criteria for the psychopath have not been done better than by Harvey Cleckley. The first edition of his book, *The Mask of Sanity,* in 1941, up to the latest edition in 1955, listed the major features believed diagnostic in an overt sense.[67] They are listed in terms of an end-result for which there is still an insufficient explanation in terms of genesis and developmental components. Further discussion of childhood features will be given later. The descriptive features of the psychopath listed by Cleckley are used as a basis for discussion.

Unexplained failures are considered in the absence of disturbance in intelligence. The adult psychopath, like his juvenile counterpart, has a history of chronic failure with only spotty successes. Failures and irrational acts are not explained by deficits in reasoning ability.

There is a paucity of powerful affects, such as guilt or anxiety, a lack of crippling neurotic manifestations, and a lack of apparent motivation for antisocial conduct. There is gross inconsistency with respect to responsibilities and obligations: while being able to convince many people of utmost sincerity, a commitment may be renounced with impunity at an opportune moment. A lack of remorse or shame are then present.

He does not care whether the truth will be detected or not. If found out there is little upset, and a lie or insincerity may continue to be maintained. This is most interesting since many consider those with emerging psychopathic tendencies deficient in role-playing skills, and thus the falsehoods are often detectable. Detection, however, has little impact on modifying the lying role.[68] In fact, the very series of foster-home, residential, or correctional placements that these youths have had, has reinforced short-term role playing. When they cause suffering, blame is not accepted for their role. Rather, responsibility is projected onto others or casual indifference is seen.

Classic formulations of "failing to learn by experience" are often cited. This does not mean an inability to learn in a learning-theory sense, nor does it mean an intellectual deficit. Rather, it is the inability to explain why the individual so behaves, and the lack of a desire for an explanation by psychopathic individuals. Patterns of getting into repetitive difficulties under almost exactly similar circumstances, followed by promises to never do it again are typical. The pattern gives little concern to the individual, and it appears not only in plausible excuses given for exculpation, but in the general mockery of standards of justice and law which have no personal meaning for them. A cognitive take of the standards has not taken place. They are viewed like those raised by the standards of one civilization viewed by another. A typical example among adolescents is the recurrent failure to perform in school, a failure arising not from a lack of intellectual ability or neurotic conflict, but from a lack of desire. Nor is this a purely cultural phenomenon of a lower socio-enconomic class. Adolescents make all kinds of promises to reform, not be truant, do their work, just as their slightly older counterparts do who have committed illegal acts only to repeat the pattern. Obviously this does not mean that all such failures indicate budding psychopaths, since many diagnostic possibilities exist.

An incapacity for love was noted by early workers who referred to a peculiar lack of genuine attachment to others. Affection was eloquently verbalized, with protests of undying devotion. Yet, when these maneuvers were challenged, a series of petulant and rageful responses was elicited. People with pain-dependency conflicts were most likely to be caught up in relationships with these individuals, and most likely to become victims of exploitation. One need not look to the middleaged con artist who milks widows of funds. Such relationships can be seen in love relationships of adolescent boys and girls. More commonly, exploitation is observed in relationships whereby the gullible, or those with a high need for acceptance, are exploited by those whose psychopathic insensitivity permits them to read victims. There is little compassion for the victims, who are regarded as weak and perhaps contemptible.

An example is a sixteen-year-old boy whose extracurricular activities were peddling drugs and pimping girls in his local high school. He was pleased when a girl showed interest in him. A relationship was soon established where he became upset in other sphere of his life, such as when his competitors bested him, or he was on the losing side in an athletic contest. The girl was then available to absorb his physical beatings. No sexual intercourse was involved between the couple, but he physically beat her on innumerable occasions to the point of broken ribs and black eyes.

A contrast was an attractive adolescent girl who carried on a series of affairs with boys and promoted physical fights between them. Her excitement mounted as blood was let and several boys sustained lost teeth and scars. When in time a group of boys caught on and abandoned her, there were plenty of fish in the sea, which permitted her to continue her predatory ways.

Closely related are shallow and impersonal relationships—sexual and otherwise. Although sexual activity may be promiscuous, the impersonality and indifference are striking. Sexuality, like many other acts, is used in the service of exploitation or power-seeking.

The lack of insight is colossal. What is again most impressive is their indifference to this lack. It is not that they do not mouth facile explanations for their behavior, but that their efforts are so aimless. Experience with juveniles and adults appears congruent. An example is a seventeen-year-old engaged in predatory activity for several years who submitted the name of the sentencing judge with the address of the court as a reference when he applied for a job.

Problems of persistent self-defeating behavior cannot be adequately explained in a descriptive framework. In appraising the long-range histories of psychopathic individuals, there is often a pattern of defeat and disappointment going back to early childhood. The activities such as deliberate failures, provocative insults to authority figures, and disasters wraught upon themselves with a full cognizance beforehand of what they are doing are all self-destructive, but are usually overlooked by the institutions with whom they are in contact.

An inability to handle alcohol is a familiar phenomenon in psychopathic adults. This may be seen in the young adolescent, although it becomes more difficult to evaluate because of the lability of their responses to alcohol. A similar pattern, however, is seen in their responses to drugs. Minimal amounts may provoke widely exaggerated responses or release aggression already in a state of jeopardy.

Finally, although suicidal gestures and manipulative efforts are frequent, a desire to die by these efforts appears lacking, (in contrast to the suicidal patient, whose primary problems lie in the realm of depression). Their depressions are more related to the immediate deprivation, and their efforts are directed to manipulating others to lessen their plight. Some have confused this with primary depressions and unfortunately see all depressions as reinforcements of secondary gain. Although it does not seem that any suicidal effort operates in a vacuum (outside of a communicative effort directed at someone), the motives and feelings which operate in those who are deeply depressed or genuinely remorseful about their behavior seem lacking in those with psychopathic tendencies. Even in the midst of extreme limit-setting as in institutional or correctional placements, they show a lack of remorse. Even when a suicide occurs their acts have the element of an overt attack or manipulation. Great risks are taken to accomplish ends, risks which can misfire from their reckless audacity. Suicides appear more related to poor planning and miscalculation.

The Validity of The Concept of Psychopathy.   The historic use of the concept of psychopathy for 150 years in different contexts and with different meaning does not in and of itself establish its validity or invalidity. The merits and demerits of utilizing a diagnosis needs appraisal apart from its usages. Unfortunately, much writing is confined to the level of case description or repetition of frequently cited symptoms and signs. Varieties of psychodynamic constellations for different types of psychopathic manifestations, clinical antecedents of childhood psychopathies, and the developmental problems of psychopathy, all remain in need of clarification. Almost every symptom and sign listed as one of the characteristics of psychopathy raises questions as to whether these characteristics are limited to this one diagnostic category. Is psychopathy a weighting of characteristics that determine whether the diagnosis of psychopath should be used? Contrast this with a viewpoint in which psychopathic personalities as a generic group are made up of those who live primarily on an instinctual level.[69]

An indispensible condition for clarity is to avoid confusing the commission of an antisocial or illegal act with the diagnosis of psychopathy. Such thinking is not confined to lay people, but is an error frequently committed by workers in schools, correction centers, mental hospitals, and community mental health centers. The most flagrant error is behavior not in accord with the moral standards of the clinician being diagnosed as psychopathy—an error which produces a chaotic effect when recommending treatment. It has a further adverse impact on socio-legal situations. It is necessary to see all types of antisocial behavior as compatible with different diagnoses or even situational occurrences. Such behavior can be responsive to psychological realignments wherein the ego permits impulsive or regressive activities to occur. It is not inconsistent for adults or adolescents with neurotic or psychotic disturbances to engage in blatant antisocial conduct, nor is it inconsistent for a young child with similar problems to lie, cheat, steal, or be physically assaultive. Rather than using conduct as diagnostic the criteria should involve appraisal of defects in socialization processes and ego functioning.

Certain deficits over control of impulses can alert observers to developmental disturbances. In some children, such socially responsive affects as guilt and anxiety are seen not to develop with a control-exerting function over behavior. An unbridled egoistic and uninhibited quality emerges with a prominent element of scheming and deception involved. The dominance of self-serving at any cost begins to dominate motivation.

A recurrent issue is the status of psychopathy as a disease. To focus on acts of an antisocial type as diagnostic criteria hardly suffices to establish anything more than the presence of unsocialized behavior. Similar arguments could be raised with respect to the whole framework of emotional disorders The type of debate evolved during the 20th century during a shift from symptoms being presented in a somatic context, reflecting a disturbance in bodily functioning, to a viewpoint of emotional symptoms reflecting a disturbance in psychosocial disequilibrium. When this happened, confirming a disease concept in terms of the physical disease model became nebulous, and it also gave rise to formulations about the sick society. The blur gave rise to questions about the real difference between the individual who steals because of its symbolic significance, and the person who steals because he is hungry. Are they not all caught up in some type of meshwork of psychosocial pathology?

Psychopathy is not an illness simply because physicians try to treat these people, or because they are placed in "psychopathic hospitals." Almost all deviant human behavior can be encompassed under the atomized microscope of the psychopathologist. One solution is to view psychopathy as the degree to which an abnormality in personality functioning afflicts an individual—apart from whatever social friction he engenders.[70] A statistical concept of personality then slips in so that psychopathy becomes a type of abnormality which deviates from a norm without necessarily getting into antisocial or legal difficulties. The psychopath then becomes a personality type—rather than being diagnosed as ill. The virtue is holding to a diagnostic standard that does not argue in an ex post facto manner that because a deviant act has occurred, the perpetrator must therefore be a psychopath.

A heuristic analogy to intellectual defect is of value. While an original model grouped those believed intellectually deficient for legal, educational, and administrative purposes, only more recently have specific subtypes, with their varying etiologies, been established. In the absence of clinical criteria confusion was engendered, since knowledge and decisions were based overwhelmingly on nothing but the nature of the social inconveniences. Once criteria for studying clinical and biological aspects of intelligence were present, it was possible to distinguish pathological development as well as subcultural variants. Only when this becomes possible for the group called psychopathic, will the argument get closer to resolution regarding psychopathy as disease. It may be that a parameter akin to distribution of individual differences of intelligence will be found and permit an answer to the question of whether psychopathic personalities have a disease or rather a behavioral peculiarity.

A sad example of continuing word games is seen in the revised diagnostic manual of the American Psychiatric Association.[71] Attempts to distinguish *antisocial personality*, defined in terms of a few standard descriptive items from *dyssocial behavior* are made. Dyssocial behavior is defined as an individual who is predatory and follows more or less criminal pursuits, but is considered not to have a manifest psychiatric disorder. The presupposition is that we possess sufficient discriminatory techniques to make such categorical assignments. It presumes such individuals are psychiatrically normal, but socially abnormal. The distinction is either so completely obvious that it is unnecessary, or alludes to a basis for making such a distinction beyond the tautological which clinicians do not have. Logical possibilities are that the diagnosis of dyssocial behavior should be abandoned entirely, or that it be viewed as one variety of antisocial personality to encompass cultural variants. The presupposition that psychological factors can distinguish between antisocial personalities and dyssocial behavior is considered moot, if not a misfit.[72].

Etiological Theories on Psychopathic Personalities. Before extending the consideration of personality disorders beyond the strict limits of psychopathy, there are relevant theoretical formulations regarding dispositions. Consider the following major contributors.

1. Genetic factors
2. Cerebral dysfunction
3. Parental losses
4. Intrafamilial and group influences
5. Learned behavior

Genetic factors pose a problem in a causative model of psychopathic behavior—as they do with any behavioral variation. Contemporary theory discusses these in the context of dispositional tendencies rather than in terms of absolute manifestations. The environment acts on dispositions. The paradigm of a definitive genetic study is that of uniovular twins who are separated at birth. In 1931 a study by Lange investigated thirteen criminals who had a uniovular twin. It was found that ten of the partners were criminals as well.[73] However, the study was naive as the twins were raised together. Such a study with twins reared separately from birth would be necessary for significance..

The substantive issue of *criminality* not being a diagnostic entity is relevant. Such studies really tell us only one thing—that a person has been convicted of a criminal act. Rosanoff et al. described 340 pairs of twins divided into adult and youthful criminals and disturbed children.[74] They were able to show that chance environmental factors often accounted for criminal propensities in discordant members of uniovular pairs. Kallman, in an investigation homosexuality in forty uniovular twins, found a 100 percent concordance rate, while in forty-five binovular male pairs a 42 percent concordance rate was found.[75] In a study not specifically concerned with criminal behavior, Slater analyzed 300 twin pairs.[76] Eight uniovular and forty-three twins had a psychopathic or neurotic twin. Only two of the uniovular and eight of the binovular had similar disturbances, reflecting the complexity of factors that may be operating in the environment to induce criminal behavior.

If genetic factors are extended to physique, the influence of rates of development must be considered. The athletic habitus of Kretschmer or mesomorph of Sheldon are cited most frequently as having higher correlations with criminal behavior. Glueck's study using Sheldonian types of 500 juvenile delinquents did find a predominance of mesomorphs.[77] In turn, the criticism is that other groups in a nondelinquent population may have as high an incidence of mesomorphy.[78] A girl who is in the earlier group of physical developers will accumulate more tempting opportunities to deviate. Another example is the boy whose early physical maturity does not find a niche, or who becomes the target for scapegoating by his peers. In this regard there are studies which indicate the stability of behavioral characteristics over time.[79]

Some extend this as an argument for the primacy of temperament based on intitial reactivity and environmental factors in contrast to the significance of factors, such as parental loss.[80] These points reveal how complicated a process drawing inferences about genetic influences and psychopathy is. Permeating these approaches, is the recurrent problem of diagnostic confusion. If diagnoses are unreliable, all the sophisticated inferences are questionable. Further, genetic predispositions do not negate the influence of environmental action both in the genesis of these conditions and for types of treatment and prevention.

Organic dysfunction in the central nervous system contributing to psychopathy has long been raised as a possibility. Naive forms of this theory seized on early physical illness or head trauma, and represented a common-sense approach where physical illness or chronic disabilities produce a diathesis toward taking it out on society. Yet common sense does not explain those who view disabilities as an extra stimulus to overcompensate. Plaguing questions remain as to whether there are significant differences in psychopathy as a personality diagnosis from those with organic loadings. There is little evidence that physical conditions differ when delinquents are compared to nondelinquents.[81] There is also common knowledge that physiological states, such as physical exhaustion or mentstruation, raise the potential for antisocial behavior.[82] Some feel so strongly about the physical diathesis thesis that they recommend plastic surgery for delinquent youths with bodily disfigurements as a prophylactic step.[83] A plethora of interpersonal and environmental responses can occur in response to physical insult. Not only does this refer to physical limitations, but to the idiosyncratic disappointments in a family. Parents who place high hopes on a particular child to fulfill their needs which do not materialize, convey failure. A repercussion may be a displacement of conflicts dealing with pride, ambition, and power out of the family circle.

Brain damage is one of the most overused diagnoses among those with behavioral problems. The over diagnosis results from the naive application of biological reductionism to behavioral problems. It takes the form of reasoning that since the brain is the basis of behavior, disturbances in the latter must be due to disturbances in the former. The psychological and philosophical fallacies in such reasoning do not require elucidation. That a child has a brain, and that something may go wrong with it, does not exclude learned conflicts and responses. Having raised these caveats about the overusage of the concept, let it now be appraised in an overall perspective as one type of disturbance that may be present and need consideration in any differential diagnosis with persistent delinquent conduct.

Behavioral changes of an antisocial type that should alert the clinician to further investigation are: a history of recent personality change and mood liability with sudden and unexplained variability. The significance of these changes lies in their development in contrast to previous personality functioning, and if explosive or violent outbursts are an accompaniment. Low frustration-tolerance and irritability, poor concentration and distractibility, difficulty in abstraction, perceptual dysfunction, and learning disabilities are also factors.

The history of personality change is so often cited as being indicative of organically induced impairment that it warrants investigation. It attains greater significance when it occurs subsequent to some infectious process or physical trauma. Early studies cite huge percentages of delinquents as having had encephalitis or meningitis—up to 60-70 percent. Two examples are illustrative. A 1931 study reported 72 percent of delinquents had histories of possible brain injury or abnormal neurological signs. A 1945 study reported 60 percent of 500 juvenile delinquents had some type of unspecified neurological lesion.[84] These studies almost always omit basics such as control groups, as well as an investigation of environmental difficulties that could be present in a causal nexus. Another limitation is the weight given to traumas—many of which are almost universally experienced in the course of development.

The interpretaion of *soft* neurological signs presents another dilemma. There are pervasive methodological difficulties in evaluating such hypotheses. Witness a study of criminal psychopaths by Stafford-Clark in which 54 percent were reported as having sustained head injuries or epilepsy, but a control group automatically excluded those with such a history—prejudging what was to be evaluated.[85] There are choices between a view in which only extreme neurological disorder may be conducive to delinquency versus a theory which resorts to a continuum of pathology of increasing severity. The former is seen in the Cambridge-Somerville study by the McCords in which only distinct neurological disorders were correlated with delinquency at a significant level.[86] The latter is represented by theories such as that of Pasamanick, in which a continuum of reproductive casualty was related to prenatal complications, prematurity, and previous fetal loss.[87] Among the casualties were: abortion, stillbirth, cerebral palsy, epilepsy, mental defect, behavior disorders, reading and learning difficulties, and tics. These were correlated in some studies with a higher incidence of later delinquency. Yet in the McCords' study no significant relationship was found between delinquency and prematurity, difficult labor, Caesarean sections, the general health of the child, or enuresis. The Newcastle study of 1,000 families evaluating all of these factors found only psychological stress in pregnancy to be significant.[88] The finding is elusive in view of the eluctable nature of stress, and the further likelihood that factors contributing to it may continue after delivery.

The question of a specific deficit from epilepsy related to psychopathic behavior is often raised. The hypothesis has been subject to virulent debate. In some studies environmental factors intrude as revealed in those by Gruenberg and Pond.[89] Three groups of children were seen at the Maudsley Clinic in London. The first two groups were composed of fifty-three children, each of whom had epilepsy, but only in the second group were behavior problems present; a third group had behavior problems without epilepsy. The second group were found to have a significantly higher incidence of adverse social environments, such as broken homes, familial disturbance, intensive sibling rivalry, and adverse parental attitudes.

Critical questions are relevant: Are the findings due to subtle organic difference in the type of epilipsy? Are they due to differences in personality structure of the given child who will respond differently to epilepsy and in turn induce different parental responses? Are the differences due to parental personalities who respond differently to physical limitations in their offspring? Or are the differences due to emotional conflicts in the child which are relatively independent of the incidence of epilepsy? Further doubt about any direct correlation betweeen organic cerebral injury and behavioral difficulties was raised in a study of thiry-two patients with head injuries which necessitated hospitalization.[90] They were compared to thirty-two patients with head injuries attending psychiatric clinics. Neither the severity of the injury, nor its location, were dispositive toward the degree of behavioral disturbance. The latter was more related to pretraumatic personality, family setting, and an adverse environment continuing after the accident.[91]

Particular brain lesions as related not only to psychopathy, but to specific types of psychopathy, are an open question at this time. Theories involve the role of areas in the limbic system, such as the hippocampus, hypothalamus, anterior hypothalamic nuclei, and cingulate cortex. Lesions in the hypothalamic nuclei, medial frontal cortex, or temporal lobes (Kluver-Bucy Syndrome) are held to lead to personality disturbances for which psychopathy is one possibility.[92] Again, the question of why psychopathy arises in some individuals is ascribed to the pre-existing personality traits. Case reports from the neurological and neurosurgical literature have dealt with cases where brain lesions or tumors have been associated with belligerent, aggressive, hypersexual, or perverse symptoms.[93] Surgical extirpation of the lesion is then the treatment. Again, questions are left hanging about whether the symptoms either abate or persist. The same has been reported for temporal lobe epilepsy or tumors associated with agressive hypersexuality.[94]

Electroencephalographic (EEG) abnormalities in those diagnosed as psychopaths have remained variable both in their form and in estimates of incidence. Rather than any specific EEG pattern which would permit identification of psychopathy, a variety of patterns can be found which are present in nonsymptomatic populations as well.[95] Three explanations have been offered related to EEG abnormalities when psychopathic behavior is predominant:

1. Specific pathology may be present and related to organic lesions, such as in epilepsy or encephalitis.
2. Maturational immaturities or physiological alterations in brain functions may present as a developmental phenomenon of the nervous system.
3. Dysrhythmic patterns believed related to psychopathy are in the nature of low-frequency wave abnormalities. These are an excess of theta rhythms (four to seven cycles per second). This rhythm is actually comparatively common in young children, which raises the question of maturational lag in the central nervous system when the pattern persists beyond childhood.

Aging itself contributes to a decline in the prevalence of abnormal theta rhythms in both psychopathic and neurotic individuals, but the rate of decline is more rapid in the neurotic. By age forty, there is a pronounced disappearance of these waves in all groups, viewed as significant since the incidence of psychopathic behavior declines prominently by that age as well. This is the oft-cited phenomenon of psychopathy burning out toward the end of the fourth decade.

Plaguing questions such as the methodological difficulties cited above regarding psychopathy investigations remain. More specifically, not all psychopaths have EEG abnormalities, many have such an abnormality without psychopathy, and the maturational question needs clarification in view of our limited knowledge of developmental changes which occur in the human brain.

Parental loss as a disposition to psychopathy specifically, or delinquency in general, is another theory. Far more is involved in the formulations of object relations theory, attachment behaviors, and losses than encompassed merely by measuring incidences of deaths of parental figures in childhood in a delinquent versus a nondelinquent population. Again, methodological questions permeate interpretations, involving such questions as retrospective versus anterespective studies, ages of the children at death, family configurations, responses of others in the child's environment after death, and ages of respective parents at death when two populations are compared.

In its original form, the impact of losing a parent was raised in the context of what might happen to a child without parents. Extreme but provocative cases were used, such as Itard's "wolf child" in the late 18th century.[96] The child lived alone in the forests of Aveyron from age five to twelve. Though he was often regarded as retarded, it would seem no easy task to be able to survive in a forest for seven years. In more recent times, Gesell reported on two Indian girls believed to have been succored by a wolf from nine months to being rescued at eighteen months and eight years respectively.[97] In these cases, the conclusion with respect to socialization processes was that the children were not able to overcome the deepest animal patterns and act by the norms of the remaining population. The thesis is that the impact of parental loss or separation induces similar defects in socialization in children.

Antisocial or asocial theories of development soon became entangled in complicated, yet related, arguments involving the spectrum of early experiences. All the arguments dealing with the consequences of parental deprivation have been raised with respect to delinquency in all its forms. These arguments have been explored—the material dealing with depressive phenomena particularly—and will not be recapitulated. This is one of the bases on which the hypothesis has been attacked, since it attempts to explain too much under rubrics of asocialized development. Therefore, only some of the studies bearing directly on later psychopathic trends will be cited as illustrations.

An early study of Bowlby's outlined the concept of the affectless and affectionless psychopath related to the effects of deprivation and repeated changes of parental figures.[98] The hypothesis was that young children, deprived of mothers, were likely to suffer serious handicaps in their character structure. In quantitative terms, the greater the deprivation, the more isolated and asocial the result. The early Bowlby position—that prolonged separation from the maternal object in a child under five years was one of the foremost causes of delinquent character formation—has been modified over the years by others and Bowlby. The clinical explanation is that the ego and superego of structures subjected to severe deprivation have not developed in a manner conducive to regulating expression of impulses. "Their capacity for inhibition is absent or impaired...they are ineffective personalities, unable to learn from experience and consequently their own worst enemies."[99]

Early emphasis on maternal deprivation was subject to criticism and attempts made to demonstrate that fathers also had a significant role.[100] Findings in 316 delinquents who did not have a father or father-substitute available while only seventeen of them had failed to have a mother or mother-substitute available were significant.[101] Empirical studies support this. An examination of 200 women prisoners concluded paternal loss in childhood was a significant factor for them.[102] An English study found that of 500 male Borstal admissions only ninety-two had not been separated from either parent in childhood.[103] Using age-group corrected census figures, the incidence of paternal and parental death was both significant. Brown and Epps investigated 546 women prisoners and found a significantly higher incidence of paternal loss compared to the general population of a comparable age group.[104] A significant finding was also made with respect to 168 consecutive male prisoners.

Caution of the most stringent kind must be applied in these studies when drawing inferences.[105] Few confine themselves to a diagnostic grouping which meets clinical criteria for psychopathy. Rather, they deal with a motley collection of offenders—at best categorized by the offense for which they have been convicted or sentenced. Thus, in the Brown and Epps study most of the women appeared to have been thieves or had committed property offenses. About 10 percent were charged with prostitution or forgery. Twenty-three were alcoholics and twenty-one were sentenced for child-neglect. We really know nothing of their clinical status even on a descriptive level.

Caution must also be used in interpreting the meaning of loss. Is it a situation of unresolved bereavement that gives a clinical impact, or rather the socioeconomic events that are set in motion subsequent to a parental loss? Is it the unavailability of consistent parental figures, or the multitplicity of care-taking figures which has an adverse effect? The parent who is lost may have an adverse impact by the social role that is left void in the family. The warning about not confusing correlations with causality is relevant. Findings which indicate data on incidence, such as relative rates of paternal or maternal losses or separation, merely suggest that fathers more readily abandon families than mothers, primarily from psychological and legal reasons.[106] Therefore, it would be fallacious to assign etiological significance to factors such as paternal absence.

Intrafamilial and group factors are based on a particular interpersonal constellation while learning influences provide a basis for how particular types of psychopathology originate. Theories on the role of the family, or on broader cultural units, on the development of delinquency easily extend into sociological theorizing on delinquency. Therefore, the comments made here are directed to empirical referents that have often been seen as contributory—apart from any psychodynamic formulations. Attention is again called to the evaluation of possible causal relationships as factors in psychopathy, since more often heterogenous groupings of multiple possibilities occur.

It is axiomatic that most psychopathologists believe the family plays a major role in the emergence of delinquent trends. This is so even for those who believe genetic loadings may predispose toward traits conducive to the development of psychopathic behaviors. While the factors of broken homes and poverty are contributors, most psychopathologists would probably hold that the most accurate predictor of psychopathy among the group of social variables is to have a father who is either a psychopath, an alcoholic, or antisocial in some respect. The problem is to determine which factors have the greatest significance in a given case, and to assign a relative degree of weighting to different factors. Not only have factors of parental loss or separation been observed, but components such as inadequate parenting, and subtle forms of parental neglect and rejection have been singled out. This is unfortunately vague, since it is difficult to appraise how these terms are used in empirical studies. While psychological conflicts can be pointed out if there is an opportunity to engage in therapeutic work with an individual or family unit, there is still a large remainder for whom such knowledge is not available.

Detecting these factors for large groups on a predictive basis, once an attempt is made to go beyond major signs of family disorganization, presents difficulties in appraising covert factors in family functioning which contribute to delinquent behavior. Although the predicament is present in all situations of research in which isolation of one variable is attempted, it presents a striking problem when causal factors cannot be agreed upon. As an example, while some may object to a proposal to evaluate eye color of delinquent youths as absurd, it is conceivable that a statistical significance might be found and explanations then offered on the basis of some neurophysiological vulnerability, since eye color is chromosomally determined. Think of the complexities when less remote variables are considered, such as large families, sibling relationships, income level, degrees of crowding in households, types of parental discipline, degrees of parental hostility, types of family acting out patterns, and value of academic, social, or vocational attainment and its achievement within any given family. All of these variables very likely play a contributory role in delinquency or psychopathy. The problem is that they play a role in everything else as well so that specificity is elusive.

Certain family configurations are seen more frequently in families of delinquents. Conscious parental attitudes appear to be only one subtle influence operating, but they cannot be ignored in a search for covert or unconscious motivations. Old formulations of parental rejection have been given more specificity in reports of the impact of parental hostility, minimal interest in child-rearing, lack of attachment to the child, an atmosphere of muted violence, or the promotion of vicarious acting out behaviors. The impact of different types of parental conflicts on children is germane. We do not know which children will be able to cope with problems adequately and at what developmental level. It is in keeping with our knowledge of development that a child is more vulnerable to certain forms of acting out or impulsive behaviors not only from constitutional influences, but in response to experiences at vulnerable periods.

Hilda Lewis studied 500 children in terms of family attitudes.[107] The children had been removed from their families to a reception center and removed once before this as well. One of her findings from these children who presented with social difficulties was that only those removed from their mothers before two years of age had a significant correlation with types of personality disturbances. Psychiatric examinations, psychological testing, and social workers interviewing families were conducted. Forty-five percent of the children had a disturbance in family relationships with ninety-nine fathers and 180 mothers disturbed. Statistical correlations of adverse family attitudes related to "personality disturbances" were significant in the following areas: maternal neglect, lack of affection, overindulgence, dullness, mental disorder, a mother long dead, paternal neglect, and the factor of maternal separation when under two years. One hundred who were found with some degree of abnormal mental state were given a psychiatric follow-up three years later. Of twenty-five who had been rated initially as having an abormal mental state, sixteen were rated normal at the time of follow-up. Seventy-five had a marked or moderate personality disorder, and twenty-three were rated normal on follow-up.

Besides the intrinsic interest in these figures, there is the inference that children show a great deal of variability in response to parental difficulties. It now seems to be necessary to raise hypotheses as to which particular type of parental influence most adversely affects different types of antisocial outcome. This is congruent with the observations of Anthony in dealing with children who had a psychotic parent in which a spectrum of responses was possible.[108] The responses varied in terms of four high-risk groups in which there were three responses of the children: antecedents of adult psychosis, disturbances associated with parental psychosis, and reactions to the parental psychosis that could be situational, neurotic, or antisocial. The latter two groups actually responded favorably when separated from the psychotic parents.

Not all studies have found significant correlations between parental attitudes and offenders who show personality disturban-ces. In study after study the methodology is so defective as to negate much confidence in the findings. Consider a study by Zuckerman et al., in which children at a child guidance clinic were divided into five groups based on symptoms and diagnosis.[109] An attempt was made to assess the type of psychopathology in the child by parental personalities in terms of which types of symptoms would be most likely to be induced in the child. A failure to make an accurate prediction, such as which parents would have delinquent children, occurred. However, the authors admitted to the doubtful validity of their study since many parents gave untrue answers or responses in terms of social acceptability. Another study dealt with 100 habitual offenders.[110] Fifty were detained preventively, and fifty were recidivists who were selected on the basis of a four-year remission followed by two further convictions prior to a prison sentence. Diagnostically, the group was classified into 12 percent "non-deviant professional criminals," 36 percent "aggressive, emotionally indifferent criminal psychopaths," and 52 percent "passive, inadequate personalities." Yet how much credence can be given to a study in which the last group, considered inadequate and comprising a majority, were classified on the basis of their wishing to be caught and punished, as described in the study? Further surprise is registered when 28 percent were listed as having perfectly normal homes—the source of the information being a direct question to the prisoner. Perhaps the time has come to question research conclusions based on direct question-answer interrogatory or inventory approaches.

Data from the Glueck studies on 500 juvenile delinquents and 500 controls utilized a multifactorial approach for descriptive items about family attitudes.[111] Both paternal and maternal attitudes were found to correlate adversely with later delinquency and reconvictions. Attitudes referred to hostility, neglect, indifference, erratic approaches to discipline, and mental disturbance in a parent. A positive correlation of these attitudes with traits in the delinquent were found: tendencies to fantasize, wandering, and truancy. These findings are in agreement with the work cited earlier in the Cambridge-Somerville study.

In addition to the facts discussed here as adverse familial or group influences, broader contributions may be operating. Surprisingly, correlations appear insignificant between hostility and antagonism to parents, and antagonism toward law and agencies of social control.[112] Families of delinquents are often characterized as having punitive parents.[113] There are also such influences as illegitimacy, adoptive status, socio-economic level, and families with a high incidence of antisocial or criminal conduct. Integration of these multiple factors into any comprehensive theory is obviously desirable but is most difficult. A high degree of correlation between socio-economic status and these stigmas raises many questions related in general to the nongeneric nature of delinquency and psychopathy.

Learning influences are difficult to evaluate as an independent set of dispositions related to antisocial behavior or psychopathy. Nor can they logically be considered as a separate category. Only in a more restricted sense can the theory of learning and antisocial conduct or psychopathy be validly appraised. The learning emphasis in a broad sense is that psychopathy is not a disease or defect but rather a set of learned responses which do not equip one for conforming to the rules of society.[114] Nor can one learned model be assumed for all cases. One formulation stresses repeated childhood experiences which reinforce a pattern of verbalized contrition after a transgression rather than receiving punishment. Successfully avoiding punishment then reinforces contrite behaviors while extinguishing fears of punishment attached to transgressions.

Parental traits may make the carrying out of punishment difficult. Some parents find it difficult to let children wait or endure delays for gratification. Delay is experienced as tantamount to a deprivation or something punitive, so parental efforts are directed toward not permitting such situations. Apart from the difficulty that life may not continue to be so gratifying, what are the difficulties from such child-rearing practices for the child? One difficulty stems from parental failure to punish, or permitting manipulation. Such failure is taken as a sign of love by the child, with all the difficulties this will later cause. From this distorted route love is seen as something contingent upon being able to manipulate others. In the absence of manipulative success, an absence of love is experienced. In the course of development the child feels pride in his manipulative abilities, which secure love. Since the goal is to avoid the painful consequences of acts by manipulation, little genuine concern is experienced for other people. Rather, others are used to alleviate one's own discomfort.

From the paradigm of how psychopathic behaviors are learned, empirical and experimental findings follow. A low level of painful affects such as guilt and anxiety would be predicted since hope rests eternal, from previous reinforcements, that one can escape the consequences of transgressing. The psychopath would be someone whose conditioning of anxiety to inhibit certain responses based on previous punishments for acts is impaired.[115] Further, once such an act is committed, the anticipated punishment in those so conditioned does not operate. Anticipations of requiring punishment for purposes of restoring a feeling of well-being do not hold. Nor is there the meaning that love will be withheld until one is punished. Since being loved means being an operator who controls others, being punished as a condition for acceptance back into the good graces of authority figures is not needed. Rather than inner controls being based on strong inhibitions of punished responses, control is dependent on momentary external guides and sensitive readings of situations. Guilt, as a manifestation of anxiety which accompanies an expectation that one will lose the love of those upon whom one depends, is vitiated in its effectiveness.

The possibility that the psychopath conditions less easily to anxiety means the capacity to acquire and utilize conditioned anticipatory fear responses will be in jeopardy. Avoidance learning is poorly developed as a consequence. Experimental work offers support for an altered sense of time in psychopaths.[116] It is believed related to a lack of cogency of the future as a conspicuous element— the usual quip that the psychopath lives only for the moment. The link to the lack of efficacy of punishment is seen in the lack of anticipation of the future. Hence, time seems to pass quickly for them and is not evaluated as lasting as long as it objectively does. More immediate adversive events in the near future are generally more fear-arousing than those distant in time—described as a "temporal gradient" of fear arousal.[117] It is postulated that the temporal gradient is much steeper for psychopathic personalities. In fact, the slope may be so steep that an adversive event in the future may have little emotional significance for the psychopath; it is the whole matter of integrating present and future rewards and punishments that goes awry for him. Anticipation of adversive consequences which seem remote do not take at the moment of performing an act.

A fascinating question is why there is a failure of the pleasure principle to operate in the course of development to a significant degree. Is this an inborn deficit at the level of neural integration— presumably at least partially determined by genetic factors? These questions verge into the physiological and autonomic correlates of psychopathy in which the findings are consistent with an autonomic hypo-responsiveness to provocative or stressful situations.[118] Such a deficit need not be restricted to the autonomic nervous system for critical under-arousal and a high sensory threshold may contribute. The hypothesis is that what is an optimal level of arousal for the normal person is insufficient for the psychopath. Hence, the restless search for excitement, drugs, and novel experiences until they start to burn out in their forties, which may correspond to a cortico-sensory realignment in the course of aging. From this diathesis an attenuation of sensory input occurs, and many cues in the environment could be missed. Hence, input information, or social and emotional cues, needed to modulate behavior are not registered. A correlate would be less regulation by the approval or disapproval of others. However, the hypothesis of intrapsychic components or defenses which distort and repress on the basis of selective learning processes are not irrelevant. The closeness of intrapsychic conflict, learning experiences, and psychophysiological correlates is nowhere better illustrated than in unraveling the nature of psychopathic behavior.

Explanations based on learning theory are subject to the same limitations as other explanations. That learning processes play one crucial part in emotional reactions including delinquencies is unquestioned. The hypotheses put forward regarding the learned aspects of delinquent behaviors are valuable. The limitation is their lack of generalizability; we do not yet know how sufficient such explanations are for large numbers of individuals. Nor do we know if these findings are present in a varied quantitative distribution. Perhaps sufficient details are still lacking about the kinds of learning that must go on for different types of antisocial conduct. We would not necessarily expect that the learning experiences and processes involved for a group which meets one set of diagnostic criteria, such as for a psychopath, need be the same as for more minor types of antisociality or for someone who periodically resorts to such behavior under stress.

Since the psychological mechanisms behind many delinquent acts often have a commonality, there should be a carry-over by degrees for antisocial lapses. As an example of vulnerability from the generalized model, a question may be raised about whether the potential psychopath has, in reality, been nurtured in an environment where he was subjected to less deprivation and protected from punishment or fear rather than the opposite. While no one is completely protected, the implication is that the psychopath could have been relatively less exposed to a punitive environment so that anxiety for behavior was not conditioned properly.

There is an argument that proper schedules of punishment to inhibit behavior have not occurred. Yet this type of limitation squares with the backgrounds of few psychopaths on the one hand, but is actually quite prevalent in the backgrounds of a great number of children who do not emerge as psychopathic. Many more psychopaths appear to come from backgrounds of gross neglect on both a social and personal level. Explanations centered on children who have not had adequate limits set are more relevant to reinforcement of ambivalent tendencies with a difficulty in establishing self-imposed delay. The neurotic character problem appears to be sui generis from psychopathy, and explanations which fail to make such distinctions further confuse appraisal of developmental antecedents as well as treatment recommendations.

There is also the phenomenon of certain behaviors which continue despite a conscious awareness of their self-destructive nature. Learning theory formulations have often put this in terms of animal and human experimentation, showing that a triad of excessive punishment, difficult discrimination, and confinement may lead to behaviors which are maladaptive and stereotyped.[119] For children, this is seen in punitive parents, inconsistency, and a capricious inability to take a firm position on what behavior is expected—all within the confines of the intensity of contemporary family living. If this suffices as an adequate explanation of those driven to destroy themselves in some form, rather than being deterred by any amount of punishment, is another question.

PROBLEMS IN THE CLASSIFICATIONS OF PSYCHOPATHY

Typologies of delinquency and psychopathic behaviors vary somewhat by profession or discipline, but classification systems vary more by theoretical orientation, background, and values than anything else. There is also a viewpoint that advocates elimination of all classifications on the basis that diagnoses and classification may be an impediment to treatment. Others believe the undesirable social consequences of diagnoses mitigate against their use. Abandonment of diagnosis is not advocated here, but mentioned in what is seen as a sincere but misguided effort by those who believe in the primacy of the relationship above all else. A more prevalent group, scattered among innumerable agencies and resource individuals who come into contact with those with antisocial tendencies, is composed of those who lack adequate training and sophistication in the details of antisocial behaviors. The majority of offenders have no classification made of their personal and social predicament beyond the terminology of a legal category based on conviction.

Before considering forms of classification within a standardized nomenclature, other approaches will be examined. A difficulty is presented even by those who recognize that, despite the heterogeneity and chaos of much antisocial behavior, some logical basis is desirable. One difficulty is presented by those who feel that only broad classifications are possible. This is seen in operational approaches which hold delinquency should be seen as nothing more than "what the law says it is." It is also observed in approaches which view antisocial behavior as equivalent to the study of personality or human behavior itself. Another view is held by critics who continue to insist that only if delinquency is a medical problem is it proper to view it as falling within the province of a "disease entity."

Several efforts at classification of psychopathy have been made. Table 16 illustrates the diversity of criteria that have been employed:

TABLE 16

Bases for Classification of Psychopathy

I. *Legal:* Based on commission of a delinquent or criminal act.

II. *Social Class:* Correlated with types of antisocial conduct.

III. *Developmental Approaches*

    A. Based on when acting out patterns are believed to begin
       1. Genetic studies
       2. Parental/constitutional
       3. Family influences
       4. Subcultural

    B. Stage of overt delinquency—when behavior begins to deviate in the community

    C. Classification at point of formal contact:
       1. Seen by clinicians for complaints about conduct
       2. At juvenile court level
       3. Delinquency institutions
       4. Reformatories or prisons

IV. *By Type of Treatment Employed*

    A. Treatment strategies
       1. Mode of treatment
       2. Setting of treatment

    B. Type and character of treater

    C. Outcome approach
       1. Symptoms change
       2. Social change
       3. Recidivism—post-treatment, post-probation, or post-parole

Behavioral classifications utilize overt bases for a typology, such as a criminal act, or an overt personality characteristic. There is an overlap with descriptive psychiatry on one hand, and legal classifications on the other. The acts vary, such as stealing, truancy, absenting, aggressive conduct, or sexual delinquencies, to name a few. Behavioral ratings may be in terms of manipulative, demanding, complaining, conforming, defensive whining, etc. One difficulty in both legal and behavioral approaches is the failure to give cognizance to the reactive quality for many behaviors. It leads to the fallacy of the continuing quest to detect significance when comparing populations of "delinquent/criminal" and others unless subtle differences in nervous system functioning are confirmed. Reactive responses are often in response to some personal or interpersonal situation in the predisposed individual which elicits antisocial behavior in contrast to synthesizing personality types out of general delinquent populations.

However, when population groups are studies, such as comparing delinquent and nondelinquent groups in toto, differential features become clearer. These provide an additional dimension for the clinical assessment of the way a particular individual or family differs from others who have committed similar acts. Hence, the Gluecks distinguished between "core" and "fringe" types of offenders based on 500 delinquents and a control group of 500 nondelinquents already discussed.[119]

The search is for a continuum in which antisocial attitudes emerge from massive and varied data to make a useful definition of clinical types. The hope is for interlinkages of traits and factors rather than for idiosyncratic classification. The Gluecks did not view criminal or delinquent acts as exclusively social reactions, although they are so dealt with by a legally organized society. "They occur in the minds and conduct of individual human beings who vary in genetic equipment and early childhood training. That is why there are variations in responses of individuals to the pressures and enticements of home, neighborhood, society, and general culture."[119] The requirement is for both an adequate and sufficient selectivity of background and developmental factors to avoid the fait accompli type of classification based on legal convictions, such as rapists, robbers, murderers, and so on. More recently some have advocated an ecological approach emphasizing environmental variables as they interact with personal characteristics in contrast to a dispositional or trait approach.[120]

Conversely, a classification system of psychopathy cannot limit itself to the "personality disorder" diagnosis of psychiatric nomenclature, for among people with the same diagnosis, some are delinquent and many are not. Hence, a specificity for delinquent acts is required. Clinical insights are required along with the use of a typology by traits or factors in groups. Only in this manner can valid treatment and preventive approaches be instituted in contrast to the typical pattern utilized in communities which can at best only be described as hopes that good will and compassion will suffice.

Attempts to classify by psychometric devices have proven helpful. When personality tests are used to compare delinquents and nondelinquents, no significant differences are found.[121] Tests of cerebral dysfunction can help, as can personality inventories, in describing individuals and groups. Again the question is whether the distribution is different from that of the general population. If not, these measures do not have validity as predictive devices, although with any individual they may assist in understanding his personality structure.

Inconsistency of discipline has been cited so often as undesirable that it is now taken as axiomatic. However, appraisal of the subtle forms that inconsistency takes challenge the most sophisticated clinicians since they go far beyond simple consistency in external rule-following by parents. There is the matter of overt condemnation of behavior which is covertly or unconsciously sanctioned. Particularly cogent is the realm of acting out, aggressive, and sexual behaviors within families and in our culture. There is the further situation of different individuals in a child's life presenting different sets of norms and models which may be inconsistent with each other. Once the child is into the latency, he quickly becomes aware of the gross inconsistencies between what people say the rules are and how they behave. Discrepancies in consistency are observed most conspicuously in situations which threaten an individual. These permit inconsistent behaviors to emerge which justify a model if it appears to be important enough to a particular individual or to his own anxiety.

There is a need to go far beyond measures of consistency in terms of such generally accepted behaviors as those seen in routine rules for living. This has relevance for cases from strict, law-abiding families who manifest delinquent behavior. There is also the inconsistency in parents who overstimulate a child and then become lax when he is on the upswing. When he is on the downswing the parent is strict, withdrawn, and perhaps punitive. Such instability has added consequences if the parent responds to the child's overstimulation by further punitive means when the behavior was a response to the parental mood in the beginning. Lack of confidence in one's ability to perceive others accurately is a consequence.

Hence, a connection with the matrix of low self-esteem, depression, and defective images concerning one's body can be seen.[122]

Several studies on the contribution of inconsistency to delinquency have been done, such as the early work of Healy in 1915 and Burt in 1929. In addition, the Glueck's work, that of Bandura and Walters in 1957, and Andry's study—all referred to—are relevant. In the McCord study of delinquent boys intra-parental inconsistency contributed to delinquent behavior in addition to lack of warmth.[123] In a subsequent study of nondelinquent boys, the mothers were found to be more consistent in discipline for nonaggressive than aggressive boys.[124]

While considerations for treatment are not the main issue here, a few points are necessary in view of the way treatment or rehabilitation programs are recommended on the basis of the classification or diagnosis used. This is true for those who make administrative decisions for assignment to institutions or programs without ever seeing the individual, and for those who pursue a clinical course of therapy related to a classification. Despite millions of dollars in time, money, and effort expended, it is only fair to state that when all the variables are mixed, a far from adequate basis for making treatment recommendations exists. The situation will become more confusing from the pressure to develop services with a minimum of critical evaluation. Presumably, it is hoped that something better-than-chance relationships exists between type and treatment. Working out the specifics of the relationship and recommendations is badly needed. When the treatment is carried out, by whom, the different characteristics and background of treaters, types of follow-up and criteria employed, all need evaluation.

Consider a few of the variables involved: treatment within an institution or not, type of treatment, use of punishment, open versus closed units, degree of permissiveness, type of affection available, single rooms versus group dormitories, an educational or vocational program or neither, assignment of jobs, type of security, duration of stay, age range, use of psychopharmocological medications, recreational possibilities, and the qualifications of those listed as carrying out treatments.

From this complexity what emerges, once the evangelism about new approaches or programs dissipates, is routine, stereotyped reports, such as:[125] "He manipulates—surround him with controls." "He's hostile and aggressive—tranquilize him." "He's a homosexual—keep him segregated." "He's psychotic—send him to a hospital." "There's nothing the matter with him—give him a trade." "He's sick—don't stir up anything because he won't be able to handle it." "He's delinquent—try a group approach." "He's stealing—give him behavior mod."

CLINICAL NOSOLOGIES

Group for the Advancement of Psychiatry (GAP) Classification. The value of having a workable, descriptive classification system has been stressed. Hopefully, those dealing in psychopathology should have something more to offer than simply descriptive categories. One useful working approach has been made by the Group for the Advancement of Psychiatry (GAP) with a developmental emphasis.[126] The diagnostic system from the American Psychiatric Association handbook is another approach. The GAP categories have the advantage of combining different perspectives and approaches. These, along with other sources, will be used to elaborate character types, which are seen in relationship to different kinds of antisociality.

TABLE 17
Types of Personality Disorders

1. Compulsive (obsessive-compulsive) personality
2. Hysterical personality
3. Passive-dependent (oral) personality
4. Passive-aggressive (oppositional) personality
5. Narcissistic personality
6. Overly independent personality
7. Schizoid (isolated) personality
8. Paranoid (mistrustful) personality
9. Tension discharge disorders (antisocial or explosive personality)
   a. Impulse-ridden character
   b. Neurotic character
10. Sociosyntonic (dyssocial) personality
11. Cyclothymic (depressive) pesonality
12. Masochistic personality

These character types are discussed with the degree of psychodynamic formulation believed necessary to provide a basic understanding. Clinical usefulness, explanatory power, and a basis for clinical investigation, are the essential criteria.

General Features. Individuals with a personality disorder rarely experience personal discomfort or anxiety if their traits are in good working order. In contrast are those with neurotic or psychotic conflicts who develop symptoms. Particularly is this so for a child or adolescent whose characterological features still have a greater degree of malleability. Rarely is intrapsychic discomfort experienced in the character problems to the same degree as neuroses or psychoses because the traits are ego-syntonic. Symptomatic manifestations occur in some of these disorders quite early in life. It is one of the areas most in need of intensive exploration, as is longitudinal research with a view to determining the antecedents that lead to different character problems. Both an adequate developmental theory which explains such vulnerabilities, and a viable theory of symptom development, are required.

Signs of taking it out on the environment or alloplastic behaviors, have frequently been observed in young children. There has been a long-felt need to be able to detect these individuals at the earliest possible age. When Bernard Glueck, Sr., studied 608 prisoners in Sing-Sing Prison and found 18.9 percent diagnosed as psychopaths, a significant finding was that 86.8 percent had a history of childhood behaviors viewed as a harbinger of later psychopathy.[127] These childhood behaviors were truancy, backwardness in school, lack of interest, disciplinary problems, trouble-making, and extreme mischievousness. Recent studies are congruent indicating that the more severe and extensive the early history of antisocial behavior (repeated truancies, repetitive episodes of fighting, and running away overnight) the more consistent this behavior remains over a period of eight to nine years, and as part of a general sociopathic picture.[128]

Attempts are made periodically to set the groundwork for detecting children who will emerge as characterological difficulties. A 1933 study by Ackerly compared thirty delinquents with thirty nondelinquent children.[129] The former were found to be extroverted, overactive, restless, and were described as persistently infantile. Their records revealed more health problems, poor school performance, and emotional unbalance. An interesting aside was made regarding their rebelliousness which was seen as an accompaniment of physical, mental, and environmental handicaps. Ackerly believed that rebellion and delinquency went hand-in-hand with a healthy ego integration as a means of escaping social isolation or resolving conflict by lowering social standards.

In the mid-1930s Healy and Bronner compared 153 families with delinquents to 145 controls.[130] They believed a reliable prognostication of outcome could be made if groupings utilized the importance of frustration, insecurity, inferiority feelings, rejection, denial, jealousy, guilt, and responses to family disharmony in relationship to delinquency. Lowrey saw the crucial difficulty rooted in disturbed love relationships within the family.[131] Parents who mutually adored each other to the detriment of the child, parental fixation on the child, sibling rivalry, permitting the child excessive degrees of expression, and overprotective devices were seen as contributory.

Karpman always argued for a restrictive and tight definition of psychopathy. He believed the childhood of the psychopath was not merely overindulgence, since so many children are overindulged.[132] Instead, the unbending nature of the child was the core problem in the potential psychopath. The child's behavior was seen as progressively outraging the family to the point where they reacted defensively or resorted to excessive repressive measures in an effort at socialization. The potential psychopath is seen as someone who lacks sufficient capacity to defer pleasure and sacrifice immediate gain. One is reminded of the analagous controversy regarding schizophrenia where some maintain that disturbed family relationships are a response to the schizophrenic rather than schizophrenic behaviors emerging as a product of family disturbance.

Longitudinal Follow-ups.   Robins performed a thirty-year follow-up on 524 child-guidance patients which included 100 controls.[133] In adulthood ninety-four of the 524 children were diagnosed as antisocial personalities. Significant pre-existing childhood signs were persistent thefts, lying, chronic patterns of disobedience to authority figures, truancy, absenting from home, attaching themselves to children or adolescents older than themselves who were manifesting antisocial conduct, staying away from home overnight, outbursts of physical aggression, impulsive acts, and general recklessness. These are almost synonymous with the general list of offenses listed on petitions for minors seen on intake in a juvenile court system.

In addition, several symptom patterns which did not appear to be antisocial in children were present. Yet, they were later found to be present in a varying number of those diagnosed as antisocial in adulthood. Thus, 32 percent of their sample of antisocial adults were neurotic as children, 32 percent had been described as dirty in appearance, 31 percent exhibited sleep-walking or talking in their sleep, and 29 percent were irritable children.

These interesting findings are disturbing. Assigning significance to when such symptoms are a manifestation of a developmental disturbance, neurotic conflict, or tokening the possibility of future psychopathy is difficult. In the Robins study, not a single one of the adults independently diagnosed as antisocial, without knowledge of the childhood symptomatology, lacked at least one of the childhood antisocial behaviors listed. The number of symptoms becomes important as a prognosticator. The presence in childhood of ten or more of the behaviors listed was found to have a 43 percent chance of acquiring a diagnosis of "antisocial personality" in adulthood. If less than three signs were present, only 4 percent were given the diagnosis. Two other significant correlations were in the data: (1) positive correlations existed between later alcoholism with these symptoms, and a significant inverse relationship in terms of an absence of anxiety neurosis, (2) no significance between the number of childhood antisocial symptoms and a diagnosis in adulthood of schizophrenia or hysteria was found.

In addition to quantitative implications from these childhood manifestations, a host of less tangible implications remain in the child's life. More disturbances are present in the relationship with parents and peers, school problems, and a general discomfort from a chronic state of being at war with representatives of authority. Personal discomfort appears related to their struggle with aggression to a degree beyond that with which most children have to cope.

Provocative questions arise from the Robins study. Not all the children, even those with ten or more antisocial symptoms and behaviors, ended up in adulthood with a diagnosis of antisocial personality. The thirty-year follow-up showed 90 percent of them to be "psychiatrically ill." Yet, this type of phraseology is nebulous. In the Midtown Manhattan epidemilogic survey an equally high incidence of mental symptoms was found.[134] While such a study does inform us that a greater number of such symptoms in childhood increases the adult risk of antisociality, it does not tell us why such an eventuality emerges in some, nor can it tell us which individual children will have such an outcome. It does tell us on a statistical basis that it is undesirable to have these symptoms in childhood if later antisociality is seen as an unfavorable outcome.

As mentioned earlier, the environments of antisocial individuals are cited as having high rates of family psychopathy, parental rejection, alcoholism, broken homes, or loadings from the lower socio-economic classes. Both retrospective and anterespective studies with children carry such data. To what degree is the presence of these social factors the sina qua non for psychopathy? If they are simply contributory, are they so general that specificity cannot be attained? Are these symptoms in childhood necessary in the sense that, in their absence, antisocial personalities could not develop? Data from the Robins study are only suggestive. If a group of children with six or more symptoms were considered, only two environmental factors appeared present in a contributory way, and then at a slight degree of significance. One of these was the factor of being a boy—hardly a profound finding; the other was a lack, or inconsistent amount, of parental discipline—an oft-mentioned contributor to childhood problems of all types. In children with less than six symptoms, only one environmental variable appeared significant for later antisociality which was the presence of a father who was himself antisocial or an alcoholic.

Difficulties in appraising the impact of broader socio-economic factors are related to their status as independent variables. It is a fallacy to assume that listing reasons for a particular path of development is equivalent to establishing a casual nexus, let alone a necessity for a given outcome. If a family has an absent or alcoholic father, and antisocial conduct develops, is it due to the former as an independent variable or because of some connection with psychopathy? The factors may or may not be independent, but in any event they have to converge on the child as agent. Therefore, we cannot determine how much weight to give to what variable. To complicate matters, children from the lower or middle classes are not different from each other to the extent that they later emerge as antisocial when presenting originally with the same degree of antisocial symptoms and behaviors.[135]

Although a parsimonious interpretation is that environmental factors themselves cannot be assigned causal status, there is another possibility. It may be that the absence of sufficient environmental adversities in the middle class are balanced by more subtle intrafamilial forms of psychopathology which contribute to development of antisocial tendencies. Confirmation of this hypothesis would require a sample of lower-class children from intact families who were not subject to the adverse factors listed. It would also require that they be appraised, along with the children from a middle-class group, to determine whether covert intrafamilial patterns promoting antisociality were present. Lower-class intact families without covert factors operating could then be compared to middle-class intact families with covert factors present. A lower incidence of antisocial development in the former would be confirmatory evidence that environmental background factors may be predisposing but do not qualify for causal status.

REFERENCES

1. E. Kretschmer, *Physique and Character* (New York: Harcourt, Brace, 1926).
2. W. H. Sheldon and S. S. Stevens, *The Varieties of Temperament* (New York: Harper and Row, 1942).
3. C. G. Jung, *Two Essays on Analytical Psychology,* trans. by H. G. and C. F. Baynes (New York: Dodd, Mead, and Co., 1928).
4. W. Bromberg, *Crime and the Mind,* p. 54. (New York: Macmillan, 1965).
5. A. Brigham, Journal of prison discipline and lunatic asylums, *American Journal of Insanity* 2(1845):175.
6. C. Lombroso, *Crime: Its Causes and Remedies,* p. 14 trans. by H. Q. Horton (Boston: Little Brown, 1911).
7. A. Meyer, *Reports of the New York State Pathological Institute* (Attica: 1904-05).
8. A. Thomas, et al., *Behavioral Individuality in Early Childhood* (New York: New York University Press, 1963).
9. A. Thomas, S. Chess, and H. Birch, *Temerament and Behavior Disorders in Children* (New York: New York University Press, 1968).
10. C. D. Broad, The nature of a continuant, *Readings in Philosophical Analysis,* ed. by H. Feigl and W. Sellars, p. 472-481 (New York: Appleton-Century Crofts, 1949).
11. W. Mischel, *Personality and Assessment* (New York: John Wiley, 1968).
12. H. Hartshorne and M. A. May, *Studies in the Nature of Character, 3 vols.* (New York: Macmillan, 1928-30).
13. A. M. Platt, *The Child Savers* (Chicago: The University of Chicago Press, 1969).
14. W. Healy, *The Individual Delinquent* (Boston: Little Brown and Co., 1915).
15. W. Healy, *Pathological Lying, Accusation, and Swindling* (Boston: Little Brown and Co., 1915).
16. W. A. White, *Insanity and the Criminal Law* (New York: Macmillan, 1923).
17. C. Darrow, *Crime, Its Cause and Treatment* (Chicago: Crowell, 1922).
18. B. Glueck, A study of admissions to Sing-Sing *Mental Hygiene* 2(1918):84-139.
19. B. Diamond, Psychiatry and the criminal *Postgraduate Medicine* 36A(1964):46-54.
20. W. Richmond, *The Adolescent Girl* (New York: Macmillan, 1925).
21. B. B. Lindsey and W. Evans, *The Revolt of Modern Youth* (New York: Boni and Liversigh, 1925).
22. W. Stekel, *Peculiarities of Behavior* (New York: Horace Liveright, 1925).

23. A. Aichhorn, *Wayward Youth* (New York: Viking Press, 1935).

24. L. P. Clark, *A Psychological Study of Stealing in Juvenile Delinquency* (Washington, D. C.: Nervous and Mental Diseases Publising Company, 1925).

25. R. G. Gordon, *Autolucus—The Future for Miscreant Youth* (London: Kegan Paul, 1968).

26. C. Burt, *The Young Delinquent* (New York: Appleton, 1925).

27. S. Freud, Some character-types met with in psycho-analytic work, *Standard Edition* 14:309-333.

28. H. Kohut, *The Analysis of the Self* (New York: International Universities Press, 1971).

29. E. Jacques, *Work, Creativity, and Social Justice* (New York: International Universities Press, 1970).

30. S. Freud, Beyond the pleasure principle, *Standard Edition* 18:7-64.

31. S. Jones, The origin and structure of the super-ego. *International Journal of Psycho-Analysis* 7(1926):303-311.

32. W. Reich, The need for punishment and the neurotic process, *International Journal of Psycho-Analysis* 9(1928):227-246.

33. F. Alexander, The neurotic character, *The Scope of Psychoanalysis, 1921-1961*, pp. 56-73 (New York: Basic Books, 1961).

34. L. Bender and P. Schilder, Suicidal preoccupations and attempts in children *American Journal of Orthopsychiatry* 7(1937):225-234.

35. P. Greenacre, The imposter, *Psychoanalytic Quarterly* 27(1958):359-382.

36. J. S. Chapman, Peregrinating problem patients: Munchausen's Syndrome *Journal of the American Medical Association* 165(1957):927-933.

37. R. S. Stoller, *Sex and Gender* (New York: Science House, 1968).

38. D. M. Levy, On the problem of delinquency *American Journal of Orthopsychiatry* 2(1932):197-211.

39. J.Masters, *Casanova* (New York: Bernard Geis, 1969; Macmillan Co., 1931).

40. F. Alexander, and H. Staub, *The Criminal, the Judge, and the Public* (New York: Macmillan Co., 1931).

41. R. V. Sampson, *The Psychology of Power* (New York: Randon House, 1965).

42. W. Richmond, *The Delinquent Boy* (New York: Holt and Rinehart, 1933).

43. P. Hoch, *Rip Off the Big Game: The Exploitation of Sports by the Power Elite* (New York: Doubleday, 1972).

44. A. A. Berle, *Power* (New York: Harcourt, Brace, and World, 1969).

45. S. Halleck, *Psychiatry and the Dilemmas of Crime* (New York: Harper and Row, 1967).

46. E. Sanders, *The Family* (New York: E. P. Dutton, 1971).

47. E. Jacques, Death and the mid-life crisis *International Journal of Psycho-Analysis* 46(1965):502-514.

48. O. Fenichel, Trophy and triumph, *The Collected Papers of Otto Fenichel*, 2nd series, pp. 141-162 (New York: W. W. Norton and Co., 1954).

49. *Diagnostic and Statistical Manual of Mental Disorders,* 2nd ed. (Washington, D.C., American Psychoanalytic Association, 1968).
50. E. Kahn, *Psychopathic Personalities* (New Haven: Yale University Press, 1931).
51. J. D. Noshpitz, The antisocial or asocial adolescent: on the etiology of adolescent delinquency *Pediatric Clinics of North America* 7(1960):97-114.
52. J. Bowlby, *Maternal Care and Mental Health* (Geneva: World Health Organization, Mono. no. 2, 1951).
53. S. Maughs, A concept of psychopathy and psychopathic personality: its evolution and historical development *Journal of Criminal Psychopathology* 1(1941):329-499.
54. J. C. Prichard, *A Treatise on Insanity and Other Disorders Affecting the Mind* (London: Sherwood, Gilbert, and Piper, 1835).
55. P. D. C. Bonfigl, Moral Insanity, *American Journal of Insanity* 36(1879):476-496.
56. J. Gouster, Moral insanity, *Journal of Nervous and Mental Diseases* 5(1878):181-182.
57. C. E. Rosenberg, *The Trial of the Assassin Guiteau* (Chicago: University of Chicago Press, 1968).
58. D. H. Tuke, Moral or emotional insanity, *Journal of Mental Science* 31(1885):174-190.
59. M. E. Wolfgang, Pioneers in criminology, Cesare Lombroso (1835-1909), *Journal of Criminal Law and Criminology* 52(1961):361-391.
60. A. Meyer, *Collected Papers, Vol. I and II* (Baltimore: Johns Hopkins Press, 1951).
61. K. Birnbaum, *The Psychopathic Criminal* (Berlin: P. Laugenscheidt, 1914).
62. F. Froukel, The psychopathic constitution in relation to war neuroses, *Archives of Neurology and Psychiatry* 5(1912):82.
63. E. Kraepelin, *Psychiatric* (Leipzig: Barth, 1915).
64. A. E. Johnson, The constitutional psychopathic inferior: a problem in diagnoses, *American Journal of Psychiatry* 2(1923):467-473.
65. B. Karpman, The problem of psychopaths, *Psychiatric Quarterly* 3(1929):495-526.
66. F. Wittels, The criminal psychopath in the psychoanalytic system, *Psychoanalysis Review* 24(1937):276.
67. H. Cleckley, *The Mask of Sanity* (St. Louis: Mosby, 1955).
68. H. G. Gough, A sociological theory of psychopathy, *American Journal of Sociology* 53(1948):359-366.
69. B. Karpman, The myth of the psychopathic personality, *American Journal of Psychiatry* 104(1948):523-534.
70. R. M. Mowbray, The concept of the psychopath, *Journal of Mental Science* 100(1960):537-542.
71. Diagnostic and Statistical Manual of Mental Disroders, op. cit.
72. K. Stojanovich, Antisocial and dyssocial, *Archives of General Psychiatry* 21(1969):561-567.

73. J. Lange, *Crime and Destiny* (London: George Allen and Unwin, 1931).

74. A. J. Rosanoff, L. M. Haudy and L. A. Rosanoff, Criminality and delinquency in twins, *Journal of Criminal Law and Criminology* 24(1934):923-1000.

75. F. J. Kallman, *Heredity in Health and Mental Disorder* (New York: Norton, 1953).

76 E. T. O. Slater, *Psychotic and Neurotic Illnesses in Twins, Special Report Series no. 278* (London: Medical Research Council, 1953).

77. S. S. Glueck and E. T. Glueck, *Family Environment and Delinquency* (Boston: Houghton Mifflin, 1962).

78. B. Wootten et al., *Social Science and Social Pathology* (London: Allen and Unwin, 1959).

79. A. Thomas et al., *Behavioral Individuality in Early Childhood* (New York: New York University Press, 1963).

80. S. Glueck and E. T. Glueck, *Unraveling Juvenile Delinquency* (New York: The Commonwealth Fund, 1950).

81. K. Dalton, Menstruation and crime, *British Medical Journal* 2(1961):1752.

82. R. S. Banay, Physical disfigurement as a factor in delinquency and crime, *Federal Probation* 7(1943):20-24.

83. A. W. Row, A possible endocrine factor in the behavior of the young, *American Journal of Orthopsychiatry* 1(1931):451-475.

84. G. N. Thompson, Psychiatric factors influencing learning, *Journal of Nervous and Mental Diseases* 101(1945):347-356.

85. D. Stafford-Clark, D. Pond and J. S. Lovett-Doust, The psychopath in prison: a preliminary report of co-operative research, *British Journal of Delinquency* 2(1951):117.

86. J. McCord and W. McCord, *The Origins of Crime* (New York: Columbia University Press, 1959).

87. B. Pasamanick, R. E. Rogers, and G. M. Lilienfeld, *American Journal of Psychiatry* 112(1956):613-618.

88. S. Brondon, An epidemological study of maladjustment in childhood, (M.D. Thesis, University of Durham, 1960) cited in Delinquency, by P. D. Scott, *Modern Perspectives in Child Psychiatry*, ed. by T. G. Howells (Springfield: Charles C Thomas, 1965).

89. F. Gruenberg and D. A. Pond, Conduct disorder in epileptic children, *Journal of Neurology and Psychiatry* 20(1957):65-68.

90. J. A. Harrington and F. J. J. Letemendia, Persistent psychiatric disorder after head injuries in children, *Journal of Mental Science* 104(1958):1205-1218.

91. D. A. Pond, Psychiatric aspects of epileptic and brain-injured children, *British Medical Journal* 2(1966):1377-1382, and 1454-1459.

92. H. Kluver and P. C. Bucy, Preliminary analysis of the temporal lobes in monkeys, *Basic Readings in Neuropsychology*, ed. by R. L. Isaacson, pp. 60-86 (New York: Harper and Row, 1964).

93. W. Haymaker, *Bing's Local Diagnosis in Neurological Diseases*, 2nd ed. (St. Louis: C. V. Mosby, 1968).

94. P. C. VanReeth, J. Dierkens and D. Luminet, Hypersexuality in epilepsy and temporal lobe tumors, *Acta Neurologica et Psychiatrica Belgica* 58(1958):94.

95. D. Hill and G. Parr, *Electroencephography* (New York: Macmillan, 1950).

96. R. M. Silberstein and H. Irwin, Jean-Marc-Gaspard Itard and the Savage of Aveyron: an unsolved diagnostic problem in child psychiatry, *Journal of the American Academy of Child Psychiatry* 1(1962):314-322.

97. A. Gesell, *Wolf Child and Human Child* (London: Methuen, 1941).

98. J. Bowlby, *Forty-Four Juvenile Thieves* (London: Bailliere, Tindall, and Cox, 1946).

99. J. Bowlby, Maternal race and mental health, *Bulletin of the World Health Organization* 3(1951):334-335.

100. R. G. Andry, Paternal and maternal roles and delinquency, *Deprivation of Maternal Care* (Geneva: World Health Organization, 1962), pp. 31-44.

101. M. W. Warren and T. B. Palmer, Community treatment project: an evaluation of community treatment of delinquents, *California Youth Authority, CTP Research Department, No. 6,* 1965.

102. F. Brown, Depression and childhood bereavement, *Journal of Mental Science* 107(1961):754-777.

103. A. Little, Parental deprivation, separation and crime, *British Journal of Criminology* 5(1965):419.

104. F. Brown and P. Epps, Childhood bereavement and subsequent crime, *British Journal of Psychiatry* 112(1966):1043-1048.

105. *Perspectives on Human Deprivation: Biological, Psychological, and Sociological* (Bethesda: National Institute of Child Health and Human Development, 1968).

106. W. McCord and J. McCord, *Psychopathy and Delinquency* (New York: Grune and Stratton, 1956).

107. H. Lewis, *Deprived Children* (London: Oxford University Press, 1954).

108. E. J. Anthony, A clinical evaluation of children with psychotic parents, *American Journal of Psychiatry* 126(1969):177-184.

109. M. Zuckerman, B. H. Barrett and R. M Bragiel. Parental attitudes of parents of child guidance centers, *Child Development* 3(1960):401.

110. D.J. West, *The Habitual Criminal: A Psychiatric Survey* (London: Heinemann, 1963).

111. S. S. Glueck and E. T. Glueck, *Physique and Delinquency* (New York: Harper and Row, 1956).

112. N. Watt and B. Maher, Prisoners' attitudes toward home and the judicial system, *Journal of Criminal Law, Crime, and Political Science* 49(1958):327-330.

113. M. A. Merrill, *Problems of Child Delinquency* (Boston: Houghton Mifflin, 1947).

114. B. Maher, *Principles of Psychopathology* (New York: McGraw-Hill, 1966).

115. D. Lykken, A study of anxiety in the sociopathic personality, *Journal of Abnormal Social Psychology* 55(1957):6-10.

116. A. W. Siegman, The relationship between future time perspective, time estimation and impulse-control in a group of young offenders and a control group, *Journal of Consulting Psychology* 25(1961):470-475.

117. R. D. Hare, Acquisition and generalization of a conditioned-fear response in psychopathic and non-psychopathic criminals, *Journal of Psychiatry* 59(1965):367-370.

118. R. D. Hare, Psychopathy: Theory and Research (New York: John Wiley and Sons, 1970).

119. S. S. Glueck and E. T. Glueck, *Toward a Typology of Juvenile Offenders* (New York: Grune and Stratton, 1970).

120. J. Monahan and L.C. Monahan, Prediction research and the role of psychologists in correctional institutions, *San Diego Law Review* 14(1977):1028-1038.

121. K. F. Schuessler and D. R. Cressy, Personality characteristics of criminals, *American Journal of Sociology* 55(1950):483-484.

122. E. Kaufman and L. Heims, The body image of the juvenile delinquent, *American Journal of Orthopsychiatry* 28(1950):146-159.

123. McCord, *The Origins of Crime*, op. cit.

124. W. McCord, J. McCord, and A. Howard, Familial correlates of aggression in nondelinquent male children, *Journal of Abnormal Social Psychology* 62(1961):79-93.

125. M. A. Grant, Interaction between kinds of treatment and kinds of delinquents, *Inquiries Concerning Kinds of Treatment for Kinds of Delinquents*, Mono. 2 (Board of Corrections, State of California, 1961).

126. Group for the Advancement of Psychiatry, *Psychopathological Disorders in Childhood*, vol. 6, rpt. no. 62, 1966.

127. B. Glueck, A study of 608 admissions to sing-sing prison. The psychopathic delinquent, *Journal of Mental Hygiene* 2(1918):149.

128. S. B. Guze and D. W. Goodwin, Diagnostic consistency in antisocial personality, *American Journal of Psychiatry* 128(1971):360-361.

129.S. Ackerly, Rebellion and its relation to delinquency and neurosis in sixty adolescents, *American Journal of Orthopsychiatry* 3(1933):147-160.

130. W. Healy and A. Bonner, *A New Light on Delinquency and its Treatment* (New Haven: Yale University Press, 1936).

131. L. Lowry, The family as a builder of personality, *American Journal of Orthopsychiatry* 6(1936):117-124.

132. B. Karpman, The myth of the psychopathic personality, *American Journal of Psychiatry* 104(1948):523-534.

133. L. N. Robins, *Deviant Children Grow Up: A Sociological and Psychiatric Study of Sociopathic Personality* (Baltimore: Williams and Wilkens, 1960).

134. L. Srole, *Mental Health in the Metropolis: The Midtown Study, vol. 1* (New York: McGraw-Hill, 1962).

135. P.O'Neal, Y.N. Robins, L.J. King and J. Schaefer, Parental deviance and the genesis of sociopathic personality, *American Journal of Psychiatry* 118(1962):1114-1118.

Chapter Eleven

Antisocial Behavior: Neurotic and Characterological Aspects

THE ROLE OF NEUROTIC CONFLICT

In contrast to the sociogenic perspective or descriptive types of psychiatry, the areas of neurotic conflict and characterological structures present a different emphasis. While trait theory was presented in the last chapter, the emphasis in descriptive psychiatry is customarily on phenotypic characteristics—that is to say, their externally manifest and overt symptomatology. On the other hand, the traits and behaviors associated with neurotic conflict and characterological aspects deal with genotypic dispositions. While phenotypic dispositions are not particularly consistent, underlying neurotic conflicts and character structures maintain a certain consistency and endure over time. It is necessary to clarify how the concept of *structure* is used with reference to neurosis and character problems.

There are hallmarks of neurotic conflict which can give rise to antisocial behavior.

1. Unconscious conflicts are involved in the expression of desires or impulses.

2. Defenses are maintained by the ego to deal with these impulses and their associated affects.

3. A superego system functions either in an ego-supportive manner, or on the id side of a conflict.

4. Internalization of conflict occurs in contrast to transient reactive states.

5. Although the expressions vary, the conflict tends to persist and be expressed repetitively in different settings. It is this component which merges into the relatively fixed and ingrained traits in a personality.

6. If neurotic symptoms emerge, they are often seen as a symbolic expression of psychological conflict whose origins are in the developmental period.

7. Certain stresses may be so sudden, or overwhelming, that they induce a traumatic neurosis which taps pre-existing conflicts.

Neurosis is difficult to define. It is a concept used not only clinically, in terms of different kinds of symptoms which go with neuroses such as conversions, phobias, obsessional symptoms, etc., but also it becomes impossible to avoid discussing the entire theory of neurotic conflict and their varying modes of expression. Psychodynamic theory itself evolved as a way of offering explanations of how unresolved conflict gives rise to anxiety which in turn leads to a host of defensive efforts on the part of the ego. Disturbances in behavior, the emotions, or cognitions, make evident the types of defenses employed. Symptoms are seen as compromises between repressed ideas or wishes and defensive operations. The ego distorts the repressed ideas so they are not easily recognizable. Hence, the compromise—the unconscious wish and the defensive alteration leading to a derivative expression. These derivatives of the repressed, in turn, become the object of new defensive measures, since the unconscious remains active in terms of exerting constant pressure.

The symptomatic expression may be perceived by the adolescent as something painful and unacceptable (ego-alien), or the conflicts may be subsumed as part of personality trends and traits and not perceived as a source of distress or anxiety (ego-syntonic). By adolescence the personality structure is altered enough so that neurotic conflicts lead to certain kinds of adaptational patterns. The adaptation is what permits antisocial tendencies, or possibly criminal acts, to occur with minimal anxiety, even though they may have symbolic significance.

Although there is a cliche that says conflict is universal in human life, it does not tell us how to deal with it. Interposed is the central reguatory functioning of the ego, which serves to deal with particular kinds of conflicts in ways specific to the individual. The daily devices employed reveal a plethora of options. Some conflicts are resolved because the environmental situation is altered, others because the value system of the individual shifts. A competitor for a girl moves, for example, and the immediate conflict is resolved; a girl decides that being a member of a high school swimming team is not as important as some other use of her time, and again the conflict is resolved. Ideally, conflicts are handled by sublimation, in which the adolescent engages in certain acts or fantasies which are socially acceptable. The conflicts then consciously lose their original connection with sexuality or too direct expressions of aggression. For example, an adolescent with anxiety over sexuality may teach a course on sexual behavior to those a few years younger. Hate for a person is handled by painting war scenes of blood and carnage.

Repression solves the problem on one level, but it leaves the conflict functioning in the nonreporting unconscious system. Some conflicts are handled by identification. A boy, unsure of his role, begins to emulate someone he admires. If his anxiety involves feeling weak and inferior, he may identify with the aggressor and display his bravado by feeling identified with powerful people or causes. A sixteen-year-old in a massive authority conflict with his father engages in a chase at ninety miles per hour down a highway to see "if the cops can really nail me." The conflict is displaced from home so that overt expressions of aggression there are kept under control. A need to hurt and destroy may be handled by a reaction formation of oversolicitous concern and helping others. Direct aggressive attack may be modulated by a host of verbal and behavioral methods, such as verbal putdowns or challenges, teasing, taunting, and belittling. Sexual conflicts find disguised and substitutive outlets. The adolescent, anxious about sexual desires, finds a replacement in endless discussion about sexuality, or intellectual formulations about the role of sexuality in modern life.

The possibility of symbolic expression of neurotic conflict has been mentioned. Since entire treatises from the perspective of different disciplines have been written on symbolism, it is mentioned here to note its ubiquity as a developmental phenomenon associated with the way a person actually experiences something at the time. Hence, the capacity for distortion is immense. The significance is that by the time adolescence is reached there is a storehouse of symbolic representations available to the individual, which appear in fantasies, daydreams, drawings, stories, and ultimately, perhaps, in symptom formation or acting out defenses. Along with symbolic experiences, there is a growing capacity of the ego, which becomes more capable of abstraction, complexity, and associations. The work of Piaget has dealt with the diversities of thinking, fantasy, and communication developmentally years after language per se has been attained.[1] All kinds of contradictions and incompatibilities exist side by side with reality-based presentations. These incongruities are what gain symbolic expression. During adolescence, the potential for symbolic recreation of earlier childhood symbolizations gains new momentum in vividness, along with the increased potential for internal and external conflict.

In a psychodynamic sense, contradictory impulses striving for expression press for immediate gratification. In a theoretical vein, the contradictions exist even before there is a clear delineation between somatic representations and external reality. The analogy is often made between how a dream occurs—or the manifest content—and the symptomatic expression from conflict. Since primary and secondary processes operate in everyone, the distinction is between the primary products which are under ego control and those which are not. The ego, also by way of regulating drive expression, reduces the occasions for internal conflict. This is part of the synthetic function of the ego, which reduces the amount of dissonance and conflict within the personality. But since certain impulses are allowed gratification and others not, the potential for conflict always looms. Conflict in life is then not solely in the environment where humans live, but exists between the ego and the id.

As ego development progresses in terms of the reality available to a person, reality and ego development hopefully become more congruent. If the threat of an eruption or breakthrough of id impulses emerges, acute anxiety may ensue. Under such situations, panic-stricken acting out can occur. Homosexual panic, which may have an accompanying act of violence, is one possibility as an outcome. Therapeutic implications exist since an adolescent, feeling overwhelmed, needs to rely on the supportive role of the therapist to help with his drive life. The ongoing role of the therapist, which becomes introjected, is another therapeutic gain. Therapists with unresolved acting out problems of their own give a major impetus to an adolescent who is already displaying potential in this direction. The other extreme is the overprotective therapist; the adolescent feels that the regulation of his impulse life is beyond his control. A variation of a symbiotic relationship then develops.

The role of the superego in conflict is equally significant. All of the developmental phenomena associated with early parentified prerogatives operate.[2] What emerges is a personalized version of moral and ethical principles with some type of priority listing. While this gives stability in terms of knowing what is accepted or not, it contributes to potential conflict once the norms become more fixed.

The advent of guilt and remorse—feeling bad—has been discussed in earlier chapters in terms of contributing potentials for conflict. The human who grows up with minimal superego controls has unique problems, discussed under sociopathic lack of regulation. We are speaking of the idiosyncrasies of superego development in terms of feelings of badness and unacceptableness. The opposite, over-developed superego controls, eventuates in a moral uprightness and rigid rules and formulas for control. The potential for conflict becomes immense and often gives rise to classical neuroses of the depressive or obsessional varieties.

The idea of the persecutory superego is relevant. Persecuted elements are tied into a distorted control system which is magnified, not only to control, but to dominate, intimidate, and, if necessary, browbeat. Herein lies the potential for another variety of violent aggression. An act of suicide can occur from a total acquiescence to the judgment of the internalized persecutor. Another possibility is to externalize attack on the tormentor in an act of homicidal aggression. Cases which achieve notoriety in the news media where a "previously well-behaved" youngster commits one or several acts of violent homicide, perhaps followed by a suicide attempt, are often in this category.

Another facet of superego development with great importance for neurotic conflict is the role of the ego-ideal (see also chapter 8). The potential for conflict lies in the component of unreality in the ego-ideal. In neurotic character problems the ego-ideal has attained a level of grandiosity for the self that guarantees frustration and all that ensues. Since much narcissism is tied up in the emergent ego-ideal, many early and unrealistic goals and fantasies become part of it. During adolescence, the failure to achieve, grow physically, be sexually appealing, good in terms of norms, all become sources of conflict. Inflated and distorted pictures of parental figures feed in more conflict, since the parental image bears only a minimal relationship to how parents actually see themselves or behave. The roles and trumped-up heroes of our media-ridden world become involved in the incorporative process of the ego-ideal, and they become twisted into something that few people in a civilization could ever attain. Punitive or self-punitive trends result in which even worthwhile achievements are viewed as minimal. From such distortion, unrealistically accepted, all manner of desperate acts can occur. If an adolescent views his achievements as contemptible, why show restraint from whatever primitive impulses and fantasies are possible?

While ego regression takes the form of mechanisms to deal with possibilities for being a bad or evil person, superego functioning can regress as well. How? In part, destructive behavior is possible from continuously poor self-appraisals. If it goes to the extent of the adolescent feeling not only a failure by way of a superego appraisal, but also projects his superego so that he feels persecuted, massive superego regression is a possibility. In turn, the ego begins to defend itself against threats which are highly exaggerated, and anxiety mounts. Since no one part of the personality remains isolated, drive regression occurs as well. Repressed impulses are then permitted the possibility of expression. While not all acts are necessarily violent, many are tinged sufficiently with aggressive and sexual components to be borderline in sociality, and some will breech legality.

DEVELOPMENTAL PROBLEMS

Conflicts from earlier periods predominate in those who are predisposed toward character problems. The following are some major areas in which these are in evidence:

1. Difficulties in the areas of expressing attachments and dependency needs, fluctuating between needs for deeper attachments opposed by anxiety over getting too close, with resultant anxiety
2. Low frustration-tolerance when environmental sources are not meeting the adolescent's demands
3. Difficulties in mastering the anxieties attendant upon separation-individuation processes
4. Conflict involving strivings for autonomy
5. An inbalance between the expression and control devices utilized for handling aggression or sexuality
6. Developmental arrests, fixation, and conflicts, which relate to matters differentiating gender identity

A diversity of overt behaviors are witnessed in mixed neurotic and character problems. These vary from manipulative behaviors or sucking-up techniques to expressions of impulses which are poorly modulated. Although it may be convenient to view these as a continuum, in some cases it is invalid to do so. A similarity is present between some of the behaviors in neurotic conflicts and those ascribed to problems associated with personality disorders. The customary distinction that those with character problems suffer little personal discomfort may be quite erroneous. This may be especially invalid for neurotic characters, who express their conflicts by various interpersonal expressions of aggression, since they may be just as uncomfortable personally as any pure neurotic. In both neurotic conflict and character problems experiences of painful affect, such as anxiety or guilt, may dominate: by adolescence overt and covert manifestations of petulance, defiance, and attacks on the environment provoke counter-aggression. On the other hand, developmental manifestations of being demanding, controlling, testing limits, or seeking narcissistic indulgence, can be seen in the relatively nonconflicted child as part of his development.

Some behaviors represent a form of developmental deviation. The age at which the behaviors become manifest, as well as the sequence of events, and the degree to which the behaviors persist are the key. Reactive possibilities need to be kept in mind, where a particular situation or set of events induces symptomatic disturbances. Attempting to assess children with an eye to future characterological disturbances presents challenges. The diagnostician must be able to obtain material from the child, family, and others in the environment concerning the way the child is feeling and reacting. By adolescence feelings will have expanded to include institutions and their representatives.

Continued primacy of the six predisposing influences listed above and weighting of them in the personality, suggests a solidifying character disturbance with symptom formation in the offing. Qualities of guardedness and suspiciousness are indicative of difficulties in the realm of trust. However, psychotically vulnerable youths present such traits as well. In those with more narcissistic impairments, a feeling of personal hurt or suffering is conveyed with an additional component that others, perhaps the therapist, are somehow at fault for their predicaments. Manipulative techniques of poutiness or procrastination are one turn that challenges to authority can take as part of a general picture of testing others.

Affect varies from a likeable sense of buoyancy and excitement to a sense they have formed few genuine and enduring attachments during their development. Although their external behavior and general appearance are tailored to current norms, it may represent a purely cognitive adaptation without further personal meaning, so that norms have not become internalized. While useful in terms of necessary environmental adaptations at a particular time, it has no permanence. In others, a quality of flatness or affectlessness is present. The result is a blunting of feeling in terms of interpersonal relationships. They have learned to recite the right answers on the basis of having learned what to say. It is surprising how even young children unfold quite elaborate and sophisticated techniques of manipulation and extraction from others.

In some cases the pride of the parent in their child conning someone is noticeable to those involved in the diagnostic process. Family interviewing techniques assist in providing a first-hand manner of confirming how power plays are used in family units, as well as with vulnerable individuals outside the family. When used outside the family projective devices are more easily employed. Rather than multiply endlessly the diversities detectable in any thorough psychological appraisal, consideration will be given to specific diagnoses.

The significance of dealing with separation in mixed neurotic disorders cannot be overestimated. While a great number emerge from early childhood without the burden of a symbiotic psychosis, they still have problems dealing with degrees of separation. Physical separation itself as a problem always has integral psychological components. The common example of homesickness, with its anxiety about separation from a parent, can mean many things, and generalizations are unwarranted. One girl with a mother recently diagnosed as having a malignancy became acutely homesick at camp while the past two summers at the same camp were asymptomatic. A fifteen-year-old girl was sent away to school since her divorcing parents felt this would spare her the turmoil in the year of dissolution. The result was a flurry of nightly phone calls, a half-hearted capacity to study, great concern that the mother would become sick and die and acting out. A thirteen-year-old boy expressed concern he could never do anything without the presence of his mother, much to the conscious chagrin of both parents. He then began to steal, without his mother being present.

These cases illustrate what is an area of psychological development not given enough emphasis for subsequent antisocial behavior in adolescence. As part of the more general picture of object development, the child becomes aware of separateness from parents and other objects. The stages appear to be: (a symbiotic union)-(cognitive registering of separateness)-(degrees of distress)-(a sense of self with delineated ego boundaries)-(differentiated object concept)-(object relationships). It is important to note the early work in this area came from clinical settings with young psychotic children in which the difficulties of differentiation of the self from the mother-infant attachment were overwhelming.

Locomotion is also connected with mastery of control over oneself. Mahler discussed the importance of locomotion in the practicing phase of the separation-individuation period.[3] For purposes of autonomy and control the child progresses from pleasure of carrying out locomotion per se to seeking out a comforting object when it is needed. Hence, a mother or a transitional object, such as a teddy bear or doll, are sought. Later, testing occurs by separating from parents to see what will happen.

Disruption of early mother-child symbiosis allows awareness of separateness, but it also raises the potential for separation anxiety and nostalgia for past gratifications. In an earlier theoretical framework discussion was in terms of the child's nostalgia being related to weaning and missing the breast. It is now conceptualized in a broader manner: separation anxieties are mastered by expansion of ego strengths and functions. From a more generalized and primitive association of well-being with a need-satisfying object and the converse, the infant progresses to a specific attachment in which separateness and differentness are present. With greater specificity, anxiety about the object is more specific, i.e., by learning processes the child associates emotional discomfort with the absence of the mother and consequently attempts to avoid distance. All manner of direct, substitutive, and symbolic ways of reassuring himself are developed. These vary from ritualistic reassurances that "everything will be all right" if one has a talisman or article, to societal mechanisms for gaining reassurance against the anxiety of aloneness. Involvement in religion is one way of adolescents feel they will not be alone but someone can be with them "to the end of the world," group attachments on a peer level are another.

ween eight and ten, a girl remembered lying in bed at night when her

Between eight and ten, a girl remembered lying in bed at night when her parents went out and not letting herself go to sleep until they returned. If she could muster the energy, she would then greet them. By age fifteen, when she went out her mother would repeat the reversed pattern of not permitting herself to sleep until the daughter was safe. When asked what the danger might be, the mother could only mention some vague feeling that she should be available in case something bad did happen, as her own mother, in turn, had been. Remembrances of the anxiety attendant upon separation have fused with remembrances of the associated pleasure on return.

capable of greater modulation of affect along with the capacity to do things in their own lives, rather than being helpless. Hopefully, the defenses to deal with anxiety work better and are more structuralized than with the infant faced with the absence of the maternal object. Pine has discussed individual variations in boys from four to eight years of age with respect to the separation process.[4] In work with adolescents these same variations are encountered with more potential for the recurrence of explosive regressions and antisociality.

1. Reliance on internal processes versus external support to reduce anxiety is one dimension involved in separation. The need for the physical proximity of parents can be seen on the one hand in the overly quiescent young adolescent. Everything seems to be progressing until the point is reached where separation is needed. A common example is the senior year in high school. At that point, challenges to authority, complete flip-flops in personality, and a good deal of acting out may ensue. In fact, the dramatic change alerts us to the degree of distress. Some adolescents find going away from home to college is impossible because of the associated anxiety. In fact, some unconsciously sabotage the possibility of going to college, by provoking conflicts within the family which lead to the parents' withdrawal of support. In other cases, the degree of acting out militates against their leaving home; they may involve themselves in social or legal difficulties, for example.

The need for the physical proximity of a family, coupled with the parallel limitation intrapsychically which would enable them to handle the anxiety, leads to overt disturbances. The cause actually appears to be the limitation of techniques to tolerate the separation. Somehow, cognitive ego functions such as memory images of family members and home are not sufficiently developed to cope with absences. Nor is the capacity to tolerate delay sufficient to forestall anxiety, if not panic, anticipating an eventual reunion. While the younger child may work this out in fantasy and play, the adolescent tries to handle it on a peer level, but the effort may be insufficient. Faced with the lowering of self-esteem from not leaving home, or continued anxiety the way is paved for neurotic symptom formation or some other maladaptive pattern.

2. Another variation in dealing with separation involves confrontation versus evasion. In adolescence these are both employed with full vigor. Some adolescents try active mastery, but others retreat into variations on the theme of postponement. Variations in styles of defense evolve. The need to try an immediate resolution is balanced by a need for withdrawal to recoup defenses. A thirteen-year-old, homesick at camp to the point of barely eating and listlessly going through activities, devised a plan to hitchhike home. This required some ingenuity, since he had no funds and the campsite was 300 miles away from home, yet he succeeded. While the

immediate anxiety was mastered, it did little about resolving its sources, or its potential to re-emerge.

Other adolescents continue their withdrawal behavior. They seem more devoted to denial, isolation, and repression defenses. But while these defenses work in the short-run for situations not too threatening, they do not in the absence of more stabilized internalizations. A variation is a counterphobic turn in which an adolescent, fearful of separating, leaves on his own to prove he can do so. Some teenage girls leave with friends to live in a different city. A few days or weeks later, they call home. A previously very close relationship with their home and mother often existed. It is as though these girls are saying it is too difficult to dilute the relationship, and it is an all or nothing affair. A nineteen-year-old girl married a twenty-nine-year-old instructor and dropped out of college. The couple played the role of nature lovers while continuously calling home for funds which were provided by her father. Five years later they were still living a nomadic existence and berating her middle class parents.

3. Some miscarried attempts at mastering the anxiety connected with separation lead to diffuse discharge. The ego experiences the anxiety as though overwhelming. The experiential state is helplessness. A result can be panic, diffuse motor discharges, hypomanic states, or a flight into escapades involving sex, drugs, or alcohol. These activities are in the service of allowing the adolescent to experience less conscious anxiety. It is also less painful than passively feeling helpless. In many situations the behavior takes on an impulse-ridden quality which conflates developmental, neurotic, and characterological aspects.

DIFFERENTIAL DIAGNOSTIC PROBLEMS

The differential diagnoses when antisocial behaviors are present in the adolescent and youth age groups can be summarized as follows:

1. Until proven otherwise, one should start with an initial approach of assuming behavior to be a type of response to a *developmental or situational crisis* in which antisocial conduct is occurring on a transient basis, and not in itself indicative of a psychopathological type of adaptation. This means we do not necessarily ipso facto stop here, but if there are specific indicators, we examine other possibilities.

2. The same behaviors may indicate a *reactive disorder* which is a response to a particular situation. Such behavior is a product of

conscious conflict between adolescents and others in their environment.

3. *Developmental deviations* manifest themselves in an alteration of social development beyond transient responses as well as those based on conscious conflict. The persistence of such behavior, its appearance at a certain time, and a pattern of uneven development in social relationships in terms of autonomy, capacity for control over impulses, difficulty in expanding tolerance for separation, inhibitions, marked shyness, and disturbances in the realm of aggression, are relevant diagnostic indicators.

4. Neurotic disturbances are reflected in interpersonal or environmental difficulties but represent internalized conflicts. When the behavior is directed outwardly, or has alloplastic elements, it is a *neurotic character* disturbance. The theoretical background given at the beginning of this chapter provides a framework for such symptomatic expression. While some antisocial behavior takes discrete monosymptomatic form, such as kleptomanic behavior, more commonly a range of personality types are present.

5. *Cyclothymic tendencies* or mood swings may lead to interpersonal difficulties or contribute to acting out behaviors. The relationship of a depressive personality to antisocial personality is seen as significant enough to warrant separate listing.

6. *Borderline* adjustments or *psychotic reactions* need diagnostic consideration when antisocial behavior is present. These can be prodromata ushering in a schizophrenic process, or they may occur as an accompaniment in a more general regressive process. Young children who have persisted in unsocialized conduct up to adolescence may be reflecting a psychotic process. Differentiation of highly regressive behaviors with a bizarre quality, or exaggerated or uncontrolled affect and language, makes differentiation challenging. These behaviors are often classified initially as developmental deviations on the basis of some biological, psychological, or social lag. The capacity of those with impaired ego functioning to tolerate painful affect may be an important factor in determining regressive responses. They find it difficult to perceive situations and people accurately and accept the limitations of reality, which makes them more vulnerable to acting out behavior.

7. *Organic cerebral dysfunction* or *mental subnormality* contribute to behavioral disturbances by way of cognitive and interpersonal disruption. The behavior may be misdiagnosed as psychopathic. Secondary reactions to frustration, feelings of inferiority, teasing, etc., contribute to the syndrome.

SPECIFIC CHARACTER TYPES

Discussion has focused on the *neurotic character*. What follows is a description of the major features of specific types of character structures, as they relate to antisocial behavior. While none of them by necessity exhibits antisocial conduct, conflicted parts of their character structures with respect to developmental problems gives them such a potentiality.

Compulsive Personalities. These individuals are chronically preoccupied with concerns about neatness, cleanliness, and conformity to the demands of those in authority. Vulnerability lies in their potential for overthrowing the exaggerated compliance to authority figures which they possess. These young children struggle to deal with their anxiety over impulses by compulsive measures—especially when their cognitive functioning is precocious. Qualities of tenseness and difficulty in relaxation are present, along with a system of overcontrol. Overcontrolled young children may sit contentedly with their hands folded during an hour-long interview. Their great seriousness and premature psychological development leaves an impression of intensity with a lack of the free spontaneity usually present in young children.

Anxiety is experienced when the overcontrolled system fails, and they cannot carry out their customary orderly behaviors. When that occurs, others in the enviornment may be perceived as responsible for their distress. A possible outcome is an intrapsychic realignment; when their obsessive-compulsive traits do not relieve anxiety, more overt neurotic symptoms of an obsessive-compulsive type develop. Another possibility is to take things out on false gods or authority representatives with whom they have been struggling. From the rigidity of the system an abundance of aggression is available. Contrary to a frequent picture of the compulsive personality as a rigid conformist, periodic releases occur by acting out. Dynamically, a release from the severity of critical internalized authorities occurs.

It is puzzling to those appraising the phenotypic aspects when such breakdowns in defenses can occur. Previously conforming and obedient youths have an eruption of petty acting out, such as kleptomanic activities. If a massive regression occurs, the overcontrolled hate and aggression break through, and a serious act of violence occurs. Despite strong moral convictions and opinions about right and wrong, they are influentiable by those in authority and liable to go along with activity covered up under facades of intellectual rationalization or commands. Atrocities by troops or political corruption are examples.

Peer pressures in adolescence to join in escapades are one situation. Periodic needs to relieve internalized overcontrol can be a source for acting out. Adolescent males may succumb to the challenge of a girlfriend to engage in certain acts. A sixteen-year-old boy with overt hand-washing compulsions planned a cab robbery with his girlfriend to obtain vacation money. While holding a gun on the cabbie, who refused to stop, his girlfriend urged him to shoot. When he hesitated, she screamed he was a coward. After some hesitation, he did. Certain sexual perversions are expressed compulsively and may also lead to difficulty.

Hysterical Personalities.   While not too long ago only women were believed to become hysteric, the degree of antisocial potential those with predisposed hysterical character problems have is still largely ignored. Histrionic trends give rise to dramatic and flamboyant behavior. These trends accentuate the labile emotionality present in adolescents. At times an extreme oversuggestibility in responding to others or group situations exists. This gives a capacity to be manipulated and to manipulate others. The young hysteric is often coy and engages in seductive behavior even at a very early age. While seductiveness is an over-used term, it has a significant meaning in the context of an individual who, quite early developmentally, uses and perfects techniques of luring and enticing others for ulterior motives.

A variation is the practical joker or hoaxer. In the course of inducing anxiety in others, a sense of control is speciously gained; the joker sets up the hoax and reveals it as well.[5] The difficulty is that even acts such as pulling fire alarms or ordering merchandise under false pretenses can become a great nuisance to the victim. Others act the role of the imposter or perpetrate crimes under assumed identities. Difficulties in delimiting themselves from their environment, or to overattachments to objects, is prevalent.

In addition, problems of sex-role identity with fixed feminine aspects for males is part of hysterical traits. A quality of psuedosocial poise or attractiveness to a great many boys and girls is added. The attractiveness is strikingly noticeable by early adolescence and is registered by many people. Present at a young age, it gives an ability to capitalize on it, and attain yet more reinforcement by their behaviors. Despite this, there is clinical evidence that a great deal of repression is operating with respect to many of these impulses. Confusion in gender identity and roles is an integral part of the picture, particularly in the course of adolescence and adulthood.

Another quality in the hysterical personality which gives trouble relates to pain dependency. Prominent trends with respect to the need to experience suffering are present. It is more precise to say these adolescents wish to portray themselves as suffering, and masochistic elements occupy a sector of their personality. They operate both on a conscious and unconscious level. At times of increased stress, more overt symptom formation of a conversion or dissociative nature may temporarily appear and be followed by a spontaneous cure. In childhood, conversion symptoms manifest themselves as recurrent abdominal pains, headaches, or dizziness. In adolescence, more classical hysterical symptoms appear.

When overt conversion symptomatology persists, particularly with accompanying psychological invalidism, it is an indication of a deeper disturbance of body–image. Combinations of personality traits give rise to manipulative and demanding traits accompanying dependency demands. When these demands are frustrated, acting out occurs. The most blatant acts of dissimulation and deception can take place. When confronted with their acts, denial operates to mitigate cognizance of how they have in reality been highly manipulative and dishonest with others. The potential for a psychotic regression remains possible, and is associated with difficulties in knowing what the adolescent is expressing or conveying.

Individuals who are carried away by their own narcissistic needs so they act in isolation from consequences, cannot help but run into interpersonal difficulties—if not legal ones. While overt acts of physical violence may be minimal, antisocial acts which involve property thefts are more common. Most common of all is the confusion and blundering which result from ambiguous interpersonal relationships, and lead to personal disagreements and difficulties with others. Repression and ego splitting can operate so that the degree of lying or deviousness are not consciously registered. Obviously these major personality limitations in any group situation lead to factions, feelings of being used by others, and eventual chaos. The pattern tends to be re-enacted throughout life.

Passive-dependent (Oral) Personalities. These individuals are viewed as helpless, clinging, and demanding. Their behaviors point to difficulties in achieving independence and asserting initiative. The indicators point to problems in separation and individuation. In some, passivity is part of a clinical picture involving efforts at control of others or demandingness.

Their overly inhibited control system gives a quality of passivity. Some are seen as manifesting *pathological shyness*. Both a lack of psychological initiative or assertiveness and an inhibition of motor expression are part of the picture. Impairment in interpersonal development suffers as a consequence. Because of reticence, these adolescents give a false impression that their affective contact with others is minimal. It is more beneficially seen as a style of adaptation which is a compromise between conflicting needs and which has secured rewards.

When oppositional tendencies are present, the silent approach may be utilized. However, they are distinguishable from schizoid personalities. As young children they wish for human relationships but are too constricted to achieve them—in contrast to such a lack of desire in schizoid children. Their inhibitions appear related to difficulties in maintaining control, or at least a fear of losing control should they not retain their passivity or gross inhibitions. In many areas they are able to function independently, so it is rather in the area of lack of assertiveness and overt dependency that they are impaired. Consequently, they may have difficulties in other areas, such as in academic learning or in competition. While occasionally an eruptive act of violence occurs, more often antisocial trends take the form of petty pilfering or quiescent ways of covertly asserting themselves in dealing with anger. Passive trends in girls are appealing to many boys. Until they become quite involved they miss the facade of passivity concealing potent power needs which can be used to control others.

Oppositional Personalities. A descriptive nosology calls them passive-aggressive personalities. Developmentally, they have a common stem with compulsive traits. The main difference is the more open expression of hostility in the form of negativism, in contrast to the blunting seen in compulsive defenses. The combination of oppositional patterns, with occasional breakthroughs of more open aggressive assertiveness, raises the prior probabilities that these individuals will engage in acts which take on or challenge authority. The more successful can sublimate impulses into competitive pursuits or those dedicated toward change; the unfortunate pursue borderline or clearly antisocial acts.

Under a guise of conformity, these youths subtly provoke conflicts. Exaggerated conformity can make rule-following a reductio ad absurdum. The most prominent symptomatology besides negativism and stubbornness include dawdling, procrastination, and covert measures which betray the aggression. The need to undermine authority by dawdling may show up in the realm of learning disturbances. Failing to hear or needing to battle authority figures constantly interferes with learning.

If their defenses are attenuated, they may act out their feelings aggressively in tension-discharge types of disorders, such as physical assaults or periodic vandalism. Power battles which elicit stubbornness are perfectly tailored for difficulties with parents and schools. What is commonly overlooked is that the same opposition can take the form of opposing many other problems in life. While some of these complaints may be just, the emphasis is on the personality structure which finds a need to keep fighting. If anger goes beyond simply opposing, acts of vandalism or provoking fights are seen.

The Narcissistic Character. Narcissistic character structures have a proneness toward antisociality based on potentialities toward disappointment or defeat. Traits associated with this personality structure are: a reserved haughtiness, smugness, vanity, conveying a quality of specialness, an oozing of arrogance, and a general attitude of superiority. Concomitant is a high degree of aggressiveness which is not too thinly concealed.

The developmental procursors of this personality have conflicts centered around rage and envy. While we do not have information of sufficient depth and quantity to confirm the early type of parental relationships, the confused image of an overprotective mother, who is yet cold and narcissistic herself, predominates. In learning theory terms, the conflict is one of seeming overnurturance encouraging closeness but with avoidance when the child seeks to get close. One or both parents have narcissistic traits, which the children experience directly, and then take their own particular role. Under the armor of being special lies a self-concept of unworthiness, and a fear that they may be left alone and abandoned. Despite genuine talents they believe they are fraudulent and not worthy of respect or decent treatment. Their demeaning treatment of themselves parallels their treatment of others. Since others are in positions to grant esteem or affection, they are often objects of envy for they can make or break one. Ambivalence is thus quite prominent.

Yet, in a developmental context are not such conflicts played out in every child? In general, the answer is yes, but by adolescence both quantitative and quaiitative differences have emerged. Distinctions need to be drawn between *pathological narcissism* and *adult narcissism* as well as normal *infantile narcissism*. It is not simply that adolescents who have emerged with a narcissistic character structure have overinvested in themselves, but that they do it in a particular way which does not really make them feel good about themselves. A qualitative difference exists between maintaining what is basically a psychopathological self and one that has narcissistic distortion. If the pathological elements predominate, there is a need to protect against early incorporated representations which threaten from within. Since these early object representations are defective, both ego and superego deformations occur. Both the narcissistic (self) investment and the object (other) investment are involved.

Bear in mind the differences which exist in younger children with respect to narcissism, versus the narcissistic character as it has unfolded by adolescence. In younger children, we expect overt efforts to control others and anger if the efforts fail; by adolescence we do not. In a context of basic trust a child is able to tolerate degrees of separation and deprivation. Their ability to believe in others, and their reliability, take precedence over doubts. They are able to tolerate the failures and criticisms that occur since the overall atmosphere is one of support with warm affect.

A narcissistic character leaves an adolescent plagued by doubts. There is no inner reassurance that adults will be available when needed. In a similar vein, pathological narcissism makes demands on the developing personality which appear insatiable. These demands are not only toward others, but on themselves, since they cannot ever reassure themselves that they are doing all right. There is a sharp distinction between the self-centeredness of the young child, and the aloof disdain which exists in the narcissistic character. By adolescence a quality of ruthlessness has been added. Again, this is quite different from the destructiveness of the frustrated child.

Nor does the grandiosity of the child have the same driven quality for power, possessiveness, and exclusivity as seen in the narcissistic character. The wishes of the child are attuned to acceptance rather than conquering. Aggressiveness can be used in a derisive manner when threatened, or it can be seen in acts of courage or foolhardiness. Outbursts of rage can take place, especially when control or dominance are threatened, or when the adolescent is no longer able to maintain a facade of superiority.[6] The need to depreciate, seen an integral part of their functioning, may not succeed—which also leads to rage.

During adolescence and beyond, narcissism expresses itself in the form of a compulsive need for conquests. One subgroup is the *phallic-narcissist*. To maintain such a narcissistic balance is precarious, since minor insults or traumata can so easily upset it. Since adverse experiences with attendant humiliation always do occur to some extent in the course of any child's development, there are many risks taken to avoid them. Those with such a character structure seek to anticipate criticism. An abrasive or defensive quality is thus added. If they possess sufficient talent, many are able to get adequate compensatory rewards to keep their defenses against rage intact. Those with less talent, but whose narcissistic power needs are as prominent, are eventually more likely to resort to institutions such as the military, academia, or the church, in an effort to insure a framework in which they can play out their needs for superiority over others. They conceive of relationships in terms of one participant being at the mercy the other.

In the face of narcissistic injury, the vulnerable adolescent is prone to react with transient depressive spells or direct aggression. The depressions have a transient quality, since resort is had to direct expression of aggression or acting out as a solution for the painful affect of depression. Since they are threatened by their failure to control others, as well as fear of being controlled, no price may be too high when seeking to guard their precarious well-being.

Herein lies the potential for a variety of antisocial behaviors. As mentioned, they are most vulnerable with respect to the threat of separation. To tolerate separation means that respect and affection for the missing object is present. For someone whose narcissism sees themselves as self-sufficient or a prized object, the threat of dependency is very great. Hence, emotional contact with others is blunted, though not to the extent of their accepting others as more talented. Envy, with its concomitant need to deride others, always lurks in the background. Envy is fed by an expectation of receiving more.[7] The aloof coolness and disdain appear reactive to the underlying dependency needs.

Without pursuing all the developmental ramifications, the grandiosity and exhibitionism of the young child have not been integrated. A consequence is that ambitions are not handled in an ego-syntonic manner. Instead there is a persistence of grandiose aims. While they have an inflated image of themselves, they actually are quite beholden to others for admiration and applause. Their failure to differentiate an idealized version of themselves from the de facto representation leads to perpetual seeking of a fictionalized self-image. More precisely, it is an inability to gratify themselves by realistic possibilities which are worthy of attainment in their own right. Many property offenses occur from this persistent vulnerability, which in adulthood may take a form of white collar crimes. On occasion, blows to self-esteem of sufficient magnitude result in acts of violence. While such a push may occasionally lead to some outstanding achievement, the price paid is high, in that success seems to gratify briefly and need repetition. Examples are legion. The movie star or athlete who will not quit are two common possibilities. Yet, the spite and hate in anonymous millions burdened by an overgrandiose self-image, which they feel driven to pursue by hook or crook, bears witness to the prevalence of the problem.

Overly Independent Personalities. As children these individuals exude active and ebullient behavior. Such drive is not the drivenness of physiological hyperactiveness which is another difficulty. From their overactivity and drive level, it is difficult for the overly independent young child to accept limits set by authority figures. The behavior may have a pseudo-precocious character from the zest and enthusiasm present. In turn, this is not primarily an aggressive or destructive type of behavior. It is rather that impatience leads to impulsive acts. The child pushes to take on activities and responsibilities beyond a given ego capacity.

Behaviors can be reactive to helplessness or dependency. In that sense these traits develop from the pain experienced as part of antecedent states. An overcompensatory quality is present in their assertiveness, which leads to overlapping with narcissistic traits. This can be in response to some fantasized defect, or to conceal anxieties involving threats of harm, injury, or sexuality. Physical illness is experienced as a great handicap. They react to such occurrences by becoming difficult to manage and driving themselves to recuperate too quickly or to take on activities prematurely which give a counterphobic quality. These dispositions can verge into behaviors which are deviant socially or illegal. Their genesis and maintenance are not so much in the service of committing a crime but rather to maintain a personality in balance.

Schizoid Personalities. These youths exhibit distance and detachment in interpersonal relationships. They are shy and loners; some seem withdrawn and cold even toward those whom they know best. Difficulties exist in the areas of expression and competition. However, unpredictable competitive ventures may be undertaken with respect to one particular area of involvement while the remainder of their life remains uninvolved, inhibited, and isolated.

Their desire not to become intimate with others is detectable early in childhood in a preference for being alone or with one or two friends. The quality of reserving commitment to relationships is puzzling to others unless others in the family are similar. They have a restricted capacity for experiencing affect, and limited ability to form warm and emotionally meaningful attachments. Preoccupation with daydreams and autistic reveries are normally kept well-concealed from others. Intellectual success may come to those so endowed. However, many of the children begin to show difficulties in concept formation or cognitive aberrations when under stress.

The theoretical argument persists about whether individuals with schizoid traits are actually preschizophrenic. Although some say the schizoid personality is only preschizophrenic in a small minority, this does not negate the theoretical viewpoint that what we are dealing with may actually be *schizotypes* who under a combination of certain internal and external stresses may decompensate into an overt process of schizophrenia. This is particularly so when these unobtrusive individuals have an occasional, and unpredictable, outburst of violence, at times of homicidal or sexually perverse proportions. The relationship of these personality traits to schizophrenia is discussed more thoroughly in the chapter dealing with psychosis. It is mentioned here from the limitation on personality development which gives the potential for isolated antisocial acts in the context of a psychotic regression and disorganization. It appears that some suicidal shoot-outs involve such a regression. However, the great majority of schizoids do not engage in antisocial acts, but continue their lives of quiet desperation.

Paranoid Personalities. A degree of overlap exists between paranoid and schizoid personalities. Paranoids are listed to call attention to another personality with the potential to resort to antisocial or illegal acts. Their patterns of brooding and suspiciousness, a paramount feature, give a proneness to misinterpret or misread others' comments or acts. Their own intentions become confused with others. The danger lies in their acting on misperceptions.

Unfortunately, a marked rigidity is present in their thinking together with an inability to out-argue themselves into losing their mistrust or changing their pattern of thinking. Use of projective mechanisms is prominent. When these traits become prominent or persistent, they are referred to as paranoid or experiencing an acute paranoid state. Many of the points made about the general nature of schizoidia and schizotypal traits hold for those who emerge in adolescence with solidified paranoid traits.

Tension-discharge Personalities. These individuals act out their feelings directly on other people in their environment or society's representatives. In contrast to personality structures of overcontrol, which appear in the form of schizoid, constricted, or obsessional types, tension-discharge personalities exhibit chronic behavioral patterns of expressing aggressive or sexual impulses in a more overt manner on others. Many of the characteristics and diagnostic terms discussed in the chapter on psychiatric aspects of antisocial behavior have been applied to the tension-discharge group. Such a grouping blurs important distinctions between the manners of reducing tension. As a minimum, two groupings need to be distinguished:

1. *Impulse-ridden Personalities.* These individuals have shallow relationships with others, accompanied by a low frustration-tolerance. A need to discharge their wishes and impulses without brooking delay is a hallmark. Discharge occurs more in response to whatever the need of the moment is, with little regard for consequences. Acts are carried out with a minimal amount of anxiety or guilt. Nor are postulates requiring internalized conflict needed to lead to such a discharge pattern. The conflict is externalized between these youths and their environment. Varying degrees of neurotic conflict are present, but even then a basic defect is present in their control system, with a deficit in superego development and a lack of insight about their difficulties which are rationalized as others being at fault.

Their intolerance of tension, and difficulty in delay, are conspicuous. Denial of dependency needs, strong reaction formations against these needs by exaggerated independence, projection of hostility onto others, and rationalizations for their behavior are rampant. In their longitudinal histories, one obtains data about types of emotional deprivations. As we have noted, they are not restricted to overt neglect, abandonment, poverty, or physical deprivation. The hurts can be subtle and occur in settings of material affluence. Questions have been raised about dysrhythmic electroencephalographic tracings even though epileptic seizure patterns are not in evidence.

A subgroup has a high prevalence of enuresis, fire-setting, stealing, vandalism, destructive outbursts, and other antisocial acts. At adolescence, the use of drugs and alcohol with habituation and addiction patterns become more prevalent. Many unsophisticated approaches are used to work with these adolescents, focusing on the problem of drugs or alcohol as primary rather than as simply byproducts of a severe defect in personality development. Their overall intelligence appears adequate, but defects in judgement and time concepts prevail.

2. *Neurotic Personality Disorders.* Although the behavior of this group is superficially similar to the impulse-ridden type, they act out or discharge their tension in different manners. Their behavior appears more characteristic of repressed neurotic conflicts, in that they repeat a pattern of unconscious conflict. Rather than tending toward pure discharge phenomena, symbolic meaning may be in evidence. A greater prominence of disturbing affects, such as anxiety or guilt, are present. A subgroup appear unconsciously to be seeking limit settings or punishment, and their behavior becomes progressively more challenging unless some type of intervention is instituted. Their acting out has a quality of reacting to intensified conflict rather than being a sudden discharge or a basic lack of superego development. Interpersonal relationships are warmer and more meaningful although tinged with ambivalence. This is the grouping referred to earlier as neurotic characters.

Sociosyntonic Personality Disorders. Different subgroupings are possible here as well. The American Psychiatric Association in their *Diagnostic and Statistical Manual* attempts to segregate individuals who are predatory, and pursue minor or less criminal pursuits, into a category called *dyssocial behavior*. There is an effort to segregate this diagnosis by stating it is a condition without manifest psychiatric disorder, such as is seen in racketeers, dishonest gamblers, prostitutes, or dope peddlers. One of the essential points made repeatedly throughout these chapters is thereby bypassed: any one type of behavior or act by itself rarely provides a valid basis for any adequate diagnosis or personality assessment. The only possible exception might be that of a well-developed delusional system being pathognomonic of a psychotic process. However, the above examples of behavior can all be seen in multiple diagnostic areas.

These controversies frequently spill over into the forensic area, where the meaning of particular diagnoses is debated. Often the controversial problems pertaining to responsibility for criminal acts is involved by virtue of debate about the meaning of diagnoses. It is a theme discussed in terms of what substantively constitutes the presence or absence of mental illness. The problem stems in part from the official *Diagnostic Manual* which lists diagnoses based on varying criteria, such as etiology, or a certain symptom (running away, hyperkinesis, etc.), without seeing the place of these behaviors developmentally and in terms of what place and meaning any bit of behavior has. In the Second Edition of the *Diagnostic and Statistical Manual of Mental Disorder* in 1968 a special category was created for dyssocial behavior under the rubric of "without manifest psychiatric disorder." *Antisocial personality* is still retained under "personality disorders" and presumably under mental disorders. A third edition is in the offing which has been under debate and discussion for years.

The distinction in the dyssocial group appears based on introducing a cultural or sociogenic basis into diagnoses to distinguish those who are antisocial based on what was normative in their childrearing experiences and continues as such in their current cultural setting. Some show aggressive and destructive trends consonant with their neighborhood group, gang, or family, although incongruent with the demands of society at large. Another group is composed of those who deviate from the culture because of development outside that of the majority. They may have been nurtured in isolated rural settings or exposed to subcultural influences of a religious or pseudo-religious type which permit them to behave in ways different from the society at large.

Sexual deviation is another category that could be included under personality disorders. It will not be discussed further here since it was covered in an earlier chapter. Again, symptomatic sexual deviation is possible with any number of diagnoses, such as neurosis, psychosis, cerebral dysfunction, and different types of personality disorder. It may reflect subcultural influences from the group in which a person has developed. Developmental deviations or transient sexual disturbances during adolescence should be distinguished clearly from internalized and persistent conflicts which indicate a more entrenched personality disorder and not something developmental or reactive.

Cyclothymic (Depressive) Personalities. These individuals have a particular diathesis toward occasional antisocial behavior. Again, caution is needed. It cannot be said that the majority of individuals with depressive tendencies engage in delinquent or criminal acts, unless we take a psychodynamic perspective and realize that psychologically we are all delinquents. If anything, the depressed adolescent is likely to resort to borderline social conduct at times or periodically utilize acting out defenses. What are the general personality characteristics that emerge in the depressive-prone during their development? Observationally, they appear conscientious and serious. Qualities of reliability, somberness, and a low mood tendency are conveyed. There is a tendency to worry, revealed in their demeanor. It appears difficult for them to join in with humor—particularly if it is at the expense of someone else. When these predisposing traits give rise to a more overt clinical picture, a diagnosis of some type of neurotic or psychotic depression is made, although I have indicated elsewhere that this is the most widely missed diagnosis in childhood and adolescence.[8]

From the development of overcivilized qualities which predispose toward depressions, a compromise is sought by adolescence. An increased possibility of reacting to rejections or overreacting to losses, failures, frustrations, and disappointments then exists. Some emphasize antecedent developmental problems in the areas of object loss, attachment, and dependency. Others stress failures in self-esteem systems. While there is an overt interest in helping others and self-sacrifice, a parallel wish to be a recipient is present as well. Needs to receive are often denied and concealed. In its place ideas of self-reliance, autonomy, and a need to demonstrate superiority are consciously emphasized. When these wishes are thwarted, the entire self-esteem system is thrown into disarray with mobilization of anger and rage. Nor should the high guilt level in the depressed person be ignored. Guilt may be related to the diverse ways they have sought alleviation, coupled with a need to be critical of themselves and their achievements to an exaggerated degree. These factors guarantee the maintenance of a high level of frustration, and also aid the control of hostility when the right occasion arises. Repression of hostility and aggression operate indiscriminately by overgneralization.

An adolescent who feels inferior compared to others behaves in a manner befitting such a feeling. Unfortunately, if they brood about their plight, depressive moods are sustained. While others see these youths as compliant, polite, decorous, subservient, conciliatory, or even ingratiating, the clinician is more realistic in seeing these behaviors as serving the function of denying the amount of hostility and countering it by reaction formations. Sincerity is not challenged. If things do not go too far awry, their great dependability and literalness lead their peer group to give them positions of responsibility, and if they are not too self-effacing, these commendations can be enjoyed. Having the respect of others is important, but, as with so many aspects of the depressive-prone, it can feed disappointments. When their dependency needs are thwarted, or self-esteem becomes deflated, they are faced with the threat of outright aggression or extractive demands laid on others for emotional support to an increasing degree. If there are breakthroughs of aggression, the expression can vary from petty pilfering to more sophisticated offenses, such as embezzlement, forgery, or bribery. At the same time, the occurrence of such acts, in someone whose personal standards have typically been so high, is particularly humiliating. A vicious circle results with increasing discrepancy between the ego-ideal and behavior.

One last compromise exists in the young depressive. When younger, the child handled the situations giving rise to depression either by hyperactivity and motor discharge as one alternative or emotional withdrawal as a defense. When depression emerges in adolescence, the pattern of acting out motorically is again present as something that will give immediate relief. While this need not involve delinquent acts, it does have the threat in it of hopes that drugs, alcohol, sex, or exciting escapades will relieve the discomfort.

Masochistic (Pain-dependent) Personalities. These individuals have personality components which can co-exist in all the personality types discussed. Unresolved theoretical problems abound when inquiry is made into the ontogenesis and nature of masochism. The question of why people often act against their own best interests remains preplexing and fascinating. Such theoretical issues as the primacy of love over sadism, and masochism as a reflection of some biological urging toward destruction and dissolution (the death insinct) are relevant.

Operationally, those with masochistic tendencies are said to seek unpleasure for the sake of pleasure. However, developmental observations with children reveal that rather than pain being experienced as pleasurable, the pain is a necessary condition for the experience of pleasure. These tendencies are not confined to any one area of life. Masochistic tendencies in the sexual sphere are seen as only one minor grouping which can result. Nor are formulations of females as innately masochistic, in some presumed biological way, seen as other than a cultural compliance and rationalization of a set of attitudes which have developed in response to masculine anxieties.

The historical term for individuals who develop the anomaly of pain-dependency is that of *moral masochism*. Moral masochists court disappointment, defeat, and self-punishment in diverse ways and settings. Some patterns gain a tenacious hold. By adolescence, a smooth-functioning masochistic character may be experiencing minimal guilt. When things go too well, discontent and anxiety become manifest and lead to a need to provoke others. When the provocation is responded to, a feeling of being hurt followed by self-righteousness occurs. Being humiliated or punished alleviates anxiety, but it also serves as a source of power over others. The technique is that of provocateurs enjoying the power which forces others to punish them. By that route the victim actually becomes the one controlling the perpetrator. It is important to keep in mind that there are masochistic components present in many personalities, and what attains clinical attention is often a matter of degree. They can all induce megative therapeutic reactions.

Masochistic tendencies have the potential to become directly connected with antisocial behavior. They do not simply provoke it, but they display a correlative need to be victimized. Their tendencies to complain and whine make them unpleasant, and on occasion others take the invite and put them down. The putdown may involve physically assaultive behavior, sexual or otherwise, or be confined to others humiliating them by verbal and social devices of ridicule, shame, and exclusion which man has perfected. Pushed to an extreme, acting out behaviors function as masochistic provocations. Consider the rebelliousness of adolescents in this regard. In some cases masochistic gratification is obtained by courting punishment, such as in the commission of a crime. More subtle forms occur, such as living outside the mainstream of society, which provides a comforting sense of being excluded—the "poor little me" syndrome. The attempt to make others feel bad, is an elaboration of tendencies to make others feel they are the oppressors. The adolescent girl who repeats cycles of letting boys use her is a classic, often rationalized as due to social forces, which may contribute but is not sufficient as an explanation.

DISSILLUSIONMENT AS PART OF NEUROTIC CONFLICT

Manifestations of Disillusionment. Disillusionment plays a key role in adolescent turmoil. The main antecedent is the role of idealizing others. It is apparent to those who deal with adolescents that —in contrast to the picture of moral laxity which is often presented—they are often struggling with a harsh set of moral demands. The prominence of manifestations of greediness, noisy chaos, messiness, and preoccupations with bodily sensations and pleasures, makes this difficult to accept. Experimentation with drugs or alcohol, wild racing of cars on highways, promiscuous sexual activity, or overt expressions of aggression and fighting, elicit condemnation by those in positions of authority—teachers, parents, clergy, judges, attorneys, and physicians—who experience concern over these behaviors.

Open displays of primitive aggression and sexuality, which adults have struggled with in terms of taming their own desires, reinvoke what has been precariously socialized and long repressed. By understanding the struggle with disillusioned figures, adolescents can best be assisted to resolve conflicts which lead to personal turmoil of a self-destructive type. The most vitriolic adolescent conceptualizes adults as those who possess the power which they must struggle against. Verbalizations are in terms of struggles for freedom, equality, and individuality. A parallel theme is the disillusionment which occurs with adults whom they know, or to causes they once embraced. In the course of therapy, a quiet, lonely, isolated, and perplexed individual exists for whom intimacy between adults and themselves has broken down.

In the context of confusing developmental stances, the role of disillusionment gives an explanatory framework. A prominent idealization of parents has occurred in the course of the child's development. Throughout childhood, parents are not experienced as fully loving, nor are they necessarily kind or attentive. In fact, parents can be angry, aloof, and depriving. When children feel alone and overwhelmed, they have to tolerate deprivations without the presence of a parental figure to support and comfort them. At times the threat of abandonment or death arises. The parent is appraised cognitively and affectively as omnipotent. The ego defends itself from these threats by a process of ego-splitting. While some feel this concept is a slippery one, it does have descriptive meaning in the sense of the good qualities of the parents being retained while dissonant aspects are ignored. More is conveyed than repression, which is actually an intersystemic process between the ego and id. The split is intrasystemic within the ego, which permits reality to be disavowed so that only idealized elements are accepted. The result is an idealization of parents as just, and who, with benevolent omnipotence, control those under their rule-giving.

These processes are not confined to the realm of psychopathology. They are part of normal child development where adults are idealized as those available to take care of them and possess unlimited knowledge and power. This puts an unbelievable burden on parents, who often respond by denying this role. The overt refusal of the parent to play such a role by expressed disclaimers offers little relief. During the elementary school years the idelization begins to dissolve when the child becomes aware of the split between the idealized and some of the actual behavior, which often falls far short. There is the general duplicity present in parents who uphold cultural norms. Common examples are preaching morality and honesty, while ignoring the gross discrepancies before their eyes. When younger, these discrepancies are not noticed by children because of their enormous need to idealize. At best, in the course of empirical experiences, the idealization diminishes. When children have a strong need to continue such idealization—despite a growing contradiction by reality—they enter adolescence in a vulnerable state. Their need to maintain love and affection for their parents, and avoid hostility toward them, means that if idealization is lost it will be very painful but will heighten the probability of ego disorganization. Efforts at denial may eventuate in desperate efforts to avoid seeing imperfections in one-time heroes. A grossly exaggerated adaptation is based on desperate efforts to maintain outworn figures. What results is a conflict to maintain parental norms, minimize avoidance of the stress of peer identification, and bypass adolescence by being overly good. Developmentally, the behavior is either arrested or regressive.

Maintenance of narcissistic idealizations at such a price has become psychopathological. Rather than struggling to maintain the idealizations, a leap into nonconformity may emerge. A dramatic change from a previously well-behaved and conforming preadolescent into one whose reputation spreads as that of an acter-outer begins. Reality contact is maintained, as these adolescents are not in the midst of a psychotic process, but psychotic episodes can occur. Most common is an abandonment of the idealizations including the good aspects of the parental objects. All that has previously been held good now is viewed as stupid and hypocritical, and a general feeling of being oppressed by authority figures or institutions is experienced. An angry, bitter disillusionment is experienced by the ego.

Disillusionment is not just conscious disappointment. In young children, the beginnings of disillusionment are seen in derivative expressions that they are not being treated fairly, or being unjustly criticized or put upon by authorities. They are conveying not being perceived as they truly are, but rather as someone who is worse off than they believe they are. In contrast, the previous idealization has seen the adult figures or institutions as much superior or more perfect than they truly are. Subtle psychological processes occur in families where the parents project their own unacceptable impulses or hates onto the child. In turn, conflicts sensed in the parents are seen in the children. Gathering such insights can be extremely helpful to clinicians working with adolescents since it permits a degree of tapering of the disillusionment.

The more disparity exists in reality, the greater the potential for disillusionment. Nor is this confined to a conflict between the conscious conveyances of the parent to the child; many covert and unconscious attitudes of people and institutions which are transmitted to a person in the course of his life also become sources of disillusionment. Conflicts exist between sheltered, overmet dependency gratifications within a home in the course of rearing, and the harsh reality of the world and peer group during adolescence who are unwilling to meet such demands. The situation can become complicated by the permissiveness currently present for obtaining sexual gratifications or early narcissistic endowments. While a parent adapts to openness in terms of accepting sexuality or aggression, this is too simple a formulation in terms of the need to synthesize diverse components. A sexually enticing daughter is not just an object of beauty for a mother who is declining in her own attractiveness along with a diminishing sense of capacity. Similarly, the athletic prowess of an adolescent son may not solely be a matter of pride for a father who feels his own physical abilities diminishing.

Adolescents sense the attitudes and feelings. They may verbalize statements about how parental emphasis on ideals is used to criticize them. An almost unlimited variety of experiences within families is seen clinically. In many situations parents project their own unresolved anxieties, depressions, and disavowed impulses which are then seen in their adolescent offspring. A few examples: a widowed mother represses her own sexual desires, but her children during adolescence arouse great anxiety in her by their open sexual expressions; an unhappy woman survives marriage by affairs and then experiences anxiety about her adolescent's sexual behavior. The adolescent feels unjustly accused and engages in altercations— verbal or physical—with her parents without knowing why. In some cases, a parental marriage has survived on the basis of a neurotic interaction when discontent with a spouse is displaced onto the children. Of course, when the child becomes an adolescent and is no longer willing to continue as the butt of parental discontent, the marriage shows signs of trouble. Many of these marriages have involved unresolved problems between the parents of acquiescence versus assertiveness. Strivings for dominance between them have never been resolved. The adolescent caught up in the situation senses a feeling of injustice and is readily aware of parental inconsistencies.

Without therapy things continue at this level and are not resolved. While the parent may disparage the attempts of their adolescents to receive therapy, and many of them refuse personally to involve themselves in treatment, the adolescents are puzzled once the situation of not necessarily being the culprit is clarified. They are puzzled by the attempt of parents to undermine therapy or to ridicule it as something that only weak people or people who need people seek. On the other hand, youths may be puzzled that their parents have sent them for treatment. Such an adolescent is caught in the midst of parental pressures to remain the same, i.e., weak, and if therapy begins to progress so that many of the axioms begin to be questioned, the parents move in more aggressively to challenge the therapeutic process. Some of these adolescents under such stress regress into utter conformity and acceptance of parental norms. Their need to maintain parental idealization proves the overwhelming victor.

CASE ILLUSTRATIONS

Case 1. In a typical manner a seventeen-year-old youth with a scholarship at a leading university proceeded to blow it. During his first several months much time was spent drinking, using drugs, and driving to adjacent schools where girls he knew attended. At the end of the first semester, he failed two courses. Both parents expressed disbelief when informed since they had not previously witnessed such behavior. In reality, the boy had been chafing during high school and experiencing anxiety not communicated to the parents; nor did they wish to see it on the few occasions in high school when it erupted. Their strict conformity, an emphasis on will power and hard work as providing solutions to life's problems, eventually led them to heap scorn on their son when they realized such rules were not working. Their reliance on this professed creed had kept them from examining the brittleness of their own value system. Its manifest failure in their son mobilized their defenses and aggression to preserve their security.

Expulsion from college and a profound depression led to a psychiatric referral. Once home the boy sought out and settled down into his pre-existing state of a preoccupied and anxious youth. From the day of his return his parents urged him to get some spine and go back to college and conquer it. Evenings, when sitting with his parents in their home, the boy found himself slipping up to his room for a drink out of a bottle of liquor "to be able to tolerate my parents." After a few interviews he expressed his own ambitions and ideals, which were quite at variance with his parents. Plans had been made on his own to live apart from his parents, continue therapy, and decide in the future if he ever wished to return to college. His next appointment was then cancelled by the parents, who stated he had finally straightened up. The father had taken his son to a Marine recruiting office where he had enlisted. Some months later while on a return leave, the boy presented externally with many of the mannerisms, carriage, and speech inflections of his father, which left a stilted impression. He mouthed platitides similar to those of his parents about contempt for those who were weak and sought to pursue their own strivings rather than engaging in pursuits of value to society or their country.

Approximately a year later a long-distance telephone call from a psychiatric hospital in a different part of the country related that the boy had received a discharge from the Armed Forces after committing a robbery. He was currently in the midst of an acute paranoid psychotic episode, being unable to differentiate a friend from an enemy, and would let no one into his hospital room. He alternated between abject pleading for forgiveness and haughtily walking about the ward with a disdainful look. The parental attitude at that time, as conveyed through staff at the hospital, was that their son had finally demonstrated he was without the substance needed in their family, and they were now disowning him.

Case 2. A different disillusionment was seen in a fifteen-year-old boy who came from a strict religious family. Developmentally there were difficulties with bed wetting until he was nine years of age. His rebellious behavior had been crushed. At the commencement of preadolescence, unruly behavior re-emerged and was first handled by pharmacological attempts to control him by his family physician. The next approach used was aversive conditioning. An episode of taking the parent's car and having an accident led to a boarding school. While there the behavior continued, and he was described as being defiant and challenging to teachers. Pranks, such as tipping over the janitor's buckets, were committed with boys who had similar problems. His initial approach in therapy was to say that he saw psychiatry as "just another type of establishment set-up" and that attempts to get him to shape up would meet with failure. A great fear of losing his autonomy and personal integrity by submission to adults was apparent. Deep attitudes of provocation, pointing to a profound need to prove that others found him intolerable, unacceptable, and would eventually try to get rid of him were recurrent.

An unfortunate secondary consequence in these youths is that they see their attacks on authorities as justified. The conflict between early verbalized ideals, such as those conveyed by strict parents, and the need to deal with the anger from disillusionment with the way parents, among others, have acted, is crucial. Therapy necessarily takes time. The suffering and anguish in relinquishing idealized images is a slow and painful process. The need to disappoint, or perhaps disillusion, someone else is extremely prominent. A person or agency who is seen as corruptible or false provides a match. A byproduct is a generalization in which ideals which can be realistically used are rejected along with the more unrealizable elements. The indifference, resentments, and standoffishness in many of these adolescents seem to be signals of a disillusionment process. An intriguing question is why it is so difficult for the human to relinquish his early idealizations and why they adhere with such tenacity. The need to separate, betray, and punish the disappointing objects of their idealization is relevant.

DEPRESSIVE CORE AND ACTING OUT

Special consideration is given in this section to the relationship between depressed adolescents and acting out behaviors because it has been so neglected in clinical and criminogical literature. The problem is not rare. While actual criminal acts may constitute a small percentage of the overall group, adolescents are developmentally in a state where needs for separation and individuation leave them more vulnerable toward mourning. When in a state of reactive depression, they are more likely to be dealing with the consequences of pathological mourning, which raises the threshold for acting out behavior. The adolescent is more likely to have exaggerated and inappropriate mood responses, compared to both older and younger population groups, so this age group should be considered a high-risk category. As we have discussed in other parts of this book, the ego uses many devices to come to terms with the pains of disappointment. In fact, experiencing depressive affect as a reaction to loss is usually distinguished from a full clinical syndrome of depression or as part of an entrenched depressive character structure.

While the younger child manifests hyperactivity or apathy in dealing with disappointments, the adolescent utilizes action. This is particularly so with boys, because a passive solution to their problems seems equivalent to a blow to their masculine self-esteem.[9] Hence, apathy and depression stand in contrast to assertion and activity. While the former approach acquiesces to what seems a dismal reality, the latter carries the threat of harming the self or others by way of assertiveness or aggressiveness to modify an intolerable situation. They justify their behavior by stating they choose not to participate, compete, or strike out for new successes. The pattern is seen increasingly in young women, who no longer see their self-esteem contingent primarily on being loved and pleasing others rather than attempting to alter their unhappy situations.[10]

Since depressed adolescents are usually not psychotic, they are painfully in contact with the world. The defenses employed by the psychotic, such as delusional compensations, are not available. The situation of powerful contact with others where one feels depleted or diminished continues to be experienced. Even brief episodes of flighty activity, corresponding to hypomania, are all too intimately tied to the pain with which one is attempting to cope. Especially with the adolescent, a good deal of impulsive behavior and agitation can be seen. In fact, there are several phases to the depressions of adolescence, and what makes things confusing diagnostically is the seemingly rational basis for their acts. Some protect themselves against losses by projecting responsibility onto the environment; others intrapunitively assume responsibility for all that happens to them, but they behave as though hard work and dedicated service will avoid depressions. The former appear angry and attacking, while the latter are seeking to please to the point of sacrificing their own best interests to others—a form of altruistic surrender. The former have their defenses directed against helplessness, while the latter have their defenses directed against hopelessness.[11]

If either of these defense systems break down, the feeling of being helpless emerges with a parallel state of despair. Faith and hope as reaction formations give way. In the type of cognitive deficit present in the depressed, the self-depreciatory capacity becomes vastly overexaggerated, just as the despair about the world ever changing persists. It is not only that they feel worthless, but that they formulate the problem in terms of their own deficits being responsible for the predicaments of others as well as themselves. While suicide occurs as a possible option, a more probable solution is to act out. The depressed state with a lowering of self-esteem is a predisposing state for the commission of acts which can take on a criminal element. In fact, most every type of criminal act is possible within a depressed ego state. This can vary from petty pilfering to homicide.[12]

> One boy, aged sixteen, lost his mother due to a malignancy. He began to drink liquor quite heavily with boys about two years older. However, in contrast to the drinking which began as a group phenomenon, he would wander off alone once drinking. It was during one of these intoxicated episodes that he attacked and raped a woman in her twenties.
>
> Another boy of sixteen had become quite apathetic and withdrawn, accomplishing little in the way of school work for over a year. His life became brighter when a friend of his deceased father, who had once been in prison with his father, recruited him to participate in burglaries. A mixture of identifications, pride in taking on a role his father once had, and a lifting of the state of apathy, all provided sufficient rewards. While this boy was viewed as a typical case of a juvenile on the path toward an adult criminal career (which might be so), what was missed in this case, and so many like it, was the background of loneliness and sadness from which no escape seemed possible. A good deal of anger and resentment about a potentially hopeless existence was simply seen as an anger based on social class disparity.

Many examples are possible of a minor yet more prevalent type. The depressed adolescent girl who seeks reassurance against loneliness through sex is one type. Neurotic character structures may handle depression by symbolic means. One girl alternated between overeating when depressed on some occasions and shoplifting on others. After either type of binge she felt terrible and condemned herself as a bad and worthless person. Some of these situations appear related to the alterations of some idealized figure who is found to be human rather than some type of supermoralistic model which the adolescent is trying to emulate. When a sixteen-year-old girl realized her father was not happy with her mother, as he had falsely been reassuring her, she first became depressed. Then, with a devil-may-care attitude, she began to carry on sexually with a large number of boys she knew only slightly.

One type of depressed adolescent who begins to act out, sometimes involving direct criminal acts, is the individual we have mentioned who has suffered a severe disillusionment as a precipitating factor in a depression. The disillusionment can function to allow anger to be expressed against others, and in this manner it limits the amount of heightened self-criticism which exists. The exaggerated perfectionism and goodness ascribed to certain adult figures, whereby they are all good and the youth all bad, is transferred into a reversed pattern.

The parental figures, or their equivalents, are seen as responsible for their plight. A sudden clarification occurs, so they feel wised up. All that their former idealizations stood for begin to be attacked. Lacking faith in former commitments, they act contrary to accepted norms. Property offenses such as robberies or burglaries occur, or they can commit precipitous acts of a homicidal nature. Such acts can be interpreted as an immature ego unable to integrate the ambivalence toward others with the ambivalence of others toward itself. The ego defect is in not being able to perceive the same object as being both good and bad. The overidealization on the one hand and the need for reformation on the other signify disturbances in object relationships.[13] Actual object losses function as a contributing variable, since the capacity to mourn is impaired.

THE SIGNIFICANCE OF SPECIAL OFFENSES: PROPERTY

Incidence. Among the various behaviors which bring the neurotic character into legal difficulties, the category of property offenses is particularly suited for their problems. This is so not only for adolescence, but also during adult years if the conflicts are not ameliorated. It is for this reason that special consideration is given to illustrate some of the possibilities in which conflicts with regard to possessions, power, control, and manipulation of others are played out. The types of property offenses are almost legion. Table 18 illustrates some of the major possibilities which vary in frequency, depending on the age and conflicts of a particular person.

TABLE 18

Major Types of Property Offenses
Other than Intended

A. Property Transferred (Involuntarily)

1. Burglary

2. Robbery

3. Larceny-Theft

   a. shoplifting
   b. sneaking objects from stores or offices
   c. stealing from hotels and apartment buildings
   d picking pockets
   e. jewelry counter substitutions
   f. returning goods fraudulently
   g. buying or receiving stolen property

4. Auto Thefts

5. Shakedowns and Extortions

It is desirable to ask what special contributions psychiatry can make to the many criminological works extant about such offenders. In fact, it is particularly because of many works which discuss property offenses in great detail but omit the clinical components that this particular area is given special consideration. Only a brief resume will be given of the descriptive aspects of this group. The stage will be set for some psychiatric perspectives to give additional degrees of insight. Unfortunately discussions often end once the legal categories of offenses are given, coupled with data about the incidence of different offenses, or the percentage increase in offenses from year to year.

Theoretical Differences. There is no intent to recapitulate the material put forth in chapter nine, which dealt with the sociogenic aspects of delinquency. As noted there, whatever methodological flaws exist, the data are highly persuasive when one notes the figures with reference to property crimes. Figures of 84.6 percent for auto thefts, 85.2 percent for burglaries, 77.0 percent for robberies, and 77.4 percent for larceny-thefts are the incidence of arrests for those offenses perpetrated by those under twenty-five years of age. The message does seem clear that these are primarily adolescent offenses.

There are many ways to view the significance of these statistics. The historical emphasis was on the importance of protecting the vested interests of the commercial classes in a capitalistic society. Jerome Hall has treated this problem in a very scholarly manner.[14] He traced the development of the law of theft in the history of English law dating from the "Carrier's Case" in 1473 through the Industrial Revolution in the 18th century. However, the problem of why certain individuals engage in such behavior, and why a predominance of these individuals are in the younger age brackets, remains.

are rarely emphasized today since that theory has not received documentation as the predominant motive for thefts. In the absence of such documentations, what has emerged is a sophisticated version of the theory. The sophisticated approach views the commission of property crimes as related to the high value placed on private property in our society. The theory stresses the inherent contradictions existing in a society that cherishes and protects its property while at the same time enhancing the desires to an intolerable degree for individuals to acquire property.[15]

Differences must exist between those who violate the law to acquire such property and those who do not. Data are offered in support of this: offenses such as check forgery, department store pilfering, and juvenile car thefts are actually committed by adolescents who espouse the predominant values of the society which they violate. But if this is so, why are property offenses carried out? One theory is that the juvenile delinquent drifts between delinquent and nondelinquent stages of life without completely rejecting the dominant values of the larger society.[16] As he emerges into the youth culture, particularly if he lives in an area of poverty and gangs, the youth becomes identified with a criminal style of life.

It is here that Cohen's theory of gangs is important, or possibly the theory that a theft subculture is emerging, particularly when there are limited conventional and criminal opportunities to achieve successful goals. Theft then provides an institutionalized subcultural means to attain desired success status.[17]

Repeating offenses, more arrests, convictions, and sentencing, with an accompanying societal stigmatization, complete the criminological model of explanation. Committing theft instead of burglary is not seen as particularly significant. Amounts of money or property taken to obtain money are seen as the significant variable, and the search is not directed toward special variables which contribute toward being a robber or a pilferer. In support of this general theory, data are cited which show that young offenders have backgrounds of arrests in different types of property offenses.

Such criminological theorizing is not offered with the goal of entirely rejecting it. It is an appealing, if not elegant theory, in its search to integrate diverse areas about why this age group has such a high rate of property offenses. What is lacking from a psychiatric perspective is the degree of specificity to satisfy a psychological criterion for such behaviors. The discrepancy between desires and capacities goes to the point where a psychiatric explanation begins. It is unsatisfying in a clinical framework, although perhaps not in a criminological, simply to stop within a generalized framework and not to be able to explain why a particular individual behaves the way he does. The clinician who has an opportunity to evaluate and work with property offenders, juvenile and otherwise, is impressed by individual differences between those who carry on one type of property offense over another. Although someone who shoplifts may have joined in an auto theft at one time, what seems important is not the overlap so much as the one pattern being preferred or having salience.

Pursuing this argument further, persistent patterns of robbery behavior are not the same as for shoplifting. Even though the same youth might, at times, carry out both, what seems important is to find an explanation for why he deviates into carrying out a different type of property offense when he does. It might be that a youth joins a peer group to carry out an auto theft and is apprehended, but this is quite different from his more typical patterns of property offending. It is this type of specificity-seeking that gives cogency to the contribution a psychiatrist can make to the problem of crime. For, even if a high percentage of arrests for property offenses are in the under-twenty-five age category, as all the evidence bears out, the problem why all youths are not conventional criminals is not answered. While almost every adolescent commits some minor delinquent or even criminal act, it is still difficult to account for why all in this age group do not, in fact, commit the same crimes. We are left in the position of offering an explanation for why some adolescents become committed to property violations and to a particular pattern of preference. We must go on to ask why the majority do not go this particular route on more than a sporadic basis.

Robbery. This is the property crime par excellence since it combines two features: use of violence along with theft. It is usually perpetrated on a stranger, in contrast to other types of violent offenses such as homicide, assault, and rape. The classical example of crime in the streets is a mugging. Yet, a good deal of ambiguity persists on a descriptive level about the offense. Our knowledge is minimal, and the absence of viable critical studies of robbers along with relevant psychodynamic formulations are much needed. If we do not even have basic descriptive data, how can we hope to go beyond and attempt more microscopic investigations on individual robbers to understand the factors in their personalities which lead in this direction?

Robbers themselves are a heterogenous group. While some carry a weapon, others assiduously avoid it. Some use toys or sham weapons. Since the elements of an act of robbery involve taking property or a thing of value in the presence of a victim by the use (or threat) of force, the elements of fear and anxiety in the victim are high. The perpetrator may make a distinction with a good deal of pride that he never carries a weapon during a robbery. However, the victim does not know whether he will be harmed or not. While robbery is largely a city crime, with two-thirds of all robberies occurring in cities with more than 250,000 inhabitants, there are subvarieties.

In terms of frequencies, half of the robberies occur in the streets.[18] In addition, robberies are classified into six categories based on the site of occurrence: commercial houses, service (gas) stations, chain stores, houses, banks, and a group for the miscellaneous. Even these categories omit details about the quality or kind of act. A street robbery can vary from a single youth without a weapon grabbing an elderly woman's purse to a gang of youths with weapons accosting a couple at gunpoint and taking their money. A liquor store may be robbed at gunpoint with liquor and money both being taken, in contrast to the furtive, hurried snatching of money from the till of a confectionary. Armed robbers are responsible for 66 percent of robberies while 34 percent are strong-arm types. Again, psychiatric formulations see these as reflecting different personality features. If an armed robber carries a firearm, as 66 percent do, this has a different significance than relying on a knife, as 24 percent do. Is it important to seek explanations for such differences? It is to the extent that we lack basic knowledge about these offenses, and we are even more restricted in formulating hypotheses about the choice of offense.

In a gun-infested culture such as in the United States, possession of guns not only becomes part of male gender identity, but it has ramifications in terms of exerting control over others. In one study, manliness was seen as equivalent to forcing others to do their will by utilization of a gun.[19] The acquisition of money was not seen as the most important element, but rather the brief moment in forcing others to follow commands. The sense of omnipotence over others rather than a desire to hurt people appears as one of the chief characteristics. The males were not large physically, nor were they overtly aggressive. Being able to possess a gun was the means to meet power needs. An interesting consideration is what would happen if handguns were restricted.

If these formulations are correct for males, what can be said about females, who make up 7 percent of arrests for robberies according to the Uniform Crime Reports? Is this a power device, or are additional components operating? These formulations can be pursued in clinical work with the perpetrators as well as with the victims. While obtaining money is one motive, it is obviously not the only one. Among other things, the victim not only loses money or property, but runs the risk of serious personal injury. The emotional reaction to a traumatic situation cannot be ignored, since a panoply of reactions is possible, depending on the victim. Emotional consequences may be seen many months later in predisposed victims of crimes, in the form of continuous reworking of the episode in the form of anxiety attacks, nightmares, and ruminations.

From this amorphous mass of possibilities regarding robberies, typologies are created. Most criminological approaches focus on the role and location of the victim of a robbery. A classic English study developed a classification of robbery incidents utilizing the following:[20]

1. Robbery of persons who were in charge of money and goods as part of their employment
2. Robbery in the open following sudden attack
3. Robbery on private premises
4. Robbery after short associations such as for heterosexual or homosexual purposes
5. Robbery in cases of previous association of some duration, such as between friends, lovers, and workmates

As might be predicted, the first two categories constituted about 75 percent of robberies in London during the time of the study (from

1950-1960). These categories are similar to those employed by the FBI in the Uniform Crime Reports. However, they tell us little about the individuals perpetrating the robberies. When further information is sought, we are forced back to the level of description, such as incidence among youth age groups, and rates of apprehension related to socio-economic class.

There have been attempts to classify robbers, but these rely on variables such as extent of commitment to crime, degree of planning in executing the crime, and the reasons for carrying out acts. One typology utilized sixty-seven inmates who were serving time for robberies committed in Boston between January 1, 1968, through June 30, 1970, although twelve of the group claimed to be innocent at the time of the study.[21] Robbery offenders were classified into four groups: the professional, the opportunist, the addict, and the alcoholic. The professional robber was classified as the public stereotype of the committed robber. Robberies were planned by him, carried out with accomplices, and large sums of money were obtained to support a hedonistic lifestyle.

The opportunist category was more frequent. They are younger, without a long-term commitment to robbery, and commit other forms of theft such as larceny and shoplifting. The sums obtained by robbery here are small—often less than twenty dollars. In contrast to the commercial establishments targeted by the professionals, they choose elderly ladies with purses, drunks, cab drivers, and people who walk alone on dark streets. Their desires are for more spending money, nice clothes, or cash in their pockets to impress their peers they are doing all right. Weapons are rarely carried, and the group presence itself functions as a weapon to pressure the victims in many cases.

Addict robbers comprise a group which varies from hardline narcotics users to a mixture of those using psychotomimetic drugs. Some of these robberies are related to needing money for drugs, while others are connected to the impact on their behavior from taking the drugs. The last category is similar to the fourth category—the alcoholic robber. Some of these youths commit robberies to obtain money for alcohol, some commit an assault and robbery in the context of being intoxicated, and other robberies appear to be impulsive acts which lead erroneously to impressions that robberies occur randomly.

These descriptions illustrate the gap that remains despite the best of such studies on robbery. Many deficits exist for what a clinician feels are essential components in understanding behavior. As valuable as many of the criminological studies have been for classifying robbers and their victims, they do not give us a picture either of the internal psychodynamics of particular robbers, or of the milieu they were in at the time. In that sense, they leave us devoid of depth understanding of the motivations which amalgamate into a final common pathway for different types of robbery.

To extend our psychiatric understanding of youths who commit such crimes, we must keep in mind that an element of violence has an equal role in the act of taking in a robbery. We have a confluence of psychological motives which go beyond monetary reward as part of the act. The physical aggression involved in putting a victim in fear is an essential psychological motive. Again, keep in mind that the legal distinction for an act of physical assault—to threaten or harm another person or to strike out at him—is also present in robberies. The need is to understand the act as stemming from degrees of conscious and unconscious conflicts. If the victim is not put in fear of harm, the psychological significance of the act is missed. In the absence of putting the victim in fear, we are in the realm of more concealed or sneakily performed property offenses which have a different psychological meaning.

Similarly, youths who carry weapons are reacting to different motivational components within them than those who do not. Utilizing a pocket knife carries a different significance than carrying a pistol, and in turn a dime-store toy pistol is different from an actual pistol. The distinction about whether an actual pistol is loaded or not is also significant. It does not require a depth inquiry to see that a young male who has to put someone in great fear, by way of possessing a weapon which can maim, is reacting to more than a simple need for money. If an individual feels confident in his power needs and assertiveness, the need to challenge another with a weapon is minimized. Yet, how inconsistent with the conscious image of the robber as well as that of the general public. For, far from being a powerful and feared person, on clinical investigation, we begin to see these youths as threatened human beings whose anxieties are so great they need a weapon to confront another person rather than facing him man to man. Hence, a corollary is that the more potentially destructive the actual weapon carried by the robber, the more threatened and inadequate he feels, and the more need he has to defend his image of strength as a reaction formation by actually carrying out an act of violence.

Is this line of psychodynamic thinking consistent with the external referents for this group of offenders? In many ways it is. If we ask why the young robber feels such a great need not only to put others in a state of fear, but to take their money or possessions, we enter the realm of his strong social needs—to belong, to have status, or machismo. It can be accomplished by buying expensive things such as bikes, motorcycles, cars, clothes, drugs, and eventually graduate to the level of expensive apartments and women—the hallmarks of the super-male. Within this subcultural group, he remains an utter conformist, just like the supposedly deviant adolescent within his group.

Another component in acts of robbery is exhibitionism. Since there is a connotation of daring in the act, status accrues. The risk-taking involves components of histrionic dramatization, self-display, and a supposed degree of individual courage. That many of these acts are counterphobic in nature is not known to those perpetrating the robbery or to those who adulate. The open and daring qualities of the robbery, in contrast to the stealth of the burglar, are what give these youths their status. The connection with unresolved needs for applause and approval at almost any price in some robberies is related to a grandiose component. Unresolved problems in the realm of narcissism need to be dealt with if any effective resolution is to take place short of waiting until they reach the fourth decade of life and begin to burn out. The popular image of male sexual identity connected with the risk-taking youth is consistent.

In many ways the bandits of old, with the endless myths about them, conveyed a similar model. Some of these were hidden under the Robin Hood mythology of taking from the rich to give to the poor. Bandits have been investigated and found to have a degree of violence which was often perpetrated to a hideous degree. Violence was used partly as a technique of terror, and partly for vengeance. In many cases, acts of violence connected with banditry were rationalized under some form of doing their own thing. In one of the most scholarly historical treatises dealing with banditry, the author comments on the physical deformities or ugliness which existed in many of the bandits.[22] They were often weak, lame, or had lost an appendage. This gave them more of an aura of being fearsome, and also contributed to their need for elegance or ostentatiousness in dress and manner.

These personal characteristics also permit an explanation for the adulation by the general public in their quest for someone else to handle their desires to acquire the possessions of others or to place them in fear. Bandits are allowed much vicarious acting out. The ambivalence witnessed in people with respect to notorious bank robbers, about whom legends and folksongs grow, is not by chance. The identification is especially possible if the robbery is enacted against a large and impersonal organization such as a bank or national chain store. The dash of the romantic bank holdup portrayed in the movie "Bonnie and Clyde" was criticized by some because the couple was portrayed at the end as being shot in swirls of blood. There was far less criticism of the falsely romanticized version of the life they were leading.

The types of psychopathology among youth engaging in robberies are multiple. While some youths are seen in the course of court evaluations prior to hearings or trials, or later in prisons, a cooperative defendant is required as well as a psychiatrist sophisticated in criminal procedure and psychopathology who is interested in acquiring research knowledge about these youths. Diagnostically, the range of standardized diagnoses vary from the neurotically conflicted to those acting out diverse unconscious needs. In some of the more bizarre cases, psychosis has been found.

> An eighteen-year-old girl, with a previous episode diagnosed as hebephrenic schizophrenia, appeared at a bank teller's window with a toy pistol. She had purchased the pistol two hours earlier at a dime-store after brooding several days on how to take a vacation with her boyfriend (a fifteen-year-old boy). Not having funds to take the elegant vacation she wished, she decided that robbing a bank would be the quickest way to accomplish it. Accordingly, she entered a bank at 2 P.M., in the midst of the peak business hour, demanded and obtained several thousand dollars. She walked out despite the automatic camera which recorded the entire event. Later that evening, when her roommates saw her counting packs of money and heard the evening news about the robbery, they connected the events and called the police. Not all females who rob banks are of this variety, but the case is mentioned to illustrate the diversity possible.

On a psychological level, the daring involved in these acts has been seen and mentioned in terms of its counterphobic quality. To take the degree of risk a robber does often requires a good deal of denial in terms of ego functioning. At times the process extends so that selective repression occurs for parts of the act, which is regarded as convenient forgetting by courts since other parts of the act are remembered. It is by way of such selectivity, coupled with ego-splitting, that the risks can be taken. The splitting allows the degree of sadism or aggression shown in some cases. Although beating a victim or pistol-whipping are possibilities, the most nonsensical is the felony murder in the course of a bank robbery. As one example, in the course of executing one of several robberies, a robber turned and simply fired at one of the helpless bystanders or guards who are standing passively by, observing and fearful. The passivity of the victims in these cases raises the anxiety and hatred of the robbers about the possibility that they might be caught in such a predicament themselves.

The denial of the event is related to the shame and humiliation of being caught, since this is quite at variance with their self-image of a powerful figure. In other cases, the aggression is so open and abrupt that parts of the picture become repressed. Sometimes behavior is so extreme as to make them appear psychotic or retarded. When seen over a period of time, hysterical defenses appear involving denial and reversal into the opposite. A violent act of aggression in the youth is followed by becoming a jester for other prisoners or engaging in clowning behavior.

Burglary. Burglary, like robbery, is a criminal behavior overwhelmingly performed by the adolescent and youth age groups. Nationally, persons under twenty-five years accounted for 83 percent of arrests for burglary in 1972.[23] The criminal law reference to "breaking and entering" to take property is now broken into three subclassifications: forcible entry, unlawful entry without force, and attempted forcible entry. Again, as with robbery, categorizing offenses gives an idea of where the crime is committed, by whom, with reference to age and location. One shorthand classification refers to "bubs" and "bobs." The bubs are "burglarizing unoccupied buildings," while bobs are "burglarizing occupied buildings." Yet these data tell us little about why which pattern of behavior has been chosen. As a segment of property crime, burglary comprises 46 percent of the total. One person may account for innumerable burglaries, but at times a group of participants account for only one. Seeing these offenses as a homogeneous statistic in terms of a standardized offense blurs the significant differences between them.

As a psychological component, the elements of stealth and opportunity are highly significant. Forcible entry accounted for 76 percent of the burglaries, while 18 percent did not involve force, and only 6 percent were attempts. Slightly more than 60 percent of robberies involved residences. As a group, night-time entries represent 61 percent of all burglaries. This distinction is significant since, by the common law, burglary in the daytime was more significant than entering a dwelling under the cover of darkness.

The psychological significance is the more open display of aggression needed for someone to enter a dwelling in the daytime.

Again, to assume that obtaining money and property is a sufficient explanation for burglary does not come to grips with why the pattern is acted out in preference to legitimate means of acquisition. If economic arguments are used to justify the acts, we must ask why all those who wish to obtain property do not do so in this particular manner. Inquiry again leads into the personality functioning in these individuals which may offer some hypotheses.

The amount of research on burglars, just as with robbers, has been minimal. That done by clinicians has been almost nonexistent. The work that has been done from a criminological perspective seems primarily interested in the professional thief who is defined as someone carrying out burglaries for monetary gain. The good burglar among his colleagues is seen not only as proficient in his work, but competent by those who are knowledgeable about burglary. Part is the code of honor among thieves whereby they do not violate the rules of professional thievery such as squawking or burning on their partners. This perspective utilizes criteria established by Sutherland in his classic work forty years ago where an attempt was made to provide a systematic analysis of the profession of theft and how it persisted as a product of social disorganization.[24]

Criteria for the professional thief is listed to illustrate two points. On the one hand, they show how scholarly a sociological analysis can be conducted with interactional implications. On the other hand, the criteria still leave us devoid of knowledge about the types of psychological structure and functioning that are present. Again, based on clinical work, burglars are not a homogeneous group any more than robbers are. Another limitation of the criminological studies is their omission of the non-professional burglar.

The following criteria are given for the professional thief: (1) The professional thief makes stealing his livelihood and regards it as an occupation. (2) A body of knowledge is utilized for planning and executing burglaries and the expertise allows one to look with contempt upon amateurs in the field. (3) It is assumed that along with specialized skills and experience, the burglar has acquired attitudes, and a working philosophy which makes him a member of the profession. (4) By processes of identification and success he becomes a member of a professional subcultural group with its own standards of integrity, recognition, and security, the professional burglar wants to belong to such a group and hold membership in it. (5) Burglaries are committed in a skilled manner so that the risks of apprehension or going to prison are minimized while the monetary gains are maximized.

What is interesting is how comparatively rare a burglar who meets all of the criteria is. In one study, a good burglar was classified as such if he received four thousand dollars or more on his largest score, and either entered a place by cutting a hole in the roof or wall, or opened the safe by drilling. Of forty-seven incarcerated burglars interviewed, only two achieved goodness.[25] First of all, the skills required to be a good burglar are not widely disseminated. To avoid being apprehended or confronted requires knowledge of how to thwart the criminal justice system by use of bondsmen and attorneys, for example. There are so many protection devices in use these days, from alarms to security guards, that the sole performer is becoming rare. To be successful, the burglar must obtain advance knowledge about what is available at a particular place and time. Not to prepare in advance can mean failure, and consequently one or more tipsters are usually involved, to increase the success ratio. Finally, if a burglar is successful in all of the above preparations, and valuable merchandise is obtained, he must have a way to dispose of the loot. Contact with criminal resources or fences is required. The relationship on a personal, social, and professional level between burglars and fences is another fruitful area for psychological investigation which has barely been scratched. In fact, stealing to order is more profitable since it eliminates the middleman as fence.[26]

It becomes apparent that most burglaries do not belong in an elite class of work done by professionals with all of the systematization and organization that requires. While the process of recruitment for professionalized burglary goes on from the group of adolescents and amateurs who come to the attention of older thieves, varieties of burglary transpire which have different motivations and contexts. Consider the following burglaries in terms of their diversities:

1. A group of adolescents scan middle class neighborhoods seeking houses that look dark, suggesting the occupants are out or on vacation. While some are seeking money, others seek goods they can easily sell, such as radios and television sets.

2. A lone house-breaker enters residential dwellings looking for check blanks to steal. An effort is made to disturb nothing in the dwelling, but to take stored check blanks since these might not bskscovered as missing for weeks or months by the owner.

3. Variations on the blank check theme are credit cards taken from homes, hotel rooms, and resorts.

4. Specialized types of stores are sought out. The more the activities verge toward organization, such as being able to dispose of the material, the more specific goods such as jewelry, are looked for in dwellings or business establishments.

5. The excitement and challenge of being able to enter a place and leave without detection takes on a meaning in its own right. While some of these youths take money if it is not concealed well, not all do so. The variations on this theme are endless. One youth on entry simply stood alone for hours on end in homes when the occupants were all asleep. Another sought a home where the occupants were gone where he would sit or explore the house or business establishment. It is interesting in this regard that Charles Manson and his followers in the Sharon Tate-LaBianca killings were reported to engage in games of breaking into homes at night and crawling around in the dark, which they called "creeping."[27] Another boy spent the night concealed in the closet of a bedroom, an act which has obvious sexual and voyeuristic implications. Another would stand near the bed of a sleeping woman without doing anything, hoping she would not awaken. A twenty-year-old entered countless apartments, usually of single working girls who he knew would be gone during the daytime. While there he would put on their underclothing and masturbate. He would leave without making it look like a burglary had occurred. If the possibility of being caught arose while he was in the dwelling, he would take some money in an effort to make it look like he was trying to escape and had dropped some money accidentally. He felt guilty about taking money although he needed to disguise the true nature of the burglary.

6. Sexual components enter into burglary in different ways. Some have been discussed earlier. A special category is a burglary in which a woman victim is on the scene. The burglar decides to take something from her sexually besides the goods he was originally seeking.

7. For historical purposes, the old fashioned safe burglar should be listed. He would enter banks or business establishments and blow off the door of the safe. Currently, it is so difficult to do this for any large establishment that such a burglar has almost become extinct, with the exception of small business or home safes. Most modern bank safes are so complicated that for practical purposes they are seldom bothered with.

What type of personality development is conducive to these of behaviors? One of the most impressive psychological features is the use of denial mechanisms, not only with respect to getting caught, but also with respect to criminally and directly taking things. In addition, there is also the element of chance, similar to gambling, in which the criminal does not know if the odds will turn out in his favor or not. In some form or another, the odds are being played out in most property offenses. It would be interesting and valuable to test whether most young burglars do not become professional burglars, but continue to handle their unresolved personal conflicts in adult life by way of more subtle property offenses, such as embezzlement, fraud, confidence games, and other types of white collar crimes. Some are able to handle these needs within the letter of the law by manipulating others as a form of taking.

Different personality traits are displayed when a victim is confronted directly with the threat of force, with or without a weapon, and the threat of losing something, as opposed to an act with more obvious skulking qualities where the burglar tries to ayoid being seen. In that sense, there is a crucial difference in the performers. The more removed nature permits the perpetrator to feel that he is not actually committing a crime. Ego-splitting is the device which allows intellectual knowledge and performance, but the appropriate degree of affect that should inhibit the behavior is lacking. Diagnostically these youths are not all sociopathic; here we are talking about types of neurotic conflict in which the degree of emergency emotions to prohibit the act are not operating to a degree sufficient to overcome the other gratifications or resolutions sought.

TABLE 19

General Differences Between Burglary and Robbery

Burglary	*Robbery*
1. The act is sneakily performed.	1. The act is direct.
2. The act avoids direct confrontation.	2. The act involves face-to-face confrontation between perpetrator and victim.
3. A closed unit (home or building) is entered.	3. Victims are usually encountered in the open.
4. A weapon is usually avoided.	4. A weapon or simulated weapon is often carried.
5. The symbolism involves the act of entering and taking	5. The symbolism is connected with putting someone in fear and then depriving them.

The ego-splitting device is reflected in depersonalization. It is clinically detected in youths who commit burglaries and are then able psychologically to explain it as though they were observing themselves perform the act. Some are aware of a surprising degree of calmness or passivity during the transction: "It was as though I wasn't doing it but someone else was." Some of these youths lack the appropriate affect with respect to taking others' possessions since they feel that the objects were actually theirs. Some degree of rationalization is requied so that their deprivation gives them special rights to take. Unresolved dependency problems loom large. An allied position is that since the objects taken are of small value proportionate to the entire value in the house, the extent of the act does not measure up to a full-fledged crime—perhaps a bit of deviousness or prankishness at best. It is amazing how this device persists through the third decade of life even when a loading van is backed up to empty the contents of the house. The persistence of underestimation of the crime is an indicator of the degree of the removal from conscious awareness which many aspects of the act have.

While the act of burglary rarely goes to the extent of a full dissociative state, the element of depersonalization is more frequent that is usually appreciated. To detect the psychological mechanism requires psychiatric sophistication. It requires a perspective and desire to discover the mental state of the burglar at the time of the act, and to see his act as more than just seeking financial gain. Some degree of not acknowledging that it is truly the person in question doing the act is present. This involves verbalizations in terms of psychological distancing from the act. Descriptions of the act as automatic or observed are part of the picture.

Variations on the theme are numerous. Some youths complain of a numbness accompanying the automaton phenomenon. Again, they are a participant in the sense of being a passive and indifferent spectator to what is going on. Despite this deadened inner state, there is no impediment to the motor component of the act. A degree of persistence to maintain the split affect is required, so that the full impact is usually not experienced by the ego during the course of the act. (When that occasionally does happen, a good deal of anxiety is experienced, which leads to feelings of doubt about identity which are valid since they are not fully integrating all aspects of their personality into a cohesive self. It is analogous to a dream state from which only fragments remain clear.)

From the degree of repression required, there is a fear of lack of control. The youth typically seeks reassurance by being close to those he knows. If the burglaries are carried out in a group, being near the group make him feel integrated. Repetition of burglaries can be counterphobic as well. The psychodynamic meaning is related to the threat being overwhelmed if the cognitive nature of the act is registered. A severe narcissistic mortification from the accompanying feeling of having lost active control and feeling helpless in terms of the repetitive behavior may be present.

A few comments are needed about the symbolic aspects of these acts, beyond specific acts of a sexual nature that are committed in the course of a burglary, such as the examples mentioned above of seeking females' underclothing, or youths who are surprised by the unexpected return of a woman during the course of a burglary and then rape her. The specific symbolic aspects are viewed in terms of the male component of breaking and entering—of going into a forbidden place—where one is not supposed to be—and taking something. The acts are categorized in terms of symbolic penetration of an unwilling object, an act equivalent to rape which is why burglary is a relatively rare act for females.

What needs emphasis is the diversity of personality types and conflicts possible in burglaries. It is one more means resorted to by an individual trying to come to terms with diverse conscious and unconscious needs and conflicts. As a final illustration of this thesis, the case of William Heirens is used.[28]

> In June, 1946, a seventeen-year-old college student, William Heirens, was arrested in Chicago after an attempted burglary. He was identified as the murderer of six-year-old Susan Degnan, who had been kidnapped and dismembered, and of an ex-Wave who had been brutally murdered in her hotel. A third murder (of a woman) was proved to have been committed by him. The killings had been savage, the bodies mutilated; on the wall of the apartment of the young Wave a message was written in lipstick: 'For heaven's sake catch me before I kill more; I cannot control myself.' A ransom note had been left in the room from which the child had been taken; parts of her body were found in sewers and drains. The citizens of Chicago were horrified by these murders, particularly because the police were powerless to identify the murderer.
>
> William Heirens' arrest was accidental. He was intercepted by an off-duty policeman when he tried to make a getaway after an attempted burglary. It turned out that the boy had a police record, having been arrested for burglaries at thirteen and fifteen. He also was arrested for carrying a gun

when returning from rifle practice at the university after the perpetration of the murders; at that time his record was not checked. He was dismissed as just a kid with a gun, and told to register the weapon.

At the age of thirteen he was apprehended by the police trying to break into a basement storeroom. Subsequently he admitted nine burglaries during the preceding six months. He was committed to a reform school where he stayed for a year. Two months after his release he was again arrested. In Juvenile Court the judge acceded to the wishes of the family, and the young criminal was placed on probation and sent to an academy. He had a satisfactory school record, was in no way conspicuous in his environment, and showed himself a devout Catholic, going to confession regularly. He visited home frequently, and his probation was terminated in January, 1945. In September, 1945, he entered the University of Chicago, where he shared a dormitory room with an older student. During the weekend leaves from the academy and during the time he stayed at the dormitory or at home he committed innumerable burglaries and three murders without those in his environment being aware of anything strange or conspicuous about him. Some loot from the burglaries was recovered from his room at the dormitory and parents' home.

The burglaries were committed in a pattern. He climbed over the fire escape into a window and frequently completed his criminal action by defecating or urinating at the place of the crime. He did not sell any of the loot but cached it away. According to his own story, he felt sexually excited before his burglaries and found a sexual release through breaking into strange apartments. When discovered in the act of breaking in, he had to kill. Apparently he became panicky since he could not make use of his usual outlets and the archaic impulses were gratified by the killing and either dismembering or mutilating victims.

The case of William Heirens is reported for several reasons: (1) the attitude of his environment up to the time of his last arrest; (2) the public reaction—general and specific—after his arrest, and (3) the reaction after his conviction.

It seems strange that a young boy could commit innumerable burglaries and three murders without anyone becoming aware of any indication of the youngster's psychopathology. It seems incredible that his parents, teachers and priests had no suspicions after his first two arrests and commitment to the academy. From twelve to fourteen he was eager to earn his own money and took odd jobs. He did not spend much money on himself, but gave expensive presents to his family out of proportion to his earnings.

Neither did anyone question the origin of the objects cached away in his room at the dormitory and at home. He was described as a likeable fellow but withdrawn; he did not have close friends, although he participated in the social activities of his club and had dates with girls. How was it possible that nobody sensed anything pathological in this severely sick boy? There is only one remark allegedly made by his mother and reported by one newspaper which, if true, may indicate her unawareness of Heirens' criminality was only a seeming one. After the discovery of the murder of Susan Degnan, she asked her son: "You would not have done such a terrible thing, would you?" How could such a question come to a mother's mind regarding a son of whose murderous impulses she is not aware?

The newspapers played up the murders to a high degree before identification of the murderer, pointing to the helplessness and inefficiency of the police and arousing a near panic in the population of Chicago. After Heirens was arrested his handwriting showed similarity to the one on the ranson note; the general concern seemed to be to elicit a confession from the boy. The confession seemed to be of tremendous importance and was obtained by methods which are of interest in connection with this topic. The newspapers reported Heirens has been subjected to an injection of sodium pentothal (truth serum) by a psychiatrist in the presence of the State's Attorney and that under the effect of the drug, he confessed to the three murders. The report was never repudiated or denied, so there is a strong possibility it is correct. Confession of the murders was deemed so important that, although a confession induced by a drug is not admissable in court according to American and British law, the method was nevertheless applied. A tremendous relief was expressed in the press and the subsequent reporting of the Heirens case for awhile showed an almost sympathetic tone. After the drug-induced confession, however, when the murder suspect refused to give a voluntary, written confession, the attitude of the newspapers changed into one of hostility and vindictiveness and again showed signs of alarm.

In early boyhood Heirens showed all the indications of a severely disturbed child. What means were employed to help him? Arrested after his burglaries, he was sent to a reform school and dismissed after a year. He was then re-exposed to his home, which must have had some part in his development. He promptly resumed his delinquent acting out, was arrested, and, on the insistence of his family, was placed on probation and sent to an academy from where he continued his criminal career. There is no mention of any attempt to have the boy treated adequately and his environment professed not to have been aware of any pathology. He entered college and still received no intervention. The collection of stolen objects in his room must have been conspicuous. Is it credible that a young boy can be so clever in deceiving everyone to such an extent without others having part in the deception?

The writing on the wall after the murder of the ex-Wave, "For Heaven's sake, catch me before I kill more; I cannot control myself," seems a genuine cry of despair. Certainly he is not the first case in history to commit murder after murder where the environment was oblivious to the situation in spite of many indications of the reality of the crimes.

Larceny-thefts. Definition and Distribution. The various larcenies and thefts constitute the largest group of felony offenses. The list includes diverse acts such as shoplifting, purse-snatching, pickpocketing, auto theft, and bicycle theft. The essential element is the unlawful taking of property or articles of value which belong to someone else with the absence of force, violence, or fraud. The intent is to deprive another of possessions.

In the days of the common law, prior to criminal codes, larceny was the only crime of theft, and robbery was one subdivision of it (classified as "larceny by force"). Types of property crimes like embezzlement, forgery, worthless checks, and con games are now viewed as separate offenses. Many legal elements and distinctions have been delineated. What constitutes unlawful or trespassory taking, carrying away of personal property, or even what constitutes another's property, are subject to legal distinctions. Similarly, to establish the element of intent to deprive another permanently has raised a host of distinctions beginning with simply borrowing. Once into modern history, distinctions of larceny by servants shifted to employees and all of the varieties of white-collar crime. The following table illustrates the distribution of larceny by type and the setting in which it occurs.[29]

For larceny thefts, the police clearance rate ("solving by arrest") is only 20 percent. Seventy percent of the adult age group prosecuted were found guilty, 6 percent were found quilty of a lesser charge, and 24 percent had their cases dismissed or were acquitted. The data are significant since even these figures are a gross underestimation of the overall incidence of larceny. First of all, police clearance reports

TABLE 20

Larceny Analysis by Type and Area (1972)

(Percent Distribution)

Area

Classification	Total United States	Cities Over 250,000	Suburban	Rural
Pocket-picking	1.0	2.0	0.4	0.3
Purse-snatching.........	2.2	4.3	0.7	0.4
Shoplifting	10.8	10.5	9.4	4.0
From motor vehicles (except accessories) ...	17.3	18.8	15.7	14.7
Motor vehicle accessories...........	17.5	20.1	18.1	13.6
Bicycles	16.5	12.1	17.5	4.9
From buildings	17.0	18.6	14.9	16.5
From coin-operated machines	1.4	1.1	1.3	1.5
All others...............	16.3	12.5	22.0	44.1
Total	100.0	100.0	100.0	100.0

Source: *Uniform Crime Reports,* 1972, p. 22.

only deal with offenses brought to their attention. Data obtained from community surveys indicate that this is only a fraction of the true incidence. Second, the *Uniform Crime Reports* deal only with larcenous offenses involving fifty dollars or more. The quantity of petty pilfering would be expected to outweigh those crimes in terms of frequency. Also note that the *F.B.I.'s* annual report does not categorize many white-collar crimes. Of the seven offenses included in the "Crime Index" (murder, forcible rape, robbery, aggravated assault, burglary, larceny over fifty dollars, and auto theft), the larceny category accounts for 45 percent of the arrests. Of these arrests, 50 percent involved individuals under eighteen, while 66 percent were under twenty-one. Another interesting facet about larceny is that it is a crime of preference for women, who are involved in 30 percent of all arrests for larceny-theft. This is a higher rate of incidence than for any other offense in the Crime Index.

Developmental Antecedents. More diversity is present psychologically in larceny thefts than in robbery or burglary. The examples could be extended endlessly, but different legal categories of larceny share a common thread of dishonesty. The objects sought and the means to acquire them reflect different developmental lines and regressions as well as different symbolic components. Taking goods off the store counter is different psychologically from chronically taking articles from an employer; in turn, they differ from devising complicated schemes for embezzling funds. Stealing a car taps different aspects of the personality than arranging a fraudulent insurance claim. The possible ways people play out their acquisitive needs to possess property, or its symbolic equivalent—money—are endless.

Two things are predominant in the cultural matrix to which children are exposed: an enormous emphasis on acquisition coupled with exhortation to be honest and not take from others. The strength of wanting to possess or take something does not reflect just socially acquired needs, important as that mode of reinforcement is. Early patternings of nourishment, attachment, and survival, as discussed elsewhere, make possessions seem vital to survival and integrity. While the chain of logic—from acquiring possessions early in childhood to anxiety about their availability to later varieties of the theft—may seem tenuous, it is a reality. The following table illustrates derivative forms of acquisitive needs:

TABLE 21

Types of White Collar Crimes

A. *Crimes by Persons Operating on an Individual,* ad hoc *Basis:*
   Tax violations, buying on credit without intent to pay, credit card frauds, bankruptcy frauds, frauds on insurance companies, etc.

B. *Occupational Crimes by Those Inside Business or Government in Violation of Their Duty of Loyalty and Fidelity to Employer or Client:* Commercial bribery or kickbacks, bank violations by employees, embezzlements, securities frauds, employee petty larceny, frauds by computer, violation of fiduciary relationships, etc.

C. *Crimes Incidental to Furtherance of Business Operations but not the Central Purpose of the Business:* Tax violations, antitrust violations, commercial bribery, food and drug violations, false weights and measurements, housing code violations, deceptive advertising, fraud against government, etc.

D. *White-Collar Crime as a Business:* Medical or health frauds, advance fee swindles, phony contests, bankruptcy frauds, security frauds, home improvement schemes, merchandise swindles, land frauds, charity and religious frauds, personal improvement schemes, fraudulent applications and/or use of credit cards, varieties of insurance frauds, etc.

Source: H. Edelhertz, *The Nature, Impact, and Prosecution of White-Collar Crime,* Washington, D.C.: National Institution of Law Enforcement and Criminal Justice, U.S. Government Printing Office, 1970, pp. 73-75.

On a basic level, it is incongruous to view all acts of taking as the same. Some acts of taking represent failure to attain and integrate aspects of personality functioning; other acts are related to a breakdown or regression in functioning; yet others are defensive, in response to psychological assaults on the developing personality.

When do we begin to think of a child's taking as tantamount to thievery? When does the act attain such a distinction? In psychiatric terms, when do we begin to see the act as a symptom reflecting psychological conflict and not the act of a developmentally premature person? Or, what if the act in question is committed by someone of legal majority but whose development in this sphere has been blocked? What significance does this have in a theoretical and practical manner?

Many stages are passed through in terms of object development related to "me" and "you" and "mine" and "thine." The notion of possession is not clear at any precise psychological point. Fantasized wishes and pleasure-seeking, as early elements in the mental life of children, begin the process of seeing the entire world as "theirs." Some developmental steps in perceiving objects as separate, individuation, cognitive development, distinguishing inner wishes from outer limits, and reality testing, are all necessary to acquire a realization of what is theirs and not theirs for children.

Based on these ideas, the concept of private property in terms of possession emerges. If the inner desires are not distinct, as they are not for the young child who is pleasure-bound, there is no inner sanction against taking whatever is available. Taking in infancy is usually connected with mouth and hand-to-mouth coordination (oral possessiveness). Later, taking as a personality trait is seen in the need to incorporate as a prominent characteristic. In the ego struggle for differentiation of the self from others, anything not pleasurable, or contravening infantile demands, is relegated to "non-ego" so that only the pleasurable is considered part of the ego— the "purified pleasure ego." Part of the process involves the use of projective mechanisms, where food is either swallowed or spit out.

An extension goes beyond the confines of immediate bodily fusion for mine and not mine. Although cognitive separateness emerges, the child still equates possessions with his own ego influences. Hence, even if an object is not in their immediate perception, it is felt to be theirs by means of wishes. When they are older, things are invested with their own ego qualities. Possessions seem as though things actually were the child's, who treats them as the ego's possessions even though the child knows they are not.

Early psychoanalytic formulations gave a good deal of emphasis to bodily products not retained through the anal orifice. Symbolic elaborations were detectable. The feces, initially part of one's own body but which become not part of one's own body, are the model. It is another way of perceiving that something that is "mine" can either be lost or given up. Again, something that is external can be invested with ego qualities in terms of being retained. These intrapsychic mechanisms include the entire social framework in which they occur and the opportunities which exist for re-enforcing trends. The possibilities for conflicts about sharing, conformity, anger, and rage, which can persist and be acted out in the area of possessiveness, become enormous. An example is leaving stools in various locations outside of toilets. Anyone who has done school consulting is aware of angry and disappointed children so behaving. Similarly, there are reports from burglary scenes where a stool is left at the site with a fairly obvious message of what is being conveyed. Yet in developmental terms a part of the self is also being left as a fecal calling card. In the Middle Ages, those who were bankrupt or unable to pay their debts were given strong purges.

The connection between money and stools has been elaborated in clinical publications. Its significance is an additional paradigm for confusion about possessions of the self and others. Ferenczi presented a developmental model in terms of displacement from feces to money.[30] The excrement is regarded as the first savings account, and has to do with later collecting or hoarding. The process is one of deindividualization, in that feces, like money, are not distinctive from one person's possessions or another. Feces and money seem to lose the ego quality of belonging to one person. Yet this contributes to their devaluation as well, for the stool no longer possesses its pristine qualities. Filthy stool is like filthy money later on. The quest for distinctiveness is not given up, as witnessed by the fascination with special or shiny coins. A formulated developmental sequence goes like this:

1. Playing with stool as an infant
2. Playing with mud (deodorized stool)
3. Need to avoid "getting dirty" with mud marks
4. Interest in sand (cleaner and dehydrated) or clay
5. Play with sticks, stones, pebbles, and other earth objects
6. Marbles and coin collection as hobbies
7. Shiny coins
8. Interest in things that signify value or possession (paper money, stock shares, bankbooks)

The emotional reactions accompanying these progressions raise the potential for acting out in antisocial ways, but more specifically in terms of distorted needs for possession. If one feels "cleaned out" but yet in need of the "filthy stuff," conflict is imminent. If one is to do one's duty by giving up "dirty habits," one must be able to find other outlets for feeling deprived of things to possess and manipulate. Of course, taking from others is only one possible outcome. To manipulate others—their bodies and property—is another.

Along the pathway from interest in one's own body and its possessions to others, the formulation of transitional objects has relevance.[27] The formulation is based on the well-known observation that in infancy, parents give the children some special object along with the expectation that they will become attached to it. The significance is that it is the first "not-me" possession. Hence, a doll, teddy bear, or soft toy replaces the fist-in-mouth activities and eventually leads to a hard toy. But intermediate between the thumb and these toys—between oral activities per se and true object relationships—are transitional phenomena and objects which at first arise on the level of illusion. The illusion arises in the context of the thumb in mouth, or hand around the mouth, where the child takes an external object such as part of a sheet or a blanket into its mouth with the fingers. The object is often what is most readily available, such as a napkin or handkerchief, and accompanying the taking are humming sounds. When a particular object is singled out as vitally important, such as a blanket in going to sleep as a reassurance against anxiety, we have a transitional object.

The object continues as important and especially so during times of loneliness and when depressive moods threaten. Special qualities in the relationship exist. The infant asserts rights over the object which is not supposed to change or be altered. It is affectionately cuddled but can be banged around, hence it must survive loving and hating. The child views the object as not necessarily outside of him, as adults do, but he knows that it also does not come from within. Over time it gradually loses its intense emotional investment. Without progressing into all the ramifications of transitional objects, they are mentioned because of their significance not only in object development but in their potential for behavioral ramifications about possessions. By way of the mother's special adaptation to the child's needs, the child develops the illusion that what he creates really exists. Developmental pathology is seen in the areas of fetishism, origin and loss of affectionate feelings, drug addiction, obsessional rituals, and in lying and stealing. Stealing is a psychopathological outcome in terms of the difficulties an individual has in bridging the gap in the continuity of experience with respect to a transitional object.

The Psychodynamic Aspects of Theft. The differential diagnostic possibilities of anti-social behavior in the adolescent have been considered earlier. In essence, the clinician first appraises whether stealing is associated with incomplete or arrested growth involving areas of what is "mine" or "not mine." Questions occur: Might certain cognitive or intellectual abilities be limited? Are certain pathways of object development involved and limited and, if so, at what stage? Are there specific deficits in superego functioning? Beyond this, there is the possibility that initial development may be intact, but some type of regression has occurred. The question of what degree of balance exists between desires to possess versus degree of ego control is relevant. The balance can be phrased in terms of effective socialization models, but clinically it is a deficiency in ego dominance over desires. Finally, is the act of theft a compromise formation—meaning that neurotic symptom formation has occurred?[32]

Given the initial diagnostic perspective, there are categories to be considered for theft on a neurotic basis.

1. Theft as an expression of aggression is initially considered, since some of these aspects have already been dealt with in discussions of robbery and burglary. Yet a distinction does exist between putting someone in fear of harm by way of a direct confrontation with a weapon, or breaking and entering into a dwelling and taking something from them, and the other ways that stealing is the act of taking something from another. Emotions of envy and accompanying rage are relevant. An adolescent boy without a bicycle takes one from a ramp. A girl without the jewelry she wishes pilfers from a dime-store. Although the acts of larceny conceal aggression, by virtue of their hidden and deceptive qualities, the aggression in taking from another is always present. The most direct formulation views stealing as having satisfactions akin to those achieved in perpetrating a homicide. "Whether based on a symbolic unconscious need or analyzable as a contest of skill and finesse, the psychological fact is this: success at larceny provides ego gratification closely akin to those creative satisfactions postulated to underlie the impulse toward homicide."[33]

2. Stealing as a reflection of unresolved dependency needs from parental figures is another major grouping. This taking should be distinguished from the types of antisociality discussed in connection with sociopathic personality disturbances or those seen in "affectiveless psychopaths." This is not simply a developmental arrest, where mothering and caretaking have been grossly deficient. In the neurotic category, there are often symbolic equivalents for what is being taken. One adolescent girl, whose mother had been intermittently depressed most of her life, alternated between eating binges and stealing. As expected, her thefts were often food and candies from supermarkets or department stores. A variation leaves the child potentially liable to have difficulties with drugs or alchohol. While the degree of impulsiveness is impressive in these adolescents, their unresolved depressions appear more important. In that context, stealing is a defense against experiencing the full brunt of depressive symptomatology. Since many of these adolescents are quite likeable, radiating a need for attachment, they seek ways to parentify relationships. Unfortunately, if they feel slighted or rejected, they act out their anger.

Alice was an attractive sixteen-year-old who most teachers at her high school liked. She was a good student, and participated in extracurricular activities. She was aware of feeling sad when her favorite woman teacher was occupied with other students, but was usually able to handle her lowered mood within a day or two when her good performances would be rewarded. Over the course of a school year, the situation changed. The teacher became engaged, other students were also successful in their own ways, and factors outside the school raised her need for approval. The teacher began to notice small objects missing from her desk or the school room, but believed they had been misplaced. When an expensive fountain pen disappeared, an investigation revealed the situation. A humiliated and depressed girl abjectly confessed to school authorities and asked to be sent away to an institution for delinquents. This request was not granted, but her need for therapy was accepted.

3. Symbolic stealings are listed separately even though it might be argued that all of these categories include some symbolic takings. Caution is called for in trying to fit every act of theft into one or another category. A confluence of multiple motives and overdetermination are the perspectives to utilize. Only two are selected to illustrate the material.

Hence, while a teenage girl stealing a fountain pen may well represent specific symbolic components, it is also an aggressive act. In any clinical context, the symbolic meaning of the act for the individual should be sought. A routine case of a fifteen-year-old apprehended for taking articles from a sports store seems almost monotonous to the juvenile division of a police department. What the psychiatrist can contribute from his clinical evaluation is that the boy is in the midst of trying out for his high school athletic team and is quite anxious about it. There is anxiety about the competitive aspects (he might not make the team), and also about some of the physical contact aspects of the game. In this respect, the seemingly nonsensical aspects of why a boy would risk his future to steal an athletic supporter and cup become more comprehensible. The material presented gives reasons for certain behaviors, and the explanatory model should be distinguished from exculpation. What society chooses to do about youths caught up in these dilemmas is a different question. However, it does say something directly about how society deals with its youth.

Consider a sixteen-year-old pregnant girl. Things seem to be coming to a practical resolution since she will continue her schooling and then make a decision about whether she wishes to marry, a decision which is agreeable to all concerned. A hardware store proprietor is rather startled one day when he observes this

attractive and pregnant young female shoplifting small garden
and spading tools. When seen for a clinical evaluation, she was
humiliated, tearful, and as puzzled as everyone else. In the course of
therapy, many aspects were revealed about the symbolic feelings of
cultivation, fruition, and to have or not to have a good result with
the pregnancy. While this particular adolescent had not had a
previous history of overt delinquent activities prior to her
pregnancy, she could recall an occasion during one of her mother's
pregnancies when she was nine years of age and took various
objects out of her mother's purse. This case is reminiscent of one
described by Edward Glover in 1922.[34]

> Up to age four, a little girl had been regarded by her parents as a good-
> tempered and well-behaved child. At that time a baby brother was born, and
> she began to steal cucumbers from fruit shops. After being severely scolded by
> her mother, she stopped, and was again exemplary until age nine when she
> was expelled from school for stealing money and pencils from lockers. The
> money was kept in her school locker where it was easily found. The birth of the
> baby brother had elicited acute jealousy, and her amenable conduct
> disappeared after giving up the cucumber episodes by an attempt to murder
> the infant in his cradle by stiking him with a hammer, and on another
> occasion, twisting his penis between her finger and thumb. Otherwise, she
> remained a good child, but the hostile jealousy and envy remained unchanged
> unconsciously. Glover's explanation was that the girl was attempting to
> compensate to regain parental love by turning herself into a boy through
> collecting the stolen pencils. In a similar vein, money would replace her lost
> love. While seeking admiration from children at school, her behavior made
> her a black sheep, and also caused mortification to her parents. It was
> reported that only a few interviews were necessary to delineate these factors,
> and after a vacation and transfer to another school, her behavior remained
> uneventful. In fact, a follow-up revealed no symptomatic recurrence at the
> point of marrying after college, having five children, and becoming a
> grandmother.

4. Unresolved guilt as a contributor to theft is mentioned with
the realization that guilt has many possible outcomes. Criminality
which stems from a sense of guilt was mentioned in other
discussions. The result is to act out in a self-defeating way which
seeks punishment. Depression and masochism are related aspects.
When thefts occur under these conditions, the act often has such an
obvious lack of concealment or sophistication, under a seeming
veneer of trying to execute a theft, that the question arises as to why

it seems to take the community so long to apprehend these people. Without digressing too far, the type of explanation used in the past—that business establishments deal with the parents and wish to avoid involvement—is no longer valid. On one hand, the quantitative aspects may be higher than official data indicate. What contributes in part to the perpetuation is the game of cat and mouse enacted between the parties. It is repetition for both of them, with nothing resolved for either side. The acts often have such an exhibitionistic or flamboyant quality as to function as a form of masochistic provocation. Sources of guilt exist on many levels, but rarely does guilt seem confined to conscious sources alone. If this is so and the unconscious sources of guilt remain, we would expect repetitions of the behavior. Nor would deterrence be achieved by way of either parental or community sanctions. In fact, this is exactly what we do find, which is another contributing factor to the unresolved problem of crime which never seems to abate from generation to generation.

5. Stealing as a direct expression of sexual impulses is, again, not a separate category from all of the others. Attention is given here to some of the acts being more directly connected with stealing. Recall that when discussing burglary, it was pointed out that some burglaries involve directly acted out sexual fantasies. Boys or girls who take pencils, fountain pens, guns, jewelry, underclothing, or swimming suits, often seem to fall in this category. Sometimes the act takes on compulsive components, so it achieves recognition as kleptomania. It may take on specific components involving excitement and risk to see if it can be pulled off. One variety of this is the youth who achieves sexual excitement by compulsively stealing women's undergarments from apartment clotheslines. Not all of these youths are aware of sexual excitement at the time, but are focusing on the act of taking. Some afterwards use the garments in connection with masturbation. Others simply accumulate them in a hoarding manner. One youth had accumulated a trunk full of women's undergarments. The articles then take on a fetishistic quality which acts either as a necessary precondition for sexual activity or in some cases as a substitute.

6. Depression and masochistic phenomena have been mentioned in connection with unresolved guilt. From the ego side of a depression, the feeling of a loss of self-esteem coupled with helplessness are paramount. Such basic human needs as feeling worthy and loved by others and the need not to be seen as weak and insecure are interconnected.[35] These painful affective states need

not have any objective correlates, and we are examining the experiential state of an individual. Narcissistic aspirations which are part of the ego-ideal are balanced by the ego's pain about its real and fantasized helplessness and inadequacy about ever changing the status quo.

To alleviate painful ego states, many devices are possible. What we are dealing with is stealing as a means of altering a depression. Why some individuals stay depressed and suffer, while others use drugs or alcohol, manipulate others, or court punishment, are questions that can only be resolved in terms of individual life histories. In a broad sense, there is the distinction between the giving up complex, with its vulnerability toward physical illnesses, versus attempts to extract and take from others.

Individual propensities and symbolisms operate. Youths may react to a "B" school grade when they are working as hard as they can for an "A" with the feeling they are a failure. Many pathways are open once depression sets in. Among adolescents, the acting out route is not infrequent. However, which acting out pathway? While one boy steals, another becomes involved with a group dedicated to high religious principles in a reversal from his former life pattern. Both function to ward off depression temporarily. A girl rejected by a boy becomes reactively depressed. If she has had a relatively good ego growth before that, she is able to mourn and grow. If not, she experiences this as a severe blow to her narcissism and may resort to acting out to lighten her depression. Again, a distinction is needed between a temporary state of reactive depression versus a reaction as though it is such a fatal blow that a commitment to a new life based on antisociality results.

It is not frequently mentioned that in more extremely depressed youths, the degree of risk-taking increases. The challenge of excitement becomes addictive. Intermingled are breakthroughs of depressive affect. Under the guise of excitement and thrills, risks are taken. Some of these begin with stealing and eventuate in shoot-outs or high-speed chases in cars with resultant accidents and sometimes death. Again, some of these youths subsequently become aware of their death-seeking at those times, while others still need to use a good deal of denial and are not aware of how depressed they are. Hence, continued restlessness and need to externalize their problems persists.

7. Stealing in connection with family secrets is another category.[36] Secrets such as adoptions, illegitimacies, extramarital affairs, or, mental illness in a family are some of the themes about

which children become aware. Levels of awareness operate with respect to these secrets, but the secretive nature is what has the major impact on coping difficulties. A parent may share a secret with a particular child or both parents connive to keep it secret. When a child steals in reaction to a sensed family secret he is acknowledging to himself and to the world that something clandestine has occurred. The taking is tantamount to calling the attention of others to the secret, and it raises the possibility of the community discovering the secret. The adolescent is then relieved of the burden. The need to expose deceiving parents should not be underestimated. When these adolescents are removed from their homes, the family secret is maintained. If they are not sent to correctional facilities, the family may try and send them away from home to friends or relatives.

8. Stealing as an act of revenge has been labeled the Monte Cristo complex, taken from the need to gain justice that the Alexandre Dumas' hero achieved in *The Count of Monte Cristo*.[37] The appeal of the story is the pursuit of justice by someone who has been wronged. It involves identification by the reader with the oppressed and insignificant person who reverses the tables on someone who is big and powerful—a classic theme of the weak and exploited child getting his revenge. Yet there is more to the theme of Monte Cristo's revenge than simply taking from the powerful being analagous to the appeal of taking from large and impersonal business organizations seen in white-collar crimes. The theme of taking what one feels entitled to implies that the property was originally one's own. If that is so, no wrong has been committed. On an emotional level, there is not only a taking but a vindictive quality of getting something back. It is like repossessing an object that was once stolen from the taker in the first place.

A youth working part-time in a hardware store was not given more than a paltry discount on an expensive bicycle. This was seen as a justification for arranging to take one of the new bicycles when they arrived at the warehouse from the manufacturer. The rationalization was that he was entitled to a better deal than had been offered by his employer. Not only is guilt not operative as an ego signal to negate such acts, but there is a feeling of accomplishment. An isolation defense operates so that the emotion is not connected to the behavior which is cognitively registered as wrong.

Perhaps a better word than revenge stealing is restitutive stealing. It conveys not just the angry component in the taking but re-taking something felt as rightfully theirs. Hence, there is no need for guilt signals, since the act is experienced as ego-syntonic. Yet to maintain the absence of guilt in such taking requires that other defenses be kept constantly on the alert. Isolation has been mentioned, but projection of greed and envy need to be perpetuated.

Auto-thefts. Taking of cars is discussed separately in view of the special characteristics it has, and because of the wide prevalence. As with other property offenses, auto-theft is primarily a crime of the younger age population. In 1972, 54 percent of all arrests for the crime were under eighteen years of age. If the computations include those under twenty-one years, we are up to 72 percent. Sixty percent of all those processed for auto-theft are referred to juvenile court jurisdictions. No other crime listed in the Crime Index has such a high rate of juvenile referrals. Automobiles make up 90 percent of the stolen vehicles, motorcycles 4 percent, trucks 5 percent, and other vehicles 1 percent. In 1972, the most popular year vehicle to be stolen in terms of frequency was the 1964 model. While geographically the volume of auto thefts is highest in the Northwestern states, with 31 percent of the total, the Western states have the highest auto theft rate per 100,000 inhabitants. As might be predicted, auto-theft is an offense committed most often in cities with a population over one million. One interesting figure is that arrest rates of girls under eighteen for auto thefts increased 110.3 percent during the 1960-1972 period, while for boys under eighteen years, it increased only 37.8 percent.[39]

It is interesting that "borrowing" a car by adolescents, has not been found to be weighted toward any one social class. Rather, it has been seen as a "favored offense" across different social classes. It could be considered a juvenile form of white-collar delinquency.[40] In contrast to auto thefts by those in the older age groups, the younger offenders do not seem interested in stripping cars or selling them for profit (which smacks more of organized crime). They are more interested in using them, in the sense of borrowing, for temporary excitement. Unfortunately for the youths, the owners have not borrowed their cars, and the unauthorized use of their vehicles is simply regarded as stealing.

A subgroup who steal cars are looking for the excitement of a cops and robbers chase. Excitement may be so prominent a component in some auto thefts that it leads to direct provocation in the hopes of eliciting a chase.

One group of adolescents often stole cars for an evening's use. They would drive at extremely high speeds, but were chased only once. At other times they would simply use the cars to pick up girls. One night after trying valiantly to be sighted speeding on a freeway without success, they spotted a police car in the parking lot of a drive-in eating establishment. They proceeded to pull into the lot directly opposite the squad car. To their further disappointment, the officers were busy enjoying their dinner and did not take the bait despite attempts to draw attention to the stolen car and themselves by cursing and making noise.

Speeding on superhighways carries realistic risks. It often gives rise to chases, in which not only those in the stolen car but those pursuing or innocent bystanders are injured. Car thefts also illustrate the interlocking of many facets. The ease of taking a car is known to all adolescents which does make one wonder why so many individuals leave expensive and prized possessions so readily available for the taking. Some of these elements minimize the labeling of taking autos as actual thefts and perpetuate the view of car theft as a prank.

Many levels of motivational meaning operate in these acts. Challenges to authority by the adolescents, coupled with parental ambivalence, operate with respect to the act itself. Contemporary symbolization of the auto as the epitome of power, class, and status capitalize on both the sexual and aggressive elements. These are reinforced by way of constant exposures to the mass media. Such attributes as forcefulness, intrusiveness, slickness, and ease of mobility appeal to adolescents struggling to harness their own ego engines without sacrificing power.

Vandalism. Two last categories need discussion from a psychiatric perspective: vandalism and arson. Neither are reported in the *Uniform Crime Reports* as part of the Crime Index list of offenses, meaning that only arrest information is reported. In fact, vandalism is defined as the willful or malicious destruction, injury, disfigurement, or defacement of property without the consent of the owner or person having custody or control. The word stems from the Germanic barbarian tribes who captured and sacked Rome in 455 A.D. As part of the sacking, monuments were destroyed and literary works burned. Currently, the arrest rate for vandalism is primarily a measure of police activity, particularly with respect to juveniles. Hence, a figure of 129,724 arrests for vandalism for all ages must refer to a small number of those who engage in such activities.[41]

Similar to the other property offenses we have discussed, 86.6 percent of those arrested were under the age of twenty-five, 79.9 percent were under twenty-one, 70.6 percent under eighteen, and 44.3 percent were under fifteen years of age. Ninety-two percent of those arrested were males, and 8 percent were females.

What surveys there are indicate that individuals, businesses, and public service institutions all suffer extensive damages. Destruction may be vented against public housing, street light systems, transit systems, and schools. Public school glass breakage alone was estimated several years ago at four to five million dollars national-ly.[42] Estimates for the business world are more difficult to determine, but could be estimated to a minimal extent through insurance claims. Individual households suffer by way of fences being torn down, cars damaged, garbage cans overturned, recrea-tional equipment destroyed on playgrounds or in yards, auto tires slashed and aerials broken. The ingenuity put into such acts of vandalism at times borders on the creative. The theme is played out in many ways, indicating the innumerable ways the aggressive-nesss is released. Consider the following diversities: public park stands are destroyed, the opening of new buildings or landmarks are sacked for souvenirs, pet animals are sprayed with paint, bombs are planted, cars are released from gear to run down an embankment, windows of cars are bashed out, lawns are cut up—the assortment and variety seem endless.

The only thing as impressive as the diversity of the acts is the absence of studies of such acts by those in the behavioral sciences. Explanations are offered in terms of the behavior simply being part of the pattern of normative behavior of young people. Such denial places the behavior in the realm of pranks. However, reacting to the behavior by minimizing it, in contrast to directly viewing it as a conscious expression of a mixture of aggressive trends, does not assist in appraising it realistically.

One study from the Bronx juvenile court classified vandalistic acts into three groups: predatory, vindictive, and wanton.[43] The predatory group was described as doing the acts for fun and as sport. In effect, this denied the more blatant aggressiveness which the perpetrators possessed. Vindictive activities were seen as express-ing hatred and antagonisms, especially of minority groups. This seems closer to the idea of the collective violence of groups (such as racial or anti-war protests). In contrast, only the wanton group was described as a type of nonutilitarian behavior of frustrated individuals. Seeking explanations for vandalism based on class differences is one of the more pervasive theories. Some explain this in terms of challenging the emphasis on private property in the middle-class cultural background. To account for the fact that vandalistic acts are not confined to one class against another, studies resort to explanations that middle-class patterns are not necessarily absorbed by those in the middle class. [44] Psychiatry should begin to get interested in such explanatory voids for it should be able to pursue questions of why acculturation has supposedly not occurred for certain individuals. Again, the diagnostic framework illustrated earlier in this chapter is relevant for gaining perspective on different types of vandalistic acts.

The explanations offered for vandalism often stay on the level of the superficial and the obvious. Hence, asking adolescents why they engage in such activities, and then assuming replies that they were bored with school, or felt affronted by teachers who are equally bored, give only a vague intimation of the degree of discontent and hatred which erupts and without any specific explanation in terms of personality functioning.

One of the few investigations of vandalism that has been done omitted the personality aspects of the perpetrators entirely. The study was a confirmation of the prevalence of vandalism. Two cars were parked, one in a New York City street and the other near Stanford University with their hoods up as though abandoned. [45] In the densely populated area of New York, within ten minutes a middle-class family of three raided it, followed by twenty-three attacks in the next two days. The California car went unnoticed except for a woman stopping to put the hood down in the rain. The impression of who these vandals are is not that of poorly trained minority groups but a heterogenous group who act out their acquisitive and destructive urges on whatever is available. While this study focused on why the situation in New York elicited many more predatory incidents than California, the same experiment could be demonstrated within given cities if one knew something about the areas to begin with or the people who live there.

Can anything more be said about these adolescents, or should the behavior be viewed as typical for this stage of development? That it is not specifically stage-related appears refuted, since the majority of adolescents commit juvenile offenses at one time or another, but they do not all vandalize. Those who vandalize appear to suffer from an ego deficit with respect to the modulation or direction of their aggression. While they are a step removed from assaulting people, although this may occur, they are attacking the goods and property of people who are usually adults or authority representatives. In that sense their capacity for expressing their anger verbally, or reflecting on it, is deficient. Rather than relying on fantasy or cognitive trials for handling their predicaments, they attack.

Many of the youths seem provocative in other ways. They may have had passive-aggressive learning problems, and then become more directly involved with challenges to teachers as adolescence gathered momentum. When they adopt an attitude of pseudo-sophistication or coolness, they provoke anger and rage in those who have to deal with them, including therapists.

There is another component that sometimes enters into acts of vandalism. A distinction is made between a solo vandalizer versus a group. Group interaction among these youths is based on many variables. In some ways it is determined by challenges within the dynamics of the group. In other ways there is a group callousness and collusiveness to deny the impact of their behavior. Many times nonverbal elements predominate, and vandalism becomes like a bit of an outing, with mirth, gaiety, and occasionally a chase by the "stupid police." The type of ego-splitting described for other types of property offenses results in participants in vandalism describing the event as though they were observers who happened on the scene.

Many aspects of childhood developmental components are relevant in terms of impulsive aspects of putting thought into acts without sufficient mediation or delay. In some respects the lack of parental figures to restrain them from taking dangerous risks contributes by way of perpetuating the risk-taking. At the same time, the environment and things in it may seem quite threatening.

> A fifteen-year-old in trouble with the juvenile court for destroying the nets on public tennis courts was involved in several other vandalistic acts. While carrying these out with one or two other boys, who differed on most occasions, no particular feeling of loyalty to these others was noted. Despite an absence of guilt about the acts, there was a strong feeling of sadness about other things in his life. An aunt reported a pattern of reckless behavior and destruction of things since an early age. What was interesting was the perplexity his mother registered about his behavior—as though it was a new problem for her. But the absence of maternal restraint to direct or interfere with the boy's destructiveness was longstanding and prominent. The mother was divorced when the boy was three years old, and the father had moved to another city, but no material deprivation ever existed. The lack of control was confirmed in clinical work with the boy who conveyed feelings that he had to look out for himself usually, since he did not feel a sense of reliance in terms of what his mother would do.

Arson. In a legal sense arson is willful or malicious burning, with or without intent to defraud. As such, it also includes attempts. Again, as with so many other property offenses, arson is also an offense of the young. In the under twenty-five-year-age bracket are 76.4 percent of arsonists; in the under-twenty-one-year group are 68.1 percent; under-eighteen-years of age are 58.3 percent; and 39.9 percent are under fifteen. Interestingly, 9.5 percent of the arsonists arrested are females.[46] The criminal act of arson comprises a polyglot of activities ranging from the burning of houses, business establishments, and cars, to forest fires, in which the estimate is that about one-fourth of all forest fires are deliberately set.[47]

One of the biggest surprises in researching the subject is to find that most criminology resources and texts entirely omit any discussion of arson. Nor do criminal law casebooks deal with it. At first this might be thought due to an implicit assumption that everyone views the behavior as so pathologic as to fall within the realm of the psychiatric. However, in practice nothing could be further from the truth. Certainly, most insurance companies are not willing to see this behavior as psychiatrically disturbed. Nor are most of the individuals coming before courts. Data based on a survey asking 300 adults of upper socio-economic status what they would do with a child who set fires support the impression. Only one-third thought of mental health professionals as a resource.[48] My hypothesis is that the omission of dealing with the subject beyond a definitional level is due to a gap in understanding on one hand versus a need to view it as a responsible act. As such, the behavior is viewed as something akin to vandalism, in which property is simply destroyed. The complexity of motives for such conduct is left unexplored.

To begin with, no common diagnostic grouping is valid. Arson has multiple causes. While some of these individuals are reported as being mentally subnormal or overtly psychotic, are they more easily apprehended because of such limitations?. Some display an obsessional neurosis clinically or an "irresistible impulse" legally. The latter are referred to as "true pyromanics."[49] In yet other youths, deep anger is acted out. The source of the anger varies, such as from a parent, girl or boyfriend, teacher, or coach. The objects against which the arsonistic tendencies are enacted touch a host of neurotic conflicts. Burning of churches contains some rather obvious suggestions, as does that of school buildings. The direct expression of aggression by destroying the building or property is similar to that in vandalism.

Freud offered a cultural theory about the origin of the use of fire based on clinical work and from his readings about mythology.[50] He related the excitement connected with fire to urethral eroticism. Freud asked why it was that, not only in the Greek myth of Prometheus stealing fire from the gods, but among the most diverse people, the acquisition of fire seemed inseparably connected with the idea of some crime? By an act of instinctual renunciation Freud viewed man giving up his desire to extinguish fires by urinating on them. Man was then able to gain mastery over fire. By way of repressing these impulses other impulses were also controlled, such as those of a sexualized type connected with burning passion. However, aggression and competitiveness are still present in the act of putting a fire out by way of a stream of urine. Witness the aggression present in telling another person, "Piss on you." Sexualized components can gain prominence, such as needing to start a fire as an antecedent to sexual arousal—equivalent to young children engaging in forbidden play with matches. In one case a youth placed ladders against houses to window-peek. He would become sexually excited and masturbate while standing on the ladder. Following his descent he would start a fire, as though consuming the act in one great flame. In some youths the hurt narcissism of those sensitized and in need of affection comes through. When they do not get what they feel they deserve, a retaliatory fire occurs.

Severe ego disturbances are seen when evaluating latency age children or young adolescents who set fires. In one study of thirty boys, a majority demonstrated severe rage reactions and two-thirds showed chronic hyperactivity.[51] Difficulties in control were manifest on many levels. In addition, some were assaultive, others exposed themselves, and others pulled women's skirts up—all of which had not been brought under control from earlier childhood. Learning difficulties were an accompaniment. A syndrome of enuresis, firesetting, and cruelty to animals existing in childhood is seen by some as predictive of later violent crimes.[52] More specifically, firesetting in the context of maternal deprivation, poor father identification, nocturnal enuresis, violence toward animals, and brutalization by one or both parents is seen as a predictor of homicide.[53] In all of these attempts at prediction, the limitation is the presence of such behaviors in many who never commit a homicide or any act of violence.

Not only are the motives in firesetting complex, but steps exist in carrying out different types of fires. Hence, it was early observed that an essential part of the act consists of staying around to assist the firemen to put out the fire. In addition, other parts of the overall behavior are significant. Hence, the "game of playing fireman" includes: turning in an alarm; excitement in hearing the screeching sirens; the arrival of the big trucks; the gathering of the crowd; firemen pulling out their long hoses; water gushing from the ends of the hoses; entering the scene as a passive observer and progressing to the level of an assistant; forming a type of comraderie with the fire-fighting team.

It is obvious that a fair degree of planning and foresight by the ego to carry out these acts is required. Beyond the above, many other impulses are expressed. The sexual and destructive aspects have been noted, and the restitutive function should be sought. An adolescent boy who felt a comfort and security in joining up and working with the firemen to gain control of a blaze is an example of the function. This seems to serve as a restitutional act with a parent. In some cases the act appears as a distress signal and a call for help to quell desires. It is a call from an overburdened adolescent to bring an absent parent to the rescue.[55]

Although providing temporary relief from tension in this manner, arson does create anxiety from the degree of aggression involved in the act. All in all, incendiarism is a complex and multiply determined act. Like so many other property offenses carried out by youths, it tends to be discussed casually as just another bit of acting up which will pass with time. Depending on the types of impulses, conflicts, and defenses which are operating, this may or may not happen. In contrast is the administration of direct penal sanctions against the behavior when it occurs in adulthood.

REFERENCES

1. D. Elkind and J. D. Flavell, ed., *Studies in Cognitive Development* (New York: Oxford University Press, 1969).
2. C. P. Malmquist, Conscience development, *The Psychoanalytic Study of the Child* 23(1968):301-331.
3. M. S. Mahler, On the significance of the normal separation-individuation phase, *Drives, Affects, and Behavior,* ed. by M. Schur, pp. 161-169, vol. 2 (New York: International Universities Press, 1965).
4. F. Pine, On the separation process: universal trends and individual differences, *Separation-Individuation,* ed. by T. B. McDevitt and C. F. Settlage, pp. 113-130 (New York: International Universities Press, 1971).

5. T. A. Arlow, Character perversions, *Comments in Psychoanalysis*, ed. by I. M. Marcus, pp. 317-335 (New York: International Universities Press, 1971).

6. H. Kohut, Thought on narcissism and narcissistic rage, *Psychoanalytic Study of the Child* 27(1972): 360-400.

7. O. F. Kernberg, Further contributions to the treatment of narcissistic personalities, *International Journal of Psychoanalysis* 55(1974):215-240.

8. C. P. Malmquist, Depressions in childhood and adolescence, *New England Journal of Medicine* 284(1971):887-893.

9. P.A. Waters, Depression, *Counseling and the College Student*, ed. by D. Farnsworth and G. B. Blaine, pp. 169-180 (Boston: Little, Brown and Company, 1970).

10. M. M. Weissman and E. S. Paykel, *The Depressed Woman: A Study of Social Relationships* (Chicago: University of Chicago Press, 1974).

11. A. Schmale, Depression as affect, character style, and symptom formation, *Psychoanalysis and Contemporary Science*, ed. by B. B. Rubinstein, vol. 1, pp. 327-351 (New York: Macmillan, 1972).

12. C. P. Malmquist, Melancholic murderers, *British Journal of Medical Psychology* 44(1971):267-271.

13. B. M. Cormier, Depression and persistent criminality, *Canadian Psychological Association Journal, Special Supplement* 11(1966):208-220.

14. J. Hall, *Theft, Law and Society*, 2nd ed. (Indianapolis: Bobbs-Merrill Co., 1952).

15. R. Quinney, *Criminology-Analysis and Critique of Crime in America* (Boston: Little, Brown and Co., 1975).

16. D. Matza and G. M. Lykes, Juvenile delinquency and subterranean values, *American Sociology Review* 26(1961):712-719.

17. I. Spergel, *Racketville, Slumtown, Haulburg: An Exploratory Study of Delinquent Subcultures* (Chicago: University of Chicago Press, 1964).

18. Federal Bureau of Investigation, *Uniform Crime Reports for the United States, 1974* (Washington, D.C.: U.S. Government Printing Office, 1975).

19. W. C. Reckless, *The Crime Problems*, 5th ed. (Englewood Cliffs: Prentice-Hall, 1973).

20. F. H. McClintoch and E. Gibson, *Robbery in London* (London: Macmillan and Co., 1961).

21. T. E. Conklin, *Robbery and the Criminal Justice System* (Philadelphia: J. B. Lippincott Co., 1972).

22. E. J. Hobsbawn, *Bandits* (London: Weindenfeld and Nicolson, 1970).

23. *Uniform Crime Reports,* op. cit., p. 21.

24. E. H. Sutherland, *The Professional Thief* (Chicago: University of Chicago Press, 1937).

25. N. Shover, Structures and careers in burglary, *Journal of Criminal Law, Crime, and Political Science* 63(1972):540-549.

26. J. A. Inciardi, *Careers in Crime* (Chicago: Rand McNally, 1975).

27. V. Bugliosi, *Helter Skelter—The True Story of the Manson Murders* (New York: W. W. Norton, 1974).

28. K. S. Eissler, Scapegoats of society, *Searchlights on Delinquency*, ed. by K. R. Eissler, pp. 288-305 (New York: International Universities Press, 1949).

29. *Uniform Crime Reports,* op. cit., p. 22.

30. S. Ferenczi, The ontogenesis of the interest in money, *First Contributions to Psycho-Analysis* (London: Hogarth Press, 1952).

31. D. W. Winnicott, Transitional objects and transitional phenomena, *Collected Papers* (New York: Basic Books, 1958).

32. A. Freud, *Normality and Pathology in Childhood* (New York: International Universities Press, 1965).

33. W. Bromberg, *Crime and the Mind*, p. 242 (New York: Macmillan Co., 1965).

34. E. Glover, *The Roots of Crime,* p. 14-15 (New York: International Universities Press, 1960).

35. E. Bibring, The mechanism of depression, *Affective Disorders*, ed. by P. Greenacre (New York: International Universities Press, 1953).

36. H. Schwarz, Contribution to symposium on acting out, *International Journal of Psycho-Analysis* 49(1968):179-181.

37. P. Castelnuovo-Tedeso, Stealing, revenge, and the Monte Cristo complex, *International Journal of Psycho-Analysis* 55(1974):169-177.

38. *Uniform Crime Reports,* op. cit., p. 25.

39. Ibid., p. 124.

40. W. W. Wattenberg and J. Balistrieri, Automobile theft: a 'favored-group' delinquency, *American Journal of Sociology* 55(1952):575-579.

41. *Uniform Crime Reports,* op. cit, p. 128.

42. The President's Commission on Law Enforcement and Administration of Justice, *Task Force Report: Crime and Its Impact—An Assessment* (Washington, D.C.; U.S. Government Printing Office, 1967), p. 46.

43. J. M. Martin, *Juvenile Vandalism: A Study of Its Nature and Prevention* (Springfield: Charles C Thomas, 1961).

44. B. Spiller, Delinquency and middle class goals, *Journal of Criminal Law, Crime, and Political Science* 56(1965):463-478.

45. P. Zimbardo, The Human Choice, *The Nebraska Symposium on Motivation*, 1969.

46. *Uniform Crime Reports,* op. cit., p. 128.

47. President's Commission, op. cit.

48. C. N. Winget and R. M. Whitman, Coping with problems: attitudes toward children who set fires, *American Journal of Psychiatry* 130(1973):442-445.

49. N. D. C. Lewis and H. Yarnell, *Pathological Firesetting* (Washington, D.C.: Nervous and Mental Disease Publishing Co., 1951).

50. S. Freud, The acquisition of power over fire, *Standard Edition* 22:187-193.

51. I. Kaufman, L. W. Heims, and D. E. Reiser, A re-evaluation of the psychodynamics of firesetting, *American Journal of Orthopsychiatry* 31(1961):123-136.

52. H. Hellman and N. Blackman, Enuresis, firesetting, and cruelty to animals: a trend prodictive of adult crime, *American Journal of Psychiatry* 122(1966):1431.

53. M. Goldstein, Brain research and violent behavior, *Archives of Neurology* 30(1974):1-35.

54. D. Scott, *The Psychology of Fire* (New York: Charles Scribner, 1974).

55. L. B. Macht and J. E. Mack, The firesetter syndrome, *Psychiatry* 31(1968)277-288.

Chapter Twelve

Antisocial Behavior: Psychotic Development

Any adequate discussion of psychoses and antisocial development in the adolescent requires a contrast between psychotic manifestations in younger children compared to the older age group. The manifestations of psychosis in younger children and adults share behavioral elements with those in adolescents. Yet, except for continuity types which commence in early childhood, the manifestations are different as is the antisociality. A guiding principle is that the manifestations of psychosis vary according to the developmental sequence and level attained by the individual. Whatever basic etiological model is espoused, disturbances in several areas of ego functioning are customarily present. It is especially evident with regard to functions such as cognition, affect, motility, language development, and reality testing. Most important are difficulties in separation-individuation within the context of how object relationships have progressed along these lines. Many times difficulties in individuation are masked until adolescence, when they become conspicuously present.

Disturbances in any one of multiple areas can have severe adverse consequences on how an adolescent relates to others over a period of time. Antecedent arrests or deviations of development in these youths can be seen when a longitudinal perspective is taken. Psychotic processes and reactions in adolescence must also be distinguished from continuing forms of infantile psychoses, such as early infantile autism, or symbiotic psychosis. In younger children there is a diagnostic need to keep questions of cerebral dysfunction and mental subnormality in mind as alternative possibilities. More difficult diagnostic problems arise in attempts to distinguish other disorders of personality development within the fluctuations of adolescence. Psychotic reactions can also emerge as an integral part of other syndromes in a secondary sense. Table 22 gives a differential breakdown of types of psychosis seen in childhood by descriptive characteristics.

TABLE 22

Psychoses of Childhood and Adolescence

I. *Psychosis without Known Impairment of Brain Tissue Function*
    A. Autistic psychosis
       1. Early infantile autism (EIA)
       2. Symbiotic psychosis (Mahler)
    B. Schizophreniform psychosis
       1. Simple
       2. Acute undifferentiated (confusional state)
       3. Paranoid type
    C. Psychosis associated with developmental deviations
       1. Childhood schizophrenia
       2. Atypical child
       3. Childhood psychosis
    D. Psychotic depressive phenomena

II. *Psychosis Associated with Impairment in Brain Tissue Function*
    A. Associated with Intoxication (atropine, bromides, cortisone, stramonium, psychedelic drugs, marijuana, etc.)
    B. Associated with Metabolic Disorders (pellagra, amaurotic idiocy, etc.)
    C. Associated with Degenerative Disorders (Schilder's disease, *dementia infantilis*, etc.)
    D. Associated with Infections (juvenile paresis, encephalitides, etc.)
    E. Associated with Convulsive Disorders (temporal lobe epilepsy, dysautonomia, etc.)
    F. Associated with Trauma
    G. Associated with Neoplasms

III. *Psychoses of Adolescence*
    A. Continuation of Types with an Earlier Onset

B. Acute Confusual State
C. Related to Organic or Toxic States
D. Psychotic Depressive Episodes
E. "Pseudo" types of Schizophrenias
F. Psychotic Reactions Presenting with An Adult Clinical Picture (seen in late adolescence)

HISTORICAL PERSPECTIVES ON NOSOLOGY

Recognition of an overtly psychotic adult is not difficult for someone with minimal clinical skills. Due to publicity and the impact of mass media such individuals are often recognized even by laymen. Unfortunately, many of the signs and symptoms which are taken as pathognomonic of a psychotic process are end-stages of a confluency of forces; hallucinations, illusions, striking peculiarities and mannerisms, posed attitudes, or caricatured speech are examples. However, many of these symptoms are lacking in an adolescent caught up in an emerging psychotic process. These blatant signs and symptoms may actually be secondary signs of schizophrenia or a psychotic reaction, and are not necessarily present in any given adult. In fact, in the great majority of those with a schizophrenic process, these symptoms do not emerge.

Even more cogent is the larger group of individuals who have a tendency to develop psychotic disturbances. Depending on a host of variables, they may or may not ever emerge from this latent potential. If schizophrenia is conceptualized as an actualized state, the population with such a latent potential is composed of a relatively large group of schizotypic people. From this population emerge those who develop the potential for an overt psychotic decompensation. Caution must be further exercised with respect to the assumption that all psychoses are manifestations of schizophrenia. It is an unwarranted assumption, especially with regard to the adolescent population. The majority of decompensations result either from slowly emerging processes in which the secondary signs appear over a period of several years (or never), or there are intermittent, florid psychotic episodes which quickly subside but have a tendency to recur under stress or trauma.

Early reports noted the onset of "stupidity" in adolescents who previously performed adequately. In all probability these were the early forerunners of a clinical description utilizing the concept of *dementia praecox*. The early idea was that a premature form of dementia resulted—perhaps based on some metabolic or degenerative disease process. Although Morel formulated the dementia concept in 1856, it eventually lead to a distinction between "dementias" and "amentias." A distinction had been reported by Thomas Willis, in 1674 who observed that the apparent deterioration in the dementias did not remain fixed in all cases.[2] Equirol (1772-1840), the great French clinician and successor to Phillipe Pinel at the Salpetrière, sensed the intermittent nature of the disturbances, especially when an adolescent psychotic process was in question.[3] In fact, Esquirol actually viewed the processes in terms of a developmental defect—a striking insight that many have not yet attained. He formulated the defect as due either to iatrogenic causes, such as excessive purgations performed for an illness, or pubertal phenomena, such as irregular meneses or masturbation. Morel's later work applied the concept of degeneracy to adolescents who showed deviant behavior. Although environmental insults could still operate, they were precipitators at best.

By 1868 Kahlbaum differentiated a symptomatic clustering within a group of psychotic individuals which he labeled "katatonia."[4] One of Kahlbaum's assistants, Hecker, delineated "hebephrenia" as a disorder of adolescents with silly, inappropriate mannerisms eventually leading to a deterioration.[5] These were seen as descriptions of separate disease entities at the time and were not integrated until Kraeplin's grouping into heberphrenic, catatonic, and paranoid forms of dementia praecox in the late 19th century. Apart from the more systematic classification based on observations of thousands of patients over decades, Kraeplin solidified Morel's earlier notions of dementia praecox as basically a hereditary disease with an onset in adolescence and culminating in a progressive pattern of deterioration. Since Kraeplin's influence remained dominant throughout the international psychiatric world for decades, by virtue of his reputation and *Handbook*, his ideas about schizophrenia as a disease with and onset in adolescence and a subsequent deterioration gained a strong foothold.[6] Ineffectual and adverse approaches administered under the guise of treatment also contributed to the idea of irreversibility.

Not until the 20th century did qualifying alternative formulations emerge. Adolf Meyer referred to patients "adolescent deterioration." He stressed a genetic-dynamic group of factors about the reactive nature of such disturbances. Jung extended the approach in the course of his work on introversion-extroversion, word association tests, complexes, symbolization, and folklore.[7] His work led to some

astute insights into the experiential components in young schizophrenics.

At the same time in Switzerland, Bleuler developed his ideas on
the "psychology of schizophrenia."[8] However, it is inaccurate to
view Bleuler's theory as primarily a psychological one in contrast to
an organic model. At least originally, he believed that the
"splitting" process was due to a toxin which caused cortical gliosis.
A major contribution was to see that the main diagnostic symptoms
which had been stressed were actually "secondary" to a basic
disturbance of association and affect. Hence, individuals with such
basic defects never deteriorated into manifesting the secondary
symptomotology (see Table 23).

TABLE 23

Primary and Secondary Symptoms of Schizophrenia

I.   Primary Symptoms in the Cognitive Realm of Schizophrenia

    A. Logically related ideas
    B. Condensation of ideas
    C. Symbolization used in preference to real objects
    D. Abstract notions used in preference to concrete notions
    E. Alliteration

II. Secondary Symptoms in Schizophrenia

    A. Autism
    B. Delusions
    C. Hallucinations
    D. Illusions
    E. Negativism
    F. Stereotypy
    G. Catatonic Symptoms

Source: Bleuber, *Dementia Praecox or the Group of Schizophrenias*, 1950.

CURRENT ETIOLOGICAL THEORIES

A recurrent issue, still in the forefront of debate about schizophrenia and psychotic processes, is the issue of hereditary influences.
Boldly put, the issue is: Do genes determine the emergence of

schizophrenic symptomatology? This is too simple a formulation, considering the present state of our knowledge. It is probably true that a predeliction for one theory over another by a particular therorist is determined by many features in their own personality and experience. However, such a predeliction is irrelevant to appraisal of the validity of the theory which must stand on independent criteria for the acceptability of any scientific theory. Those who prefer an epidemiological approach utilize populations. The significance of differences between samples from different populations are utilized and their validity is assessed in the context of the differing incidence of overt signs of schizophrenia in one population versus their absence in another. Different rates in consanguinous relationships is one target population. A favorite approach is to study concordance rates in twins.

A contrast is an environmental emphasis on child-rearing practices. Reliance is placed on the crucial role of psychological conflict with regard to key figures. An added emphasis is the role of key figures, which are perpetuated internally within individuals by way of introjective mechanisms—the perpetuation of introjects. An intriguing exercise in the history of science is to review the myriad theories put forth to explain schizophrenia and how often they contradict one another. Nor do we yet have agreement on the natural history and outcome of schizophrenic processes over a lifetime. One view is that schizophrenic episodes which commence during adolescence run a natural course in which a degree of residual alteration can always be detected if the clinician is skillful enough. Others hold to a position that there is a tendency toward improvement and resolution which slowly emerges. Those who adhere to this position believe that emotional warmth and affective contact can be established, no matter how deep the regression has been.

One basic weakness in any discussion about etiological models is the absence of a common nosological grouping. If questions of etiology are to be settled, it is presupposed that a common diagnostic entity must be utilized for different investigators. In actuality such a common grouping does not exist, except for the most blatant symtomatic cases. In adolescence the confusion is even more rampant, since psychotic episodes occur for brief periods of time. The episodes appear in the course of frequent upsurges, with or without manifest symptoms. Some clinicians classify these as schizophrenic episodes while others do not. Despite such problems, the majority of investigators in the field tend to adhere to a viewpoint that heredity plays some significant role in schizophrenia.

Although ordinary Mendelian models do not suffice for explanation since almost no families with 25 percent or 50 percent segregation ratios are found, other models are viable contenders. The main ones are dominant gene models with incomplete penetrance, genetic heterogeneity, and a polygenic model.[9] To say that hereditary factors play a role is not equivalent to maintaining that schizophrenia is inherited. As elaborated above, genes give a potential for certain developmental lines to be pursued, or tendencies to emerge. The most rigidly controlled twin studies, using adopted children, do not show a one hundred percent manifestation. Rather, large numbers of discordance are present. Such findings contribute to the abandonment of seeking out phenotypic schizophrenic individuals who would conform to a Mendelian distribution.

A more sophisticated theoretical model seeks to elicit manifestations of neural-integrative defects. Some individuals are either blessed or cursed with an inherited defect with respect to certain behavioral traits and functions. They have been described as *schizotaxic* individuals, and the resultant personality organization is *schizotypic*.[10] It is from this population group that *schizophrenics* emerge—the more limited grouping of those with diagnostic signs and symptoms textbooks describe.

If the schizotaxic individual develops a potential for a bout of schizophrenia, it may well be determined by a host of environmental factors—not the least of which are the biological and social stresses associated with the onset of puberty and all that follows in its wake. Arguments invariably arise. For example, some maintain that even if a genetic influence for schizotaxia is demonstrated, and one monozygotic twin becomes overtly schizophrenic and the other does not, schizophrenia should not be viewed as an inherited disease. Only the twin who develops schizophrenia with clinical phenotypic signs would be entitled to such a diagnosis as a result of the environmental factors which have given a necessary weighting.

What emerges is a theoretical model in which the emphasis is on types of adverse environmental or developmental factors that promote a schizophrenic outcome. If a schizotypic population can be identified genotypically, what are the factors leading to the emergence of an overt decompensation? It is at this basic level of identifying schizotypes that there are difficulties. The difficulties do not refer to the problem where clinicians have had inadequate training and do not know the issues and subtleties of diagnosis. It is the problem, given adequate and competent clinicians, of those who differ as to what should be included in the group. It is not easy to get pure culture cases who have emerged in childhood or de novo at adolescence with schizotypic features. Everyone has been exposed to noxious interactional experiences.

It appears valid to postulate a type of gene that acts in a similar manner in all of its possessors. Multiple genes may be involved for polygenic transmissions, or the degree of expressivity may vary. Further, those opposed to a monogenetic theory are opposed to a two-gene theory with one dominant and the other recessive, or to a single gene plus modifiers. However, multiplying genes as a theory of schizophrenia or psychosis is so open-ended that it may extend beyond the degree needed for disconfirmation for the testing of a scientific theory. This is raised by the dilemma of schizotypic or pseudo-types of schizophrenia presenting with such a variegated picture that genes can be multiplied endlessly. The hope is that a genotype can be identified on some crucial measure either as a behavioral configuration or by some biochemical or physiological measure. However, at this time we do not even have a set of standardized procedures for obtaining clinical data on patients or in a general population. Furthermore, measurements vary widely. Precautions about clinical bias and pre-existing knowledge about individuals or families that give a selectivity to the diagnostic process must be considered.

Can environmental factors contributing to the transmission and emergence of schizophrenia be identified? Among the many antecedent factors are adverse biological loadings of a non-genetic sort.[11] Some of the factors that have been considered are prematurity, birthrate in the mother, soft neurological signs, neonatal disturbances (colic, cyanosis, distorted rhythmic patterns in sleep, eating, and motility), and biochemical shifts (low protein-bound iodine levels, increased lactate/pyruvate ratio). Some theorize that mothers who are overtly psychotic may transmit some factor inducing change in their offspring. In fact, the broader group of children classified as high risk on the basis of certain signs are frequently so classified on the basis of these types of antecedents. But these factors do not account for the clustering of psychotic-proneness in certain families unless environmental precipitants are added onto genetic hypotheses.

Other environmental factors considered have been sibling position and roles within families. Rather than ordinal position, it is the significance of a person in regard to the development of autonomy which is a pathogenic factor. Hence, twin studies have considered the significance of a finding that a twin more submissive has a greater diathesis toward psychotic development. Somewhat different is the position that passivity or submissiveness are signs of disturbance which exist on some other etiological basis rather than the pathogenic factor in schizophrenia. Similarly, it may be that the presence of certain traits or child-rearing practices in families leads to psychotic lines of development in children rather than the existence of parental psychopathology in itself.

This quandary permeates environmental hypotheses. For example, is the range of schizotypal behaviors found in families in which one member may be overtly schizophrenic a reflection of the same biological or genetic loadings which in different members lead to differing degrees of expressivity? Or is it a response of other family members to the bizarreness with which they must cope? Wider-ranging hypotheses involving familial interactional patterns, role conflicts, and a confusion in sex identity have all been raised as causal links. However, while some see these as causal, others see them as a result of the disabilities of initially possessing schizophrenic traits.

Deep-seated attitudes involving emotional distance or closeness in families are as important as styles of communication, cognitive styles, and linguistic usage. Specific etiological issues which remain unresolved at this time are the degree to which environmental factors are necessary for the emergence of a psychotic adolescent. While some argue that they play a minimal, or insignificant, role compared to biological or genetic factors, the evidence is almost impossible to assess. To substantiate a genetic theory would mean that at least schizotypal traits should emerge with relatively the same incidence in families who appear emotionally intact compared with those who are not. That amounts to substantiation of the null hypothesis, yet this does not appear to occur. We find that fewer than half of monozygotic twin pairs are concordant for the illness, so that environmental factors must be of equal importance to the genetic.[12] If the psychopathological background of a family is higher in those who emerge with a psychosis, but it is argued that this background is not contributory to a significant degree, a circular argument is present. In this argument all disturbed factors in a family are held to be products of a disease, which is a theory not subject to disproof. Complicating matters further is the variability in the natural unfolding of schizophrenic patterns, and other psychotic manifestations in the period of adolescence and beyond. Not all psychoses are schizophrenic nor are all those with schizotypal personalities psychotic.

Clear-cut, overt cases which conform to textbook descriptions are rare. Nor is this primarily a matter of the influence of the introduction of antipsychotic types of medications. Even without such drugs the pattern is variable. This not only complicates studies but challenges the validity of influences and etiological hypotheses. The very nature of generic groupings is in question. Symptoms and signs vary—but so do the onsets, the durations of acute distress, and the outcomes. Some of these adolescents eventually have only a minimal amount of residual impairment: others have a neurotic complex or ego distortions, while only a few remain in the category of the classically unfolding dementia praecox.

PRODROMAL SIGNS AND SYMPTOMS

Withdrawal. Perhaps one of the earliest signs of a regression in ego functioning is withdrawal from the environment. Although some of these individuals have never been sociable, when they begin to withdraw their isolation is even more conspicuous. Their marked passivity, limited contact with others, and lack of initiative may heretofore have not been as noticeable. Typical occurrences in adolescents are dropping out of school, failure to report at a place of work, brief contacts with multiple jobs which last only a few days or weeks at the most, or spending large amounts of time doing nothing. They may stop seeing friends or withdraw into their homes with a pattern of eating, sleeping, watching television, or spending increased amounts of time in bed. In the contemporary milieu, many of them spend much of this idle time on drugs. A striking factor is the groping and denial in parents who seek naive preventive measures of drug education in schools while their children are in the midst of a severe regressive process.

Prior to the commencement of an overt psychotic state, a progressive state of despair occurs. The despair can go to great depths, giving a feeling that the promises and aspirations once held will not be fulfilled. Along with that, a feeling of hostile threats from the environment is experienced. It is as though one lives among hostile powers and as if there is a threat to survival—and, even more important, to the self-concept. The experiential state is feeling not loved and—worse unlovable. The adolescent feels unwanted, inadequate, and inferior. The self-concept is shifted in the direction of perceiving oneself as awkward, clumsy, and as someone who says and does stupid things. There is a pervasive feeling of not belonging, that one is strange and an outsider. In this context more overt paranoid mentations may occur.

Bodily Preoccupation. In time, an increasing preoccupation with the body commences. This parallels a heightened state of narcissism—focussing on expansive images about the self. Strange hypochondriacal sensations occur which often, particularly in the adolescent, take the form of a preoccupation with problems of sexual identity.

Lack of Impulse Control. A breakdown in modulation over impulses is another manifestation of increasing impairment in personality functioning. The breakdown may be by way of outbursts of rage or merely an accentuation of irritability which becomes progressive. At other times, inappropriate or impulsive sexual gestures occur.

Cognitive Difficulties. Parallel to these manifestations are difficulties in thinking. Most conspicuous is a difficulty in concentrating since thinking requires a high degree of ego integration. There are many kinds of thinking disturbances beyond the classical descriptions of loose associations or cognitive slippage. A blocking in mid-stream of thought processes, criss-crossing of thought patterns, the sudden injection of thoughts which do not seem connected, and automatic recollections which are a consequence of the early stages of regression in object relationships are examples. Because of the high degree of integration and abstraction necessary for thinking, cognituve difficulties are one of the most sensitive signs of impaired ego functioning.

In a gross psychosis, there is a regression of ego functioning to a level where the differences between internal thoughts and perceptions are confused, as well as what is experienced from external stimulation. At such a transitional stage the distinction between the self and the non-self loses its differentiation. In some of these individuals the prominence of persistent thoughts begins to replace object relationships in the withdrawal processes. It then becomes more conspicuous, and for some, even audible (in the form of hallucinations).

Dependency Cravings. A heightening of inordinate demands for dependency gratification may become conspicuous. The demands are toward family members, friends, and sometimes individuals they have hardly known. It includes increased insistence that others meet some of their needs, a process which conveys impairment in reality testing. Sometimes these demands for attachment or body contact take the form of peculiar or brash sexual approaches which are a desperate effort to mobilize new relationships, or the caricature of affection through group experiences where hugging and touching go on, often under drug influence.

Misinterpretations. At some point in this prodromal stage, an experience of significance occurs. The adolescent begins to attach symbolic meaning to perceptions which actually are quite innocuous. Chance associations and connections occur. Sometimes fantasic elaborations of a highly complex nature are developed involving symbols, numbers, and intuitions. When this happens meanings become so multiple that the youth becomes confused. If pushed further, meaningless gestures take on special meaning.

Loss of Ego Boundaries. Loss of ego boundaries is manifested in the illusion of transitivism.[13] It represents a regression of ego development toward an undifferentiated phase, specifically of separation-individuation. Adolescence has enormous demands for separation and individuation which requires a fair degree of emerging competence. Investigators agree on seventeen as the high risk age for the onset of schizophrenic psychosis—the first post-high school year.[14] Lack of clear separation of which ego functions belong to the self or another occur. The handicap is that the sense of integrationa dn separateness of an individual is impaired. It gives way to feelings of mutual influence, exchange, and fusion. When such a breakdown in egc boundaries occurs, there is a feeling that thoughts are known to cthers, or that one's own thoughts may be those of others. Some report the emotions of the entire world are going through them, while some say that they have been robbed of skills which they once possessed.

> A fifteen-year-old adolescent girl who became extremely withdrawn and dropped out of school a year earlier for a home tutor, reported she no longer liked to see her best friend since she was no longer able to tell what was her best friend's and what was hers. She believed that when the two of them were together the friend talked like she did and she talked like the friend and she could no longer determine who was who. There was a feeling that her own motility and gestures belonged to someone else. The internal experience of

undifferentiation was experienced as an oncoming loss of herself. It is a major source of overwhelming anxiety in individuals with psychotic reactions.

While classic descriptions place an emphasis on minute descriptions of the peculiar speech, language, and conduct, these are attempts at demarcation and delineation of the self. The hope is to prevent being absorbed into some external collective or inanimate world. Similarly, delusions of grandeur such as being some type of special person with outstanding achievements serves the same purpose of continuing to demarcate an individual so as not to be swallowed up in the masses. The extension of adolescent fantasies of power have then gone awry.

Delusions of world catastrophe appear where a person feels he is the only survivor in a world where everyone else has disappeared. Preoccupations with disasters are an example, in which a conviction arises that everything will disappear. In some cases, the suspension is resolved by provoking a violent encounter. The mechanism is an ego-split in which the world is populated with various alter-egos which are projections of self-representations. The concept of restitution is applicable. The loss of object representation is conspicuous in these individuals. Pushed to an opposite extreme we have catatonic stupors in which violence is always a threat.

Three Primary Forms of Anxiety. Laing delineates three forms of anxiety which are relevant to prodromal signs: engulfment, implosion, and petrification.[15] A firm sense of the autonomy of one's own identity is required if one is to relate to another human being and expect reciprocity. If there is no strong sense of identity most relationships threaten individuals with the loss of identity. When *engulfment* anxiety occurs, the individual dreads relating to others as such, or for that matter with anyone or anything. Because of uncertainty about autonomy, acute anxiety may arise. This is not experienced simply as an individual fearing that unless he is vigilant, he will be engulfed. It is that he experiences himself as an individual who is saving himself from drowning by having to be constantly and strenuously on the alert. Even more threatening, engulfment is felt as a risk in actually being understood, or being loved, or simply in being seen. To be hated is fearful for other reasons, but it may be less disturbing than to feel one may be swallowed up or engulfed.

A dichotomy is presented between the fear of being engulfed by another person and removing oneself by withdrawal into a state of isolation as a defense. In this type of dialectic no third option is available. Alternations do occur, to be sure. If an adolescent hates himself intensely, he may wish to lose his own identity in another. This is a form of escape from himself which is sought. However, what is most sought at one moment may become a source of overwhelming anxiety at another. A caveat can be sounded as to what may happen if two willing helpers intervene with an individual with a borderline adjustment who is regressing into a psychosis. Demands for relating place one under an obligation. There is also the adverse contribution of helping these individuals by therapists, or just plain helpers, who are trying to show how much concern or love they have for mankind.

Of course, some of the complex motivations for why any individual wants to help another enter into this picture. When the adolescents sense that another individual can "let me be," it diminishes the threat of being engulfed and permits them to commence a relationship. Panic episodes are related to fears of being buried, drowned, caught and dragged down into quicksand or water, or burned, with images of fire recurring. The end for the extreme can result in a need for resolution by self-destructive acts. Some experience a state of isolation in which they feel frozen, cold, or arid—the schizoid as frozen into a catatonic state which can explode.

Another form of overwhelming anxiety is *implosion*. It is actually an extreme impingment of reality. However, the experience is often a terror in which the person feels liable at any moment to decompensate and lose all identity. An inner emptiness is experienced, and although at times it is longed for, the possibility is also feared. An awful feeling that existance is nothing, is not simply metaphorical for certain attributes or talents, but experienced literally.

Petrification is a feeling closely related to the traditional concept of depersonalization or derealization.[16] There are a number of meanings that become associated. On one level petrification may personify a form of terror whereby an individual becomes frozen—as though turned to stone. Another meaning refers to the dread of becoming frozen. In that case the threat is a potential and not just a singular anxiety. There is the possibility of being turned from a live person with mentality into an individual who is frozen, stoned, or robotized. The implication is that these youths have their personal autonomy of choice and action and personal subjectivity has thereby been abolished. Another meaning is an individual who petrifies others. By extension, this means another person has his individuality destroyed and consequently loses his feelings or regard for him as an individual. He is then treated not as a person with any degree of freedom but impersonally.

Depersonalizing permits an adolescent to live as though devoid of feelings. What customarily happens in the regressed state in the prodromata involves aggression to depersonalize oneself and others. Consequently, there is a retaliatory fear that one will be depersonalized by others, or made into nothing. There is a pervasive anxiety that the person will be turned into something impersonal by others. Hence, the person's constant seeking confirmation of integrity. Some commentators have written about the tendency toward depersonalization which happens in a mass society which is already dehumanized and mechanized.

The threat can be subtle. If an individual experiences another as a free agent who is exerting control over him, a threat is raised that he is experiencing himself as an object of such control. Hence, autonomy and subjectivity feel drained away. He is threatened with the possibility of being no more than a thing in the world of someone else—without any life of his own and without his own being. On a practical level, the types of comments that one hears from individuals caught in the grips of petrification processes are: "I have no more self," or "I'm no longer a person," or "I've lost my identity," or "I can only react to others and not take the initiative." These are related to formulations regarding the *false self* or, the *as if* personality.

DESCRIPTIVE ASPECTS

Puberty and Onset. A crucial question with respect to psychotic processes is the influence of puberty on the emergence of symptoms. Are there descriptive features that emerge in the adolescent age not only pathognomic of schizophrenia but inherently related to this age period as well? Thus, Hecker diagnosed the symptomotology of hebephrenia and believed the clinical picture was related to that age period. It was believed to arise from a disturbance of sexual maturation which today would be ascribed to neuro-humoral irregularities.

Complicating the picture are theorists who feel it is not that the signs and symptoms of psychosis bear a similarity to adolescence, but that the normal features of adolescence show characteristics of psychosis. In turn, this has been challenged as a distortion of adolescence. It is believed that adolescents do not inherently show psychotic behavior any more than other age groups. Again, if psychotic behavior occurs during adolescence, it is often self-limited. Do we then still hold to a diagnosis under the category of a *developmental psychosis* implying that the process was the result of developmental problems and something different from schizophrenia? Keep in mind the complications this might have for epidemiological and research studies since when developmental criteria are added, the prognosis and criteria employing a disease concept are shifted.

Symptom Variation. Another complication is that classical symptoms and signs of schizophrenia vary widely in the adolescent population. The majority are in the intitial stages of psychotic behavior and show a mixed clinical picture. If we take the classical areas of impairment from schizophrenia, we would expect to see difficulties in four areas: (1) cognition; (2) object relationships; (3) altered reality testing, and (4) impulse control.

Studies and clinicians continue to emphasize the myriad manifestations of psychosis in adolescence. In one study four major types of clinical symptomology were noted.[17]

1. Hysteroid or paranoid material were manifestations of psychosis in one group. It was hypothesized that individual differences constitutionally play a role, but also pre-existing neurotic conflicts or traumatic episodes were relevent to the period of onset.

2. Schizophreniform pictures with acute confusional symptomotology or catatonic syndromes were evident. In these cases there was more hereditary evidence.

3. Depressive phenomena in adolescence—in contrast to manic-depressive psychotic reactions—were another grouping of psychotic adolescents.

4. Impulse disinhibitory states were a variety of adolescent psychosis.

In a factor-analytic study of 640 thirteen- to eighteen-year-old boys and girls with mixed symptomatology, ninety-three considered overtly schizophrenic received a high score on five of eighteen factors.[18] The high-score factors were:

1. Bizarre cognition in which the adolescents substituted or confused pronouns in conversation. For example, instead of using the pronoun "I," they used their name to refer to themselves in conversation. Their speech was incoherent and disconnected and some hallucinated.

2. Bizarre behavior included facial grimacing, postures, and engaging in dangerous behavior (putting things in their mouths and swallowing them, rocking behavior, etc.).

3. Schizoid withdrawal involved blank staring and a far-away quality. Many appeared deeply preoccupied, and were occasionally observed talking to themselves.

4. Emotional withdrawal was maintained by distance or reserve from adults and appeared to have a lack of emotional involvement.

5. Poor impulse control was exhibited when they became upset and overreacted when things did not go their way. They were subject to outbursts of anger, easily upset by peers, and reacted with anger to frustrating situations such as difficulty in learning.

These groupings illustrate no more than certain symptoms present in any age group which can become manifest in adolescence. But is there anything inherently pathognomonic about these symptoms emerging during adolescence? Various hypotheses are possible.

1. Some genetic predispositions need time before they become manifest. It may be that types of experiences cannot take place before puberty. Another complication is that psychological and physical changes take place over a period of time before the overt manifestations emerge. An example would be juvenile paresis transmitted via the mother which does not appear until adolescence.

2. Schizophrenic manifestations may have nothing to do with the developmental stage per se, but instead merely become more obvious as the child develops. The precipitating influences then constitute a discrepancy between the development of an individual's capacities and the social and personal demands being made on him.

3. Perhaps adolescence is a period of great vulnerability. Besides the social factors, it may also be related to the physical and psychological alterations within an adolescent.

4. Certain psychological conflicts and symptomatic pictures appear more frequently in adolescence. In the vulnerable individual these give a loading toward early manifestations. Such situations may be related to exaggerated mood swings, difficulties in gaining autonomy from parental closeness, regression to maintain closeness to parents, hypochondriacal manifestations, changing body image, guilt over masturbation, and adolescent neurasthenia with symptoms of increasing anxiety, irritability, and fatigue. Changing relationships between body configuration and psychological development with inconsistent growth patterns can heigten conflict.

Another complication ensues from the position of a clear-cut distinction between the psychoses of early childhood and a second grouping which does not emerge until adolescence. The position may be exaggerated or inaccurate, probably due to the lack of good longitudinal studies in the course of which early symptomatic manifestations, of a minor degree, are followed through into adolescence and beyond. It is far easier to take cross-sectional groupings in clinics for research purposes and on that basis develop theoretical formulations. The difficulty is that this method may give a false and misleading picture of the true nature of how psychotic processes emerge. It is interesting that such longitudinal investigations still come from Europe rather than the United States.

The Russian psychiatrist, Ushahov, has delineated types of schizophrenia which have a fairly insidious onset in the course of the elementary school years.[19] These are distinguished from such childhood psychoses as early infantile autism or symbiotic psychosis. Early manifestations can be seen which will not only aid the clinician in assessment but provide a research base in an area which is now quite unexplored. Some early manifestations are along autistic lines of development, but distinguished from the diagnosis of early infantile autism, in which the individuals are different from the beginning and remain preoccupied with their need to be alone and undisturbed. In contrast, early manifestations of schizophrenia in the elementary school period, are new to the previously affectionate, sociable, active, and vivacious child.

A second characteristic seen in these initial stages is described as a lowering of energy. Where these children were previously active, curious, and possessed a good deal of initiative, in time they changed to the opposite. They manifested such complaints as, "My head feels heavy," "I can't think as easily anymore," and "I read but can't remember." Some of these latency age children then begin to refuse school and are thought of as having school phobias, which is only correct in a descriptive sense.

In a third grouping are dissociative processes. Exaggerated contradictions in strivings emerge. Neurotic trends appear in terms of achievements, interests, and judgments. For some of these children disturbances in motor behaviors such as tics, or mannerisms appear. Not until adolescence do more exaggerated symptoms of emotional disturbance appear: pronounced ambivalence, mood instability, overt compulsions, and sensory disturbances. At that point a host of symptomatic manifestations occur which vary from apathy, asthenia, and lowered energy to impulse-ridden acting out, assaultive behavior, sexual attacks, aggressive activity, and vagrancy.

Fears, hypochondriacal tendencies, or fantasies slowly shift into delusions. Ideas of persecution occur in the context of a heightened self-criticism. A cognitive correspondence to the systematization of ideation occurs in preadolescent children. In the course of adolescent years the autonomy of the delusional system increases, and its discorroboration by reality testing becomes less probable. The main characteristic of the unfolding psychotic process is the episodic, transitory, and fragmentary nature of the symptomotology. While the symptoms gradually become similar to those seen in adults, such as those of a paranoid or delusional type, they seem to remain more transitory and rudimentary.

Researchers and clinicians who focus on adults miss the early manifestations. By the time patients contact them, they have already reached an established state. While the younger child shows disturbances in speech disorders or motor behavior, the adolescent shows more cognitive symptomatology. Bizarre ideation, incoherence of thoughts, confusion and derailment of thought processes, and delusions become manifest. A fixity of obsessional ideas to control anxiety is another clincal variation.

The following case history illustrates the type of material just discussed in terms of early manifestations of schizophrenia from childhood which were not seen clinically as part of a psychotic process.

A sixteen-year-old boy was referred to a clinic from school because of poor school performance and social behavior. He had few friends and his school performance was ascribed simply to a failure to do the work. His measured *I.Q.* on an individually administered intelligence test was at a superior level. His general behavior to most school personnel, such as teachers, the principal, or the school nurse, was that of disrespect. At times there was a quality of haughtiness to his behavior. He ran away from home a few times but returned after five to ten days.

On appraisal there did not appear to be any loss of contact with reality or distortion. Nor were any manifestations of thought disturbance evident. Rather, a quality of marked oppositional behavior was present, exaggerated beyond most adolescents of his age.

He first showed behavioral changes in the first and second grade. Other than that he was described as a happy child who had had friends in nursery school. A close relationship between the boy and his mother was described in these early years while the father, a salesman, was gone during the week. Because of irritability and restlessness in the early elementary school years, he was referred to a child guidance clinic which diagnosed him as having a 'hyperkinetic learning problem.' He was tried on various stimulant drugs with intermittent reports of being 'same, better, or poor.' After about a year medication stopped, and he continued a rather sporadic school performance. He was known to some of the teachers as a middle of the roader but did not manifest behavior which would lead him into further difficulties. The parents continued to remain puzzled about why his behavior had changed from his early childhood period, and were given explanations that children frequently show such differences in the course of their development.

After a few months of individual interviews at age sixteen, he terminated treatment. He was next seen at age eighteen in connection with an acute confusional state associated with 'dropping acid.' At that point he was leading a rather nomadic existence in a commune setting and though constantly surrounded by individuals he described as his friends it appeared that he was able to maintain his distance without becoming deeply attached to any of these people. He had left home a year previously, although he would appear at home at unannounced times and make demands on his parents for money or clothing. At age twenty-one he was admitted to an inpatient psychiatric unit in an acutely psychotic state with the classical symptoms of catatonic schizophrenia after an outburst of violence.

Impaired Object Relationships. Difficulty in object relationships in adolescent schizophrenia has been commented upon by many workers. An increased interpersonal sensitivity was noted long ago by Harry Stack Sullivan.[20] When coupled with a social withdrawal, an exaggerated effect occurs in terms of impaired ability to tolerate the give and take demanded in relating to others. This barrier in socialization appears related to a high anxiety level analogous to a hyperallergenic state.

Some of Masterson's work is relevant.[21] In one group of twenty-four adolescent patients, eighteen were eventually diagnosed as schizophrenic, but only seven had exhibited cognitive disturbances, poor reality testing, and inappropriate affect during their first interview. The remaining eleven presented a mixed clinical picture involving personality disturbance, depressive symptomotology, and one with a psychotic picture not seen as schizophrenia. Some appeared to have common sociopathic traits and schizoid tendencies. The group with sociopathic tendencies had background histories of difficulty in concentration, insomnia, and motor restlessness, as well as academic failure, truancy, and intrafamilial conflict. Most striking was a long-standing history of difficulty in socialization. They had blunted affect and related to others with an evasiveness coupled with suspiciousness.

The group with prominent depressive features presented with

suicidal preoccupation or an initial admission ticket based on some suicidal gesture or attempt. The conclusion was that relatively few schizophrenic adolescents present with unequivocal signs of schizophrenia. Instead sociopathic tendencies or depressive symptoms account for most of the borderline type of disturbed adolescents who emerge as adult schizophrenics.

PSEUDOSCHIZOPHRENIAS AND PSYCHOTIC CHARACTERS

Pseudo-types of schizophrenia or psychosis are particularly relevant to the adolescent age group in view of the large number who do not manifest clear-cut symptoms. These individuals have many psychotic-prone problems concealed under a veneer of neurotic traits or antisocial tendencies. Even those adolescents with disturbances in primary criteria present diagnostic dilemmas due to the ambiguities with which these manifestations can present. Disturbances in cognitive processes, general anhedonia, fluctuating social impairment, and temporary personal distress are more frequent manifestations than the oft-cited signs and symptoms of hallucinations, stupor, self-mutilation, delusional thought content, marked ambivalence, or autistic and dereistic manifestations.

When individual outbursts of aggressive assaultive behavior occur in this age group, puzzlement is great because of the lack of indicia prior to the outburst. At that point a diagnosis of psychosis may or may not be made. Difficulties arise in the grey areas with those who present few clear-cut clinical signs and symptoms. They are often able to conceal their inner states from the public, if not from clinicians, for long periods of time, particularly if they present their discontent in terms of hostility toward society or authority figures. Differential diagnosis becomes complicated when the individuals have been given other diagnoses along the way. Another difficulty arises from those opposed to diagnosis, so deviations are merely viewed as part of a continuum.

There are many ways to conceptualize individuals with concealed or covert signs, symptoms, and behaviors indicative of psychosis-proneness. At times they have been called pseudoneurotic schizophrenics, pseudopsychopathic individuals, ambulatory schizophrenics, borderlines, latent psychotics, or psychotic characters. Emphasis may be placed upon the characterlogical distortions, such as referring to their "as-if" character structures or ego distortions. Table 24 provides a classification of the primary and secondary clinical symptoms of pseudoneurotic schizophrenia.[22]

TABLE 24

SYMPTOMS OF PSEUDONEUROTIC SCHIZOPHRENIA

I. Primary Clinical Symptoms

    A. Disorders of Thinking and Associations

        1. Process (form)

            (a) Evidence of characteristics of primary process thinking

            (b) Disturbances in thought continuity and goal directed thought

            (c) Disturbances of thought flow

            (d) Disturbances of awareness, attention, anticipation, and concentration

            (e) Impairment in the process of concept-formation

        2. Content

            (a) Content dominated by stereotyped, anachronistic concepts and attitudes

            (b) Distorted concepts of self, body-image, the world, and the interrelationships of these

            (c) Rigid and distorted concepts of the meaning and utilization of intellect, emotion, and behavior

            (d) Chaotic concepts of sexuality

    B. Disorders of Emotional Regulation

        1. Process (form)

            (a) Evidence of some of the characteristics of primary process functioning

            (b) Low threshold to anxiety

            (c) Heterogeneity of emotional response; emotional volatility with dysregulation of emotional depth

            (d) Inertia in initiating, sustaining, and terminating emotional response

            (e) Impairment of ability to select and regulate aggression and assertion

            (f) Complex-bound emotional reactions

      (g) Latent period between perceiving stimulus and conscious recognition of associated emotional reaction

      (h) Somatization of emotional reactions

  2. Content

      (a) Intolerance of tension, and diffuse anxiety

      (b) Impairment of feeling tone, and anhedonia

      (c) Impairment of empathy; sensitiveness with low threshold to withdrawal reaction

      (d) Exploitation of others in effort to experience emotion

      (e) Emotional feelings repudiated; intellectualization of emotion

      (f) Craving for stimulation; craving for protection and dependency

      (g) Striving for quick, magical gratification of needs

C. Disorders of Sensorimotor and Autonomic Functioning

  1. Impairment of integration of sensory perceptions

  2. Impairment of ability to select and maintain motor responses

  3. Somatization of emotional reactions; autonomic dysfunction

  4. Impairment of sensorimotor-autonomic integration in psychosexual functioning

  5. Energy dysregulation; intolerance of sustained activity toward future goals

  6. Pursuit of sensory and motor patterns as substitutes for stimulus-appropriate thought, feeling, or action

I. Secondary Clinical Symptoms

A. Pan-Anxiety

B. Pan-Neurosis (neurotic symptoms, acting-out behavior, and character disorder symptoms)

C. Pan-Sexuality

Source: Hoch and Cattell, *Psychiatric Quarterly*, 33:491, 1959.

In a few cases many of these myriad symptoms are present. One difficulty in such a listing is the lack of knowledge of developmental processes and conflicts which reach fruition by adolescence. Some show a wide variety of behaviors which get them into difficulty with other people, community institutions, and courts, while others demonstrate a minimum of such behavior. Since adolescents are more prone to get into community difficulties anyhow, the following discussion illustrates how symptoms of pseudoneurotic schizophrenia can lead to antisocial behaviors which seem hysterical in nature.

Aggressive assaultive behavior and polymorphous sexual activity of an impulsive, compulsive, or planned type occur. Many times the degree of personal psychopathology is missed from focussing on a red herring such as drug usage. Particularly does this occur when community houses or centers staffed by minimally trained people or peers are the treaters. In other cases episodic violence appears, together with swindling, extorting, or posing as an imposter either in a socioeconomic or sexual sense as youth age approaches. Bizarre activity, or defenses against it may be the admission to a clinic or legal entanglements.

These formulations bear similarity to the ideas of Lauretta Bender on childhood schizophrenia.[23] She divided the course of schizophrenia into five variations:

1. A pseudodefective type viewed clinically as similar to the early infantile autism of Kanner
2. A pseudoneurotic type manifesting itself in middle childhood and showing symptoms similar to a psychosis emerging during that developmental period
3. A pseudopsychopathic type emerged later, during preadolescence or early adolescence
4. Psychotic episodes could be intermingled with any of the above three types
5. A pseudonormal type was seen as schizophrenia in remission

Within this framework schizophrenia is viewed as an ongoing, latent process in which psychotic states intervene periodically. In the course of the developing processes schizophrenic symptoms can shift. Antisocial manifestations can gain expression. In this connection, it is a matter of a schizophrenic process manifesting itself in diverse forms. Nor need the schizophrenic manifestations necessarily be foremost a majority of the time. Some children with developmental problems in the realm of schizophrenia use accelerated developmental processes at of puberty to reorganize their defenses against the disorganizing effect of psychotic mentation. The defensive realignment permits them to suppress disturbing symptoms. Anxiety is ameliorated and not as many defenses are needed. The result is an increase or improvement in intellectual functioning, but the child appears to be in remission.

Another possibility then looms. It takes the form of stating that a diagnosis of schizophrenia made earlier must be in error from the current satisfactory level of performance. Reinforcing this is the fact that the child may deny his former symptomatology to himself and others. However, once into adolescence there are greater demands interpersonally. He is then given less protection and is forced to become more resilient or regress. His brittle defenses again come under threat. At that point, difficulties in identifying with older adults or relating to their peer group become manifest. Impulsivity and acting out ensue.

Such behavior is often called psychopathic until it reaches explosive degrees or periodic psychotic states. A basic schizophrenic process of disorganization again calls attention to the withdrawn or autistic state. Periodic catatonic responses can do likewise. In others, there may be dramatic, panneurotic symptoms in which basic paranoid attitudes are disguised, often accompanied by obsessional trends or a precipitation of illnesses. Catatonic excitement appears determined by the severance of dependency relationships, and then misdiagnosed as hysterical outbursts. The nature of the overwhelming anxiety is related to interruptions of symbiotic attachments.

In one study three patterns of adolescent schizophrenia were seen in fifty adolescent girls who had been hospitalized at Bellevue Hospital in New York City.[24] Eleven girls showed symptomology dating back to infancy or early childhood of a bizarre nature with developmental deviations suggestive of childhood schizophrenia. They had all been regarded by their families and teachers as strange, and quite unlike other children. Eighteen of the girls had had a gradual development of schizophrenic psychosis with a childhood background of serious personality and behavior problems which included fighting, stealing, absenting from home, truancy, temper tantrums, and sundry neurotic complaints. In another fifteen girls, no serious disturbance was in evidence prior to the onset of schizophrenia during the course of adolescence. This latter group appeared to have developed in an apparently normal fashion and without prominent signs of personlity dysfunction. The group showed a sharp delineation when they began to exhibit schizophrenic states. The remaining six girls presented an acutely developing psychotic state.

A comment is needed about the primitive and archaic system of controls that develops in these children.[25] Their moral development as seen in the structural development of the superego is striking. By the time adolescence is reached, their control system is riddled with impulsivity alternating with hypercritical and harsh responses of themselves, so that a dispropotionate quantity of guilt is in evidence. Hence, similar first manifestations of psychiatric disturbance may appear in the form of depressive reactions. In turn, inhibitions or withdrawal may show up in the form of postural and characterological rigidity.

Individuals with a psychotic character structure who are prone to acting out have ego states characterized by transient, regressive alterations in consciousness.[26] States of depersonalization are present in which bizarre acts are carried out. In retrospect, these acts appear to be performed in a dreamy or twilight state. States of unreality, in which the world seems to have altered, usher in a psychotic state for a period of time. At times the adolescents describe themselves as having been caught up in a frenzy of activity and carried helplessly along—as though they had lost control over their autonomy or sense of direction. The sense of time, place, and person become vague. Many acts of a bizarre or self-destructive type accompany these phenomenological states. It is very difficult for the adolescent at those times to fix exact times concerning the sequence of events, and they are frequently rationalized by clinicians as due to the vagueness attendant upon much adolescent behavior. Many psychotic characters are viewed as having epileptic or limbic system irregularities in their central nervous system. Drug usage makes the picture even more complicated.

Most confusing with respect to differential diagnosis is the amount of anxiety seen in psychotic-prone adolescents. Their anxiety may be all-pervasive, but descriptively it appears to be closer to a non-specific type of tension rather than to anxiety, which elicits defensive responses as in a neurosis. Such defensive responses with respect to anxiety are elicited in a series of internalized neurotic conflicts. It therefore becomes difficult to obtain words accurately portraying their anxiety in this state beyond repetitions of how tense they feel, or that they do not know how to put things. Gross restlessness accompanied by a driven quality accompany the anxiety and transient phobias may emerge.

Throughout segments of intact ego functioning remain. These intact areas function for the adolescent as though he is observing his own distraught state at a distance. Control over behaviors fluctuates at times as well. Particularly in adolescents of this type, the capacity of the ego for reversibility of regressive processes is characteristic. It provides another measure of ego strength which may be missing in contrast to those with long-standing psychotic processes. The weakness of the ego in a psychotic character lies in the ease with which regression takes place; the ego strength is in the ability to reverse the regressive process. Accompanying these processes a multiplicity of symptoms can be present as well as disturbances within the environment. When regressive trends predominate, many ego functions become impaired with a prominance of denial and replacement of reality by a regressive distortion of external reality.

EXTREMES OF VIOLENCE IN THE PSYCHOTIC CHARACTER

An appraisal of extreme violent behavior in adolescents from a perspective of their developmental conflicts is essential since they may not show overt signs and symptoms of a psychosis. Further, the incidence of antisocial behavior as part of the schizophrenic process in the pre-adolescent period is not believed to be high as part of the overall complex. It is not something with a high predictive potential.

When antisocial behavior based on a psychotic character occurs it is lumped with delinquency. The reason is lack of knowledge about the complex varieties of conflicts which can give rise to delinquent acts. Since the criteria for pseudodelinquent schizophrenia are often subtle, not only for clinicians but among those working in correctional facilities, these youths tend to be placed under the legal category of delinquents, or—if of the age of legal majority—as criminals. In terms of their acts, this is correct, although it misses the clinical basis for their behavior.

Panic States. In some adolescents a panic state is experienced which precipitates an act of violence. The act may have a particularly senseless, brutal, or bizarre quality. It appears related to an inability of the ego to handle an overwhelming amount of anxiety which threatens in terms of an ultimate annihilation or destruction. These adolescents need differentiation from those whose anxiety is primarily concerned with separation fears or bodily injury.[27] In the fantasies of some there are themes of world destruction, such as burning up, falling apart, or disintegrating.

Peculiar sadistic behavior may have been perpetrated in the past or present on animals, or people. The emotionality can vary widely from apathy or flatness following such an activity to a state of frenzy or rage.

> A twelve-year-old was finally detected by the school cook in the act of putting pins in the batter for cakes. A week earlier ground glass had been discovered by some boys eating their desserts, and hence the cooks had been alerted. He talked about these incidents with a tone of nonchalance, with little visible display of affect. The only display came in a joint interview with his mother (the parents were divorced), when he related how he felt when the other boys excluded him, and when he felt they had a deliberate plan afoot to exclude him from their social, scholastic, and athletic activities. He was as firmly convinced as any adult paranoid that there was some type of elaborate plot to exclude him involving the other boys within the school and perhaps involving his mother, who vehemently denied it.

All Or Nothing Reactions. Serious acts of violence such as murder, suicide, or setting gigantic fires appear related to a kill or be killed phenomenon.[28] It is seen as exchanging a usually passive position of being vulnerable to destruction at the hands of others for a process where they become the destroyers. They describe feelings of doing to someone else what they felt had once been done to them. Mechanisms of externalization and identification with the aggressor are used to defend against fears of being overwhelmed by anxiety. Such behavior may be viewed as an integral part of a psychotic process. Another viewpoint is to see such behavior as a defense against regressing into an overt psychosis with secondary psychotic symptoms, accompanied by hallucinations or delusions.

> An eleven-year-old boy, in walking to his home through a dark street, passed a police car assigned to patrol this high-delinquency neighborhood. As the boy passed, he was called over to the car and told to get in for questioning. He was interviewed for about ten minutes and mumbled a few incoherent answers or grunts. As he was leaving the car, the police officers decided to search him for any stolen articles. He was told to lean over the end of the car with his hips 'sticking out.' A moment later he pulled out an old pocket knife and stabbed the nearest officer. When later evaluated, he recalled the incident as one where he was positive he would be attacked and felt his only hope was to strike first. He saw little inappropriateness in his behavior and thought he would do it again in 'self defense.' When others, including the judge, did not see his behavior in this manner, the boy was perplexed. He did not understand why others could not

follow his thinking processes and were even accusing him of making up ideas as an excuse to be released.

Explosive Rage. Explosive rage in these individuals often comes as a surprise to those who know them. Since the predelinquent features of a schizophrenic process may have been evidenced by autistic or inhibited behavior, uncontrolled episodes of directly acting out impulses, fits of attacking, crying, or laughing seem incongruous. Only by putting the entire clinical history together is perspective obtained.

A progressive history of brooding and ambivalence may have preceded an explosive outburst. The first such episode or unusual behavior can occur anywhere, such as at school, home, or neighborhood. It may initially be overlooked. As adolescence approaches these patterns become more frequent, but their cumulative impact may not be known. Transformations of a passive position into an active one occur with dramatic intensity when a previously passive adolescent commits a headline-catching and dramatic crime, such as shooting several people, or going on a bank-robbing spree. The destructive wishes reach a dangerous potential.[29] Some potentiating factors are:

1. When family rivalry situations are intensified due to some external factor increasing the dangerous potential.

2. Intensified rivalry situations occur which is different for a paticular child. Examples are placement in a new foster home when affectional responses are not strong enough to curb aggressive tendencies or attachments have not developed.

3. Organic factors are present as a background factor which make the child feel inferior, helpless, disorganized, and in need of love which is not experienced as forthcoming.

4. Educational difficulties become insurmountable and the child senses an inferior status, particularly when provocation and teasing by peers occurs. A type of learning problem, such as a reading disability in a child of good intelligence, may be in the picture.

5. Familial behavior patterns in which exaggerated aggressivity is present in one or both parents, and the adolescent feels threatened from them as a prime reaction pattern.

The Overly Taxed Ego. Uncontrolled aggressive behavior may be an early sign that a child is struggling with impulses beyond the capacity of vulnerable ego to handle. Temper tantrums during the adolescent years are an example, along with more open regressions, such as urinating in inappropriate places. Other examples are unpredictable outbursts against other children, or biting. If delusional features emerge, as the core of hate is projected, there is a transition to where an inner debate as to the validity of the delusional processes becomes manifest. At times there is placidity and control, but then an outburst of violence followed by a strikingly composed state. A protective setting functions as a rescuer for them. Qualities of distance and aloneness are maintined for the most part with peers. Even when in a group, they are not part of it. Their sole friend may be another severely disturbed child, a retarded one, or a pet animal. The pet may have an alternating role of physical closeness and sadistic teasing or torture.

Familial interactional patterns are significant. Young girls may prostitute or act out homosexual impulses mingled with physical violence. Signs of primitive ego and superego development are seen in their relative lack of guilt or remorse. This, coupled with their indifference and emotional flatness when they are caught, is a significant diagnostic aid. From their defective internalized control system, punishment has little meaning to them as a current deterrer or future restrainer in terms of modifying behavior.

> Robert, a fourteen-year-old boy home from a residential treatment center, was subsequently indicted for first-degree murder in connection with the strangling death of a nine-year-old neighborhood boy.
>
> Robert had had a long history of peculiar behavior and was viewed as an 'outsider' by most who knew him. To some extent he had been exposed to teasing by two older brothers who in more recent years tended to ignore him. He was the closest to the youngest sibling for whom he had adopted a maternal and protective attitude. The year before attention had been called to Robert by school authorities after he locked a boy in a closet for a whole night. What led to his admission to a treatment center was his 'play activity,' involving tying a rope around a boy's neck and then hanging it around iron bars, which would have resulted in strangulation. This was done with little affect and little insight into the nature of what he had done. No defect in intellectual performance was present when he was administered an *IQ* test. The killing resulted when a younger boy, who Robert barely knew, followed him into a store and saw him buy a pack of cigarettes. He begged for cigarettes and angered Robert when he followed him as he walked along. At one time Robert lost track of the boy but on approaching a lake the boy still lurked about a block away. At that point he motioned the boy to join him. As he and the boy walked along the side of the lake, he began to strangle him and in a state of frenzied sexual excitement while laying on top of him heard a snap in

the boy's neck. The boy gave a gasp and was motionless. The body was left lying in the lake.

Robert was apprehended a few days later after having returned to the treatment center after his weekend leave home appearing no different to the staff.

Relevance of Sullivanian Concepts.   Some theoretical formulations of Harry Stack Sullivan related to the genesis of a severely defective self-regulatory system are relevant for these adolescents.[30] The nature of their defective self-concept was referred to by Sullivan as the "malevolent transformation," or the interpersonal relationship of a child with a chronically hostile parent. Since there are ramifications of this theory, a precis of Sullivan's ideas related to psychopathological malevolence is of interest.

In late infancy a *good me* and *bad me* are postulated as evolving inner states. The former is associated with obedient behavior and wins a reward of tender handling, usually by a maternal caretaker. The bad me is associated with rebelliousness and leads to an intensive forbidding element from a maternal object. A concommitant feature is an increase in anxiety. In a broad sense this is a form of learning by an *anxiety gradient.* Two corresponding maternal images develop: a good mother who is satisfying and a bad mother who is anxiety-provoking. Another postulation is a *not-me* which comes in the course of experiencing intense and unrelieved anxiety. Such experiences are associated with uncanny emotional states and unpleasurable affects such as awe, horror, loathing, or dissociative episodes, and psychotic decompensations.

Punishment for forbidden behavior is introduced in the course of infancy and thereafter as an educational measure. This permits a progressive discrimination among authority figures as to what is, and what is not, tolerated. If authority figures are confusing, and the situations into which the child is placed are ambiguous, the oughts and musts become blurred. The experience is contradictory and an unreasonable cultural proscription which feeds anxiety. Rationalization by a child is an example of using irrelevant words in the hope of sparing anxiety or punishment.

As if behaviors are another group of devices used to aid concealment. This is seen in sequential dramatizations in which children play at being an adult by acting and sounding like an adult. They act like an adult, and finally behave as if they were an adult. Such multiple "me's" are an inherent part of normal growth processes, but they may be used deceptively. When children act as though they can get close when they really cannot deception is operating. Preoccupation with compulsive work in the course of school years is a technique to ward off anxiety by continuing a pattern which was once beneficial but no longer is. Isolation of such activities from feelings contributes to obsessional trends.

The development of malevolence is a miscarriage of anger and resentment. It is observed in children who are timid and afraid to undertake what might be urgently needed. Later, they feel mischievous and begin to take it out on pets or younger children. Rather than calling such behavior an expression of an inherent, sadistic drive, where the police power of the state is needed to keep people from tearing others to pieces, Sullivan felt that a disturbance in early learning processes had occurred. Since the dependency needs of children are not something they can choose to have or not, they must be handled in some manner.

A child associates tenderness with dependency and learns which behaviors will gain him approval (the good me) and/or disapproval (the bad me). The attitudes and feelings of those with whom the child associates intimately are uncritically accepted and introjected by way of psychological processes. The acceptance occurs without a critical capacity to appraise or reject them. If people around a youngster can express tenderness and respect, the child acquires such feelings toward himself; if they are derogatory and hateful, he similarly acquires these attitudes toward himself and carries them for the remainder of his life.

What if the seeking of emotional closeness and tenderness is rebuffed by adults with whom a child is intimate? The reaction elicited is that he has misbehaved or behaved badly. The need for closeness becomes associated with anxiety. The child is poised to strike back against provocative people who he knows. An experiential state of living among enemies is engendered which makes it difficult for anyone in contact to feel tenderly towards him. By a process of anticipation, the child attempts to beat others to the punch and conceal a need for intimacy. However, the process is extended into a pattern of provoking others to punish and ostracize. It is more comfortable to feel hated and provocative than to recognize the deep pain of an unsatisfied need for tenderness in oneself. In a broader sense, the end result can be viewed as the failure of adults to discharge their responsibility to produce a socialized human being. From such a distorted socialization experience a series of personal hurts results in which society is ultimately the loser.

"As If" Personality Components.   The as if personality structure resulting from defective object relationships has been lucidly described by Deutsch.[31] A characteristic impression is their lack of genuineness, combined with an outward facade that runs along as if it were complete. Despite normal and superior intellect, and the absence of overtly disordered behavior, an intangible feeling emerges that something is wrong. Relationships with others may seem like friendship, love, sympathy, and understanding, yet a formality is present which excludes warmth. A plastic passivity to blend into the thoughts and feelings of someone else is present, and gives an initial impression of loyalty. Such ties are in reality fragile, as noted in a sequence of ties in which their ideals and convictions merely reflect those of other people. As the models are chosen by qualities of suggestibility and passivity in the chooser, antisocial criminal acts can occur due to a passive readiness to be influenced. These were once attributed to an erotic bondage and involve sado- masochistic relationships. The potential readiness of such individu- als later in life to accommodate to group corruption is obvious.

The type of controls over their impulses appears to be like a conforming individual. Yet there is more of the clinical quality of a conditioned character type than consistent set of internalized values. Another person can come along to whom these people will relate as they have before and merely exchange their values. Acquiescence to the acting out of any group will take place with little protest, varying only somewhat by circumstances and individuals. Their vulnerability lies in their readily changing loyalties to diametric opposites. While such fluidity may be transiently present in adolescence, in the "as ifers" it is more rather than less enduring over time. A history of participating in diverse groups seeking ever- new experiences is common. Sometimes the twist taken is to quasi- religious or moral groups. As adolescence passes into youth political or activist organizations of widely varying philosophies or artistic endeavors gain appeal. An end result is often a facsimile of the originality of others. In such seekings, a potent intellectual grasp of the subject is possible, along with a firm knowledge of the forms and acts required. These are devices to externalize conflict by permitting the ego a series of temporary identifications with external authori- ties who never become introjected. There is a lack of guilt or responsibility for antisocial behaviors, since they are dependent on shifting allegiances which occur in the course of exposures during their lifetimes.

Other conditions indicative of personality conflict have similarities. These are conditions such as fugues, amnesias, hypnoid states, multiple personalities, dissociative states, and depersonalization experiences. Such phenomena are usually regarded as defensive maneuvers to handle conflict. Drugs, sensory deprivation, and hypnotic phenomena can also induce states during which antisocial behavior occurs. In all of these, numerous identifications produce a disruption in the ego and lead to a diffusion of ego identities. In some cases the aspects which are ego-syntonic remain conscious while those connected with dystonic impulses remain more repressed. In few of these categories do issues of responsibility on a conscious level get much personal credence, although they well may be raised in a legal setting.

Bychowski reported on a form of dissociation which he called "escapades."[32] The elements of escapades are illustrated by the case of a middle-class young female who began to leave home for several days at a time after her marriage. In the course of these escapades she actually contracted two bigamous marriages.

> About a year prior to the time of her being seen clinically, she began to leave home for several days at a time. During one of these periods, a second marriage was contracted to a man of her own social class. They both knew she was married, but this did not prevent them from going through with the ceremony. This double existence rapidly came to an end without further event. She lost interest in the man. However, her second escapade took a different twist. After a brief affair, she married a simple working man who at the time was separated from his wife, but the father of several children who were still living with him. She moved into his house and assumed all the chores of a simple housewife, as well as taking care of his children. She even acquired a few simple dresses in keeping with her new social class.
>
> When questions were raised concerning the awareness of her actions, it appeared she had never forgotten her personal identity. She was doing her best to make herself forget about being Mrs. X, so she could find herself in her new role. She succeeded for long periods of time. 'Did I know what I was doing?' She then explained that in a 'sick way' she knew what she was doing and that she was aware of marrying another man and committing a criminal act. She described herself as attempting to become absorbed in detail so as not to think about it. This involved reflection as to how she could have gone through with these things, but she recognized a striving on her part to 'go down to the bottom' and not think about it. Sex activity helped to forget by a process of immersion and putting off thinking for long periods of time.

Episodic Dyscontrol. Episodic dyscontrol is a formulation which accounts for many diagnoses and syndromes. Human personality is conceptualized and dedicated to the maintenance of a steady state, with various devices utilized to that end. Increased stress of an internal or external type requires the personality to pay a higher price to maintain a steady state. Five orders of dysfunction or dyscontrol were postulated by Karl Menninger.[33] They are gauged in terms of the extremities to which the ego goes in an effort to maintain its balance or conceal failures. In this sense, the orders of dysfunction represent varying degrees of increasing disorganization. Simultaneously, they are efforts to prevent further disorganization from taking place. A series of levels of control forestall surrender to further disorganization.

The mechanism of operation is viewed as a dyscontrol while the state of the individual personality is described as *disorganization* in terms of impaired, expansive, inefficient, or uncomfortable types of organization. The connotation of the word dyscontrol is that control has not yet been lost, but has rather been altered or impairred in contrast to the presence of a steady state.

Others have conceptualized episodic disorders in terms of precipitous interruptions in life-style which may be inhibitory or disinhibitory.[34] No fully acceptable classification exists for these disorders. The position taken here is that the primary value of a classification system is its benefit to the clinician or researcher. In that sense classifications show more or less consistency between etiological hypotheses, psychodynamic formultions, phenomenological reports, and neurophysiologic hypotheses.

While the syndrome of episodic behavioral disorders refers to any precipitously appearing behavior pattern of an intermittent or recurrent type which interrupts the homeostasis or psychological balance of an individual, terms from standard diagnostic classifications are useful. Such diagnoses as the following should call attention to this possibility: schizo-affective schizophrenia, chronic undifferentiated schizophrenia, acute schizophrenic episodes, depersonalization neurosis, explosive personality, hysterical personality, episodic drinking, psychosis with epilepsy, nonpsychotic organic brain syndrome with epilepsy, or unsocialized aggressive reaction of childhood or adolescence.

The following discussion illustrates the essentials of levels of dyscontrol without specific reference to a standard nomenclature:

The first order of dyscontrol is a state which lay people call *being nervous*. It implies a slight but definite impairment of adaptive control. There is a disturbance of personality organization, and a slight, but definite, failure in utilizing coping devices. In this context, the ego experiences a greater than average upsurge of anger, fear, or emotions which betray the arousal of aggression. Several devices and experiences accompany this first-order level of dyscontrol. One is an effort at hyper-suppression and hyper-repression. What the individual becomes aware of is a necessity to exert greater efforts to control himself or conceal internalized responses.

Another characteristic is *hypervigilance* or a state of increased alertness. This is greater sensitivity to the events and changes in the outside world. In part, the scanning function of the ego takes on greater work and becomes more aware of threats. Perceptual functioning becomes exaggerated, so that sounds are experienced as louder than normal, lights are brighter, and other sensations keener. The result is an alteration in sleep patterns during which insomnia begins.

A third characteristic of first-order dyscontrol is *hyper-emotionalism*. Increased touchiness, tearfulness, irritability, and changeableness indicate greater personality lability. Tendencies to cry easily, talk loudly, have brief outbursts of rage, and spells of moodiness, emerge.

A fourth device is *hyperkinesis*. This may vary from a generalized and mild overactivity to more impulsive and compulsive acts. There may be a generalized restlessness exhibited in mannerisms such as nail-biting, pacing, hand-wringing, or just a general inability to sit alone and reflect for any period of time. Of course, difficulties show up most prominently in difficulty in concentrating on school subjects or work.

Another phenomenon witnessed is *hyperintellection*. This is a form of overintellectualism in which a great deal of worrying and brooding take place with chronic concern. It is unproductive in the sense of being circular and repetitious, and it absorbs much energy. Obsessional thought processes are in evidence where the end results of prodigious intellectual effort are quite meagre.

A sixth manifestation of first-order dyscontrol is *hyper-compensatory* behavior. Examples are the elaboration of fantasies to compensate for disappointments or self-deprivations. A variation is seen in overzealous identification with some new cause, hero, or even affiliation with a former opponent or enemy. Since adolescents are prone to shifting identifications anyhow, this must be evaluated in the context of developmental fluctuations as well as in response to internalized crises. Indulgence in a wide spectrum of drug use may alternate with total avoidance. These adolescents require astute appraisal. Rabid espousals of any particular cause, with anger evidenced when anyone challenges or inquires into the premises for a position, is another tip-off. There appears to be an evangelistic quality of attempting to convert others to one's cause and puzzlement—if not outright anger—when another is not persuaded. All this exhibits a quality similar to the as if personality previously discussed. In some of these individuals the behavior is a manifestation of identification with the aggressor, enjoining causes to which one previously has had a strong antipathy. Such signs as elaborate denials of the obvious, overstaunch partisanship, and frantic protests or gestures for patriotism, peace, salvation, or martyrdom fall within this category.

Somatic discomforts can be expressions of first-order dyscontrol and should not be ignored. Somatizations vary from vegetative signs of autonomic discomfort to impairment in sexual functioning. In almost all of these beginning signs of discomfort and dyscontrol, classical formulations regarding symptom formation can be seen. Some type of pleasure-seeking may be present, as well as wishes to do with aggression. The actual attainment, or an act of indulgence or aggression per se, is not crucial. Instead, the desires and impulses for attainment are important. Contrariwise, there are wishes to undo any kind of damage which can occur from the expression of such desires which may be colored within the individual personality by self-punitive tendencies or the utilization of reparative devices.

Individuals in a state of second-order dyscontrol manifest overt discomfort. A chronic and gnawing sense of failure, uselessness, incompetence, or disappointment in themselves and others is present. These may alternate with flashes of envy, jealousy, and resentment, but an impairment in pleasure capacity is present. In descriptive nosology many of these reactions have been classified as neuroses. Rather than argue about whether this is a disease of the central nervous system, a severe illness of some type, or a purely psychological response, devices are focused on the quality of painfulness, expensiveness, and inefficiency to the organism. Commonly, there is a clinical syndrome representative of secondary dyscontrol summarized by Menninger as follows:[35]

Aggressive discharge blocked from consciousness by dissociative withdrawal (fainting, dissociation, sleep-walking, phobias and counterphobias); aggressive discharge displaced to the body (self-imposed restrictions, self-mutilation, somatization, intoxication and narcotization); aggressive discharge through symbolic and magical modifications (public and private rituals, symbolic doing and undoing, compulsions, kleptomania, pyromania, obsessional thinking, perverse sexual modalities); frozen emergency reactions which are personality deformations (inadequate, infantile, cyclothymic, narcissistic, negativistic, addictive, and fraudulent personalities indulging in lying, check forgery and malingering).

By the time third-order dyscontrol is reached, undisguised manifestations of aggression are present. Some acts may be socially condoned, although there are premonitory evidences of ego tension. Devices of displacement, projection, and paranoid interpretations lurk. Two forms of *ego rupture* occur: a chronic, repetitious occurrence of serious aggressions, or a sudden, explosive outburst. Although some individuals feel an ego rupture is imminent and seek help, they are often ignored or laughed at. This is because they do not present a dramatic picture in their request for help and do not appear overly psychotic. One eighteen-year-old who had been in contact with a community clinic murdered an unidentified bystander. A few weeks prior to this, he appeared at a local hospital after having consumed a bottle of wine. The alcohol on his breath lead the examining house officer to have him brought to the county jail, where he was booked on a charge of inebriation. This followed an altercation at the hospital in which he insisted he was afraid he was going crazy. When the physician examining him did not take him seriously, the patient struck him. He posted bail the same evening and continued his borderline adjustment for a few more weeks prior to shooting an individual in cold blood outside his house one evening.

Syndromes of third-order dyscontrol are divided into chronic aggressive behaviors, episodic impulsive acts (homicidal assaults, demoralizing or delirious status, excited syndromes) and episodic disorganized violence (seizures, brain damage syndromes, psychomotor equivalents).

When we come to fourth-order dyscontrol, extreme states of disorganization, regression, and repudiation of reality are present which usually receive psychotic diagnoses. A person at a fourth-order level still makes an effort to hide behind facades of quasi-normality. Hence, this represents a penultimate effort to avoid fifth-order disorganization. In the latter anxiety and depression are so overwhelming that death often results by suicide. The following are some of the syndromes of fourth-order disorganization also following Menninger:

A. Pervasive feelings of sadness, guilt, despondency, and hopelessness which are usually described as manifestations of some type of psychotic depression.
B. More or less continuous erratic and disorganized excitement, accompanied by an excessive verbal and motor production with states of elation, excitement, and irrascibility. Diagnostically, these are usually considered hypomanic or manic states.
C. Schizophrenic episodes in which autistic regression and self-absorption predominate as well as other mannerisms and overt cognitive defects.
D. Delusional preoccupation with one or several themes may occur. These may be persecutory and accompanied by defensiveness, suspiciousness, grandiosity, etc. Under this heading come the manifold types of paranoid responses and paranoia.
E. Confused, delirious states with disorientation, bewilderment, amnesia, confabulation, and occasional halluncinations or hyperactivity may be covered under what is called *dementia* or delirium.

Fifth-order disorganization has physiological functioning continue although psychological functioning is at a bare level of insensate existence. Homicide, suicide, or other serious acts of violence appear as options. In all too many court cases, the psychotic ego state existing in many of these orders of dyscontrol is bypassed or ignored. On the one hand, they are ignored by a legal confusion of the criteria necessary for a criminal act with psychotic behavior. On the other hand, the disturbed mental state may be ignored by unsophisticated rescuers who see the behavior primarily in social terms. That it may involve both of these does not negate the significance of an ego which has found stresses too difficult to handle.

PROBLEMS IN THE PREDICTION OF DANGEROUSNESS

In many ways the best place to discuss issues pertaining to dangerousness is in connection with psychoses. This is not necessarily because those with psychotic processes of development have a higher incidence of actual violence or even a greater potential for it as a group. The most that can be said at present, from confusing and mixed data, is that most studies do not indicate a higher incidence of violence among those classified as mentally ill.

There have been a few contrary studies, but most do not lean in this direction.

One study was based on post-hospitalization arrest rates for all male patients over sixteen years of age discharged from all of Maryland's psychiatric hospitals except one between 1947 and 1957. Only robbery was found to be significantly higher among the mentally ill.[36] A more recent study based on Bellevue Hospital patients in New York indicated a higher incidence of violence, although the study has been attcked in terms of bias in the data.[37] On the other hand, many studies show a lesser incidence of criminal behavior by the mentally ill compared to that of the general population.[38] One of the difficulties permeating the problem of predicting dangerousness is the elusiveness of the concept of mental illness. This is not to negate the concept of mental illness per se, or trivialize it as simply a matter of labeling. Mental illness is very complex, involving not only issues of clinical reliability, but the complications attendant upon these concepts and the psychological and social spheres of behavior which are not strictly tied into organic correlations.

Methodologically, psychotic behaviors associated with diagnosed organic medical conditions raise different problems than predictions from schizophrenia. There is evidence that types of psychiatric diagnoses other than psychosis are more often associated with criminality. Conditions such as sociopathy, alcoholism, drug addiction, and hysteria are examples.[39]

What perpetually raises the issue with psychotic individuals is either the bizarreness associated with their acts of violence, or the publicity that can arise from unreliable predictive statements made by clinicians. The case of Edmund E. Kemper, III, illustrates the situation.[40] At age fifteen this youth shot and killed his grandmother and grandfather. He was then sent to Atascadero in California, an institution for criminally insane and mentally disordered sex offenders. After five years of confinement and treatment, he was returned to the jurisdiction of the California Youth Authority and at age twenty-one, he was released. Two years later he applied to the Court to have his records sealed. Two psychiatrists were appointed to examine him. They concluded he was not dangerous nor was he otherwise a threat to society. It was later revealed that he had murdered and dismembered six young girls, his mother, and one of his mother's friends, in the course of a one-year period. One of the murders took place four days before the psychiatric examination which declared him harmless.

Apart from the harm based on false predictions analogous to people after physical examinations who have coronary occlusions being declared in good health, what makes problems of prediction so treacherous is that there are few substantial criteria on which to rely. Although our predictive success rates increase if such behavior has occurred in the past, we lack a solid basis to say whether it will occur in the future. In a study of adolescents who had committed homicidal acts, the problem was examined in a postdictive fashion to see if the acts could have been predicted and therefore prevented. Despite certain signs and symptoms which appeared consistently in the adolescents, the same signs and symptoms appear in many who never commit an act of violence.[41] A Supreme Court decision allowed the problem of overprediction based on false positions to be appraised in actuality. The Court held that equal protection was denied mentally ill prisoners who were detained in hospitals beyond the term of their maximum sentence.[42] The result was that 1000 patients, considered the most dangerous in New York, were transferred to civil hospitals and communities. At follow-up, only 14 percent were seen as dangerous. Using only two variables, these 14 percent could be predicted in terms of dangerous potential, yet even here these two factors overpredicted by a factor of two those who were not violent. Similarly, a California Youth Authority study tried to predict violence among 4,146 wards by multivariate statistical procedures and came up with a false positive ratio of eight to one.[44] The ramifications of such limitations in our ability to predict dangerousness are extending beyond the realm of assessing when a psychotic regression toward violence may occur. It also involves questions of when to recommend hospitalization, when to release, parole questions and future legal liability. If other states follow California, they may impose the duty on psychiatrists to warn potential victims of threats made by patients.[45] The lack of charity and guidelines, along with threats to confidentiality, are bound to lead to confusion.

Suppose a goal is the prevention of homicides occurring in a hypothetical town of 100,000 population.[46] A practical problem immediately presents itself as to how this could be accomplished. In the real world many restrictions are present on prevention: uncooperative people, authorities who are unpredictable about data release, and legal restrictions about obtaining data associated with privacy. Therefore, we will hypothesize a world at the disposal of some type of master-preventive agency which can draw on all the highest degrees of expertise available and obtain all the information it requires. We will further assume that in this setting we will not have to pay attention to the mundane restrictions which the real world possesses such as invalid data, poor sampling, etc. However, even with such assumptions, there is the major problem of needing a valid predictive instrument. Since clinicians are obviously fallible and unrealiable to a certain degree, let us assume that a group of the most highly qualified and experienced clinicians with respect to assessment of dangerous people with the propensity to kill are available. Further, we will hypothesize that some type of psychometric device with an unbelievably high rate of accuracy exists as well. Let us say that the combination is accurate to an extent of 95 percent—a rate unheard of in actuality.

Since homicidal behaviors have a very low baserate in the population, and we are here applying prediction to a large group of people, the essential problem is that many people would have to be incapacitated who would not actually commit any homicidal act in the future and have not done so at present, in the name of prevention. But how do we fare in our magic world even with a prediction rate of 95 percent accuracy? If the homicidal rate in our imaginary town is one out of one thousand (.001), and our combined approach of psychiatric evaluation and psychometric devices are 95 percent accurate, we should be able to detect ninety-five out of a hundred who would kill at some time. However, we are still left with a population of 99,900 who would not kill. If we were to make sure our society would be homicidally free, we would have to seek out the remaining five undetected potential killers. Five percent of 99,900 is 4,995, and these also would have to be isolated to insure complete safety. It becomes apparent that no society or legal system would tolerate putting 5,090 (4,995 plus 95) people away to ensure safety. In fact, until proven guilty beyond a reasonable doubt, the criminal system puts no one away. Unless we are willing to act differently for a population of the mentally ill who might commit a rare act of violence the problem of dealing with a group who have not committed a crime remains. Some argue to put away the 95 percent and leave the risk of 5 percent.

Remember we are still basing our removing these individuals from society on a hypothetical predictive instrument which in no way reflects the state of the behavioral sciences today. It must also be kept in mind that we are talking about one type of dangerous behavior which society does not like and not the diversity which is in fact present. In conclusion, it is obvious why clinicians often err in this way, and also how a society could not tolerate something of this nature when too many harmless people would be removed. The values of society are in the direction of giving people the freedom to commit an act and then stand trial, rather than playing risky statistical games. All in all, this is a very difficult problem, reflecting differences between dealing with group data, clinical and psychiatric prediction, and desires for maximum freedom in a society versus restrictions based on predictions based on low validity. Perhaps it is best on an individual basis to aim for short-term assessments with frequent personal contacts in the area of clinical prediction.[47]

REFERENCES

1. B. A. Morel, *Traite des Maladies Mentales* (Paris: J.B. Bailliere, 1857).
2. T. Willis, *De Anima Britorum* (Amsterdam, 1674).
3. J. E. D. Esquirol, *Des Maladies Mentales* (Paris: J. B. Balliere, 1838).
4. K. Kahlbaum, *Die Katatonic oder das Spannungsirresein* (Berlin: Hirschwald, 1874).
5. F. G. Alexander and T. Selesnick, *The History of Psychiatry* (New York: Harper, 1966).
6. E. Kraepelin, *Psychiatrie: ein Lehrbuch fur Studierende und Artzte*, 8th ed. (Leipzig: Barth, 1913).
7. C. G. Jung, *The Psychology of Dementia Praecox* (New York: Nervous and Mental Disease Publishing Co., 1907).
8. E. Bleuler, *Dementia Praecox or the Group of Schizophrenias,* trans. by J. Zinkin (New York: International Universities Press, 1950).
9. I. I. Gottesman and J. Shields, Genetic theorizing and schizophrenia, *British Journal of Psychiatry* 122 (1973): 15-30.
10. P. E. Meehl, Schizotaxia, schizotypy, schizophrenia, *American Psychologist* 17 (1962): 827-838.
11. N. Garmezy, Children at risk: the search for antecedents of schizophrenia, part 1, conceptual models and research methods, *Schizophrenia Bulletin* no. 8 (1974): 14-90.
12. H. Kohut, *The Analysis of the Self* (New York: International Universities Press, 1971).
13. D. Beres, Ego deviation and the concept of schizophrenia, *Psycho-analytic Study of the Child* 11 (1956): 164-235.
14. P.S. Holzman and R.R. Grinker, Jr., Schizophrenia in adolescnece, *Adolescent Psychiatry* 5(1977): 276-290.
15. R. D. Laing, *The Divided Self* (London: Tavistock, 1959).
16. M. V. Korkina, The syndrome of derealization in adolescence *Modern Perspectives in Adolescent Psychiatry*, ed. by J. G. Howells, pp. 329-357 (Edinburgh: Oliver and Boyd, 1971).

17. D. A. VanKrevelin, Psychoses in adolescence, *Modern Perspectives in Adolescent Psychiatry*, ed. J. G. Howells. pp. 381-403 (Edinburgh: Oliver and Boyd, 1971).

18. G. Spivack, P. E. Haimes, and J. Spotts, Adolescent symptomatology and its measurement, *American Journal of the Mentally Deficient* 72 (1967): 74-95.

19. G. K. Ushakov, Trends in the investigation of clinical problems in child psychiatry, *Modern Perspectives in International Child Psychiatry*, ed. by J. G. Howells, pp. 375-390 (Edinburgh: Oliver and Boyd, 1969).

20. H. S. Sullivan, Schizophrenia as a human process, *The Collected Works of Harry Stack Sullivan*, vol. 2 (New York: W. W. Norton and Co., 1962).

21. J. F. Masterson, *The Psychiatric Dilemma of Adolescence* (Boston: Little, Brown, 1967).

22. P. Hoch and J.P. Cattell, The diagnosis of pseudoneurotic schizophrenia, *Psychiatric Quarterly* 33 (1959): 491-509

23. L. Bender, The concept of pseudopsychopathic schizophrenia in adolescents, *American Journal of Orthopsychiatry* 29 (1959): 491-509.

24. A. Symonds and M. Herman, The patterns of schizophrenia in adolescence, *Psychiatric Quarterly* 31 (1957): 521-530.

25. I. Kaufman, et al., Deliniation of two diagnostic groups among juvenile delinquents: the schizophrenic and the impulse ridden character disorder, *Journal of the American Academy of Child Psychiatry* 12 (1963): 292-318.

26. J. Frosch, The psychotic character: clinical psychiatric considerations, *Journal of American Academic Child Psychiatry* 1 (1962): 269-283.

27. I. Kaufman, Crimes of violence and delinquency in schizophrenic children, *Journal of The American Academy of Child Psychiatry* 1 (1962): 269-283.

28. S. Reichard and C. Tillman, Murder and suicide as defenses against schizophrenic psychosis, *Journal of Clinical Psychopathology* 11 (1950): 149-163.

29. L. Bender, Children with homicidal aggression, *Aggression Hostility, and Anxiety in Children* (Springfield. Charles C Thomas, 1953).

30. H. S. Sullivan, Malevolence, hatred, and isolating techniques, *The Interpersonal Theory of Psychiatry* (New York: W. W. Norton, 1953), pp. 203-216.

31. H. Deutsch, Certain emotional disturbances ("as if") *Neuroses and Character Types* pp. 262-281 (New York: International Universities Press, 1965).

32. G. Bychowski, Escapades: a form of dissociation, *Psychiatric Quarterly* 31 (1962): 155-174.

33. K. Menninger, *The Vital Balance* (New York: The Viking Press, 1963).

34. R.R. Monroe, Episodic behavioral disorders: an unclassified syndrome, *American Handbook of Psychiatry*, 2nd ed., vol. 3 pp. 237-254 (New York: Basic Books, 1974).

35. Menninger, op. cit.

36. J. R. Rappaport and G. Lassen, Dangerousness—arrest rate comparisons of discharged patients and the general population, *American Journal of Psychiatry* 121 (1965): 776-783.

37. A. Zitrin, A.S. Hardesty, E.I. Burdock, and A.K. Drossman, Crime and violence among mental patients, *American Journal of Psychiatry* 133 (1976): 142-149.
38. J.R. Rappaport, *The Clinical Evaluation of the Dangerousness of the Mentally Ill* (Springfield: Charles C. Thomas, 1967).
39. S. Guze, R. A. Woodruff and P. Clayton, The medical and psychiatric implications of antisocial personality (sociopathy), *Disorders of the Nervous System* 32 (1971): 712-719.
40. B. L. Diamond, The psychiatric prediction of dangerousness, *University of Pennsylvania Law Review* 123 (1974) 439-452.
41. C. P. Malmquist, Premonitory signs of homicidal aggression in juveniles, *American Journal of Psychiatry* 128 (1971): 461-465.
42. *Baxstrom v. Herold,* 383 U.S. 107, 1966.
43. J. C. Cocozza and H. J. Steadman, Some refinements in the measurements and prediction of dangerous behavior, *American Journal of Psychiatry* 131 (1974): 1012-1014.
44. E. A. Wenk, J.O. Robison, and G. W. Smith, Can violence be predicted? *Crime and Delinquency* 18 (1972): 393-402.
45. *Tarasoff v. Regents of the University of California,* 131 Cal. Rptr. 14, 551 Pad 334 (Cal 1976).
46. J.M. Livermore, C.P. Malmquist, and P.E. Meehl, On the justifications for civil commitment, *University of Pennsylvania Law Review,* 117 (1968): 75-96.
47. P. D. Scott, Assessing dangerousness in criminals, *British Journal of Psychiatry* 131 (1977): 127-142.

Chapter Thirteen

The Juvenile
and the System of Justice

The state of the system of juvenile justice mirrors all of the controversies mentioned in earlier chapters. Perhaps the almost impossible task of any court system is to assimilate and use such data wisely, and know how to act. Surely, it cannot be said that the system of adult justice has had a better performance record with its clients. In fact, it may be that a main justification for continuance of a separate system for juveniles is the relatively worse performance by adult courts.

Several problem areas in the functioning of juvenile courts in this century will be discussed throughout the chapter and are noted here for perspective. Changing fashions and modes of how delinquent behavior is viewed reflects an emphasis on what is seen as significant etiological sources of delinquency. Since every society, past and present, has had such problems, the continuing quest for one model has a naive ring. One must keep in mind the variations and explanations for what is referred to as deviant, aberrant, or psychopathological behavior—from which some delinquent and criminal acts spring. Hence, a viewpoint which emphasizes delinquency as a failure of the social system, and not primarily individuals, rarely follows its reasoning to the logical ultimate: abandonment of the juvenile court. If the root problem with delinquency lies in the failure of social institutions, why bother with something as paltry as the juvenile court? Yet, those who take such a stance continue to advocate changes within the existing system,

involving the 3 D's: Diversion, Due process and Deinstitutionaliza-
tion.[1]

In contrast is an emphasis on individual differences accounting
for most of the juveniles who enter the legal system. The differences
may be in intelligence, cognitive abilities, personality variables,
family conflict, or the reactions of a juvenile to his environment.
Dealing with individuals who deviate was considered a mission of
the juvenile court in its founding ideology. Therefore, keep in mind
the question of why such an approach has largely failed.

A third ideology has viewed delinquency as happenstance. Since
it is so universal, the main problem pertains to those fortunates who
chance to get caught, labeled and forced into the system against
their will. If this is followed to its logical conclusion, it would lead to
abandonment of the juvenile court, or perhaps its restrictive use for
serious felonies since the main goal would be to keep juveniles out of
the system as far as possible.

Finally, some emphasize a strict jurisprudential viewpoint in
which concepts of autonomy, free will, the need for assumption of
responsibility, punishment, etc.—the hallmarks of an adult criminal
system—are espoused for juveniles. The differences between adult
and juvenile courts would become blurred in such a framework
because from elimination of the philosophical and behavioral
distinctions based on chronological age. A few exceptions to the
fusion might be permitted, such as to reflect the degree of reason, but
the exceptions would be handled like other areas of excuses in the
criminal law, such as insanity, duress, or coercion.

Overriding all these ideologies is the question whether the juvenile
court as constituted can achieve its goals. Specifically, what are its
goals? Should the court have an idea of developmental criteria to
employ beyond chronological age? It is important to realize that
courts do not prevent crime, nor does psychiatry prevent mental
illness. At most, courts intervene after the fact as do mental health
procedures. Primary prevention, if it has occurred, has largely taken
place by social measures which need to be distinguished from
interventions once difficulties or disabilities arise (secondary and
tertiary prevention). The final question is whether the benefits
secured to juveniles who enter the system, in terms of therapeutic,
rehabilitative or social benefits outweigh the damage that is done.
Such a distinction is utilitarian in analysis and appreciates that the
system is a balancing act in which some lose and some win.

HISTORICAL ORIGINS

To comprehend the confusions in the juvenile court, its emergence as a legal and social institution need appraisal. From the beginning of history, children have been dealt with differently or more leniently than adults transgressing in a similar manner. Since the creation of the first statewide system of juvenile courts in Illinois on July 1, 1899, such institutions have emerged in every state. Creation of the juvenile courts was the culmination of preceding socio-legal changes which altered the public approach in handling problem children to emphasize reformation rather than punishment, vengeance, or deterrence. Early in the last century efforts to keep child offenders in quarters separate from those of adults had begun. In the 1820s several large Eastern cities established houses of refuge for wayward children. A further impetus for rehabilitation was the development of probation services, beginning with a Massachusetts statute in 1869 authorizing an agent of the State Board of Charities to appear at criminal cases involving juveniles and to find foster homes rather than reformatories for those who were judged able to benefit.

From the legal standpoint, note that the juvenile court is a court of law. Its historical roots lie in the criminal law as well as in equity. Originally, the English common law, following Aristotle, held that children under seven years could not commit a crime since they did not possess mens rea—the guilty mind necessary for a crime. Above seven, they were presumed incapable of entertaining a criminal intent, although this was subject to refutation since they had reached the age of judgment. This position was adhered to by St. Thomas Aquinas, who held that a child at the confessional was responsible for his behavior if he was over seven.

English rules required children over fourteen to stand trial like adults and, if guilty, to serve penalties as criminals. No distinction was made between the commission of a felony or a misdemeanor, but for children between seven and fourteen years, there was a progressive weakening of the presumption that the child was doli incapax. In the 17th century, children convicted of felonies were customarily punished by death or transportation to a colony, while those convicted of misdemeanors were whipped, branded, mutilated, or put in the stocks, since prisons were not yet available.

Impressment into the army or navy was another technique developed to maintain the personnel of the armed forces and is traceable to the reign of Edward III (1327-1377).[2] By the 18th century impressment was flourishing, not only as a recruitment device, but to eliminate the socially dangerous who might be reformed by the experience. It was an early version of giving juvenile and youthful offenders an option of joining the military rather than being committed.

After prisons developed, there was still no separate procedure or confinement for juveniles. In fact, until 1847 in England, children stood trial the same as adults for all criminal offenses.[3] The common law was extremely harsh on children convicted of crimes. Blackstone's *Commentaries* at the end of the 18th century held that the criminal law relating to young offenders had not changed since the reign of Edward III. If the child could distinguish good and evil, he was subject to capital punishment. In the case of a boy of eight who had set fire to two barns, a finding was made that "he had malice, revenge, and cunning," and after a finding of guilt he was hanged. In another case, a boy of ten confessed killing his five-year-old foster sister and as "there appeared in his whole behavior plain tokens of a mischievous discretion, and as the sparing of this boy merely on account of his tender years might be of dangerous consequence to the public by propagating a notion that children might commit such atrocious crimes with impunity," it was unanimously agreed by all the judges that he was a fit subject for capital punishment.[4]

It is of further historical interest that the legal approach to juveniles in England has never changed to the degree it has in the United States. The English courts for children continue to be modified criminal courts with established rules of evidence and procedure which deal at first instance with juvenile offenders. The French penal code under Napoleon was actually the first to provide a uniform and different treatment for young lawbreakers. In the United States, a gradual revolt against the common law doctrines took hold once the juvenile court movement commenced in the 20th century. Typically, the age of criminal responsibility was raised to sixteen or eighteen years of age, and procedures and rules of evidence were established. These changes in turn became controversial on grounds that too many legal safeguards were abolished.

English courts of chancery with their basis in equity are often cited as another basis which contributed to a separate system for juveniles. The noted jurist Roscoe Pond did not agree, holding that the juvenile court was actually a creation of "judicial empiricism."[5] In his view the initiative of a few socially minded judges established a new legal institution on the criminal side of the law since there was a need for it at the time. Pound viewed references to its origins in chancery as ex post facto legal rationalizations. Throughout much of their early history, the chancery courts had little to do with children beyond supervising the inheritance of wealthy minors, but they did provide a source for elaborating upon the doctrine of parens patriae (father of the country). By way of parens patriae, the King, through his chancellors, had the responsibility for protecting the infants in the realm. The sovereign, as pater patriae, had an obligation to attend to the welfare of children who might be neglected, abused, or abandoned by parents or guardians.

The 1899 Illinois Act, which established the first juvenile court, not only accepted this thinking but extended it. Since chancery proceedings provided protection only to children needing protection from the actions of their parents, in practice it amounted to no more than intervention for cases similar to the contemporary battered child syndrome or wasting the assets of wards. The Illinois Act provided that children charged with violating laws would be given the same assistance as "dependent" and "neglected" children—the two other main categories which involve a minor with the law. In that way equity expanded beyond the function of protecting the property of affluent wards.

PROCEDURAL PROCESSES

The Juvenile versus the Adult System. Current procedures utilized when a juvenile offender is apprehended after a possible infraction of the law are different from those in a criminal procedure with adults (See Table 25).

TABLE 25

Contrasting Procedures
Used in the Adult and Juvenile Courts

Criminal Courts	*Juvenile Courts*
1. Warrant issued.	1. Summons issued.
2. Suspect arrested.	2. Child "taken into custody."
3. Preliminary hearing before magistrate to determine validity of complaint.	3. Case "screened" by police or "intake" division of court. Petition filed "in the matter of the welfare of the child."
4. Held in jail.	4. If necessary, child detained in a Juvenile Center.

5. Has a right to release on bail.

5. No right to release on bail, but judge may require parents to give bail if child released.

6. Arraignment and formal public trial. Adversary proceeding with prosecutor *vs.* defense lawyer; strict rule of evidence, etc. The trial is characterized by contentiousness.

6. If child denies facts alleged in petition, early hearing for adjudication. Informal hearing, public excluded; judge seeks to get at facts, not to preside over adversary proceeding.

7. Right to a jury trial.

7. No right to a jury trial.

8. Standard of proof: guilt beyond a reasonable doubt.

8. Standard of proof: only since 1970, proof beyond a reasonable doubt, and the only if the act against the juvenile can lead to incarceration.

9. Finding of guilty or not guilty.

9. Adjudication of delinquency or dismissal.

10. Court may order a pre-sentence investigation.

10. If not already made, and if the child admits facts in petition, pre-sentence investigation is made before the hearing.

11. Sentence, punishment plays major role. Deterrence often cited.

11. Dispositions for rehabilitation by guardianship, or "treatment" by state is the justification cited.

12. Criminal record.

12. No criminal record.

13. Records public.

13. Records theoretically private, subject to judge's control. In practice, many reports are released by way of workers in a court system.

The contrast provides an overall picture of what happens to children, apart from the few hours in which they are evaluated, and sets the stage for presenting controversial aspects of the system of juvenile justice. Our discussion is confined to juveniles handled in the juvenile courts and not those waived to an adult criminal court for prosecution. The waiver issue is discussed separately. The juvenile court is not a criminal court, and the procedures employed are more like those of a civil court. Until 1967, when the Gault case was decided by the United States Supreme court, many of the procedural safeguards employed in adult criminal courts did not apply to juveniles.[6] Gault held that in cases of delinquency which could lead to incarceration, juveniles were entitled to counsel, to confront and cross-examine witnesses, to receive a timely notice of charges, to the privilege against self-incrimination so they could remain silent, and to obtain appellate review.

Right to a jury trial, proof beyond a reasonable doubt, bail, avoidance of hearsay evidence, indictment by a grand jury, and open hearings, are still not required. These omissions are ascribed to the alleged emphasis on rehabilitation rather than judging the child guilty or not guilty. In Gault the Supreme Court held there were certain basic rights applicable to juveniles under the Bill of Rights and specified them. Critics have argued that enforcing such legal rights reinforces a criminal atmosphere and hampers a psychosocial perspective needed for dealing with juveniles in antisocial difficulty. However, such changes can be taken as indicative of the dissatisfaction with the methods and results of the juvenile process.

Legal implications from the Gault case continue to reverberate. No one is clear on the relationship between the rights afforded juveniles and those afforded adults accused of crimes. Some believe that the rights of the two classes—juveniles and adults—are equivalent. Others feel that the rights of juveniles are more restricted while others feel they are less so. It is also not clear whether rights granted to adults become applicable to juveniles.

Once there is an arrest, the juvenile may be placed in a detention home, supposedly separate from facilities used for adult offenders; in practice it may be a contrivance such as a facility down a hallway from adult prisoners. Constitutional questions regarding the confinement of recalcitrant adolescents in penal institutions are relevant.[7] It is desirable from a psychiatric viewpoint that dependent and neglected children under the jurisdiction of the same court should be kept separate from children held for a delinquency hearing. Neither of these may occur in practice, because of a viewpoint that whenever juvenile courts intervene it is for a therapeutic function rather than law enforcement. The stay in a detention facility can vary from hours to months. The case may be heard before a referee or a probation officer, judgment may be immediate, and the child released with a warning upon promise of good behavior. In other cases, a juvenile may be released to the custody of his parents or guardian to appear at a later court hearing, or instead held in a detention home or jail until the next juvenile court session in those instances in which attendance or testimony can be guaranteed only in this manner.

The pre-sentence investigation is an effort to secure background information of a social nature before the court reaches a decision about disposition of the minor. A minority of cases have a psychiatric evaluation done in conjunction with such investigation. Of those that are done, few are carried out by those with specialization in the field of child psychiatry and familiar with diagnostic and therapeutic approaches to children and families. A conference surveyed all members of the American Psychiatric Association who were either Board Certified or eligible for taking the examination to become certified in child psychiatry as well as those who merely signified an interest in child psychiatry. Of the 913 psychiatrists who responded, only 0.3 percent were attached full time to a juvenile court and probation service, 3.3 percent part time, and 13 percent as consultants (customarily a half day per week.)[8]

Nor do these statistics give any qualitative appraisal of the evaluations. They only suggest the quantitative deficit in psychiatric personnel. It is apparent that most juvenile courts are without the services of a trained child psychiatrist. It is not unusual to find metropolitan areas with over 500,000 population who have never had such a consultant and are oblivious to a lack. In part this reflects the view of juvenile delinquency as a response to social conditions rather than individual or family psychopathology. Yet the juvenile process itself is relatively helpless to alter the social environment.

Police Screening.   The crucial step of police screening of juveniles is significant, not only because the overwhelming number of children who eventually appear in court are referred by the police, but experience with police reinforces latent delinquent trends. The knowledge, attitude, and conflicts of apprehending officers may play a crucial role in subsequent behavior of the juvenile. It is not simply a matter of applying adult rules for making an arrest or taking into custody.

Any or all of the following occur in practice which divert the youth from a court adjudication: (a) release of the juvenile, with or without a warning, but without an official record; (b) release, but filing of a report for a police juvenile bureau, or a more formal report referring the matter to the juvenile bureau for possible action; (c) turning the youth over to a juvenile bureau immediately; (d) direct referral of the case to the juvenile court; (e) admission of a youth to some type of mental health or hospital facility.

In some cases, a mandatory referral to the juvenile bureau or the juvenile court is required, such as with crimes of violence, felonies, and serious misdemeanors, or with youths on parole or probation. Hearings at juvenile police bureaus result in approximately half the cases being referred to a higher court.[9]

Part of the problem of police screening involves not only the recent right of a juvenile to have a "Miranda Warning" (that the accused is entitled to a lawyer and if he cannot afford one, one will be provided, and to be warned that he can remain silent since anything said can and will be used in court), but a correlative right to waive his constitutional rights. Indeed, since it is questionable whether adults know what legal rights they are waiving, it is even more likely that a minor does not. The result is a collection of ambiguous rulings in which different courts decide whether the waiver was done in a knowledgeable and intelligent manner. The lack of integration of developmental and clinical knowledge with legal decision-making is striking. Consider a fifteen-year-old who waived his Miranda Rights and then, after three-and-one-half hours of incommunicado interrogation, gave a confession which was held to be voluntary.[10]

However, note the common belief of police that a hearing in an authoritarian setting is desirable in its own right to impress and scare juveniles into mending their ways. The legal issues raised by these hearings are noteworthy, such as the right to counsel and to remain silent. These are rarely mentioned to the juvenile or to his family, and have been the focus of recent Supreme Court decisions in the realm of adult criminal law. Many of the procedures are carried out under the guise of a quasijudicial setting, although in fact the police have no authority to compel attendance. In practice, the leverage of the setting and police authority usually result in an appearance. Attempting to obtain a confession is a further goal. There is a belief that confession contributes to eliminating the acts as well as achieving a cleansing of the soul. Denial of guilt is viewed as evidence of recalcitrance, while a humble, polite, and obsequious manner is taken as evidence of penitence and the absence of need for a court referral. Such practices suggested to one conflicted adolescent that he take drama lessons to improve his ability to be honest, since his external demeanor and "knowing the rules" were taken as the guiding criteria.

Practices which operate with such naivete, yet have the power to condemn and punish, contribute to confirming delinquents in their dedication to delinquency. Adolescent behavior has levels of meaning within the context of role seeking. A delinquent role may be only fleetingly envisaged, or presented within a delinquent environment. However, at some point an attribution of delinquency is made in a transactional process in which juveniles consciously and unconsciously provoke and challenge adults into the utilization of coercive measures against them. A sequence of self-reinforcement of negative self-evaluations begins which easily leads to further illegal acts. "For it can happen that a youngster when committed as an official offender to a corrective procedure, decides in defiant despair to commit himself to the role of an incorrigible. One third of all delinquents are 'caught'—often having made only the flimsiest attempts to conceal their criminal intention. The autobiographies of professsional criminals of undoubted skill in their craft clearly reveal the clumsiness of their first delinquent steps—a clumsiness inviting detection and, maybe, the corrective influences of somebody who cares. Where such help is not forthcoming, there is only the world of professional crime and of law enforcement to confirm the young deviant in the role of loyal and expert criminal."[11]

Disposition Problems. In discussing the alternatives for dealing with a minor apprehended for violating a law, the possibilities were all being made at a police or court intake level (intake disposition). About half the cases which reach the latter are handled by intake workers without a judge giving the child a warning or arranging an official hearing date after arraignment. A further extension of intake disposition—which has aroused much controversy—is *informal disposition* (unofficial handling), in which a disposition recommendation is made without filing a petition alleging delinquency, neglect, or dependency. The child has thus not been adjudicated delinquent, although many sanctions may be imposed on the child and family. Among possibilities, he may be placed on unofficial probation against his wishes and his family, he may be referred to a mental health clinic or hospital for treatment, detained for a possible official hearing later, or have his case continued indefinitely. While some view informal disposition as a progressive step since it keeps many juveniles out of the juvenile court system, short of official hearings there is an implicit assumption that informal disposition gets juveniles the help they need.

Critics view informal disposition as a straightforward violation of constitutional rights. Without the petition and subsequent court hearing whereby the child is adjudicated delinquent or not, the court does not formally assume jurisdiction. Therefore, any coercive action employed against a child or family raises the spectre of violating rights since they may not wish to comply with the recommendations. To refuse to go along means a pseudo-choice, since the procedure will then move ahead to a formal hearing colored by the now apparent opposition between court workers and the family. Those who try to justify these activities are more impressed with practical administrative and political problems than with questions of constitutional rights. Their main argument seems to be based on unofficial hearings resulting in fewer children being placed on probation. But should fiscal economy be the primary criterion? Or, conversely, how formal do we want juvenile justice to get?

Another criticism is that informal disposition is an unjustified attempt to expand the intervention of other agencies or services, such as welfare departments, into delinquency. A practical dilemma for a politically ambitious juvenile court judge is that judges prefer to report low delinquency rates, yet this practice itself makes it more difficult to obtain adequate funds. It should also be apparent that shifting standards are one factor contributing to the gross unreliability of statistics on delinquency.

Formal disposition refers to the hearing before a judge or his representative after a formal petition has been entered. There are three types of formal disposition decisions: dismissal, probation, or institutionalization. The following is a list showing some of the variations within each possibility:[12]

1. Dismissal or discharge, with or without warning, and with or without a request for restitution
2. Official probation, with or without conditions imposed by the court, and with or without restitution
3. Foster home placement, with or without probation, arranged for by the court staff, a welfare department, or a private agency
4. Commitment to a public training school, a religious or charitable institution, or a residential treatment center

5. Referral to another court for a petition to commit as mentally ill
6. Waiver of the case to adult criminal court
7. Adjudication and release on suspended sentence, with or without a time limit, or imposition of sentence and suspension of execution of judgment with or without conditions
8. Imposition of a fine, if permitted, in some jurisdictions
9. Commitment to a correctional after initial placement in a juvenile institution, or transfer
10. Extension of probation upon the child's reaching maturity when the case warrants additional supervision, or when the term of probation expires
11. Temporary detention awaiting final disposition or prior to commitment to a state institution
12. Termination of probation prior to release from court jurisdiction
13. Revocation or probation and return to court prior to institutional commitment

PROBLEMS ON THE TREATMENT LEVEL

Administrative Problems. Political battles develop between divisions of government involving juvenile delinquents. Controversies arise over which programs should be instituted for children with antisocial tendencies, and who should manage the treatment facilities. It is debated whether various counties should provide their own treatment centers or whether they should be provided on a state level. A specific problem may arise over handling special categories of juvenile offenders, such as violent youths. Some argue for special institutions to house the dangerous adolescent while others argue for free mingling. These questions obviously involve administrative and financial problems. There is also the problem of what degree of responsibility should be assumed by private organizations and nonprofit foundations versus public institutions. Such controversies, coupled with the possibility of personal power struggles raise questions about the degree of delegated state power such organizations should have.

Financial problems are not the only limitations placed upon the juvenile court's weakened potentiality. In many cases, judges do not seek appointment to such office and may even decline offers. A deleterious effect upon the prestige of the related fields of probation and social work results. Judges often lack the broad social science background necessary for effective juvenile work. Until recently many law students regarded criminal law as one of the least desirable areas in which to practice and law schools omitted more than a passing reference to the juvenile court. Even today this type of work may be tacked on to the rest of a lawyer's agenda as a moral commitment for a few hours a week. Involving young attorneys may mean, given their lack of depth in the behavioral sciences, a highly legalistic orientation focused on constitutional issues. Similarly, psychiatric consultants to juvenile correctional facilities and juvenile courts are inadequate in number and quality as we have noted. When such deficits in professional expertise commonly exist in juvenile courts, individualized justice becomes a fiction. Critics have referred to the situation as the "unfulfilled promise of the juvenile court," since it has never actualized its potential.

Treatment in correctional settings has had such a broad meaning that it is difficult to distinguish what is called treatment from general activities or vocational-educational measures. It may include social maneuvers aimed at certain demographic groups with a high incidence of delinquency by attempts to alter the groups' social organization. In fact, courts may fail to distinguish between therapeutic programs and prison-like training schools.[13] In many situations, the psychiatrist serves as consultant with direct participation in the field being minimal or nonexistent. Environmental maneuvers such as placing the child in a boarding home, foster home, or group living situation are frequently used as sole treatment devices, particularly by welfare agencies or community clinics. The lack of effectiveness with these techniques is almost a moot question at present since the personnel and homes available are so far removed from required norms that a fair assessment is impractical. To argue against these on the basis of their high failure rate is no more valid than to argue against the results of individual psychotherapy or psychoanalysis performed by poorly trained or confused people who attempt to carry out such treatment. The question still remains as to the validity of these devices to alter delinquent behavior.

Institutional treatment may be ordered by the court as another alternative. Again, there are many variations from traditional psychiatric units in a state hospital. For instance, outdoor work and rehabilitation programs under youth commissions, such as camp work or forestry programs, are considered treatment. In between these extremes are residential treatment centers and aftercare community programs with different goals and orientations, such as long-term periods with multiple therapeutic approaches, halfway houses or hostels, night hospitals for adolescents, and so on. The hope has been that with more adequate extramural community approaches, commitment or involuntary placement of children in institutions could be progressively diminished. The motivation for change was the dismal result from archaic training schools or reform schools which neither trained, reformed, nor treated, but usually injured the juvenile. It was hoped these could be eliminated so that therapeutically oriented centers could be instituted.

Since there will probably always be a need for some type of institutional facility, attention should be given to the type of institutions available to the court, particularly for antisocial adolescents. Many of these barely function on a maintenance level. If adolescents are sent to a state hospital, ostensibly for psychiatric help, they are frequently placed on adult wards, managed by drugs, and released in the absence of criteria for release. Very little in the way of treatment or rehabilitation appears to go on.[14] Nor can much be said for the institutions under correctional jurisdiction. These points are made to denote the handicaps under which juvenile court proceedings labor when they deal with some of the most recalcitrant cases. Putting children away often becomes the goal in itself with minimal rationales of treatment.

Probation as treatment. Probation is considered a form of treatment developed within the administrative framework of the juvenile court. A minor placed on probation remains under court control with the possibility of plans being altered later by the court. Three elements are considered essential with probation as a device for dealing with juvenile offenders:

1. Retention of juvenile offenders in their local community, with or without a suspended sentence, instead of commitment to an institution
2. The taking of such action only after study by the judge of a report that embodies the findings of a social investigation into the offender's makeup, career, and probabilities of recidivism and reform
3. The resulting placement of the probationer under the guidance of an adequately trained probation officer

The probation worker and the psychiatrist make reports available to the judge which help to determine whether the child should remain in the community or be institutionalized. When the decision is to place the minor on probation, various arrangements are possible.

1. An inactive (irregular) type of checking-in periodically is one practice. The effectiveness of this approach for any goal whatsoever is questionable.

2. Most frequent is a form of probation where the juvenile is seen approximately once every week or two with a goal of continued contact to insure that the situations which elicited the behavior do not again do so. The length of the contact varies widely. The efficiency seems primarily to keep a record of ongoing activities.

3. The last arrangement is intensive probation. Regular weekly visits are scheduled, which involve the use of a social caseworker or group therapy work.

It is difficult to determine how the first two varieties of probation can accomplish the goal of modifying behavior; they seem to be implicitly and solely operating on a deterrence principle—the effectiveness of which is debatable. For the child or adolescent with entrenched patterns of antisocial behavior, very few of these approaches would be predicted as likely to be effective. They may in fact increase the contempt for ineffectual authority which juvenile offenders have in abundance. Evaluation of the effectiveness of these probationary techniques with respect to different variables, such as the incidence of recidivism, would require a comparison of the specific approach used in contrast to a control group where no such efforts were made and other variables were matched.

Institutional Aspects. The atmosphere of institutions supposed to rehabilitate juvenile offenders often have more of a penal cast than a treatment environment. Many of the institutions house repeaters who come back innumerable times and whose relatives horizontally and longitudinally may have gone through similar experiences. Mingled with the repeaters are innumerable types of juvenile delinquents, from the withdrawn schizoid who serves his time to the gang type who is quick to attach himself to a group as he did in his own neighborhood. High rates of recidivism, often over 50 percent, are commonplace.

Too frequently the psychiatric consultant is used as someone who is supposed to weed out psychotics. There are many well-trained persons who believe it is the job of the psychiatrist to confirm the suspicions of a probation worker that a given juvenile may be psychotic and then arrange for this small minority to be committed to a mental hospital. "Psychotic" is usually used in a very restricted sense such as "hearing voices" or other secondary Bleulerian criteria for schizophreniza. A concept of mental illness as a process in the course of which a juvenile can appear psychotic at one moment and not so a short time later when his ego is reconstituted seems neglected. The idea seems very difficult for members of many disciplines dealing with antisocial individuals to grasp, since they expect someone to be either sick or not.

In reality it is in the gray area that most juveniles reside. They are not necessarily psychotic but involved with personal, family, and community conflicts on many levels. The institutional approach views these few suspects as having a disease for which a doctor should be called in to say whether they are sick or not; even if they are not ill it is reassuring to the staff to have a doctor tell them that the child can adjust, which means he can take it enough to survive in the institution. It further puts the psychiatrist in the role of deciding whether someone can take it by adjusting to the demands of correctional living, hardly a therapeutic orientation. The psychiatric consultant is then in the role of being called in to see a child who has not adjusted to institutional life which is used as a criterion for improvement or cure.

Many psychiatrists do not choose institutional work with these children or adolescents for many reasons. Even when salaries are adequate, the low status and lack of professional prestige remain. The problem is never confronted in terms of seeing that, even given equal salaries, a capable psychiatrist will not chose to work in such settings and that greater incentive is needed. Political complications further contribute to a negative image and difficulty in maintaining staff. Since public institutions are usually state or county facilities, perennial justifications for budget requests occur. Problems with understaffing and poorly trained personnel pose difficulties. At best in-service training programs attempt to compensate for the deficit, but can rarely substitute knowledge despite good will. Many facilities are situated outside of metropolitan areas where qualified personnel can be obtained only as consultants on varying time bases.

In some cases administrators of private or semi-public residential treatment facilities seek ardently to avoid taking acting out children, before or following adjudication of delinquency, holding that these children should be the sole responsibility of correctional institutions. The practice allows residential centers to have much tamer children, with less staff, and higher "cure" rates.

Even in cases where an excellent pre-sentence evaluation has been done by a caseworker with an emphasis upon the child's conflicts and feelings, his social milieu and family interplay, once he goes to a training school, or is placed on probation, an authoritarian approach emphasizing discipline and punishment for not obeying authority to holds sway. The drawback of such approaches is that respect for authority achieved by a coercive process results in observing externals, while the seething resentment and rage are not dealt with. This fosters an immature conscience dedicated to conforming from fear of an external authority. The approach in many institutions is oriented toward the few whose behavior is of a dyssocial nature and who have never learned from their families and community how to behave in the appropriate manner. There is then a generalization to the remaining majority, where they are to be re-educated in their attitudes toward authority to become good citizens by obeying the law and holding a job. The simplification of this approach, with the assumption that acting externally normal in an institution makes one capable of community participation, make it suspect, yet it appears to be a prevailing pattern in many institutions.

Nor is the alternative one of reducing the entire problem of treatment and prevention to individual and family psychodynamics and psychotherapy. Rather, it is to educate personnel at all levels who deal with delinquents about the complexity of human motivational patterns and dynamic trends. This may eliminate the overbalance of an emphasis on superficial re-education processes and discipline as curative. The adolescent needs limits in an institution and not chaotic permissiveness, but he also needs a situation within which he can have emotionally satisfying and close relationships with his peers and adults. If his internalized controls and interpersonal relationships are disturbed, he needs specific therapy so that he can develop controls from within in the context of such relationships.

In some training schools, problem children are handled by administering tranquilizers in increasing dosages until the child's rebelliousness and lack of respect for authority are diluted. The psychiatrist is then someone called upon to write drug orders, since he is the only person legally eligible to do so. In other cases, when the psychiatric consultant is expected to see the children, his limited availability allows him to see only a few, since interviewing the child, grasping and reading the past history, dictating his opinion, and possibly talking to other staff who see the child daily, give little opportunity to see more than a few children.

This routine does not provide any time for him to meet with treatment or administrative staff. Seeing other members of the family is seldom done by consulting psychiatrists in these situations since there is not time, nor are the parents often available at the time he is there. In many cases, those psychiatrists acting as part-time consultants accommodate by feeling it is their proper job to adjust drug dosages as noted, or help enforce the disciplinary rules as the raison d'etre for an institutional program.

JUVENILE JURISPRUDENCE

Much of the confusion present for anyone caught up in the network of juvenile justice is due to uncertainties regarding the philosophy of the juvenile court itself. The duality present between rehabilitation versus community protection has existed since its founding. It is axiomatic that a legal system involves not only a mechanism for the settlement of disputes and punishment of offenders but the practices and beliefs of society toward activities of groups within it. Although not a criminal court, in recent years a feeling became prevalent that juvenile court had lost too much of its judicial character and become more of a welfare agency or administrative board as in in the Scandinavian countries.

The split in opinion is not solely between lawyers versus nonlawyers so much as between those who believe the court should restrict its activities to cases where authority must be exercised for strict violations of laws as contrasted with those who believe the court should have a broader base not only to adjudicate delinquents but to deal with predelinquents. The latter is not to determine if any specific act has necessarily been committed, but to ensure the welfare of the child. Those opposing the latter view believe this turns the court into a de facto welfare agency with policies and issues being determined at best by the behavioral sciences rather than by judicial traditions and rulings. The result is a confused status for juvenile jurisprudence as well as the juvenile population.

This ambiguous state of the juvenile court has been attacked with increasing vigor. On a practical level it has led to legal challenges. On the level of scholarly commentary the court has been dissected for the lack of a pervasive philosophy to govern the approach to juveniles.

Basic jurisprudential questions remain: Why do we handle

juveniles differently from adults? Who should be considered a juvenile?Can the continuation of current practices be justified? Should the disposition of a juvenile accused of behavior equivalent to an adult criminal offense be handled differently? Is there a need for a juvenile jurisprudence? What type of treatment standards need be set?

Five influences have been assigned as responsible for a *welfare* emphasis in contrast to a legalistic emphasis in development of the juvenile court:[15] (1) an aggressive social work orientation of the United States Children's Bureau, created within the Department of Labor in 1912, which occupied itself with matters coming before juvenile courts; (2) a broadening of jurisdiction from delinquent to neglected and dependent children (this expansion advocated the juvenile court hold sway not only over problems of maladjusted children but over those abandoned or inadequately provided for, a shift incorporated such matters as adoption, problems of illegitimacy, divorce, neglect, dependency, and family problems within the juvenile court or the broader-based family courts); (3) the professionalization of social work not only as academic department within universities, but also in organizations which led to placement of personnel in key positions; (4) court decisions which quickly moved beyond the constitutionality of the juvenile court to pursue a position of treating minors for problems rather than punishing for delinquencies; (5) the emerging influence of a dynamic psychiatry which seemed to offer more to delinquent youths than the static categories of Kraepelinian psychiatry.

obviously have a different standing in a welfare versus a legal approach. Within the judicial orientation the psychiatrist functions in a role much closer to his role in an adult criminal court. As noted, part of the problem is a reaction against the overextension of the reformative and redemptive aspects of welfare policy in the courts— an approach which has not succeeded in curtailing the incidence of minors coming before the court.

A primary suggestion relates to the juvenile court being able to function in a rehabilitative and treatment manner with children, but first having to establish that such intervention is needed. This would separate two functions of the court: the determination of jurisdiction and facts from disposition processes. Strict legal procedures would apply to the former, while the latter involves a broad framework of treatment. Increasing emphasis on legal rules of evidence regarding the truth or falsehood of facts alleged in a petition occurred. At the time of disposition planning the full psychiatric, psychological, and social emphasis would be available.

Another reform would prohibit temporary detention and not allow it to be permitted without a prompt court hearing. All the vagaries present in other aspects of the juvenile court proceedings are present in decisions to detain a juvenile pending the processing of their case. Juvenile detention has a mixture of motives. It is not only to insure that a juvenile will show up for a hearing (analogous to jail for adults) but it may also be used to control behavior or help enforce parental controls on unruly minors. The right to confidentiality of records, such as a psychiatrist's report, has also been violated too frequently in comparison to adult evaluations.

Since the Gault case giving the right to counsel, debate has centered on attempts to avoid a contentious atmosphere of the proceedings, such as those prevailing in a criminal court. Many believe that the parents and child should not only be notified of their right to counsel but that the need for counsel should be expanded to those who appear ignorant of their rights. Another issue pertains to the different interests of the child and the parents. A lawyer might question whether a child needs an attorney to look after his own best interests. Since an attorney may not be aware of many unconscious factors operating in families, he may believe that the child would achieve maximum benefit from a family attorney, yet the parents' interests may not coincide with the juvenile.

> This situation is illustrated in the case of a fifteen-year-old girl for whom the parents petitioned the court due to her incorrigibility. For some time a reported pattern of promiscuous behavior had been noted, with the local police apprehending the girl with her boy friend and bringing her home. The parents' reaction was to plead helplessness to control her behavior. When the case came to a juvenile court hearing, the girl was placed on probation. Some time later, the girl was seen for psychiatric consultation and many of the family patterns promoting acting out were noted, such as the mother's advice on where to park so as to minimize being caught, etc. In such cases, the juvenile's best interests are not served by having her adjudicated a delinquent with all of its consequences.

Similarly, the right to appeal a decision should be made clear, despite the small numbers of such cases. It may be that the child or parent is ignorant of this right, or that there is no stenographic record of the proceeding needed for an appeal from rural settings. Avoidance of double jeopardy proceedings is needed to prevent a child later being subjected to a criminal prosecution on the basis that his initial trial in a juvenile court was a civil proceeding. The Supreme Court has held that a seventeen-year-old could not be prosecuted in a criminal court following an adjudication in juvenile court since this violated the Fifth Amendment's double jeopardy clause.[16]

There are other problems of an administrative nature with respect to the juvenile court. Some pertain to matters of organization in which the court may be attached to the local probate or county district court. Thus, part-time judges may set certain times in which to hear cases under juvenile jurisdiction. In many cases, this is the part of their job which they least relish. If they are appointed or elected, it is not uncommon to find the position used as a temporary political position until better things come along. The background and training of the judges vary widely. In some jurisdictions, no legal training or experience is required, which reflects the welfare viewpoint on the nature of the court. In other areas, one judge with legal training may be necessary, while the majority of cases are seen by referees whose backgrounds also vary widely.

Many judges are dedicated and strive valiantly to do what they consider best, but this frequently represents little more than imposing their own subjective and moralistic views on how children should have respect for authority. In many ways, it is an attitude paralleled when psychiatrists trained to work with adults attempt to work with families and children. The case is similar with other personnel attached or related to the juvenile court, in which a majority may have had no specialized training.

Even more important is the prevalence of widely varying subjective views on the nature of antisocial behavior. Since many of the legal safeguards of criminal trials do not apply, the crucial significance of the ability and training of the personnel who make dispositions concerning minors is evident. That they frequently lack such training coupled with experience in the behavioral sciences to aid them in their decisions is also evident. The inner conflicts of personnel which lead them to work with this type of pathology must also be kept in mind, as in all clinical and community work.

Additional confusion may attend the position of labeling the behavior of juveniles as sick if they are referred for treatment to an independent community psychiatric clinic or one attached to a court. This is especially true in cases of lower-class or culturally deprived families when they are told their child will receive treatment. The behavior is not viewed as an illness, and they may be confused about ordering their son or daughter into treatment. Even when attempts at explanation are made, the therapeutic effort is still viewed as punishment.

With the brief number of visits and short-term approaches of most community mental health centers, the situation remains unaltered. The situation becomes complicated when the conditions subject to punishment as delinquent acts are considered, for many of these are not crimes for adults, but in reality reflect family problems or disturbed parents as much as an antisocial adolescent. Thus, such offenses as truancy, associating with immoral persons, incorrigibility, behaving in habitually disobedient ways, or using profanity, are examples of behavior for which the child may be labeled delinquent, or in some jurisdictions adjudicated, and told he is sick and in need of mental health treatment. Great inconsistency exists in using these categories of offense from one geographical area to another.

GENERAL IMPRESSIONS

Despite these specific criticisms of juvenile justice, it appears that the theory behind the juvenile court approach has not yet been evaluated; nor can it be. A deeper criticism goes beyond inadequate staffing, for even if there were sufficient personnel, it would make little difference since there is no evidence that the procedures employed have significant effect on rehabilitating the delinquent. Even deeper is that we have not articulated what the purpose of the juvenile court should be. The purpose of the juvenile court as rehabilitative may be secondary to a goal of serving as a deterrent to would-be delinquents in a process analogous to criminal courts. How effective it is in this regard is completely unknown.

The rehabilitative position has never been a testable hypothesis due to the lack of standardized procedures and competent personnel over a prolonged period so that the practices could be adequately appraised. The cessation of all delinquency would not constitute the requirement for a tested validity of the juvenile court approach. What would be required is a comparative study of the incidence of types of delinquencies when other methods were used and long-term follow-up of the individuals was accomplished. Detection for later criminality would be one outcome revealed, for juveniles would also be evaluated in terms of other ego variables, such as vocational and educational functioning, marital adjustment, self-esteem, and signs and symptoms of emotional conflict.

To what extent juveniles act illegally, or if they were capable of sublimating impulses would be another important question to determine. However, in few communities has there been anything approximating adequate diagnostic and treatment institutions needed for handling the children and families coming before a juvenile court. From the very first juvenile court in Illinois such problems were in evidence since a probation staff was authorized, but no funds and salaries to hire professionals provided. Local fiscal economy measures often view the juvenile court as a likely area in which to cut the budget, despite the long future ahead for most of the children in trouble.

Nor have crucial experiments been carried out to confirm or deny the validity of the approaches used in the juvenile court. There is much vagueness built into the dispositional system. The psychiatrist or probation worker find themselves in the position of making recommendations, but then not having them accepted or carried out. There may not be a frank acknowledgement of such rejection, with the impression given that the behavioral sciences are being utilized, while in fact they are not. In other cases, contrary psychiatric opinions may be courted to maintain the image of utilizing a behaviorally oriented approach, while the result is an attempt to buttress a preconceived notion of what should be done. The position is not that independent judgements should be vacated, but rather that there should be a specific commitment to ways of dealing with cases. When this does not happen, the result is that no specific hypotheses regarding the disposition of delinquent youths are tested, and there is a perpetual lack of clarification as to what procedures may be more effective.

What can the diagnostic appraisal of a specialist in child psychiatry be in relation to the processes employed by the juvenile court? Many points of controversy are those on which psychiatrists may differ, such as a welfare versus a judicial emphasis in the juvenile court. However, some concerns reflect the specific interest of the clinician who deals with disturbed children.

Since it would be pragmatically impossible to recommend anything like individual therapy for the large numbers coming before juvenile courts, such a recommendation would be without practical import. Even family approaches, whose results vary depending on the type of problem and the charisma of the therapist, would not be available to more than a small number. Group therapy, widely advocated a decade or two ago as the treatment of choice for delinquents, seems to have lost many of its ardent supporters. Must psychiatrists conclude that what might have had some beneficial effect is not available? Some feel the only choice is to withdraw and have little to do officially with a system whose failures are obvious. This is a dilemma rarely confronted directly by most psychiatrists. Their tendency is to treat a handful of patients without facing the overall issues and problems of delinquency in most communities.[16].

The conclusion is that in operation juvenile courts rarely abide by the goal of rehabilitation, although they continue to use rehabilitation as their justification. The overwhelming number of children seen in juvenile courts are there for the same reason as the cases seen in criminal courts: their behavior is viewed as unacceptable and possibly dangerous to the community and a judgment is made that the behavior will not be tolerated even though for status offenses no actual crime has been committed. The crucial step is to decide what may be done. Punishment as retribution per se against juveniles is neither socially acceptable nor believed effective; punishment as deterrence has rarely proved effective in acts committed against a person. Even for acts against property, which are prevalent in adolescence, the factors of unconscious motivation and the symbolic meaning of an act, such as driving a stolen car, have not been prevented by punishment. These facts lead to a resort to the rationalization of rehabilitation for whatever is done.

Increased attention has been paid to the question of whether the juvenile court and its allied agencies actually rehabilitate at all, or whether most of its activities are in the realm of a disguised protection of the public interest. The earlier discussion about lack of procedural safeguards is important, but the major issue in such theoretical confusion is the dishonesty which is present, particularly from the perspective of the juvenile. This has been viewed as one source for a pervasive sense of injustice which the juvenile experiences when in contact with the juvenile justice system. The duplicity attendant upon a procedure called civil and not criminal, which is supposedly for the juvenile's welfare, yet which may result in incarceration in an institution with poorly trained and under-staffed professionals of marginal standing attempting to help him, is obvious.

Allen noted, "Measures which subject individuals to the substantial and involuntary deprivation of their liberty are essentially punitive in character, and this reality is not altered by the facts that the motivations that prompt incarceration are to provide therapy or otherwise contribute to the person's well-being or reform."[17] The result is a generalization process leading to contempt for the legal processes. Since these proceedings occur at a time when adolescents are struggling with emancipating themselves from the authorities within their own families, and with their own crystallizing inner control system, the effect is often devastating.

An additional hypocrisy is in the attribution of causality for the delinquent behavior to some social unit, be this the family or social organization. However, during the legal process personal fault is assigned to the delinquent. Fault is not equivalent to criminal responsibility but it is a long way from blaming social institutions for their plight. Without entering into the hoary arguments as to what the ultimate etiological basis for delinquency is, the noted inconsistencies lend cogency to a contempt for the legal process, and a further lack of personal responsibility for behavior since there is a failure of the authorities to resolve their own ambivalence and call a spade a spade. It has been held that the actual basis for disposition of juvenile cases reinstates a principle of offense, tempered by the doctrine of parental and social responsibility for the juvenile's behavior, and the availability of correctional facilities.

> How do the workings of this arrangement appear to juvenile delinquents? The answer may be simply stated. It appears unjust—rampantly so. Few delinquents can do more than express a simmering sense of injustice. They cannot explain it partly because they are half-literate schoolboys, but mainly because they, like everyone else, are mystified. In addition to the normal sources of mystification, the juvenile delinquent is additionally confused because, unfortunately, he hardly understands most of the words that are used to justify that disposition. In other words, he hears that he is either being put on probation or in prison and that the reason in both cases is to help him. That is about all that he really hears in court. It is quite enough.[18]

As a result of this community confusion, the juvenile himself is not only confused but angry. The anger is superimposed on the conflicts and feelings already present. The setting is ripe for the displacement of the original conflicts to the juvenile court and its agents. The conclusion is that the inherent duplicity in the processes they are subjected to—punishment under the guise of rehabilitation, assessing individual responsibility while maintaining the juveniles are products of familial and social etiology, inadequate institutions, and personnel labeled as treatment,—promotes rather than modifies delinquent behavior.

LEGAL ISSUES

Among the multiple issues raised in dealing with the future of the juvenile process, legal issues have gained momentum since the Gault case. However, concern has been building for at least a decade.[19] Issues such as timely notice for a hearing, the content of such notices, the vagueness of statutes pertaining to pleadings, right to counsel, right to confrontation of witnesses, and the privilege against self-incrimination have now been guaranteed to juveniles under due process. Gault actually only applied to when the determination of delinquency could result in commitment to an institution where the freedom of the juvenile would be curtailed. Additional legal issues can be raised, focused on the various stages of apprehension, intake, adjudication, and sentencing. Matters like discovery, right to a speedy trial, public proceedings, jury trial, waiver, and a change of venue are related due process issues many of which remain unsettled in different jurisdictions.

Even if these requirements from the adult criminal process are met and extended to juveniles, they do not resolve the ultimate issue of juvenile rehabilitation. Despite the sharp attack on the juvenile process, few wish to revert entirely to the pre-20th century approach, which failed to make legal distinctions between juveniles and adult offenders. A system of juvenile justice must ultimately hinge on the quality of its institutions and personnel at all levels—from intake to confinement. Preoccupation with the details of due process, as necessary as these details are for the individual caught up in what can become a legal maze, may have little influence on what happens to the juvenile even when these criteria are met.

Not only does due process at the trial level not affect the subsequent processes for those found delinquent, it shifts the focus from what may be the only justification for the separate handling of juveniles. Historically, the justification was not a regard for youth per se from a legal standpoint, but rather a pragmatic effort to shift the aims of the traditional criminal law from retribution, punishment, and deterrence to a genuine effort at rehabilitation outside of adult prisons. In that sense, the last sixty years can be regarded as a prolonged pilot study in which juveniles were supposed to be treated differently and with different goals in mind than those perpetrated on adult offenders.

It is not the existence of separate procedures for handling juveniles that is under attack, but the modification of misguided products of those procedures. In fact, differences in dispositional alternatives may become the significant difference between adults and juveniles, once the juvenile is found delinquent within procedural safeguards. Even if the accomplishment of legal safeguards for juveniles at the trial level is achieved, vast numbers are still left who are perfunctorily remanded to institutions for confinement. Those remanded are then not considered punished, nor is the setting referred to as a prison.

The issue of what happens to the juvenile once adjudicated delinquent and/or confined, and the rights at that terminal stage of the legal proceedings, has to be the ultimate question for what the special handling of juveniles is all about. Relevant questions about juvenile rehabilitation are needed: (1) *Can* a given juvenile delinquent be rehabilitated? (2) What are the *measures* used to effect this? (3) Is there a *right* to treatment for the juvenile in such situations? (4) Are there any *standards* for appraising the adequacy of what is done as treatment in such correctional settings? (5) Can the proferred treatment be *refused?*

BASIS FOR CONFINEMENT

Legal Basis. The confinement of the juvenile is based on the presumption that he can be rehabilitated. The right of the state on constitutional grounds to supersede the parents for this purpose has long been established.[20] Hence, the sacrifice of certain procedural safeguards, but also the generalized grouping of offenders as delinquent on the basis of widely varying behaviors. Assignment of delinquency status to someone on the basis of their being ungovernable by their parents, in contrast to commission of overt offenses makes some juvenile offenses a status crime, like vagrancy. The social stigma of delinquency is attached to all categorized in terms of their future. It is not that the stigmatization has any negative impact from the peer group. In some cultural settings, the delinquency appellation has the opposite effect. However, the adverse consequences of the labeling extend beyond the immediate response of peers. The categorization of a juvenile as a delinquent does not disappear from official scrutiny nor do the records actually remain private as guaranteed.[21] The records may be circulated among various community agencies and, by the ever-ready copying machines available, circulate from one school or clinic to another.

The basis of detention for diverse acts lies in the position that the procedure is a civil one. While the safeguards of criminal procedure are sacrificed, the hoped-for goal is the removal of the punitive nature of the procedure and its consequences so that an incarceration does not become a de facto punitive measure. These ambiguities have rarely been resolved, since the distinction between treatment and punishment is not realistic. Detention against one's wishes in a semi-total institution violates many essentials required for a therapeutic contract. There is the double-bind situation in which something both is and is not at the same time. The juvenile is told he is committed in a civil procedure and not a criminal one, that he is a delinquent and not a criminal, that he is being detained for his own best interests and not those of others, and that he is being rehabilitated and not punished. Such statements are evasive and to a great extent untrue.

The greatest extremes in the handling of juveniles are seen when the English and Scandinavian approaches are contrasted. While the English juvenile courts are courts of law, with established rules of evidence and procedures, and have been described as modified criminal courts, the Scandinavian Child Welfare Councils are administrative tribunals not bound by rules of law and evidence. Many historical and cultural factors have contributed to the difference. The conservatism of the English approach to delinquent minors is seen in Blackstone noting at the end of the 18th century that the criminal law relating to minors had not changed for 400 years.[22] Since prison confinement had not yet developed, felonies were punished by death or exile and misdemeanors by whipping, mutilating, or exposure in the stocks. The 19th century saw the shift to imprisonment in England with minors being incarcerated with adult offenders. This is the background for disposing of juvenile deviants from which a reforming zeal of child savers arose to rehabilitate juvenile offenders rather than punish them.[23] It led to the juvenile court movement in England and the United States by the turn of the century, and only gradually to a reconsideration of what the rehabilitation measures and institutions to handle juveniles were accomplishing and how they functioned in practice.

In practice, treatment facilities for delinquents have never been able to rid themselves of a penal cast. Despite the devoted efforts of some staffs at correctional facilities, one cannot purge the penal characteristics in many even when individual staffs make valiant efforts to try and treat them to the best of their ability. In some cases the facilities are not even geographically independent of adult prisons.[24] The facilities for juveniles may be old jails or their equivalent. In some jurisdictions juveniles are held in solitary confinement before a hearing and the recalcitrant confined in cells without beds from two to five days.[25]

There is the further questionable practice of transferring juveniles from juvenile facilities to penal institutions without an intermediary court hearing. Such a procedure would seem impossible to justify by any therapeutic criteria. These are the juvenile cases which are equivalent to adults committed on a civil basis to mental hospitals as psychopaths who are then transferred to a penitentiary after refusing to admit their offense. Part of the rationale given is that they were deemed in need of being made more amenable to accept the rejected treatment offered in the hospital.[26] From a treatment vantage point, such ambivalence need not be present. The blatant anti-therapeutic nature of the procedures should be pointed out constantly.

Waiver. Although we are primarily focusing on the situation of the juvenile in juvenile institutions, the question of remand or waiver to adult criminal courts is important. It is important since, if the motion is carried and the juvenile is tried and convicted, the result is that the juvenile is sentenced like any adult. Even where counsel is appointed on request, there is rarely a provision to inform the juvenile of this right on a waiver motion. The attitude persists that the presence of counsel impedes reformation. It would seem axiomatic that a juvenile would require counsel in such situations since no pretense of juvenile rehabilitation is being made.

Waiver is an interesting social phenomenon in its own right. Granting of waiver by a judge is subject to all of the social and political vagaries of the moment. If a juvenile is to be rehabilitated, on what basis is he being sent up? The question of his treatability may not be determinable. In practice this revolves around interpretation of phrases such as the juvenile having exhausted the treatment facilities available to juveniles, or that he is not considered amenable to treatment as a juvenile.

A hearing on the waiver motion may involve argument or testimony in which correctional personnel, or other people involved from clinics or agencies, are brought in to testify pro or con. The hearing takes on the atmosphere of custody hearings in which the two sides primarily state their conclusionary pro or con positions as to whether a given juvenile is treatable in juvenile facilities. There is an unfortunate dearth of reasoning in terms of why and how a given juvenile can be treated. When demonstrations for the feasibility of treatment are called for, the evidence may be in the nature of the offender never having been committed to an institution before or that an institution feels itself equipped to handle all offenders or offenses. Caution is in order with respect to use of the word "treatment" at these hearings. In many cases specifics as to what is available, the number and quality of personnel, the various professionals involved, their experience, and the extent of their involvement are not brought out in testimony.

Waiver elicits the ambivalent foundation for much of the juvenile process, since if the transfer is effected it is purely an extra-rehabilitative move. Clinically, youths who have committed a homicide and are waived may in fact have as good a therapeutic prognosis as the more prevalent character disorder or subcultural delinquent who repeatedly commits property offenses. Waiver is a decision based not so much on legal or treatment grounds, but primarily on public clamor. It is a conclusion that a youth cannot be rehabilitated by juvenile facilities, but this is the question often never put to the test. The conclusion is made that there is no reason for exercising juvenile jurisdiction, since a youth is unamenable to treatment within the juvenile system and the case is transferred to adult criminal court.

Waiver has a limit on the lower age at which a juvenile can be certified to the adult system of criminal justice. Public outcry after a sensational act, such as strangling a younger child, or some type of sexually deviant act, often results in pressures to have a child remanded. A similar situation exists in states in which a juvenile court by statute has no jurisdiction over capital offenses, such as rape or murder. Again, this policy has little rationale on the basis of the behavior or by any treatment criteria. In Illinois, the decision to waive is solely up to the state's attorney and no hearing or standards are necessary.

In fact, few norms for transfer are utilized anywhere, since the guiding criteria are a *subjective* set of factors which tally up to not amenable. There is a direct implication for the treatment question present in the legal justifications for waiver procedures. The one referred to is a model which holds that youths are screened out who are really not juvenile in attitude. This amounts to a naive version of a developmental approach in which there is a presumption that certain personality and behavioral norms which characterize someone older than the statutory limit exist in a given youth. The difficulty is that there is rarely an adequate evaluation to appraise the hypothesis. A question-begging conclusion is that a particular youth is in fact overdeveloped for his years and should be processed as an adult (which means being indicted for a criminal offense).

A second justification offered for waiver is to confront the inadequate treatment facilities available in a community. The stress is then not on the advanced criminal tendencies of a youth, but rather on the fact that he may not be treatable in any available institution within a jurisdiction (not treatable through current existing facilities). In some cases these reasons are used in the same presumptive manner with no more than perfunctory evidence. In others, the background of criminality or expert testimony regarding a youth is available. Such situations must be kept in mind when juveniles request waiver on their own initiative. Several reasons for this exist. A juvenile might be convinced that he can present evidence in an adult court that will not result in a conviction; he may prefer to take a chance on spending a limited amount of time incarcerated if it is a minor offense by adult standards; or, he may only be fined. This would appear to be the reasoning observed in adolescent prostitutes. Many of them have learned from more sophisticated girls who pass on their styles.

Since a majority of juvenile offenders have little desire for rehabilitation, especially that offered by delinquency institutions, they opt for the technicality of the criminal law. This negates many arguments about the stigmatization of criminal procedures. Such maneuverings also belie the treatment goals promised in juvenile proceedings. While the limitations of their cognitive processes and impulsivity may predispose them not to desire to change, we must also consider objectively what is really being offered in the form of rehabilitation. If the juvenile does not have a right to demand waiver, a further question is raised about rehabilitative goals. Giving the juvenile the right to choose waiver is analgous to giving an option to an acting out patient to accept or reject treatment.

All varieties of testing, avoiding, and resistance become evident when treatment is offered to these adolescents in the most optimal of treatment settings. It is not surprising that the combination of their psychosocial problems and the frequent knowedge of inadequacies in juvenile institutions leads them to reject the juvenile process if a long imprisonment is not envisioned. In essence, the legal basis for detention of a juvenile stresses that a juvenile need not abandon his freedom under the 14th Amendment in return for what is offered as correction or "treatment" until and unless the state can prove by legal procedures that his conduct warrants such a loss of liberty.

Juveniles and Jury Trials. Before leaving the legal basis for detaining juveniles, a word needs to be said about jury trials in the determination of delinquency. This has importance in delineating which guarantees of constitutional law will be given to juveniles.

The ambiguity persists from the lack of a consistent jurisprudence applicable to juveniles, with legal guarantees at the hearing stage becoming confused with whatever the ephemeral treatment situations of the moment are like. In 1970 the Supreme Court held that the standard of proof in delinquency hearings that could lead to incarceration was "proof beyond a reasonable doubt."[27] The ruling was also made retroactive on the basis that the standard of proof utilized will substantially affect the outcome of a fact-finding hearing.[28]

However, the limit in extending the constitutional criminal provisions was set in the McKeiver case, which held that the 14th Amendment's due process clause did not require states to provide jury trials for alleged juveniles even if the acts in question could lead to commitment to state training schools.[29] This did not mean that a state could not make such a provision, but that it was not required to do so. The position was extended by a Circuit Court of Appeals which denied juveniles a right to a jury trial even if they could become incarcerated in an adult prison.[30]

By not giving juveniles the right to a jury trial, the issue of whether juvenile proccedings are basically civil or criminal was postponed in terms of a substantive examination. Reliance was placed on whether hearings were fair and orderly. The justification given for using a jury system was not used. Most court rulings have been against giving juveniles the right to a jury. It has also been noted that there is nothing contrary to a standard of justice which requires use of a jury since many systems do not use them. Some would argue further that jury trials impede the innovativeness in procedures needed for a progressive juvenile court system, so that we would be bogged down by the problems in adult courts, due to the formality and adversary emphasis.

However, these arguments do seem to bypass whatever justifications can be given for a jury system to begin with. In Kalven and Zeisel's tome on juries, the jury is seen as a protection for the individual accused. In situations where juries and judges disagree, juries are massively in favor of defendants.[31] The use of juries may initially operate in a low visibility manner by way of influencing a prosecutor whether to proceed or not. Other customary arguments are relevant: promotion of discussion of the facts among laymen, clarifying the bases for a decision by way of orders given to the jury, avoidance of sole reliance on a judge who has had previous contacts with the juveniles or the attorneys in cases, and opening up the proceedings to more public scrutiny. The issue is certain to recur in the future, and the ultimate decision will have to be made by what type of an institution the juvenile court is supposed to be.

Behavioral Basis. The subjective basis of the legal process with respect to juveniles is nowhere more clearly evident that in the behavioral basis as to what conduct will be judged as indicating a need for institutionalization. This behavioral criterion is not the sole one, nor would some hold it to be the major one. Since removal from home and community under the rationale of treatment is a major exercise of the police power of the state with punitive overtones, use of such power demands cautious application and some indications of success from the procedure.

One of the simplest behavioral criterion employed is the past record of the offender. This may be used in a quantitative fashion. Add up the number of past offenses within a given time period, and, if it exceeds a certain number, depending on the gravity of the behavior, commit the youth. If all of the cases coming through juvenile court were surveyed over a time period, this would be the most prevalent basis for delinquent commitment. In practice, it is illustrated by such juvenile offenses as car theft, riding in stolen automobiles, drinking intoxicating beverages, and simple assaults; among adolescent females it would be seen in incorrigibility, truancy, or promiscuity. The sequence is customarily that of an initial warning or informal probation, followed by formal probation, and then by a third offense at which time the question of institutionalization is raised.

This does not reveal the subtle influences which determine whether or not detention will actually be carried out. A contrite attitude—the mea culpa—often convincing to a judge or referee, is frequently viewed as the hallmark of a rehabilitable juvenile. In contrast, the surly, passive-aggressive youth is viewed as a challenge to the authority structure of the court and society. Such behavior is taken as indicia that a youth needs rehabilitation. Note that the appraisal is usually by externals and one could predict that the clever and intelligent juvenile offender, who has a certain histrionic flair, will be able to present a convincing mea culpa.

There may be additional aid coming from pre-sentence reports from probation officers, who must be evaluated on the basis of their own experience, talent, and case loads. Only in a small percent is a psychiatric appraisal at the judge's disposal before sentencing a juvenile, usually for the more serious offenses. From the large numbers of juveniles caught up in the process, few have a thorough appraisal. Recall that fully one third of juvenile judges have no probation, social work staff, psychologist, or psychiatrist available.[32] Among the remaining 10-20 percent, few of the psychiatrists or psychologists have had training or expertise in work with children and in family psychopathology, or more than cursory experience with the problems facing juvenile courts and their limited dispositional options.

Other behavioral bases employed in practice evaluate behavior in terms of offenses against property, against people, the social offensiveness of the behavior, and its potential for recidivism. The greater amount of evidence that a youth is an instigator, or using stolen property as a way of life or support, in contrast to being a follower, the more likelihood that he will be assigned to an institution. Confusion is compounded by using detention in an implicit manner as a punitive measure in some cases, while in others the juvenile is evaluated by personal and family psychopathology. In fact, once an acting out juvenile is appraised from the perspective of family psychodynamics, but disposed of by remanding him to a detention facility, the feeling of resentment in the youth is compounded.

The same rehabilitative error is made in drug or alcohol addiction programs. The individual is merely removed from a conflicted environment for a time, following which he is customarily sent back to the same setting. He is at best given brief dosages of treatment, based on whatever happens to be in use at the time in a given institution, usually some variant of group experience and confrontation techniques. This raises interesting questions. Should a family unit be ordered into a family detention unit? Out-patient treatments have had unreliable results, as most therapists predicted. Such coercive vehicles for treatment might suffice for a confinement period if organic therapies were to be applied, but they are fraught with uncertainties when the interpersonal context is viewed as crucial to the maintenance of antisocial behavior.

Capacity for Danger Basis. There is one instance in which the juvenile is either committed to a correctional institution or waived to an adult criminal court, in which the basis for detention is similar to adults. This is the case where the question of potential danger to others is present. A violent act may have been committed, or its potentiality suspected. However, even here the controlling factor for incapacitation remains cloaked under references to treatment.

All the unresolved questions of dangerousness which permeate detention of adults on this basis are present for juveniles. These issues are raised with the mentally ill who are civilly committed, and in some states they require a special label, such as "mentally ill and dangerous." This puts them in separate security institutions when so committed; it is used with sexual psychopaths and is raised with release problems for those confined after a "not guilty by reason of insanity" plea. Diagnostically, some of these individuals are psychotic, but a great number are plagued by severe character disturbances or acts of episodic deviancy. The majority of detained juveniles are not psychotic, but have varieties of character disorders or are youths responding to subcultural influences.

Issues concerning dangerousness are quite broad for juveniles. On one level there is an attempt to predict or forestall a major outburst of violence. On another level preventing repetitive but more minor aggressions is encompassed within the dangerous dimension. Opinions about the mental state of an individual, and particularly his potential to act in a dangerous manner in the future, are no better than clinical impressions. These decisions have to be made by courts, which then carry the maximum degree of restraint. The clinical signs and symptoms that are used to appraise dangerousness employ factors such as a history of overt assaultive behavior, a history of drug addiction, indices of impulse dyscontrol problems in which there have been outbursts of rage and fights, paranoid tendencies, sexual deviation, regressive object relationships, and a subcultural background which sanctions violence. The lack of reliability for predicting future violence by clinical criteria is notable.

Efforts to devise more accurate predictive measures have limitations. There is no feasible manner of developing actuarial tables to predict dangerousness for those who are before the juvenile court, or waived to adult courts, since the court must make an immediate decision with respect to discharge. To develop reliable tables would require that a certain number of individuals, who may be currently appraised as potentially dangerous, would have to be released for purposes of validating the predictive power of clinical or psychometric prediction. Without this essential step, which would have to be carried out for different offenses, personalities and social variables, we do not know what the actual incidence of dangerous behavior is. There would be many benefits if we had this knowledge. As an example, if a group of 40 adolescent rapists on a first offense were released and it was found that within two years 40 percent of them repeated a rape and another 20 percent committed some other sexual offense, we would then have a base rate of one out of five or two out of five—assuming sufficiently large numbers and other statistically reliable procedures—who would be dangerous in terms of a chance of repeating the behavior within a given time. Decision-making by those in responsible judicial, administrative, and clinical positions would have the capability of clarification. If a decision were made on the basis of this data to detain first-time juvenile rapists, we would detain eighty adolescents who appear unlikely to rape again and sixty who would not commit another sex offense. Whether this is desirable or undesirable as a social policy is something subject to debate and revision, of course, but it is true that at present we have nothing close to this type of data available, so that efforts to detain or release are at best an expression based on the insights of clinical work, and at worst a meaningless randomization based on personal guess.[33]

Nor would a set of tables suffice. Tables are invalid as a basis for predicting dangerousness before an individual has been detained because even if nothing more than a custodial stay has taken place, it is different from predicting dangerousness before antisocial behavior has occurred. If any type of treatment is carried out, the same restriction holds since this does not permit us to develop base rates for recurrence of a given behavior, which is first assembled and called dangerous for some purpose. If we are talking about serious violence, such as aggravated assaults or homicides, note that these are events with a low probability of occurence. There is thus a lack of both base rates and reliable psychometric tools.

What results is the utilization of dangerousness appraisals by one or more people—usually based on the past occurrence of a certain act. But to continue to detain a person in the future by predicting dangerousness from a past act reflects more of penal policy than a rehabilitative one. The ultimate decision should be based on the degree of social risk which society and courts are willing to take. There should be *specific* knowledge if a rational decision is to be made. Another inconsistency in the use of the dangerousness criterion is that use of a determinate prison sentence does not employ concepts of dangerousness to continue detaining an individual. Such individuals may be discharged and have a far greater potential to commit antisocial behavior than many of the emotionally conflicted or culturally damaged juveniles who engage in sundry acts of delinquency. To retain a juvenile solely, or primarily, because of an alleged or suspected social dangerousness, without specifying that he is treatable and that treatment is available, is hard to justify under the goals of juvenile justice.

THE RIGHT AND THE ADEQUACY OF TREATMENT
FOR JUVENILES

Any discussion of treatment presupposes there is such an entity, and that it is meaningful. Both presuppositions have been challenged when it comes to treating delinquent youth. The word *treatment* is bandied about ad libitum, but just as with other groups of individuals who are involuntarily detained, talking about treatment must be examined. When dealing with the detained juvenile, an immediate issue arises. Justifications for detaining a juvenile are put in terms of rehabilitation, customarily thought of as receiving treatment. Injustices are perpetrated if this is regarded merely as a word game. There are overtones of different theoretical viewpoints at stake on the nature of the delinquency process, as well as a substantive legal challenge to much of the correctional enterprise for dealing with detained delinquents.

One position is that the delinquent really has no need of treatment. This is adhered to on the one hand if there are suggestions of a medical model of diagnosis and treatment. The subvarieties of this approach vary from rehabilitative efforts, focused on broad-based environmental exposures within an institution, to resocialization experiences. The former approaches point to benefits of being removed from a noxious social environment, such as a slum or disorganized family, and being placed in an institution free from those influences. This comes close to being equivalent to custodial treatments in state hospitals for the mentally ill in which an emphasis is placed on a neutral environment. The added element with youth in correctional facilities is supposedly an opportunity to be reeducated with respect to social values—usually via some group therapy approach and a staff orientation which varies from authoritarian to buddy.

Such approaches raise questions for the treater as well as for issues related to involuntary confinement. Justification for involuntary detainment, the follow-up results available, the lumping of sundry types of diagnostic problems and ages, the length of stay, and the effect of removing the juvenile for a period while the noxious environment to which he will return usually remains constant, are problems which need study.

These same problems are relevent when more specific socialization measures are introduced to accompany a period of removal. Much variation occurs under the rubric of socialization. It may include group experiences such as physical work programs (forestry camps and athletics) and varieties of group interaction which change frequently due to what gets emphasized at a particular time or by a particular individual with an evangelistic mission to heal delinquents. In addition, other treatment approaches may be utilized, depending on what institution is involved, the personnel available, and over what particular length of time it is appraised.

Programs based on behavior modification techniques frequently have juveniles earning points, or their symbolic equivalents in the form of colored tokens, for good behavior. In an institutional setting this usually means conformity. The tokens are used to purchase objects or obtain privileges such as passes home or cigarettes. It is difficult to generalize about the results of behavior modification techniques on delinquent behavior. An immediate question is in terms of the large number of studies focused on a single behavior target. Some broader based programs have demonstrated positive results,[34] but methodological questions remain.

A primary question is the fact that we do not know whether the alleged changes would have occurred in the absence of the experimental manipulation. In 82 percent of the studies there was an absence of no-treatment control groups which are especially important at a time of life when the passage of time and changing life styles themselves produce behavioral change.[35] Problems associated with establishing the pre-treatment baseline for adolescents, and the effects of systematic variation of the treatments are needed. When something as complicated as delinquency is being treated, it is important to know how change is being measured, and how valid what is being measured is in terms of outcome. The old truism of simply going by re-arrest rates is not valid, but simple question interviews with adolescents might not be either.

Other programs place an emphasis on remedial educational techniques from the knowledge of the high rate of educational disability present in most committed delinquent youths. Other programs stress attempts to guide or counsel the youth away from his wayward ways. There may be direct utilization of efforts to inculcate respect for authority by focusing on disciplinary techniques (not physical brutality, which is a danger that can occur in any institutionalized setting, but rather the planned utilization of restriction of privileges, isolation, or loss of visitation privileges for violation of institutional rules).

Guided group interaction focuses on the attitudes and norms maintained by a group of delinquents rather than the behavior or attitudes of any one individual.[36] The theoretical assumption is that the abnormality of the delinquent resides in a peer group which supports his deviancy—hence the assumption that dealing with the values of the peer group as a unit will affect behavior. This would seem a valid underpinning for the type of subcultural delinquent in gangs as described by Albert Cohen,[37] but it would have little impact for juveniles responding to familial, interpersonal, or internalized conflicts.

A variant employs the delinquent himself as a therapist for his fellow delinquents. This is a utilization of role theory by holding to a position that a youth will learn conventional ways of behaving by acting out conventional roles with their concomitant duties.[38] This approach is similar to self-help groups as Alcoholics Anonymous, except that we must keep in mind the differences when used in a confined setting with juveniles. One difference is that a juvenile may not be given the choice to accept or reject the proffered treatment. The *Task Force on Juvenile Delinquency* has pointed out that authorities in correctional services for juveniles agree on two major principles: (1) traditional forms of incarceration in correctional institutions should be avoided as much as possible, and (2) alternatives must be sufficiently broad and diversified to provide for a wide range of treatment situations and procedures geared to the requirements of different types of delinquents.[39] In practice, these are rarely met.

> Such institutions, it is believed, are of dubious value as rehabilitative mechanisms, especially with the inadequate staffing and facilities found in most of them. Extended periods of incarceration in such institutions may prove to be positively damaging to a youth and may reduce the likelihood that he can be rehabilitated. In addition to the stigma attached to assignment to a correctional institution, which may become a serious barrier to the offender's return to a normal social life, there are such added hazards as the loss of contact with conventional society and intensified contact with such offenders. Not only is this form of treatment potentially damaging to the subjects, but the cost of such standard correctional approaches is much greater than that associated with most of the alternatives to incarceration.[40]

After these cogent points the *Task Force* concluded, "It seems the better part of both wisdom and justice to use institutional confinement only for those who would be dangerous to the community without it." The practical application is to try and eliminate as many of the traditional training schools as possible. Massachusetts actually tried this.[41] What theoretical discourse misses in attempts to change the existing structure are the political and personnel problems in carrying out change. The result of decisions to confine brings us back to the unresolved determination of dangerousness to justify such confinement for juveniles. Hence, the continuing importance of need for further explication of standards regarding dangerousness, given the present lack of validation.

Any survey of rehabilitative approaches reveals wide variations in what is presumed etiological with respect to delinquency. It is not necessarily that the workers in institutions clarify what their views are, but rather that they implicitly adhere to some view. Institutions with approaches focused on individual psychodynamics and family psychopathology exist, but they are rare and usually alien to a majority of correctional approaches. Part of this is due to the absence of sufficient numbers of personnel with psychodynamic training and sophistication who participate in the operational network of delinquent institutions. The situation is not much different from that in many other state institutions, such as hospitals where civilly committed individuals or mentally ill adolescents are detained. An added difference with delinquents is that the organic therapies have been even less effective, and hence delinquents receive less benefit from the psychopharmacological approaches which have aided the overworked state hospitals. Apart from outbursts of rage and anger during confinement, drug therapies have little use with delinquents except to put the lid on.

Another point concerns personnel. Approaches with delinquents have never emphasized the need for adequate diagnostic appraisal in terms of psychiatric nosology both at the court level or if institutionalized.[42] This is true for a descriptive and a psychodynamic approach. The result is that individuals institutionalized on the basis of delinquency hearings are a heterogenous group. In practice, the position has been to screen out or offer hospital commitment to those who are considered mentally ill.

The compensated cases of psychosis, or those subject to periodic psychotic episodes, are frequently processed as delinquents, just as adults who are processed as criminals. If regressive behavior or outbursts occur, they are handled by sedation or a temporary transfer to a security hospital and a subsequent retransfer back to the correctional facility when the acute psychosis subsides. In reality, a mixture of personality disorders and neurotic character problems are present in delinquent youths. Keep in mind the paucity of skilled personnel at the juvenile court processing and adjudicatory levels as well. The same limitation on expertise holds for institutions. Note that in many circles training and expertise are considered handicaps, so that an emphasis on using individuals without training beyond workshop levels predominates. The rationale is that these people are more in touch with delinquents.

CONDITIONS FOR A THERAPEUTIC ALLIANCE

To administer psychological treatments to anyone under conditions of involuntary confinement raises complex issues. *Legal* questions with respect to what is done to an individual under the 8th Amendment's "cruel and unusual punishment" provisions, deprivation of liberty, invasion of privacy, interference with the right to be left alone, indeterminate confinement as a violation of due process, and questions of statutory and constitutional interpretation concerning the basis for detaining a juvenile for rehabilitation, are all germane. *Therapeutic* questions regard the efficacy of treatment approaches carried out under these conditions, except for the rare juvenile who senses such a need and its justification. These limitations hold for any approach short of the coercive administration of an organic therapy to an unwilling patient, such as by holding a person down while giving him a tranquilizer or barbiturate injection or administering electro-convulsive treatments.

If a juvenile does not wish to explore reactions to his past life and family, or his internal responses and conflicts, a question should be raised about whether he can be treated successfully. This does not mean that a wholehearted acceptance of institutional placement by a disturbed adolescent must be present, without ambivalence or negative therapeutic reactions, if treatment is to be undertaken, but it does mean that in the absence of a professional collaborative arrangement to deal with conflicting wishes and feelings, with the goal of their eventual resolution, from the perspective of the juvenile little more may be present than serving time. From the perspective of the community, this may amount to a form of preventive detention to delay or postpone the opportunity for carrying out further antisocial behavior. One does not become a patient merely by living in an institution either voluntarily or involuntarily. The discrepancy between actual treatment versus occupying space is glaring if one inquires into settings for out-patients and asks whether treatment is present merely because a patient appears at the office of a therapist.

Duration of confinement under a rehabilitative framework for a juvenile delinquent needs exploration. This is particularly so with indeterminate sentencing approaches and the possibility of continued jurisdiction until age twenty-one. It has been noted that the greatest impact from an institutional placement is accomplished during the first few weeks or months of a stay and may conceivably last no longer than the first few days.[43] Those who advocate longer stays should have the burden of proof. Otherwise, time limits on confinement—if the actual goal is treatment—are desirable. If after a given time period a treatment relationship between the juvenile and his therapist in an institution is not present, acknowledgment should be made that factors are interfering with a therapeutic contact being established. To pursue detention beyond this point has more potential for affecting a situation adversely.

Arguments that the delinquent, like the criminal, really has no right of treatment but only the right to accept the freedom of an institution to offer it, reveal the blatant penal characteristics of detention at any age. Penal detention assuredly carries no overt promises of treatment, but to acknowledge this openly for juveniles portrays treatment as a thing which is offered at the whim of institutional personnel. Although this may be the situation, few would be willing to have it spread clearly upon the record, which would represent a further step in divesting the juvenile process of ambiguity.

The position advocated in this book is that therapy is a joint enterprise between at least two sides. On one side is a family containing a juvenile; on the other is a therapist in an institution supposedly geared toward treatment. Time should be provided all parties to decide whether or not they are going to work together. During this clarification period, educational influences are transpiring as to what treatment is about, the mutual demands and responsibilities of the parties, the need for treatment if indicated, and informed consent prior to its implementation.

These factors are basic in any successful therapeutic encounter. Clarifications should minimize the abrasive interactions which occur in a coercive setting. If after such exploration it is mutually decided that treatment cannot take place, it would appear futile to push the issue. Various therapeutic decisions might be needed, such as how and if to proceed with a juvenile whose delinquent tendencies are intimately bound up with family psychopathology but whose family members prefer not to become involved. At this time it is almost impossible to determine whether correctional facilities would be capable of accepting and implementing such an approach based on education, trial, and an eventual therapeutic contract.

At present there are few treatment programs operating by such standards. The few that do appear to make it feasible, but they have adequate staff and therapeutic sophistication. Furthermore, can it logically and empirically be defended that a therapeutic enterprise can proceed with hostile individuals under semi-penal regulations who are indefinitely confined and dedicated not to accept treatment? To refer to such a situation as therapeutic does not seem rational. The outcome is a therapeutic nihilism and an advocacy that delinquents be handled in their local communities.

A more difficult issue arises with cases which are viewed as untreatable by yardsticks such as lack of adequate or competent personnel or lack of knowledge as to treatment. Although some therapeutic enthusiasts argue that everyone is treatable, in practice this may not be so. Are these individuals to be sent to separate quarters for the untreatable? Again, keeping them with the remainder of the group might do little harm to others. What is the justification for keeping juveniles not receiving treatment or are not treatable in institutions? Pressing the argument returns us to the possibility of dangerous behavior occurring if they are released. [44]

As an example, an adolescent who has had a series of impulsive violent episodes has a diagnostic assessment which indicates little chance of altering his behavior pattern, even with the best therapeutic facilities over a long period. He has little desire to participate in treatment planning (even for those who do, the results are questionable). The usual phraseology used in institutional settings regarding such individuals refers to them as running a course of "slowly burning out" over a decade or more. Should such an individual be released or kept for an indefinite time? After a sufficient period of time all sides can appreciate the possibilities. Continued detention under a treatment rationalization would not be a desirable or honest option. If a need is felt to detain, it should not be under a pretense of rehabilitation. This may vary from an effort directed at retribution to deterrence of such behavior in other adolescents, or to carrying out what in effect amounts to preventive detention without categorizing it as such.

Open acknowledgment of diverse goals by detention would mean that rehabilitation as a goal for *all* juvenile delinquents would be abandoned. Those for whom the rehabilitation concept is abandoned would need the protections of the criminal law if it were felt that institutionalization was required. It is hoped that an initial screening would detect those for whom a treatment arrangement is deemed feasible. For the subgroup in which the question of dangerousness arises, there may be need for special procedures

directed to this issue. Great flexibility in therapeutic programs
would be needed if they are to be meaningful for experimentation
and as adjuncts for the use of educational and social rehabilitation
models. There may also be a need to take the risks attendant upon
shifts to part-time release or out-patient facilities. Again, the
limitation is the quantitative and qualitative deficiencies in the
triage of follow-up facilities with accompanying research to give
rationality and confirmation or disconfirmation.

VARIATIONS ON A THEME OF REHABILITATION

What are the programs and techniques encompassed under the
rehabilitative model for handling juvenile delinquents? Semantic
and substantive issues need to be faced. When the word *rehabilitation* is used in statutes and judicial opinions dealing with juveniles,
is it really meant to be taken seriously? Is it being used in the sense of
attempting to reconstruct a deformed personality of a juvenile
offender? To deal with his family psychopathology? To alter the
socio-cultural influences which have contributed to a final end-
process which has led a juvenile to be adjudicated delinquent and
remanded to an institution?

In this broad sense the rehabilitative goal is rarely achieved. It
has been argued that it is not achievable due to the radical solutions
that would be required. At the other extreme, some argue the term
rehabilitation was never meant to be taken literally, and that it is
only a euphemistic phrase expressing the fond hope of socially
minded reformers. If so, it was never meant to be used as a criterion
to evaluate what is done to juveniles placed in institutions in terms
of meeting a standard of treatment. The goal of placement is then
explained as providing more humane detention facilities for minors,
to keep them segregated from adult criminals, and to give them
moral guidance.[45] If this is so, the rehabilitative position is placed on
the level of an elective procedure, and not made the primary basis for
detention. However, this is rarely specified in clear terms. Continued
reiteration goes on that the legal basis for involuntarily holding a
juvenile under a civil commitment is rehabilitation.

Should rehabilitation be seen as equivalent to treatment?
Immediately, a problem is encountered which is not solved by a
dictionary. One of the primary ambiguities is the confusion and
outright disagreement about the nature of delinquency and the
myriad remedies proposed. Confusion extends throughout the
institutional approaches used with confined delinquents. When we

consider that the definitions of delinquency do not necessarily correspond to criminal conduct, a further mixture of social judgment, moral condemnation, sociological theorizing, and psychiatric appraisal results. Heterogenous groupings raise questions as to the basis for labelling anyone delinquent as well as treating such disparate groups. Further complications are variations between jurisdictions, as well as inconsistencies on the dispositional level, which provide an idiosyncratic emphasis to the basis for detention.

Attempts to clarify the basic nature of delinquent behaviors lead to perplexing questions analagous to those raised about the nature of mental illness. Hence, is an individual mentally ill on the basis of a cluster of symptoms and signs of a disturbance being present, or should the criteria rather be in terms of a lack of well-being, underachievement, or a lack of a creative life? When confining delinquents, a group which has passed through several stages of screening, including past efforts to deal with the juvenile in the community, the adjudication of delinquency, decisions to bypass probation, or utilization of other clinical or community facilities, is selected.

At this point, some believe a further process based on refined selection should take place. Selection would involve screening varieties of infractions, having adequate diagnostic appraisals available on which to make rational treatment and prognostic statements, and segregation of those considered recidivistic, recalcitrant, aggressive, or potentially dangerous. To accomplish this raises further problems about the current inadequacies, theoretically and practically, of making valid statements about groups. It is not that such data would not be useful, but research has been meagre in quality and defective in methodology.

Nor can efforts toward providing reception and diagnostic centers be thought of as solving the problem. They are plagued by the same shortages of staff and lack of expertise as other facilities. The same confusion about the nature of delinquency enters into such centers as well. Specific delineations of symptoms, personality structure, and family psychopathology are not the primary orientation in delinquency institutions. The orientation is closer to a broad view of mental illness in which juveniles who are involved in a variety of personal, family, and social predicaments are classified as problems in need of assistance. The latter view does not emphasize an act-focused approach, but rather emphasizes the *actor*—a distinction rooted in modern criminology in contrast to classical criminology.[46] Rehabilitation is then not conceived as primarily dealing with an infraction by a juvenile. In theory, it urges that the overall personality be dealt with instead of the act.

In practice the personality is rarely dealt with. Instead, the focus embodies environmental alterations or broad community action programs.[47] This is basically a sophisticated version of the Dickensian model that living with thieves makes thieves—a dyssocial model of delinquency. The result is a confused potpourri of techniques utilized in various institutions under the guiding theme of rehabilitation. The looseness permits almost any activity that is carried out to be referred to as rehabilitation or treatment. The effectiveness of such procedures is rarely determined. The issues are similar to those raised when adults are detained involuntarily on some basis in which rehabilitation may not even be the primary justification for confinement.[48]

Along with this confusion there is the correctional atmosphere itself, which raises questions about therapeutic efficacy. Whether the atmosphere is actually antithetical to treatment can be debated either way. Goals have been variously expressed as stopping delinquency without reference to personal and family concomitants, while in other institutions the overall remodeling of an individual is held to be the goal. In some cases there is an emphasis on institutionalization itself as rehabilitative—the transference of the custodial model to the correctional scene. In other institutions, there may be a direct acknowledgment that the mission is to protect the public, which is why disruptive youths are in custody. If there is an attempt to stress specific techniques of rehabilitation, even though many varieties are possible, in practice only a few predominate.

Predominant techniques tend to be some variety of group discussion or participation, or various educational measures. Work programs may be make-work in the sense of forest reclamation. The justification is that the adolescent has too much energy to burn up. These educational measures at best seek to give some type of job proficiency. In each of these approaches, there is a vague but implicit assumption about the etiology of delinquency, such as lack of vocational or educational skills. By a chain of events, these are held etiological by way of leading a youth to become a school dropout and then a delinquent.

Nor can the issue of pain-infliction as a reformative device be ignored. This is based on the assumption that punishment reforms. Pain infliction can become a selected therapeutic technique. Pain can vary from naive disciplinary methods to more sophisticated techniques of operant conditioning to reshape the juvenile.[49] In general terms, juvenile adjudication, as well as coercively maintaining an individual in a custodial institution, are de facto punitive measures. They are meant to be, on the theory that transgressions should not be rewarded. It is precisely in this area that confusion reigns, since the path is then open to utilize punitive measures as treatment.

Given such confusion, attempts to distinguish penal from treatment approaches break down. More specifically, the argument holds that antisocial behavior should not be rewarded by placement in a setting that is gratifying, since this reinforces such acts. As in all other approaches to delinquency, there are implicit theories in such treatment approaches. Aversive reinforcement (by painful stimuli, deprivation of freedoms, food, visitation rights, or goods) is used to program behavior. Positive reinforcement in the form of rewards or working for privileges are used. Perhaps the most widely used form of aversive reinforcement or deprivation in the criminal law is the device of taking money from a transgressor in the form of a fine. In these approaches, as in most others, there have unfortunately been major methodological defects with juveniles from different socio-economic backgrounds, intellectual and educational variations, mixing of juveniles with different offenses, absence of adequate control groups, and little long-term follow-up even in such crude terms as recommitment, let alone functioning outside an institution.

Lack of clarification of the general goals of correctional facilities for juvenile delinquents raises further problems about the evaluation of treatment programs. Like any institution in which there are involuntary inmates, deviants are incapacitated. A troublesome individual is removed from society and at least one contribution toward great harmony in society is made. Further, if such individuals are removed, the rate of delinquency should theoretically decrease. Figures which indicate this does not occur are handled by arguments that social organizations are deteriorating which offsets rehabilitative measures.

The deterrent effect is also stressed with the same unanswered arguments that are used for deterrence with adults. We do not have convincing evidence that specific deterrence operates with a single delinquent, nor that general deterrence operates with juveniles who do not deviate, are not apprehanded, or not committed as delinquents.[50] As noted, using the term "treatment" in the context of administering punishment has a further consequence of promoting ambiguity as to just what treatment is. Almost anything becomes justifiable from the lack of clear visibility as to what treatment in delinquent institutions entails.

Psychiatry and psychology do not have valid answers as to the role of punishment in affecting behavior. It is a very complex scientific question where even laboratory results are conflicting, and are not transposable to the unpredictable world.[51] We are a long way from having valid data that punishment is justified as a form of rehabilitation when administered in correctional settings. It is not known whether some punishments succeed in getting individuals to stop certain behaviors once out of an institution, or whether punishment instead leads to repetition or substitution activities. We also do not know whether a developmental phenomenon operates, so that in time behaviors are altered and become phased out; nor do we know if punishing one adolescent, say by the very act of involuntary detention, acts as a deterrent to his buddies. There is suggestive evidence from clinical work that the opposite effect may be produced in some adolescents, in that increased anger, rage, and further alienation from society result. Again, the confusion present in discussing these goals should be noted, since once we begin to talk about protection of society or deterrence, we are not making the rehabilitation of a detained individual juvenile primary.

Both a quantitative and qualitative problem are present. Quantitatively, how effective must punishment be to call it treatment? How much recidivism and relapse will be tolerated? Qualitatively, what is the justification for using procedures on a captive population in which measures mainly reflect the personal views and values of the particular staff using them? Favorite theories of criminality, as well as many unconscious attitudes regarding antisocial behavior, become fused into a treatment rationale.

These questions should not be taken as evidence for confirming an opposite point of view that some non-punitive measures, such as vocational counselling, have been validated and are therefore preferred. The effectiveness of any measure needs independent appraisal by whatever criteria are selected, such as the lack of recidivsm for delinquency, absence of certain symptoms, ability to integrate within society, vocational success, or greater freedom from personal conflict, to name a few. The failure to define specifically what a rehabilitation program involves in terms of procedures and goals gives room for perpetual argument about results. It makes discussions of right to treatment and adequacy thereof for the detained juvenile seem academic. However, such discussions do have the value of making public the predicament so that maintenance of the status quo becomes more difficult.

Maintenance of such ambiguity is functional. There are many reasons for maintaining such a state of affairs, and various groups wish to keep it so. The need for sectors of the official and unofficial public to deal with their own value systems and conflicts via correctional systems, most especially in the handling of deviant adolescents, comprises a large sector. To contain a host of conflicting values and demands, correctional programs are often a prime example of pluralism in action. In this context, both punitive and nonpunitive measures, attempts at individual treatment versus recreational and physical fitness programs, strict disciplinary measures versus permissiveness, vocational programs versus outdoor work, are all encompassed within different correctional settings with varying emphases. What is called treatment is really a measure of the conflicting values and needs of the general populace directed against a conspicuously deviant sector.

Pluralism gives the public reassurance that bad kids are being isolated from the community so that they and their children are being protected while they are simultaneously told that the setting is one in which the best intersts of juveniles are served by rehabilitation.[52] The main problem is not solely the lack of personnel in numerical terms, or the more serious lack in terms of expertise as exemplified in the approaches cited where volunteers, fellow delinquents, and ex-criminals are considered the best treaters. Since arguments exist as to what treatment amounts to with delinquents, and in institutional settings, viewing treatment proposals as serving other functions seems justified. These functions may be a rationalization of the conflicts under discussion to assure the maintenance of sameness, or they may be a covert expression of hostility via the advocacy of a treatment measure which amounts to degradation.[53] These are givens in such situations, in which an interesting question is the persistence of deficiences. That the deficiencies do not to alter substantively should raise questions about the sincerity of the wish to provide adequate treatment, and the limitations of rational thought processes to deal with such problems.[54]

Some go further and not that there is a need not to disrupt the stability in a bureaucracy. The system employs thousands of individuals and gives them not only monetary rewards but a feeling of doing something worthwhile. This varies from the lowest menial employees to the highest administrators, and would also include scholars and community agencies who continue to write reports dealing with the current status and problems of the juvenile court. All of these have a need to preserve continuity and assure themselves that no major changes will occur.[55]

All of these have a need to preserve continuity and assure themselves that no major changes will occur.[55]

From this background cogent questions arise about the inadequate techniques for appraisal and classification of delinquent activities, even if adequate personnel were available.[56] Who is to be designated as a treater? Should there be any professional standards at all, or merely the utilization of those who evince an interest in such work? Have we achieved a clarification of which measures the treaters feel can be dignified as adequate? How should adequacy then be defined? Is there any promise that the societal need for scapegoating groups in the population will change? On this basis, should a juvenile delinquent be involuntarily detained in an institution on the basis that he will receive rehabilitation? If not, what changes are necessary if it is believed some juveniles need to be involuntarily detained for some reason? Can we really pin our hopes on maintaining diverse delinquents in their communities by way of local agencies?

CONTINUATION OF DETENTION AND RELEASE

The Treatment Situation. The psychological aspects believed necessary for accomplishing therapeutic goals have been discussed. There are essentials for any therapeutic contract, depending on the nature of the relationship between the therapist and the patient or group of patients. Knowledge of the disturbances in human personality functioning and development is one essential. Without such knowledge any treater is ill-equipped to appraise deviations in socialization, personal conflicts, and social stresses that are present, and how ego functions have come to terms with them. This does not mean that many relationships and experiences are insignificant, but it does mean that if we lose our boundaries so that any human encounter begins to be called therapy, evaluation becomes more confusing and suspect.

If we assume a therapeutic relationship is present in the context used here, are there criteria to us in appraising whether a type of human relationship should be considered therapy? For thousands of youths who are confined within institutions of the type now existing, statistically few will be given therapy based on individual conflicts and family psychopathology.[57] A view that professionals are not needed is accompanying increasing skepticism that juvenile institutions fail to rehabilitate even under the best of circumstances. The argument is for the use of ex-offenders, neighbors, those who live in similar circumstances, and therapists who lack professional credentials (such as a graduate degree in social work). The result is a reinforcement of the position that it is not a series of conflicts within the delinquent and his family, in a process of mutual interaction within a peer group and society, which is relevant to delinquent behavior, but forces which permit delinquents to feel they have been wronged by a corrupt social fabric.

For the individual delinquent, a perpetuation of a pattern of projective attack of challenging others and the system is reenacted. Yet, as noted, the system somehow does assign fault to the individual delinquent, under a pretense of rehabilitation. There is little cognitive or emotional doubt in the delinquent that someone is assigning blame. The result is that little change in the community—often referred to as the inherent stability of social institutions—takes place. Fault has been assessed as residing within the delinquent juvenile by removing him from the environment and ignoring his compulsive and self-destructive ways. The antagonism continues to be played out within institutional settings where challenges to authority versus submission and conformity permeate much of the daily atmosphere.

To accept a policy of autonomy regarding personal therapeutic involvement for an institutionalized delinquent has the value of eliminating the pretense, that treatment is the justification for their being confined if they opt for no treatment. The issue is then forced as to whether detention itself should be considered therapeutic. To detain a delinquent as the sole goal runs into 14th Amendment problems in which due process would demand something beyond a pretense of treatment.

"Due process" requires that the nature and duration of the commitment be based on some reasonable relation to the purpose for which the individual is committed, as the Supreme Court said in a case involving civil commitment for incompetency to stand trial.[58] Similarly, "equal protection" of the laws under the 14th Amendment is not being effectuated if one institution falls below others in terms of quality of treaters, number of staff, or inferior facilities. A comparison of public and private facilities in this respect would find a wide divergence.

Such rehabilitative arguments as the benefits from the experiences of institutionalization itself, the adult models available for identification, and the rehabilitative effects of punishment, deprivation, and denial are questionable. They would need close scrutiny as a justification for continuation of a stay in an institution. If no therapeutic pretense about incapacitation of juveniles is made, alternative legal and jurisprudential models are needed. To continue a penal model in a context in which the justification is rehabilitative raises provocative questions. There is need for determination of the length of stay in such settings, as well as a study of procedures for release of an individual who may be repetitively acting out destructive impulses against neutral observers in his community.

Length of Institutionalization. Length of institutionalization— in practice—is determined by factors extraneous to any rehabilitative ideal. Many of the factors governing the original commitment of the delinquent to an institution govern the length of stay, such as the seriousness of the offense. Thus, an assaultive offense is considered indicative of someone who should be institutionalized longer than a case of repetitive truancy. Compare the operational similarity to the ratings of seriousness in adult courts and proportional sentences, and the focus on the act rather than the actor. Another factor is the number of times a youth has been institutionalized previously.

Conformity to the disciplinary rules of the institution by not presenting challenges to authority also counts. Since authority problems are why a large number of youths are committed to begin with, there is a strong emphasis on conformity as equivalent to a cure. If the more enterprising and manipulative youths are able to contain themselves, or even show a semblance of conformity, they are more likely to be released. Yet another factor is the mundane consideration of the pressure of new admissions. Greater numbers committed per year promotes a drop in the mean length of stay. Efforts to coordinate institutional discharge with school terms, as well as the comings and goings of institutional personnel, also influence discharge timing.

The age of the juvenile influences his stay and the approaches used. An older youth, especially if there have been several returns, is most likely to be classified as recalcitrant and in need of stricter discipline. Hence, he may be assigned to settings with stricter discipline, again with the assumption that the self-discipline required to do a work task will generalize to his behavior once he leaves the institution.

The actual composition of a population of confined delinquent youths varies widely, although the programs in use at a given institution usually do not. Somewhere in the dispositional process the few overt, psychotic juveniles who have been engaging in antisocial conduct have been screened out and either committed to mental hospitals or sent to clinics. By this process, a logical fallacy is propagated that all of the emotionally disturbed delinquents have been screened out. This reflects a type of unsophisticated thinking regarding personality development and deviation. It is mentioned to note that if perchance a youth with bizarre symptomatology is committed to a delinquency institution, he will most likely be discharged either to his home with the recommendation that he get help (with or without the help of some after-care agent) or directly transferred to a residential treatment center or hospital, if one is available. The possibility of transfer to an institution with strict discipline for a boy who is disruptive or aggressive always looms in the background, with the approach becoming more penal. There is also the matter of administrative transfers when a youth is shifted to a penal institution. [59]The word game is played to the hilt in which the reasoning is that there is no constitutional infringement of his rights, since a juvenile in a prison is held not to *be* a prisoner and, therefore, cannot be punished. [60]

Once institutionalized, little recourse exists for a delinquent apart from such traditional remedies as habeas corpus. Since the detention is supposedly for their own best interests, habeas corpus requires documentation of some major error of fact. Some states provide for the child, parents, or friends to make a motion requesting that a modification or revocation of the disposition take place. [61] Rejection may be appealed. In most cases modification hinges on the ability to show a change in the circumstances which led to the commitment. Two types of dilemmas arise.

If the alleged change is supposed to have taken place in the delinquent, evidence must be forthcoming from the staff of the institution where the juvenile is detained. It is rare for a private psychiatrist or psychologist to be retained by a family to evaluate whether a juvenile in a delinquency institution should be released. Even when this occurs, the argument is offered that the private psychiatrist has not had the benefit of observing the youth within the institutional setting. The other problem in seeking release is to argue that the environment from which the youngster became a delinquent has changed sufficiently so that he may be returned to it. This leads to ploys, such as parental protestations of reform, promises to discipline the child, motions of relatives to obtain custody and offer a new home, and so on. Any attempt to appraise the significance of such changes quickly leads to a realization of the lack of substance involved in most of them. [62]

THE TREATMENT POSITION FOR DELINQUENTS:
MEANINGFULNESS

A Viewpoint on Minors.   Because of the above limitations in the process, substance, personnel, and promise of juvenile rehabilitation, the following conclusions are offered. The main problem associated with the rehabilitative approach resides not only in the acknowledged difficulty of delivering on the promise, but in the inherent concealment of a position which fails to distinguish a hope from a promise. Jurisdiction is thus exercised under a guise. To appraise the discrepancies requires that the entire basis of juvenile jurisprudence be examined in the context of its historical origins and contemporary functional performance, which has been one of the aims of this chapter.

A court designed as an institution not to correct but to help children does not need to be viewed as one in which its population is in need of protection by such constitutional measures as the due process guarantees present in criminal procedures. In fact, there would be nothing inconsistent in actively seeking out children beyond the ken of those who had committed overt delinquencies. They could be offered the same humane services of institutions and personnel who were helping children who had violated civil rules or ordinances, as well as any treating behavior considered undesirable in a juvenile.

Precisely by the use of such language confusion has resulted. If incorrigibility, truancy, swearing, smoking, and wearing long hair reflect behaviors adults do not like on some basis at a particular historical moment, the juvenile process in effect shifts from attempting to remedy personal and social pathology in children and families to enforcing parental dictates via parens patriae power of the state. Even if intervention were limited to acts considered criminal, the approach is largely one of bypassing the pathological elements that give rise to the behavior. On the other hand, if the basis for delinquency is actually primarily in the environment, it is unlikely to change or be remedied by periodic incapacitations of the juvenile who continues to return to the same environment.

From legislatures making many acts subject to juvenile court jurisdiction, a mixture of adult benevolence and punitiveness results. The mixture is based on a felt need to control or stop such behavior. It then becomes part of an institutional process for enforcing types of socialization practices on a minor who is resistant to such conformity in the social sphere. At bottom, it is telling minors they will be made to conform, but that the change will be done in a setting called rehabilitative in which they will be socialized according to the norms in vogue in their communities. Acts considered criminal will similarly receive the promise of socialization coupled with isolation with peers who are similarly designated. Consequently, it does not really matter whether the juvenile desires such rehabilitation or not. The process is focused on conformity to the norms of a particular adult subculture, and their expectations for how they want juveniles to behave. This not only sanctions the laxity with respect to findings of fact in the juvenile process, but allows wide intrusions into the privacy and freedom of the child by the state which are far beyond criminal jurisdiction.

It is the attempt to enforce social, moral, and institutional needs in a child, beyond criminal statues, that permits the use of delinquency adjudications for a host of challenges to adult authority—direct or substitute—such as not obeying school personnel or truancy. There is a carryover implicit in these solutions that children can be, and should be, made to obey parents, treat adults with respect, and go to school. This bypasses much of what we know about behavior being based on mutual respect and integrity within a family. It does not seek the source of such deviations, which should be determined by various possibilities of conflict on an overt, covert, or symbolic level, and which may have achieved added reinforcement and promotion in subcultural groups.

Detecting these conflicts and subtleties presents a challenge to the most competent of clinicians who attempt to diagnose and treat children and families with psychological and social disabilities. There is a basic assumption regarding solutions for behavior in delinquency institutions and in the juvenile process which appears to be in conflict with a view of behavior that raises questions about psychological or social deviancy arising in contexts of disturbed development. In many ways the rehabilitative efforts are a nostalgic remnant of the Victorian ethic of child submissiveness to parental discipline. The difference is that it is called rehabilitation.

Nor should there be any equivocation about the primacy of the concern of the court in the elimination of disruptive influences. Basically, the same criteria apply to juveniles as to adults who pose a threat to the integrity and safety of the community.[63] Acknowledgment of this primacy would have the beneficial result of eliminating duplicity for the juvenile and institutional staff. To accomplish this requires that the goal of rehabilitation be limited more sharply than it has been. It means a revision of the scope of juvenile jurisdiction in line with the realistic performance which institutions are capable of achieving, although even this would be made secondary. Procedures would be viewed as coercive and applied to conduct which was not merely viewed as resistant to socialization, but for which the police power of the state is called upon to restrict. This was the original model laid down for the juvenile court in Illinois. However, by a process of accretion subsequent legislatures continued to add new juvenile violations.[64]

Restricting the coercive sanction to conduct where a specific infraction of criminal statutes has occured could have additional surplus benefits. It would eliminate some juveniles who are being sent to institutions, and avoid the adverse consequences contigent upon solidifying an antisocial identity.[65] It may thus function to affect some juveniles favorably in a preventive manner, instead of enhancing their criminal propensities.[66]

Delinquents and the Right to Treatment. What about the right to treatment of the institutionalized delinquent? Does it make sense to continue to talk as though he is being held under a justification of rehabilitation? As the word is now used with respect to those detained, our discussion has noted that procedures called rehabilitation can amount to almost anything. No one can say what treatment should or does amount to in such situations, since the word treatment gets applied to almost everything. Indeed, the delinquent is in a worse situation than someone civilly committed as mentally ill, for there are emerging some criteria for the latter case which have to be met.

Rehabilitation of juvenile delinquents admits to little restriction or measurement. It is rather a goal for which there are hopes of attainment. It appears that one of the main justifications for using the word rehabilitation is to detain an individual, since without such justification detention would likely be unconstitutional, due to the glaring penal nature of the provision.[67] Hence, confinement has to be rationalized on the basis of juveniles sacrificing other protections in exchange for treatment.

The following conclusions appear warranted:

1. A right to treatment for juvenile delinquents, although more difficult to appraise than such a right for patients who are involuntarily committed as mentally ill, is nevertheless being increasingly seen by courts as a statutory or constitutional right.[68]

2. Appraisal of treatment measures with delinquents is more difficult due to the lack of any consistent and widely accepted

theoretical explanatory model for delinquency. With mental illness, there are various theories regarding etiology and treatment, but a greater consensus on what should be done for the majority. The problem is that it may not be available. Results from any technique used with delinquents have failed to show any consistent degree of rehabilitation. This in itself would argue for questioning rehabilitation as the primary justification. The rationalization of a quid pro quo excludes denial of procedural rights.[69]

Special procedures utilized for processing juveniles prejudicially, as well as at the adjudicative and dispositional levels, can be justified only in terms of special treatment programs. There is a tone in opinions that the goal is of individualized treatment for the particular delinquent, and that if such treatment is not forthcoming, a challenge to the validity of the custody may be raised on the grounds that no special treatment is being given. This would be analagous to the Supreme Court decision dealing with a mentally ill person being involuntarily detained for fifteen years in a mental hospital without treatment which was seen as unconstitutional for violating his right to liberty.[70] No specification of what treatment amounts to is usually given. The problem of criteria for appraising adequacy becomes pivotal. A Circuit Court of Appeals has upheld a constitutional right to treatment for institutionalized juveniles under the 14th Amendment.[71] It specified that "right to treatment" includes not only the right to minimum acceptable standards of care and treatment, but the right to *individualized* care and treatment as well.

The medical model has been largely insignificant in the diagnostic evaluation or treatment of juvenile delinquents. The relative lack of psychiatric personnel in the field negates attempt to apply even the vaguest standards for treatment as used in hospitals with the mentally ill who are civilly committed. The problem is the lack of standards that would, on the one hand, hold up to critical scrutiny the validity of treatment measures, and on the other hand, the wide license that the confinement process gives to interfering with the liberty of a juvenile under false pretenses.

3. Another conclusion that appears warranted is the absence of standards to appraise the quality of the treaters. This is a criterion useful judicially to challenge what is called treatment and its adequacy, since the deficiencies are overt and classifiable. This need not only refer to the vast numbers of unfilled positions, but to sanctioning the use of relatively untrained and unskilled personnel as staff. While some of the programs amount to the equivalent of

custodial maintenance, those which attempt other types of naive interventions have little justification as treatment measures when the price is loss of liberty.

4. A basis for detention in juvenile institutions in terms of norms for treatment adequacy has little factual or psychological validity for the majority of those detained. The question is whether a rationalization of treatment is needed, or whether it would be wiser and more equitable, as well as preventive, to eliminate the guise and acknowledge that treatment is not the reason for detention. If this requires an appraisal of the basis for detention along statutory or constitutional grounds, the situation may require presenting data on the existing treatment processes and the ambiguous results and directly facing the issue. A blurring of the civil-penal distinction might result, which would raise further questions about the nature of committing juvenile delinquents to institutions. [72]

5. Juveniles who are deemed in need of incapacitation per se need to be handled like other individuals who behave in such a manner. The juvenile process, if restricted to criminal offenses, could deal with these juveniles on the basis of confronting them with the offense, and if necessary, using a correctional institution with the same hope as with an adult offender, i. e., that it may have some rehabilitative or deterrent effect on their behavior.

This is not to argue for sending juveniles to prisons which are by nature punitive. It would instead tighten the procedures by which delinquents are institutionalized, so that fewer of them would meet this fate. For those who did, all efforts would be made to deal with the juvenile in a humane and therapeutic manner. However, if the staff, funds, and know-how to accomplish this are not present, we must be wary of continuing to use the rationalization of treatment when it is inappropriate. The proposal eliminates the pretense of institutionalization, with the limitations in knowledge, staff, and approaches for treatment purposes. It is acknowledged that an occasional facility and staff do provide what would be labelled adequate treatment by most clinicians in terms of effort expended and measures used. There are also occasional relationships which emerge as genuine therapeutic encounters for the juvenile. Overall, however, these are true for a minority, and may almost be viewed as fortuitous happenings when they do occur.

6. The juvenile offender alleged to be dangerous raises the same perplexing and unresolved problems as for anyone alleged to be dangerous. These judgments require great clinical skill to marshal the relevant factors pertaining to past behavior as well as potential

acts. This is especially so when it concerns the potentiality for an act which has not yet occurred. The situation presents problems of both a predictive and clinical nature. The predictive capacity of the clinician is grossly limited, and statistical measures are similarly limited at this time, from the lack of accurate base rates on which to make such predictions valid as we have discussed in chapter 12.

Conclusions. The implication is that detention of juveniles has been on the basis of providing treatments which either do not exist or are invalid. In cases where certain treatment measures might prevail, they are often not available. A right to treatment is hard to negate legally for confined juvenile delinquents unless one wishes to specify that when the phrase is used it is to be thought of as referring simply to intent rather than results.

Our knowledge of rehabilitating delinquents is so meagre, as confirmed by investigations and results, that we are utilizing techniques on a trial and error basis. This means that delinquents are, in fact, experimentees who should be viewed in this context. This should mean that humane considerations should apply as in any such investigation. It further means that considerations about the use of human volunteers should be respected. Of course, for those delinquents who have acted antisocially on some basis for which it appears that a certain therapeutaic approach is likely to have a fair chance of success, it should be offered with the safeguards of informed consent through the parent or guardian *and* the minor. Such a right to refuse what is offered as treatment hopes to steer a path between preserving professional discretion while setting safeguards for the arbitrary imposition of intrusive or experimental procedures. The use of psychopharmacologicals or electrical treatment are on the cutting edge of challenges.[72]

To rebut inadequacy of treatment would require a resort to acceptance of the "best we can do with what we have" doctrine. Whether this justifies continuation of the practices is the basic issue. The more just and optimal solution would be to restrict admittance to the process of juvenile detention at all levels, from pre-court contacts to adjudication and disposition.

For those who are adjudicated delinquent, and are further appraised as in need of removal from the community, revisions need to be conceived of in terms of alternative paths to detain an individual until he is deemed safe to be returned to the community. Some may receive treatment if and when it is available. The need to balance concerns for public safety against the tolerance for deviation in juveniles is the junction. With our present limitations it would be desirable to limit restraint to those whose aggressive behavior seems imminent and continuing. This position amounts to an abandonment of the rehabilitative justification for detention of juveniles. Detention in delinquency institutions could be used only when the commission of restricted criminal acts has occurred, and when there are no feasible alternative dispositions available for the juvenile. What legal alterations and procedural safeguards this will require are much in need of discussion by all disciplines concerned with children and adolescents. There is always the advantage of the more optimistic and less judgmental outlook of juvenile law compared to criminal law.[73] That is why we ought to preserve the best part of it.

REFERENCES

1. E. M. Schur, *Radical Nonintervention: Rethinking the Delinquency Problem* (Englewood Cliffs, N. J.: Prentice-Hall, 1973).
2. L. Radzinowicz, Impressment into the army and navy—a rough and ready instrument of preventive police and criminal justice, *Crime and Culture*, ed. by M. E. Wolfgang, pp. 287-313 (New York: John Wiley, 1968).
3. A. Prevezer, An historical summary of the English juvenile court system and an assessment of certain of its features in the light of American practice, *Wayne Law Review* 4(1957):1-24.
4. W. Blackstone, On the persons capable of committing crimes, *Commentaries on the Law of England*, pp. 22-24 (Chicago:Callaghan, 1899).
5. R. Pound, *Interpretations of Legal History*, p. 134 (New York: Macmillan, 1923).
6. *In re Gault*. 387 U.S. 1, 1967.
7. M. E. Persig, The constitutional validity of confining disruptive delinquents in penal institutions, *Minnesota Law Review* 54(1969):101-145.
8. *Career Training in Child Training*, ed. by O. Krug (Washington, D. C.: American Psychiatric Association, p. 49, 1964).
9. Juvenile delinquents: the police, state courts, and individualized justice, *Harvard Law Review* 79(1966):775-810.
10. *State v. Melanson*, 250 So. 2d609 (La. App. 1972).
11. E. H. Erikson, The confirmation of the delinquent, *Chicago Review* 10(1957):15-23.
12. H. E. Fradkin, Disposition dilemmas of American juvenile courts, *Justice for the Child*, ed. M. K. Rosenheim, p. 126 (New York: Macmillan, 1962).
13. *United States ex rel. Murray v. Owens*, 465 F. 2d 289 (2d Cir. 1972).

14. A. Gilbert, Adolescents in state hospitals: expensive expediency, *American Journal of Orthopsychiatry* 35(1965):825-827.

15. H. W. Dunham, The juvenile court: contradictory orientations in processing offenders, *Law and Contemporary Problems* 28(1958):508-527.

16. *Breed v. Jones,* 421 U.S. 519(1975).

17. F. A. Allen, Criminal justice, legal values and the rehabilitative ideal, *Journal of Criminal Law, Criminology, and Political Science* 50(1959):230.

18. D. Matza, *Delinquency and Drift* p. 132. (New York: John Wiley, 1964).

20. N. Kittrie, Can the right to treatment remedy the ills of the juvenile process? *Georgetown Law Review* 57(1969):848-885.

20. A. V. Cicourel, *The Social Organization of American Justice* (New York: John Wiley, 1968).

21. C. P. Malmquist, Problems of confidentiality in child psychiatry, *American Journal of Orthopsychiatry* 35(1965):787-792.

22. Blackstone, op. cit.

23. A. M. Platt, *The Child Savers* (Chicago: University of Chicago Press, 1969).

24. Persig, op. cit.

25. Note, District of Columbia juvenile delinquency proceedings: apprehension to detention, *Georgetown Law Review,* 49(1960):322-357.

26. L. Frankel, Preventive restraints and just compensation; toward a sanction law of the future, *Yale Law Journal* 78(1968):229-267.

27. *In re Winship,* 397 U.S. 358 (1970).

28. *Ivan v. City of New York,* 407 U.S. 203 (1972).

29. *McKeiver v. Pennsylvania,* 403 U.S. 528 (1971).

30. *United States ex rel. Murray v. Owens,* op. cit.

31. H. Kalven and H. Leisel, *The American Jury* (Chicago: University of Chicago Press, 1966).

32. E. Lemert, The juvenile court-quest and realities, *Task Force Report: Juvenile Delinquency and Youth Crime,* 1967, p. 9.

33. J. Goldstein and J. Katz, Dangerousness and mental illness: some observations on the decision to release persons acquitted by reason of insanity, *Yale Law Journal* 70(1960):225-239.

34. R. L. Schwitzgabel, Preliminary socialization for psychotherapy of behavior disordered adolescents, *Journal of Consulting and Clinical Psychology* 33(1969):71-77.

35. W. S. Davidson and E. Seidman, Studies of behavior modification and juvenile delinquency, *Psychological Bulletin* 81(1974):999-1011.

36. F. L. Bixby and L. W. McCorkle, Guided group interaction in correctional work, *American Sociology Review* 16(1951):455-461.

37. A. Cohen, *Delinquent Boys: The Culture of the Gang* (Glencoe: Free Press, 1955).

38. D. R. Cressy, The theory of differential association: an introductioon, *Social Problems* 8(1960):2-6.

39. S. Wheeler, L. Cottrell and A. Romasco, Juvenile delinquency—its prevention and control, *Task Force Report: Juvenile Delinquency and Youth Crime*, pp. 409-428 (Washington, D.C.; the President's Commission on Law Enforcement and the Administration of Justice, 1967.

40. Ibid., p. 422.

41. L.E. Ohlin, R.B. Coates and A.D. Miller, Radical correctional report: a case study of the Massachusetts youth correctional system, *Harvard Education Review* 44(1974):74-111.

42. D.O. Lewis and D.A. Balla, *Delinquency and Psychopathology* (New York: Grune & Stratton, 1976).

43. Wheeler, Cotrell and Romasco op. cit., p. 424.

44. C. P. Malmquist, Dilemmas of the juvenile court, *Journal of the American Academy of Child Psychiatry* 6(1967):723-748.

45. J. W. Mack, The juvenile court, *Harvard Law Review*, 23(1909):104-122.

46. Matza, op. cit.

47. Y. Bakal, ed., Closing correctional institutions, *New Strategies for Youth Services* (Lexington: Lexington Books, 1973).

48. E. M. Emerson, *Judging Delinquents* (Chicago: Aldine, 1969).

49. J. C. Ball and A. Simpson, The extent of recidivism among juvenile delinquents in a metropolitan area, *Journal of Research, Crime and Delinquency* 2(1965):77-84.

50. R. Walters and R. Parke, The influence of punishment and related disciplinary techniques on the social behavior of children: theory and empirical findings, *Progress in Experimental Personality Research* 4(1967):179-228.

51. Emerson, op. cit.

52. E. Grotberg, *Critical Issues in Research Related to Disadvantaged Children* (Princeton: Educational Testing Service, 1969).

53. E. J. Vogel and N. W. Bell, The emotionally disturbed child as the family scapegoat, *A Modern Introduction to the Family*, ed. N. W. Bell and E. F. Vogel (Glencoe: Free Press, 1960).

54. D. Cressy, The nature and effectiveness of correctional techniques, *Law and Contemporary Problems* 23(1958):254-271.

55. Wheeler, Cottrell and Romasco, op. cit., p. 410.

56. Statistics in public institutions for delinquent children, *Children's Bureau Statistical Series, no. 81*, 1964.

57. *Jackson v. Indiana*, 406 U.S. 715 (1972).

58. Transfer of juveniles to adult correctional institutions, *Wisconsin Law Review* (1966) 866-912.

59. *Wilson v. Coughlin,* 259, Iowa 1167, 147 N.W., 2d 175, 1966.

60. *Children in the Courts—The Question of Representation,* ed. G. G. Newman (Ann Arbor: Institute of Continuing Legal Education, 1967).

61. Emerson, op. cit.

62. F. A. Allen, *The Borderland of Criminal Justice* (Chicago: University of Chicago Press, 1964).

63. H. Wang, The continuing turbulence surrounding the parens patriae concept in american juvenile courts, *McGill Law Journal* 18(1972):219.

64. H. S. Becker, ed., *The Other Side: Perspectives and Deviance* (New York: Free Press, 1964).

65. S. H. Kadish, The crisis of overcriminalization, *Annals* 374(1967):157-170.

66. *In re Gault,* op. cit.

67. *Morales v. Turman*, 383 F. Supp. 53 (E. D. Tex. 1974), 5357.2nd864(5th Cir 1976), 97 S.Ct. 1189(1977).

68. Note, *Parens patriae* and statutory vagueness in the juvenile court, *The Yale Law Journal* 82(1973):745-771.

69. *O'Conner v. Donaldson*, 95 S. Ct. 2486 (1975).

70. *Nelson v. Hyne*, 491 F. 2d 352 (7th Cir. 1974).

71. E. Z. Ferster, T. F. Courtless and E. N. Snethen, Juvenile detention: protection, prevention or punishment, *Fordham Law Review* 38(1969):161.

72. R. Delgado, Organically induced behavioral change in correctional institutions: release decisions and the "new man" phenomenon, *Southern California Law Reveiw* 50 (1977):215-270.

73. G. C. Hazard, Jr. The jurisprudence of juvenile deviance, *Pursuing Justice for the Child,* ed. M. K. Rosenheim (Chicago: University of Chicago Press, 1976).

Chapter Fourteen

Treatment of the Adolescent

Several questions need consideration when making a decision about whether psychotherapy should be chosen as a mode of treatment for adolescents. Even beyond the problem of delineating which type of psychotherapy we are talking about, there is a fundamental need for adequate diagnostic assessment. Several separate and related goals are possible. Since these goals vary, clarification is required between chosing a limited objective, such as providing symptom-removal or an immediate relief from pain by psychopharmacological means, and attempting to resolve causal factors. Clarifying therapeutic goals permits a more rational approach to what is essentially a problem in irrationality.

A variety of techniques are currently portrayed as therapy. Some are ludicrous caricatures of treatment carried out by self-styled therapists. Confusing a *desire* to help those with emotional difficulties with the *capacity* to carry out treatment lies at the root of the problem. It is a painful experience for a psychiatrist to witness the gamut of activities labelled as treatment being perpetrated on youths wrestling with deep-seated problems, but we will not pursue the topic of pseudotreatment any further.

Consider some preliminary defintions and classifications useful in deciding which type of psychotherapy is preferable.

1. Supportive measures rely on approaches to alleviate anxiety and discomfort. Alternatives are utilized which try to contain behavior that is personally or socially disruptive. If possible, this

can be through environmental alterations or, if necessary, removing adolescents from the source of their discomfort.

2. Sectors of conflict may be isolated and therapeutic efforts directed toward these particular areas. Unconscious conflict, or familial and environmental conflicts are major sources of problems. Multiple sources contributing to conflicts of this type may not be dealt with nor worked through; instead, one or more nuclear areas are selected for attention

3. Attempts to resolve conscious and unconscious conflicts, or achieve alterations within the personality structure, obviously demand more intensive efforts in terms of time, psychological understanding, and methods of resolution. These resolutions have additional goals of moving beyond environmental alterations, as desirable as these may be in their own right. Conflict resolution presupposes that the hallmark of neurotic conflict exists (an internalized conflict, which functions relatively autonomously from the external environment, and which has unconscious derivatives).

The techniques which should be used to accomplish the goals is a separate, though integrally related, problem. The modalities vary from a focus on verbal communication dealing with thoughts, fantasies, feelings, or impulses, to the use of adjuncts. With younger children such adjuncts as play, toys, drawings, puppets, clay, and paints are the traditionals. By adolescence, these have usually served their therapeutic time, although some may use painting. In addition, things may be done to the adolescent or other family members, such as administering tranquilizers to a particular member. Other approaches may be directed toward a unit larger than the individual, such as trying to treat the entire family unit. An outline of the types of therapeutic approaches used to achieve one or more of the above goals is given later in the chapter. The approaches and problems unique to the therapeutic enterprise with adolescents and beyond are the focus.

GENERAL PROBLEMS RELATED TO PSYCHOTHERAPY
WITH ADOLESCENTS

Therapy Values. Several principles relevant to any psychotherapeutic work with youths need consideration. Although some may question these, the need for a working philosophy is crucial if work with an adolescent is to progress beyond the level of friendship. The position here is not only that various therapeutic choices, such as immeditiate symptom-removal or not, are at least partially valued choices, but that the decision to engage in a therapeutic contract at all represents a value choice. An initial caveat is that seeking causative factors to the maximum extent is important in all diagnostic and treatment approaches. This is not to imply that diagnosis is the sine qua non of treatment, with the patient simply representing a mental curiosity or anomaly to unravel, like any good puzzle. A position of therapy as a value choice stands in opposition to a treatment approach which operates in an atheoretical vacuum. An example of the latter would be a therapeutic posture that doing something to a suffering individual, without thorough diagnostic inquiry and evaluating etiologic factors, should be primary.

In fact random helping interventions may be detrimental to certain individuals. If an adolescent is in a state of chronic anxiety, it may be of greater long-range benefit not to relieve the anxiety immediately, even if possible, without some knowledge as to what the multiple sources contributing to the anxiety are. The analogy is to the child with a chronic fever of unknown origin who might be treated by aspirin, but the preference would be for a complete physical and laboratory evaluation supplemented by the medical and social history of the child as to etiologic possibilities. We rarely feel content merely to prescribe something because it makes a child's pain temporarily disappear when we have no knowledge of why and how he is ill.

Diagnosis Is Important. Unfortunately, an overemphasis on diagnosis has had the consequence of discrediting diagnositc efforts. All too many clinical settings focus on reaching a conclusion, at which point the patient is either put on a waiting list or ignored. A reaction stresses putting the patient ahead of a diagnostic tag, as though these were mutually exclusive categories. There has gradually been a counter-reaction, utilizing developmental knowledge about psychopathology, which allows us to provide workable guidelines for classification of disorders. We wish to include not only the varieties of psychopathology seen in adults applied to younger age groups, but also the special categories needed for children and adolescents discussed in earlier chapters.

There are the ideas implicit in developmental deviations, reactive problems, and crises reactions seen in adolescents under many conditions.[1] Obviously, a knowledge of physical and emotional development is necessary as an accompaniment to knowledge of psychopathology before accurate diagnostic assessments can be made. Again the imperative to diagnose, if at all possible, is seen in the situation of attempting to treat a child with an abdominal pain which can represent anything from an organic gastro-intestinal condition, a conversion reaction, a psychophysiologic reaction, an anxiety or depressive equivalent, or part of somatizing in a psychotic child.

An openness in assessment of any symptom or symptom-picture is needed. Consequently, knowledge of adolescent development and family interactions are more important in the emotional sphere than the need immediately to select and carry out a treatment. Selection is especially important in psychotherapeutic endeavors since, with a few well-known exceptions, the situations are rarely emergencies which demand something be initiated on the spur of the moment. Chronic and pervasive adverse influences are usually in operation. Adequate diagnostic acumen is much more difficult and time-consuming in contrast to plunging in with rescue operations. Pursuing an organic analogy, it is much easier to teach and learn how to perform an incision, or give a stated dosage of medication, than to know why and when a certain procedure should or should not be carried out with an adolescent; it is similarly more difficult to learn how a lesion develops and continues to malfunction and affect the organism. The model can be translated into a metaphorical emotional anatomy and physiology for appraising psychological performance during adolescence. It is even more complex in operation, since the number of variables and their bio-psycho-social interaction is greater.

Differences from Treating Adults. Differences in the treatment of adolescents exist in contrast to adults.[2] The adolescent rarely seeks treatment on his own initiative, but is usually referred by others. This holds as much for the frequently cited "crises" in adolescents as any other problem. While on one hand almost everything is viewed as a crisis by some adolescents (and unfortunately some who deal with them), on the other hand there is a need to view problems as more than a transient phenomenon. While there are crises to be sure, many problems reflect more than an adverse environment. The involvement of parents is variable, since they may or may not see their child as having problems. It in part depends on the personal discomfort to them of their child's behavior. If the behavior pattern is in the characterological realm, the minor will more typically be ordered into treatment by court or school personnel. Some community agency may be involved from other family or socio-economic problems which the family has involving welfare or sectarian agencies. Adolescents with neurotic conflicts, or who come from families with neurotic conflict, more frequently seek help on their own than those with character problems. Their personal discomfort and suffering motivate them. It is only by adolescence that children make contact with a psychiatrist on their own intitiative, or ask their parents to arrange an appointment (although a younger child may ask to see a doctor with whom he has a good relationship). A practical problem is where those who seek therapeutic assistance end up, since there is a good deal of randomization in the process. College-age youths, with a history of conflict a few years earlier may try to counsel or advise youngsters. There are often few norms operating in these situations, and much naivete. For the majority of young adolescents, it is difficult to see themselves as needing treatment. The younger child is even more puzzled, confused, and overtly resistant to treatment in the beginning stages than an adult.

Another major difference from treating adults is the limitation of any appraisal and treatment plan confined to a solo patient. Certain types of reconstructive therapy are very difficult. Not only is the adolescent caught up in reality-based dependency situations, but his past is overtly in the present from the compression of thoughts, behavior, and the environment into a unified picture. The fluidity between the unconscious and conscious parts of the personality is not as well compartmentalized, and reaction and conflicts within the family constellation are still contributing to current personality development. Ways to involve or treat parents will not be pursued, but their involvement is seen as necessary to some degree in almost every type of treatment modality employed when there is an integral family unit.

Developmental considerations have been mentioned as essential. The presence of deviations, lags, and crests must be known not only for an adequate appraisal but for a valid treatment plan. An additional complication is the greater variability in the reaction to physical disease, deviation, or injuries in adolescence. Some react in a relatively bland manner to the same trauma or disability while others show marked psychopathology. Multifactorial processes operate which include the past and current psychological history in interaction with the state of physical and psychological maturation of the nervous system. Opportunities for secondary overlay with organic problems, especially the visual or auditory, are always possible. While a deprived youth with perceptual problems may develop deep resentments which need therapeutic focus, an injured athlete may enjoy the pseudo-benefits of being injured, such as attention and pity.

The manifestations vary, depending upon the developmental stage and the type of psycho-social stresses present. Treatment goals must distinguish conflict-resolution as part of the therapeutic process from permitting a youth to develop through ego growth or strengthening. The latter facilitates the potential to master developmental blocks by eliminating environmental interferences. To accomplish this requires that distinctions be made between developmental interferences, developmental conflicts, neurotic conflicts, and remnants of childhood neuroses. *Interferences* are viewed as situations where children struggle with demands made on them which may be excessive for their given ego capacity and functions at a particular time; *developmental conflicts* refer to the struggle inherent in environmental demands, or which accompany a developmental or maturational level; *neurotic conflicts* arise between drives pressing for discharge against internalized controls and superego aspects of negation or values. Structuralized mental systems may conflict within and between each other. *Childhood neuroses* (the infantile neuroses) persist beyond the level of overt conflict. They are seen as an autonomous type of psychopathology and as a necessary but not sufficient factor for the later emergence of neurosis.[3]

Descriptive Versus Dynamic Therapy. Descriptive diagnoses have value as shorthand indicators for cataloging the most conspicuous clinical symptoms present, but they provide insufficient information and reasons as to genesis, persistence and repetition of problem behavior. Thus, a diagnosis of hysterical neurosis (eructatio nervosa) or hyperkinetic reaction of adolescence tells us something about behavior but little else. Other difficulties associated with descriptive diagnoses are the confusing basis for the diagnosis. A boy who has been in a car accident and given a diagnosis of psychosis with brain trauma associated with his subdural hematoma does not convey the multiple physical, psychological, and social aspects of the syndrome of cerebral dysfunction with which he must struggle. In other cases the clinical diagnosis may actually be making reference to etiology, such as mental retardation associated with congenital syphilis.

Comprehension of the factors in development that have contributed to deviant development and which may be persisting, although in modified and derivative form, are essential. *Dynamic* formulations consider the current forces most significant in the adolescent's life. Intrapsychic components, such as drive activity, are encompassed but also cognitive and affective components, as they bear on overt acts; nor can the significance of fantasy be ignored. Environmental forces which impinge through the culture and family on a youth are an integral part of dynamic formulations. The genetic roots of behavior in the earlier life of the child, both as to organic-hereditary aspects and the intrapsychic and interpersonal shifts, give a developmental perspective. The combined dynamic-genetic diagnosis informs us, beyond the level of description, as to *how* a particular youth is functioning, along with conflicting motivations, wishes, and the genetic roots of the responses. It also gives us suggestive answers as to *why* difficulties have occurred. The perspective is a character structure which is more flexible than when appraising and treating adults. In addition there are symptoms, character problems, or interpersonal difficulties that begin to emerge from the interaction of these components.

Conceptualized theoretically, developmental factors need appraisal in terms of interferences or conflicts. Treatment is focused on removing arrests or deviations. This is not only important for younger children who are forming mental structures. When structuralization of mental activities becomes more crystallized, there should be an attempt to deal with drives and their derivative manifestations. These encompass sexual, aggressive, narcissistic, sado-masochistic, voyeuristic, and exhibitionistic activities with their accompanying affects and fantasies.

Ego-functioning also needs evaluation in terms of both cognitive and executive functions. The cognitive ego functions embrace many intellectual and reasoning components which require clinical and psychometric appraisal to be complete (perception, cognition, recall, reasoning ability, and decision-making). Executive functions embrace control over impulse discharge, motoric activity and defenses. The elaboration of a control agency, discussed in an earlier chapter, both inhibits and provides goals. Dealing with its deviations may be a crucial part of treatment. These superego components deal with the qualities of harshness or permissiveness toward the self, and the gyroscopic type of guidance or misguidance that occurs from the ego-ideal. The synthetic activity of the ego attempts to assimilate and compromise external and internal perceptions and stimuli into a coherent and causally related organization. All of these functions interdigitate. Synthesis is related to causal thinking, memory to is reqired for anticipatory activity, and a degree of ego development is needed for impulse control.

Besides intersystemic conflicts (between the id and the developing ego and superego), there are intrasystemic conflicts (within one of these structural agencies). In the superego, intrasytemic conflicts are witnessed as clashes between conflicting and contradictory identifications and internationalizations. Many contradictory id strivings are possible, such as passivity-activity, love-hate, and masculinity-femininity. Ego functions may clash with each other, depending on which goal takes precedence. The need of the ego to perceive accurately may conflict with a need to deny or repress impulses that lead to the experiencing of painful affect. Another is the striving for causal thinking in preference to the use of projection in attributing one's difficulties to others. Such interactions can be detected in evaluation by the type of verbal productions, fantasies, or dreams revealed.

The significance of the environment to personality functioning is pervasive throughout the above; it cannot be assigned a role of greater of lesser significance since it varies case by case. The environmental history exerts its influence due to its ongoing impact in the form of psychological representations. It does this on both conscious and unconscious levels. Factors such as past biological insults, family constellation and interaction, object losses, existing conflicts in other family members or individuals with whom the child is in contact (teachers or relatives), all have a bearing on the development of the child and what treatment plan would be most desirable.

In the course of treatment a perspective on the major conflicts within the formative personality, coupled with environmental sources of difficulty, should be clear. Such a perspective is coupled with insight about the characteristic ways a person deals with impulses and their derivative manifestations. There are also characteristic techniques for handling affects such as anxiety, guilt, shame, and rage, and pleasurable states. The defensive structure, fantasy life, and attempts to adapt or distort the environment, are part of the appraisal to guide the therapeutic process.

Illustrations of how these various processes are involved in choosing a treatment are relevant to questions about the particular difficulties which exist and what corresponding recommendations can be made. To obtain a significant amount of data regarding an adolescent requires an amount of empirical information. We must subsequently deduce and integrate the material to come up with formulations, working hypotheses, and conclusions. However, prior to application of such reasoning processes is the ability to obtain the material necessary for formulations. A combination of individual and conjoint interviews with a youth and parents may be necessary. This aspect of the therapeutic process is something that clinicians believe cannot be taught. There is a highly desirable quality of being able alternately to regress in the service of therapeutic empathy to permit and encourage the free flow of material, coupled with the realization that limit-setting is needed at times. In some cases it is relatively easier to obtain material from those who are not yet adult, since their impulse and fantasy life is less concealed. Yet it is the quality of the relationship between the therapist and the minor that permits such material to emerge. The stereotype of the barren therapeutic hour is the question and answer session, or the use of verbal material at a distance. Such sterility blocks clarification of conflicts and epitomizes the defensive use of therapy to avoid involvement on the part of both youth and therapist.

Mental Functions in Adolescence versus Adulthood.   There are some particular characteristics of immature, or rather undeveloped, functioning which make empathy with the experiential life of an adolescent different, and perhaps more difficult, for the adult therapist.

Narcissistic Influences.   The first is a degree of narcissism which leads the child to misinterpret occurrences. In the adult such phenomena raise the question of a severe narcissistic, if not psychotic, conflict. For example, an adolescent interpreting the birth of a sibling as a personal rejection would seem to be a grossly distorting reality-testing. Yet there are difficult intermediary questions which need a developmental answer. When, and to what extent, should an adolescent begin to react in a less egocentric manner beyond the repeated generalization that children become less egocentric as they age? What about the earlier social anxieties of peer rejection in latency age children? If adolescents function well in a solitary manner, are they necessarily reacting defensively from their lack of more involvements? Similar questions arise for introjective processes where the child assimilates the attitudes of the parents, not only by conscious modeling and imitation, but more significantly by the unconscious assimilation of ongoing parental moods and conflicts. Anger, rage, disappointment, and feelings of rejection are elicited when another person is preoccupied, shows more affection or attention toward another, excludes someone, or reacts to the death or illness of a loved one. Adolescents mobilize their egocentric feelings to cope with such circumstances.

Cognitive Differences. The level of cognitive functioning by adolescence and the difficulty in functioning on a level of adult sexual commitment(contrasted with performing sexual intercourse), raise further treatment questions. The situation is analogous to the utilization of the capacity of the therapist to think and feel via an unconscious route to the meaning of behavior. Only then do seemingly strange constructions become clear, such as the association of sexuality with overt aggression, and resultant conflicts about gender identity. Similar impressions hold for the sexual theories of oral impregnation, anal or umbilical birth, fears of castration or bodily mutilation, resurrected with adolescent denial.

Such constructions are related to the problem of the emergence of secondary process thinking, and the relative ease with which the adolescent utilizes or regresses to primary process thinking with its symbolizations, displacements, condensations, and transformations. These processes are basic to any good fairy story and hence are more real than meeting social amentities. Many "unexplainable" phenomena become clearer from this perspective, such as the acute anxiety in a physician's office of a fourteen-year-old girl who became preoccupied watching a nurse sterilize a pair of scissors, or the thirteen-year-old boy who watched a large fish being caught and then had a series of nightmares with fish attempting to bite him.

How Time Is Experienced. Variation in the sense of time is another difference in the mental life of adolescents compared to adults. The therapist must adjust to a different time scale. A child requires a level of cognitive development before time can be conceptualized. This is an interesting psychological phenomenon relevant to how children misinterpret parental absence, delay of gratification, or death. For example, what is the relationship between concepts of time and separation? Do these concepts have a common root or are they independent? In the therapeutic context the problem is viewed from the perspective of the experiential component which corresponds most closely not to duration measured by time units, such as minutes, days, or weeks, but rather the predominance of id or ego functioning in their respective balance at a particular developmental stage. This has developmental components in terms of a certain number of children at a given age having concepts of time and capacity to tolerate deprivation, but also the psychological implications of how a specific child reacts to an event such as hospitalization, absence of a parent, and other deprivations. Ego strength utilizes this in terms of the degree of postponement of demands or delay of gratification that is possible.

Application. Therapy with adolescents is based on applying the above data and knowledge. There is a presumption that appropriate interpretations and techniques can only be used if the therapist is sensitive to their use and possesses sufficient material by knowing how to obtain it.

> One constricted fourteen-year-old boy with an exceedingly high verbal ability (WISC of 148) sat calmly during the initial interviews and carried on conversations as though in the presence of adults. At first it seemed as though this was a preference, except that his history showed he had increasing difficulty staying in school because he felt that those in his peer group were ostracizing him. There were episodes which baffled the parents, such as temper outbursts accompanied by tears where things would be broken or torn. Interviews revealed this well-mannered boy to be well into an overt obsessional neurosis as a clinical diagnosis. The boy was noted to be extremely self-critical and exacting with himself. Little pleasure in the activity itself was experienced; compulsivity functioned as an end in itself. Impulse expression, as well as associated fantasy material, was considered a blur on his perfectionism as well as being anxiety-provoking since this was a constant threat to undo his facade of conformity.

A contrast be made between differences in therapy selection and how this could be approached. One approach would utilize permissiveness, conveying an attitude that it is permissible to possess impulses such as casualness and self-tolerance. Another would reinforce the rigidity which the boy has been exposed to in his family and which he has internalized. Similar alternatives could be considered when dealing with his family. Thus, the idea of family members that since the boy has trouble controlling himself, as witnessed by his outbursts, stricter limits should be placed on him by the therapist, parents, and school personnel could be challenged. However, some therapists would reinforce controls by suppressing behavior even further.

A contrast would be the utilization of identification with a tolerant therapist who would permit greater tolerance for his own impulses. Verbalization of forbidden impulses to and about the therapist and others would be seen as a necessary step in a treatment process to modify a self-punitive and exaggerated control system. Without a psychodynamic knowledge of the case, the therapist is likely to miss the significance of the pattern of personality development and not see the symptoms as reactions to the fear of lack of control in himself and parental rejection for imperfections. A dynamic approach would involve the use of feelings, verbalizations, and actual experiences of pleasure. The goal would be to lessen compulsive defenses and superego criticism. A contrary result would be by suppressive therapy to reinforce obsessional activities. If fewer angry breakthroughs occur and conformity is achieved, a therapeutic success would be registered.

Another example of the importance of dynamic understanding to appropriate therapeutic selection is a fourteen-year-old, white female whose mother complained her daughter "oozed sex." Asked what this meant, her mother gave examples of men staring at her daughter, the girl lying to her about boys, and having her own birth control pills. The mother condemned these activities but also with a quality of affective anticipation and pleasurable curiosity. While condemning the girl seeing black boys ("You know what happens with them"), she saw no problem in giving her daughter permission to talk to these boys on the telephone for an hour every evening. The mother would tell her never to let her father know about such conversations. Understanding the dynamic-genetic material permitted the pattern of material acting out to be used, as well as the hostile use of the girl by the mother who could point out to her behavior as perverse, while on another level the mother obtained vicarious gratification.

Such a dynamic configuration requires psychotherapeutic finesse if conflict resolution is to occur. This entails understanding such factors as the mother's involvement in the girl's behavior and the girl's compliance; nor could the passive withdrawal of the father, whom the mother ridiculed, be ignored. It also required understanding of how the girl vacillated between overtures to her father versus angry outbursts against him when he joined the mother in condemning her behavior. A pervasive sense of anger at her mother without knowing why and a past affectionate, emotional attachment to her father, were significant variables, as was the history of adolescent promiscuity in the mother which had long been avoided.

Frequently such girls are labeled and adjudicated delinquent. With the definition of a delinquent as a minor apprehended for committing an illegal act, or an act regarded as such for adolescents, the criteria are often met. All too frequently the clinician cooperates in this approach, which results in an assignment to a correctional institution as a form of treatment with no resolution of the family conflicts, but rather the perpetuation of authority problems.

A prediction could be made from the patterns operating in this case that a high incidence of repetitive behavior will occur unless a resolution of the contributory factors takes place. Some interpret such behavior as reflective of teenage rebellion, or as a variation within the limits of normal deviations for adolescent females in our culture. Unfortunately, that type of interpretaion leads to a perpetuation of the behavior individually, and often generationally, as in this case. Frequently, such girls and families are diagnosed as psychopathic, with nihilistic implications about untreatability and the hidden presupposition of unmodifiable constitutionality. As adolescence progresses, the antisocial behavior might become more dramatic, which in turn leads to commitment to an inpatient psychiatric ward and a resort to organic therapies. Ending up with severe diagnoses such as psychopathy or schizophrenia seems correlated with the social class of the girls; if they are from affluent families, they are more likely to be regarded as hysterical personalities and receive some form of psychotherapy.

The dynamics are significant in leading to appropriate therapeutic maneuvers to deal with the girl's involvement. A removal from the home might be required if necessary, or a mandatory involvement of the family. Ideally this treatment would allow alteration through permitting the girl to test out her impulses, privacy, and controls during therapy. The ultimate goal would be to internalize standards that are less corruptible. A capacity to handle painful affects would necessitate confronting her acting out and the family's role in the behavior. The purpose is modification and not condemnation, and it requires the therapist to be capable of appraising behavior from his knowledge of its genesis and maintenance. The relationship of an adolescent using acting out defenses and family resistance to alter the pattern can become quite a struggle.

Approaches where the therapist administers punishment to change behavior are viewed as inimical to resolving the origin and perpetuation of such behavior. There are occasions when the overt symptomatology can be altered or removed by punitive procedures. These are usually viewed as a punishment despite what the adults administering the treatment call them. Without a therapeutic goal of dealing with multiple aspects of personality functioning, it is too simple to think that symptoms disappearing by coercion will stay resolved. Capacities for pleasure in work, human intimacy, and utilizing potentials needs consideration to resolve many of these personality conflicts. Even if a goal of stopping phone calls eliminating promiscuous relationships, and beginning to attend school regularly could be achieved, these would be isolated attainments, although not without significance. Perhaps this is one reason why the rates of detected recidivism for juvenile delinquency are so high.

None of these comments should be construed as advocating an approach of permissiveness which therapeutically sanctions acting out behavior. Limits must be set and the problem is by what means and how rapidly. The format holds within therapy hours, as well as in the attitudes of the therapist toward acting out, and in dealing with the anxiety that emerges. Limits are needed for the protection of the patient, and to further personal responsibility for behavior. The effect is to interfere with the acting out as the vehicle for the unconscious satisfaction of conflicts. This conveys to adolescents that their feelings are genuine and honest responses to the predicaments they are caught in, but that what is required is to deal with factors that have been ignored or ridiculed in the past. The actual situation can be handled although it involves hard work and guts to chance the exposure.

An accompanying part of the contract conveys assistance and reassurance to deal with the painful feelings experienced. This places primacy on respect for the patient, and a viewpoint that behavior is symptomatic and indicative of conflict and a maladaptive attempt at resolution. What is not accepted is the attempt merely to reassure, or blame socio-economic forces, for the predicament. Reliance on such explanations facilitates the use of defenses of projection and rationalization rather than leading to behavioral and character alterations.

SPECIAL PROBLEMS IN TREATING ACTING OUT ADOLESCENTS

Customarily phases of treatment are delinieated progressing from initial involvement to the commencement of therapeutic work. Evenually nuclear conflicts are re-enacted in the context of therapy (transference) as well as in everyday occurrences which can be worked on. This is no different in adolescents than it is with adults. However, with antisocial adolescents, a preparatory phase is indispensable to any therapeutic intervention. This also holds as much for relationship therapies as for those more oriented toward the resolution of conflict on a conscious and unconscious basis.

Early psychological attempts to deal with antisocial individuals soon encounter the obstacle of recalcitrance to participate cooperatively in therapy. This is a variety of behavior witnessed in most of their social relationships as well. Some of the early efforts of August Aichhorn to establish a relationship by giving something concrete to these youths were in this direction. In the early days of therapy, gifts or candy were used with young children who came for treatment. Later this gift-giving was seen as an interferer from the expectations engendered in the youths, which in turn had to be resolved. In addition, Aichhorn emphasized letting the adolescent know that the therapist was just as clever as he was when there were attempts to manipulate.[4]

While such practices as gift-giving have been abandoned in the treatment of neurotic adolescents, the need to achieve a therapeutic bridge with those who act out still presents as an initial need. This requires preliminary activities before techniques of clarifying behaviors or interpretation of conscious and unconscious conflicts can have any meaning or be effective. Suggestions have been made about the preliminary phase of treatment. Eissler extended Aichhorn's thinking that acting out behaviors be dealt with first until they become sufficiently tapered in the context of a close relationship.[5] The initial aim is to foster a dependency on the therapist so that the patient becomes willing to restrain some of his behaviors to secure a continuance of the relationship. While this may be a maneuver to induce an object tie whose loss then becomes threatening, it is seen as a necessary step. Once the tie is established it becomes indispensable, because of the problems with separation which exist as core conflicts.

One central assumption is that a neurotic conflict will emerge in the context of the developing closeness which reactivates the original core conflict. This does not refer to conflict on an oedipal level. It is questionable whether many of these impulse-ridden adolescents have achieved that developmental level. The dependency relationship is rather viewed as the establishment of something that was never achieved in a satisfactory sense and thus promotes acting out. It is similar to the provision of a period of "second infancy" which Alpert has seen as an opportunity to repeat and relive the developmental processes which were absent or defective around new and corrective identification figures.[6] The essence of these procedures is to fill a gap which has impeded the development of necessary socialization processes and continues to operate to impair efforts at conflict resolution.

It is not contradictory to maintain that acting out adolescents can conform when they find themselves threatened by the presence of an external "big brother." Nor is it contradictory to say that such adolescents can work for pleasures or avoid physically assaultive behavior if given sufficient material rewards. It is rather that these ad hoc adaptive maneuvers reflect arrested levels, rather than permitting an alteration in existing developmental conflicts. Variations of the need to utilize dependent relationships for other types of problems, such as psychotic youth cannot be directly transposed from neurotic delinquent youth although there might be some overlap.

The initial phase of therapy fosters dependence and symbiosis to permit a regression for therapeutic purposes.[7] The therapist provides gratification and comfort to secure an alliance, but a gradual modification or corrective experience of what human relationships entail is also part of the relationship. This is not an effort to deal with conscious conflict, but to create an atmosphere of trust and acceptance. Nor is it expected that the offer is immediately seized upon with appreciation by the impulsive youth. These adolescents are customarily suspicious in most of their relationships. Consequently, testing and provocation are anticipated.

The goal of this stage is to recognize the characterological maneuvers, to view them as something that will be dealt with in therapy, and to avoid using shaming techniques to achieve discipline or conformity. Shaming perpetuates the rage of impotent rebellion. It guarantees the repetition of acting out since the patient feels different already, if not defective, rather than someone whose development and socialization have gone awry for a variety of reasons. It is unfortunate that so many institutional approaches for dealing with acting out youngsters perpetuate these behaviors by such techniques, as well as by a pattern of frequent shifting of therapists—by plan or necessity. These shifts reinforce the experience of loss and the danger of forming attachments.

Once an alliance is sufficiently established, the therapist can begin to deal with the patterns and conflicts which have contributed to acting out. It is not that self-destructive behaviors are permitted until then, but rather that they have been dealt with concretely and immediately without efforts cognitively and affectively to interpret. Throwing objects about an office is never tolerated, nor are daredevil pranks around a building such as setting fires and then using fire extinguishers. Nor is the practice used in military of letting two adolescents in conflict slug it out seen as beneficial.

Manipulative attempts by the adolescent to threaten, bribe, or intimidate the therapist are confronted. They are initially pointed out so that the patient is aware that others understand his ploys. There is the additional message that the therapist is not frightened by these maneuvers. In time, cautious interpretations are made regarding not being helpless, and that it is in fact feeling helpless which makes him feel he has to control others by these techniques. Once a therapeutic alliance is established, deficiencies in the patient are approached. Most conspicuous is their verbal lack—the inability to put affect into words. The pervasive effect is seen in deficits in interpersonal communications, and in the capacity to delay or fantasize. What they have been calling play is not play as much as it is busy-ness. Such a defensive employment contributes to a deficit in play-acting by fantasy or not anticipating consequences subsequent to impulsive actions.

As therapy progresses, the patient is expected to contribute more and not become a passive recipient. This is predicated upon a patient being able to accept more responsibility due to the rewards contingent upon having greater autonomy over actions. The facade of freedom of choice displayed by past impulsiveness is noted. A lessening of retaliatory fears is present from decreasing provocations. Pleasure in the expansion of other ego functions is present, such as in mastery over things, impossible before due to difficulty in planning. This is not to omit therapeutic adjuncts, which may be required for some youths, such as environmental modifications, remedial education, or tutors, but it does focus on what is a necessary background for personality change to take place. Those with prominent regressive features may not be capable of participating in therapy aimed at more extensive ego reorganization. For these the attainment of a relationship itself is a worthy accomplishment which takes time.

There are indicators of who has the capability of progressing to the level beyond gratification. One of the first is a lessening of overt acting out, with its destructiveness to the self and others. This occurs both in and out of therapy. Increased verbalizations begin to encompass questions or curiosity about themselves and their families. For a preadolescent, this is manifested when play activiities become more meaningful, with fantasies on a dyadic or triadic level. The utilization of fewer toys to play out fantasies, in contrast to the random use of a multitude of objects, is a further indication.[8] Less need for physical contact and gratification accompany the increasing capacity to deal with painful affect by words. There is a concomitant ability to tolerate painful affect, such as depression or anxiety. They will be more capable of dealing with material on their own initiative in sessions, or raising questions, without waiting for cues from the therapist about what to say or do.

There is a difference between giving to the youth and working together with him on a level which progressively utilizes concepts of clarification. Of course, this presupposes that the therapist has set up such long-term goals. It also means that the therapist is capable of detecting transitions and making interpretaions according to the appropriate psychological level . The therapist must have set a goal of moving beyond relationship therapy. Practical difficulties, such as those of time and money raised by a family, must be evaluated in the context of the particular setting and the type of therapeutic intervention proposed. Particularly with acting out youths, unless the parents are being dealt with therapeutically, it is questionable how far therapy with a youth living home can progress. If a disturbance is severe enough, the question of a temporary and later permanent removal again must be faced. It seems wise to consider this issue in the beginning stages of therapy if possible when therapeutic decisions can be more efficaciously made, such as for a more limited goal of tapering overt aggressive acts or dealing with the lags and conflicts present in one or more members of a family.

REGRESSIVE PHENOMENA
IN THE CONTEXT OF TREATING ADOLESCENTS

Types of Regression. Regression is not only a phenomenon observed during the struggles of normal growth and development. It also occupies a significant place in emotional conflict, when it is witnessed in developmental and defensive aspects. Regression is relevant to the entire problem of transference manifestations. In its broadest sense, regressive behavior is viewed as inherent in a biological organism striving for gratification and adaptation when they are not forthcoming. Tendencies to seek satisfaction at some level lead to a reversion to behaviors which once gave gratification. Regression may be useful as an ego mechanism to avoid painful affects and conflict situations by a return to techniques or an environment which once before gave gratification or reassurance.

Earlier formulations of regression stemmed from work on dream processes and emphasized the topographic model. Three types of regression were distinguished:

(1) *Topographical* regression used on a neurophysiological model where excitation extended backward in a motor-sensory-perceptual direction and finally to a psychological level. This was taken as the regressive model which led to hallucinatory wish fulfillment in infants in place of other cognitive processes.

(2) *Temporal* regression refers to using older, pre-existing psychological structures.

(3) *Formal* regression uses primitive methods of expression and representation in place of the ones currently being used.

All three regressions were viewed as representative of one process, "for what is older in time is more primitive in form and in physical topography lies nearer to the perceptual end."[9]

There are various ways in which regression can be conceptualized. It may be viewed in terms of *objects* utilized for impulse gratification which were more readily available and utilized at some time in the past. In a different manner the *aims* of the impulses may revert to modes which were more gratifying at an earlier period. In both of these regressive situations the objects and aims exist on a level of psychological representation with associated fantasies. It thus involves both content and process. Regression may also be conceptualized structurally. We then talk of drive (instinctual) regression, ego regression, and superego regression in which there is a return to fixation points in one or all three systems. Contrary to physical development, a one-way progression of growth and development does not occur. The exception in the organic realm is interference due to severe organic disease, with eventual deterioration. In contrast, the potential for psychological regression manifests itself in a constant vulnerability to techniques satisfactory at earlier times.

Earlier situations conducive to fixation in an adolescent involve overindulgence or excessive frustration at a particular time or with respect to certain experiences. Alternations between extremes, as well as combinations of them, seem particularly effective to fixate. For example, a situation of impulse satisfaction, coupled with reassurance against a painful experiential state such as anxiety, is particularly fixation-inducing. This is seen when satisfaction of sensual impulses gives dependency gratification as well, which may well lead to enduring preferences for these activities. Sexual perversions may become entrenched or lead to such behaviors in response to lack of gratification in other areas of the adolescent's life. Reassurance against the insecurity of losing an object tie may function similarly. Consider the following typical situations for fixation: activities associated with stages of dependency gratification, experiences associated with narcissistic activities and fantasies, pleasure from any combination of psycho-sexual phenomena with their accompanying social pleasures, as well as a variety of polymorphous perverse sexual activities which are inherent in early child development and can be reactivated.

Drive Regression.   As an example of drive regression, consider a fourteen-year-old girl with symptoms of nausea and frequent vomiting. Whenever she was in a competitive or exciting situation, the symptoms occurred. After a precocious and intensely intellectual latency period, her father's customary manner of greeting her by a kiss or enjoying periods of discussion with her in close physical contact led to revulsion, anger, and literal nausea during adolescence. Her lack of girlfriends of her own age, coupled with a close dependency on her mother, contributed to feelings of loneliness and expressions of self-pity ("No one likes me."). Episodic shoplifting began, usually taking items around school. Her vomiting was both an involuntary discharge over which she felt little control and also a more primitive representation of disgust. Hence, although providing a motoric and emotional dischaige, it was not experienced as gratifying or giving relief. Rather, it represented a predominance of aggressive components by way of vomiting. This occurred either when others tried to express affection toward her or entered directly into competition with her. Academic and social situations were the chief situations for eliciting these responses.

As in most of these situations, manifestations of drive regression do not exist apart from ego and superego adaptations. Ego regression was noted in object relations which reverted to an anaclitic tie to her mother. The patient was aware of her need to be near her mother more than she wished, and also of her relative neglect of independent peer relationships. Her object ties were not for mutual satisfaction, but rather existed for purposes of gratifying her dependency needs while simultaneously tying her mother down (which unconsciously expressed her aggression). The girl continued to maintain distance from her father, alternating with "safe" dependency demands on him, such as rides to school or requests to go shopping with him.

Striking examples of drive regression or lack of progression from fixation points occur in adolescents with borderline or narcissistic personalities. Without getting into the intricacies of the undecided issues between hereditary or environmental etiologies in such cases, the behavior of these adolescents reflects fixations of pre-object levels with "things," human or nonhuman, being increasingly resorted to for drive gratification. Varieties of aberrant dependency needs similarly reflect a less striking, yet pervasive, attachment to objects. The setting is one where ambivalent demands are placed on objects for oral gratification. It is the equivalent of, "Take care of me and nurture me, and I will be a good, conforming adolescent and never leave you." Reciprocal demands are simultaneously being met in parents who have their own security tied up in the child not becoming too independent. The point is that, developmentally, such fixated patterns of handling drives persist into adolescence. They are most typically seen in characterological maneuvers and expectations laid upon others with occasionally severe regressions at periods of crisis which interfere with the capacity for pleasure.

The gradual formation of symptoms or an acute decompensation into a psychotic state may take place. In either case the need for treatment becomes evident.

Ego and Superego Regressions. Ego and superego regressions are other phenomena which occur as developmental variations. These can be temporary regressions in ego functioning that occur along with drive regression, or as a consequence of developmental or environmental crises. They can occur in situations where there is difficulty in accepting success or in response to painful situations of a physical or affective type. These regressions show up in many ego functions, such as in speech, reality testing, reversion to primary process thinking, or forms of motoric dyscontrol. Examples of superego regression are the arbitrary condemnation of behavior, categorical black and white judgements, self-condemnatory attitudes, and perfectionistic standards which are rarely attained and which result in a chronic sense of failure or in the use of expiatory and neutralization techniques.

A crucial question remains difficult to evaluate anterespectively: How fixed is the regression in contrast to a transient type of reaction? The question has a bearing on treatment recommendations as well as prognostications. After a period, once a regression is initiated, a point of relative no return may be passed. Adequate gratification becomes attached to regressive behaviors, so that the impetus for mastery and progression, with its associated anxiety, is abandoned. There is progressive difficulty in giving up the pleasures, or those anticipated, which become associated with regressive activities. Hence, alternative ways of drive discharge are not attempted. Even when regression originates with ego or superego functioning, less control over id derivatives results in a blurring between mental structures. Further psychological damage ensues, since sensitive periods elapse when ego functions have not been mastered, and drive aims and objects remain at an early level as does superego development. Such variation is not merely regression as a part of development, nor a temporary defense, but a factor making a full contribution to the emergence of psychopathology.

Attention was called to types of ego and superego regression in the fourteen-year-old girl mentioned above. Ego regression was noted in her attempts to gain security by staying close to her mother; this functioned to keep her from situations of temptation as well as avoiding suspicions her mother might have. Adaptive techniques of being a model of good behavior to secure this reputation led to a state of social estrangement from her peer group. There was an accompanying superego regression manifested in self-criticism and disapproval, and an affective state of feeling unloved and unacceptable. Yet, for her to give up her idealistic standards presented the threat of acting on her impuses. Hence, a regression to earlier drive activities with ego activities geared to security like a much younger girl. There was self-condemnation, as though a major catastrophe occurred unless she lived up to exacting standards. Superego regression was played out in preoccupations of being a good or bad girl, or being virtuous and praseworthy versus seductive and dirty, and of having to suffer and cleanse herself by vomiting before she could again feel restored.

TRANSFERENCE

Initial Distinctions: The Past and the Present. The background on regressive processes relates to the treatment of adolescents as relevant to transference. An important distinction is between a *transference reaction* and a *transference neurosis*. Transference itself encompasses all the perplexing and misunderstood reactions of a patient to a therapist, including the patterns of responses and relating that are typical of a particular adolescent. In addition, there is a constant seeking of ways to attain gratification of wishes by placing demands on the therapist, and utilizing maneuvers with him. Demands for limits on punishment by the therapist as an authority figure are coupled with expectations of approval.

Transference reactions refer to diverse processes which take place in the course of treatment in contrast to the transference neurosis, where memories, impulses, and affects which have been repressed, are revived. These lead to a repetition of the demands and wishes as they once existed and a repetition of the defensive maneuvers employed against them. The existence of transference neuroses in children has been debated due to the reasoning and observations of continued attachments to several adults, coupled with living in a family structure which interferes with transferring these neurotic demands to the therapist. It rather leads to a continuance of making demands in the hopes of fulfilling them from parental objects or their substitutes. These unfulfilled demands from the pathogenic past, which have not yet terminated, continue to seek fulfillment in reality. Witness this in unconscious fantasies being directly acted out in existing family settings by children.

Yet in patients of all ages there are situations where a perpetuation of pathogenic relationships and object ties occurs, and in some of these, transference neuroses do seem to emerge. Nor can we assume that a pure culture transference neurosis, apart from the reality of present responses to a given therapist, exists. Obtaining an answer to the question of the presence or absence of transference neuroses in adolescents is difficult because we cannot use the same psychotherapeutic techniques as with adults. There is also a constant tendency toward aggressive discharge in many adolescent activities and verbalizations. Throughout the relationship of an adolescent with a therapist, there is an admixture of reality-based relationships with a new adult authority, coupled with a variety of demands based on neurotic conflicts and neuroses. The latter lead to a repetition of patterns of demands on the therapist. The double role of the therapist is present when treating adults also, but it does not present the same technical and theoretical difficulties. On the one hand the therapist must consider the reactions of a youth to him in the sense of a new person or object from whom affection and approval are sought. The other components which need consideration are the transferability from the parental and family objects which are brought into therapy and played out again in the therapeutic relationship.

Ways exist in which an adolescent manifests transference reactions to the therapist. Previous object relations and the constancies of objects are prime repeaters. This is seen in the manner of relating initially, as therapy progresses, in terms of the feelings and reactions which emerge along with testing maneuvers. Thus, the more enduring ties and reactive patterns can be noted for their appropriateness to the situation and a given therapist. It is here where current knowledge of the family history and dynamics are needed to interpret shifts which may be responsive to happenings outside treatment. Characterological patterns and defenses are perceived in their daily utilization.

Levels of Intervention. Therapy is approached in terms of levels at which therapeutic efforts are directed. The manifest level is symptoms which an adolescent has developed. Beneath this, defenses are recognized in their manifestations and interpreted by whatever treatment approach is being used. In terms of structure, the affects motivating defenses are explored in relationship to the drives and the potential of a given adolescent for development and to experience pleasure. The advantage in evaluating behavior in the context of therapy is that patterns which recur, or have a great deal of associated affect, reveal many of the core conflicts which point, like abscesses, to where an individual is currently in distress. This gives the therapist a freedom from relying solely on dynamic formulations or on reports from relatives about environmental reactions. It also permits dealing with material that is live rather than solely reconstructing past events.

Consider an adolescent with wounded self-esteem who reacts cautiously and guardedly. A quality of object tie is sensed that indicates caution is desired. Withdrawal is being used in the service of defensive protection as well as inducing anxiety in those with whom the adolescent is relating, since others feel excluded or responsible for inducing this constriction. This interlocking pattern often runs through various family members. As a resistance, it will impair progress in therapy unless it is dealt with. Yet the entrenchment of the resistance is fostered, since there is a threat that being more open and relating to the therapist may release a host of painful affects or impulses. This ego resistance is more prominent with children and adolescents than adults, since there is less ability to deal with the material verbally, and the younger individual is currently involved in an ongoing process of ego development. Defenses are needed more drastically for protection against the environment as well as against drives. Those with wounded narcissism may choose to maintain precarious sources of gratification with a preference for fantasy gratification rather than run the risk of experiencing the rewards and pains of interpersonal growth.

Dependency in the Transference. Dependency demands on the therapist are often overwhelming in the course of treating children and adolescents, not only because of conflicts, but because the reality of the situation may be quite upsetting. Dependency varies from wishes for a complete blending with the therapist to wanting to live with his family, be adopted by him or have his children for siblings. In many cases the countertransference wishes of the therapist coalesce with those of the patient, leading some therapists into taking these patients into their homes. Adolescents express these longings in terms of "we" instead of "I" in describing their experiences with their therapists outside treatment hours. A feeling of insufficient dependency gratification in the child's family leads to demands to receive this in therapy, or correspondingly to use the therapist as a target for aggression.

The less developed the verbal ability of the adolescent, the more brinksmanship of acting and aggression he will display. If not interpreted or handled satisfactorily, a repetition of the behavior coupled with increasing anxiety occurs. The dependency is not only a crucial developmental variable for children, but it is biologically and socially inescapable. Without this factor, the process of acculturation in the course of development would not occur. However, one of the consequences of these processes is the establishment of an internalized need for a feeling of approval by the external objects, along with progressive internalized representations. Hence the anxieties associated with fears of separation, abandonment, punishment for transgressions (in thought, word, or deed), as well as the loss of approval and guilt, mount. Such concomitants of the socialization process lead, with defects of different types and proportions, to a civilized human being—but they also raise the potential for conflict.

Psychotherapy carried out with those still developing poses the problem of conceptualizing the dependency relationship. It never seems to take place solely in terms of a recapitulation of the past during the course of treatment, even with adults. With the minor, the dependency situation is an ever-present reality with the therapist and the family, as well as involving the conflicted past. Parental involvement in therapy is thus unavoidable, since the parents are an active force not only in permitting treatment to take place, but in their conscious and unconscious neurotic entanglements with their offspring.

Applications. A few common and frequently encountered examples of psychopathology are:

1. A child may be acting out unconscious parental impulses, such as the repressed wish of a mother pertaining to promiscuity in her daughter.

2. Parents may be involved in a specific neurosis by reinforcing a given symptom and defensive posture. They do this by active, symbolic, and unwitting participation, such as an obsessional boy's need to take a bath and wash in a ritualistic manner with the mother present for certain of the steps, such as having five towels available in an exact place, and in an exact manner, as well as handing the towels to the boy in a specified manner, only on his demand.

3. The child may be accomplishing goals which the parent has failed to achieve. Also, parents may have set attainment levels based on their idealizations, and the child senses his mission is to carry out these wishes. Common examples are in the child who must achieve intellectually, vocationally, athletically, or socially for the parent. Unless the child so complies, the threat of rejection or abandonment, with its attendant anxiety, is omnipresent. This may be re-enacted in treatment via negative therapeutic reactions not to comply with the adult therapist any more than with the parent.

Unless this is dealt with, it contributes to therapeutic failure.

4. Conversely, there may be a reaching out to involve the child in the familial psychopathology associated with the parents' neurotic or psychotic conflicts.[10] A frequent difficulty is the delineation of the child's conflicts from those of the parents and how they interact. How the parents and family respond to childhood problems, be they in the physical, psychophysiological, social, or emotional realm, is quite relevant.

Some transference reactions in the adolescent are more typical of certain psychosexual and psychosocial stages of development. Qualities of lack of trust or confidence in others, which recur in therapy, point to anxieties associated with dependency conflicts. Old fears of losing identity in exchange for that of the therapist, or of being abandoned by the therapist, are similar. There may be an unfolding of efforts to obtain something from the therapist in the form of a gift, time, or attention, which leads to attempts to take from the therapist. Manipulative efforts not to cooperate, or to disparage the efforts of the therapist, his integrity, or his office may then ensue.

Guardedness may show up in efforts to relate at a distance. Some adolescents display this by a constant stream of chatter; others busy themselves with a flurry of activity about the office. One boy of thirteen with recurrent abdominal pains which began a year earlier when his parents were divorcing, announced how he had liked his previous therapist, since playing checkers did not require him to talk about himself. He communicated to his new therapist in this way his hopes to avoid dealing with painful affect and conflicts.

Other material in treatment may be more associated with oppositional qualities. Production of florid but irrelevant material, or periods of prominent negativism where the child will not give, are examples. Hostile verbal attacks or physical acting out within the therapeutic setting, as well as outside of therapy, then become more likely. Characterological traits of quick, symptomatic cures may occur in attempts to convince the authorities that his difficulties are over. The authorities may vary from the therapist or parent to some external agent such as a counselor or probation officer. A striking example of such a cure was noted with a fourteen-year-old encopretic boy whose soiling was cured in six sessions, but who was engaged in stealing compulsively when seen a year later. This was not simply a *symptom-exchange*; both problems stemmed from the same unresolved conflicts.

Therapists may come to represent different aspects of the child's conflicted personality relationships. These transactions are extremely useful for knowledge of particular struggles. An adolescent girl with conversion symptoms may feel that the therapist is a source of temptation, recapitulating her own wishes. At other times the same therapist may be a forbidden object who is disapproving of her wishes; at still other times, the therapist is viewed as a source of reassurance and help with anxieties. Each of these experiential states can be viewed as externalizations of id, superego, or ego aspects of the patient's personality. Another example is a sixteen-year-old obsessional boy who talked freely with his therapist about dirty thoughts about his mother and sister. He came to associate the therapist, as well as his office, with being dirty and forbidden. At other times, the therapist was viewed as a stern, critical figure who frightened the boy. Subsequently, he appeared to become more tolerant of himself, and the therapist was experienced as an ally against his drives and his critical, self-punitive tendencies. When an adolescent views the therapist as a source of temptation, attempts may be made to avoid or terminate therapy, or to retreat into endless discussions reflecting the ambivalent state, with a prominent use of intellectualized defenses.

COUNTERTRANSFERENCE

Diffences from Adult Therapy. Countertransference difficulties arise when treating adolescents at least as frequently as they do when the patient is an adult. The complex interactions unfortunately do not lend themselves to a statistical treatment, but the emotions involved in dealing with this age group make this a valid statement. The manifestations are different, due to the areas of conflict which are tapped in the therapist. Two striking countertransference differences occur in working with adolescents compared to adults: (1) the degree of aggressivity displayed by adolescents makes special demands on the therapist, and (2) there is often a relative lack of the positive feedback responses which are present in treating varieties of adult patients. A host of emotionally laden responses are elicited. Attempts by therapists to accommodate to the styles of adolescents often end in a caricature. While some are attempts to react in a preplanned manner to seem in tune with adolescents, others' efforts are directed at trying to be a replacement—"to be the kind of parent he needs."

There are various ways those treating adolescents attempt to use adolescents to fulfill or relive many of their own unfulfilled needs. Some of these needs stem from unresolved problems in their own childhoods, but others arise from contemporary frustrations. The play, *Equus,* dealt with the problems of a provincial British psychiatrist attempting to treat an adolescent boy who blinded several horses.[11] Despite the boy's serious difficulties legally and emotionally, the psychiatrist felt a quality of envy for the boy's sense of feeling, which the psychiatrist found lacking in himself. It is impossible to discuss countertransference problems in treating adolescents without giving consideration to the motivations of why clinicians wish to work with adolescents. In turn, this opens up the broader issue of why people chose a line of work dealing with those who have emotional problems. One must realize the wide variations present in individual therapists, their own constellation of conflicts and conscious and unconscious motivations which are resolved to different extents. The ultimate question as far as countertransference is concerned is the manner in which these aspects in the personality of the treater interfere with carrying out treatment.

Unresolved Conflicts in the Therapists. The urge to understand and become part of the life of a teenager may be related to wishes and fantasies to relive an unhappy teenage period and produce a different outcome. Many sexual and aggressive connotations can be present in fantasies which lead to prying in a manner which results in increased resistance or seductive responses by the adolescent. Genetic origins in the therapist which lead to curiosity about how children become men should, ideally, create a sublimated balance in activities between looking, listening, exploring, and inquiring without a predominance of acting out impulses. Omnipotent strivings are easily gratified in the therapist when an adolescent is in search of an idealized parental figure. If these needs are too paramount, the therapist will react with feelings of rejection when these idealization components are absent or when the patient begins to reappraise them. In many ways adults who have not resolved their early anxiety with strangers and other adults may be more comfortable with younger people. The difficulty then becomes one of overidentification with the youth and a relative exclusion of the parents. This may lead to attempts at sabotage by the rejected parents in the form of withdrawing their offspring from treatment. It may be a replication of a situation for the therapist where misunderstanding adults ruin things by interfering with gratifications or attachments.

An adult may re-enact with the families he is involved with many family situations from his own past as a child or adult. This can occur in mixtures, with the therapist developing identifications with different family members. The capacity to do this on one level contributes to a successful treatment; on another level it produces regressive consequences by indulging in situations from the earlier life of the therapist. The intense emotionality engendered in work with adolescents and their families leads to a host of withdrawal and protective maneuvers on the part of everyone involved.

Lacking confirmatory data on the validity of neurophysiologic techniques of treatment, such as electroconvulsive treatments or a well-established armamentarium of drugs for adolescents, a quest for less time-demanding techniques may ensue. This results in adolescents being placed on treatment regimes of a series of alternating drugs, or in desperate efforts to maneuver their environment, such as using a succession of foster homes, with the hope this will resolve their problems. Acting out adolescents, in particular, elicit great frustrations in the therapist and in his attempts to deal with the manipulative and demanding qualities which such families demonstrate. This gives rise to a host of countertransference behaviors to escape what seems to be unresolvable problems. The most frequent forms of this predicament are witnessed in telling a family that character problems are untreatable, or automatically labelling such adolescents delinquents and insisting that their treatment be carried on through a correctional approach. Community acquiescence in these facile explanations contributes to the lack of quality facilities for treating severely disturbed adolescents.

Countertransference Toward Parents or Other Authorities.
Those who wish to treat and help the sick and suffering are responding to demands in themselves to rescue those in pain or helpless. For those whose aims are directed toward adolescents, wishes to rescue them from a disturbing situation are prominent. The therapist confronts the frightened but angry child, as well as assists confused and conflicted parents. However, countertransference responses develop as easily and frequently with parents as with their children in such situations. Competitive or rivalrous strivings between the parents and therapist may emerge. An example is that of the male or female therapist attempting to be more maternalistic than the parents. Another pattern is the therapist whose wish to have grown up differently himself takes the form of straightening parents out. The result may be kindly and supportive efforts to rectify parental conflicts, but it can also lead to less desirable

consequences. When narcissistic gratification is present to the degree of viewing therapy as an opportunity to give lecture sessions and instruct parents on how to raise children, we are either witnessing a naive therapist or countertransference under the guise of guidance. What complicates the picture these days is the number of self-appointed groups and individuals who seek to mold adolescents to a particular style of life.

The therapist may literally try to replace one or both parents. In some cases resolution of the child's conflicts is camouflaged under a guise of submission, with everyone emphasizing improvement. Such accommodation by submissive family members typically results in a few brief sessions during which the psychopathology is concealed or ignored. The family equilibrium is retained on the level of maladaptation that was present before some acting out episode. The frustrated therapist recreates situations where he teases or provokes the adolescent. Insecurities in the therapist are evidenced in his taking a stern, oedipal role as someone who intimidates or frightens patients. Occasionally the hate of the therapist toward himself is displaced onto the adolescent, who represents the therapist's infantile self. A progressive series of attempts at guilt-expiation by the therapist is the outcome. Eventually, a sterile relationship with little affect or empathy results, with patients and parents given intellectual explanations for the disturbing behavior. A variation is the therapist who identifies with parents to condemn the behavior of the adolescent. Approaches based on lectures, stern warnings, or appeals to personal moral dictates becomes the modus vivendi of therapy. While the relationship with the parents progresses smoothly, reinforcing their needs to moralize, increasing resistance and acting out is seen in the adolescent.

A major source of countertransference difficulties is the pressure to do something—anything—to stop behavior. This is more threatening when dealing with juveniles than with adults, especially for the beginning therapist or one who feels he must get results. With adolescents there are frequently accompanying demands from parents, schools, and courts that something be done. Three examples are illustrative:

1. A mother requested therapy for her sixteen-year-old daughter whose problems had become overt during the preceding three years. During evaluation it was evident the problems had been developing for over a decade. On the initial presentation for therapy, demands were made that something be done immediately to stop the situation of blatant acting out. When the mother was asked what she had in

mind to accomplish this, her not unpredictable response was, "That's for you to decide and handle since you're the doctor." Such a stance usually puts the beginning therapist into a mild anxiety state since his training, especially if he is a physician, has emphasized he must do something when a patient or guardian demands it. This type of pressure may lead him to fall back on the ever-ready prescription pad. Acting out families often seek advice from clergymen, community resources, or teachers. They frequently fall into the trap of taking almost any advice to do certain ad hoc things and when they fail, as they customarily do, the advice is to take the matter into the juvenile court. An adjudication of incorrigibility may result, a vacuous conclusion meaning no more than the minor is recalcitrant to parental authority—which everyone knew to begin with. The situation ends as it began several months or years earlier, with therapeutic intervention still required. If the pattern persists, the girl may be committed as a delinquent to a correctional facility after incidents of repetitious behavior.

2. Schools also place demands on therapists for results. School personnel are frequently in the predicament of having to deal with frustrating situations of conflicted children and families, coupled with socio-cultural deprivation and lack of facilities and personnel to give such teenagers the type of emotional and learning experiences they require. Again the demand is put on the therapist to do something immediately, particularly when the behavior pattern is becoming progressively more aggressive, or when a preadolescent is behaving restlessly and not achieving. This may take the form of "Just tell us what to do when he does X, Y, or Z."

3. Families which select one member for scapegoating are trying to avoid dealing with many of their unconscious conflicts and wishes. They often present a unified front against any outsider. The outsider may be a therapist or social agency which attempts to intervene. Once more we are presented with a situation in which the demand is made that something be done to fix up the transgressor. The initial request may seem vague or refer to removal of the child from the home. In many of these situations it appears the individual is not content to remain in the perpetual role of a scapegoat. This leads to family attempts to re-establish or maintain the equilibrium which has been operative for some time, and when resistance is encountered, the child becomes more symptomatic or aggressive. Therapy is usually requested in order to re-establish the child in the previously established interactional position as a scapegoat. The scapegoated child is in an inescapable position: He can either

comply with the covert requests to stop protesting and go back to the old alignment in the family, or continue his efforts to extricate himself. If he persists in the latter, it may lead to his removal from the home. Community sanctions are then placed against him, including the confirmation to the school and community that he is in fact the family black sheep.

In all of these cases either community or family demands are placed upon therapists. Each therapist will react differently, depending on his own conflicts, training, and therapeutic orientation. The dependent therapist may feel he has to acquiesce to the urgent demands to do something. An endless chain of maneuvers and interactions may commence which rarely resolve the situation. The problem of setting limits exists not only with individual patients and their families, but with the multiple community resources and agents with whom the adolescent comes into contact, and who become involved like an extended family. The guilt-proneness of the therapist may be part of this picture, particularly when the people involved have perfected techniques of inducing guilt in others through displacing their own anxiety that not enough is being done. Although limit setting may be needed at times, it is merely a preliminary step to resolve many of the problems in these narcissistic families.

PRELIMINARIES IN THE SELECTION OF A THERAPY

At this point a consideration of the general types of therapy as applicable to the adolescent age group is needed. Table 26 distinguishes between approaches where the main effort is directed toward an individual patient versus an approach geared toward a larger unit. A further subdivision divides treatment directed primarily toward the individual adolescent, his environment, or organic treatment measures. Making a decision about where to direct the therapeutic emphasis, and the selection of which techniques to use, are probably the two most difficult initial tasks in therapeutic intervention. Lack of knowledge and effort in these directions are areas often overlooked. A third problem is the failure to match personalities of adolescents and families with the types of therapists and therapeutic techniques with whom they are most likely to get along. This must surely contribute to many of the failures and criticisms of what is done in the name of therapy.

TABLE 26

Therapeutic Procedures Used with Adolescents

I. INDIVIDUALLY ORIENTED TREATMENT

  A. Direct Involvement with the Adolescent
    1. Primary relationship therapy
    2. Directive approaches
      (a) Persuasion
      (b) Guidance
      (c) Attitude modification
      (d) Suggestive approaches
      (e) Rational therapy
      (f) Reality therapy
      (g) Existential therapy
      (h) Logotherapy
    3. Abreactive approaches
      (a) Ventilation
      (b) Drug-induced catharsis
      (c) Hypnosis
      (d) Release therapy
      (e) Activity therapies
      (f) Sensitivity groups
      (g) Est
    4. Drama types of treatment
    5. Conditioning therapies
    6. Ego-oriented therapies
      (a) Sector therapy
      (b) Adaptational therapy ("reparative psychotherapy")
      (c) Crisis interventions (situational, developmental)
      (d) Transactional therapies
    7. "Working-through" therapies
      (a) Psychoanalytically oriented therapies
      (b) Classic psychoanalysis
      (c) Nonclassical psychoanalytic approaches

  B. Environmental Treatments
    1. Hospitals
      (a) Daycare
      (b) Evening units
      (c) Mental hospitals—adolescent units
    2. Residential treatment centers
    3. Correctional institutions
    4. Group-living arrangements
    5. Foster homes
    6. Treatment in schools
      (a) Special classes
      (b) Counseling in school settings
      (c) Boarding schools
    7. Camps
    8. Therapeutic camps
    9. Milieu approaches

C. Organic Treatments
   1. Tranquilizers/Anti-depressants
   2. Sedatives
   3. Stimulants
   4. Megavitamin therapies (orthomolecular psychiatry)
   5. Electro-convulsive types of treatment
   6. Sleep treatments
   7. Psychosurgeries
   8. Genital reconstructions

II. TREATMENT AIMED AT LARGER UNITS
   A. Collaborative Therapy
   B. Conjoint Family Treatment
   C. Family-Centered Treatment Combinations
   D. Group Therapies
   E. Parent Education Training
   F. Socio-cultural Approaches
   G. Variations of Religious Cults (Western, Eastern, Altered
      Consciousness, Occult, etc.)

Under the guise of economy, or the belief that large numbers must
be treated, policies are adopted in treatment centers to utilize
uniform approaches. Hence, one clinic resorts to group therapy for
all acting out adolescents; another resorts to tranquilizers for
anxious children and amphetamines for hyperactives. In some
settings, intensive exploratory treatments are utilized indiscriminately for a small number of patients. Such indiscriminate practices
contribute to the failure of empirical evaluations to reveal any
preference between one type of therapy and another, or the
possibility of no treatment at all. This is seen in research which
compares an experimental group of those receiving treatment to a
waiting list where no treatment has been received. In practice the
treatment has often been carried out by multiple personnel of widely
varying background, experience, and training, with randomized
patients or, at best, utilizing semantic groupings such as neurotics.

Random treatment and assignment of adolescents or their
families to whomever is available for a patient may prove harmful.
An extreme example of this mass production approach to therapy is
seen in drug clinics for those with emotional disorders. It would
never be decided, as a treatment approach, to give a sedative to a
patient with acute abdominal pain, to recommend immediate
surgical exploration, or merely to tell the parents that something is
wrong in their attitude toward the problem; nor would we
automatically classify any student with learning problems as
retarded. Yet in the emotional sphere, one witnesses psychotherapeutic efforts of an exploratory type with adolescents whose
capacity to relate, have effective object relations, and distinguish

fantasies from reality, is extremely limited and who are exposed to a type of therapy tailored for those with internalized neurotic disturbances. In some adolescents the lack of satisfaction of primitive needs and deficits in earlier nurturing have been so monumental that these must first be met before interpretive therapies have relevance.

Reference has been made to the *hyperactivity syndrome.* Unfortunately, there are many preconceptions operating that many view these behavioral manifestations as reflecting organic cerebral dysfunction. A contrary position views such behavior as a possible manifestation of many disturbing emotions in the absence of positive independent findings regarding organicity. Problems arise when there is a lack of confirmatory organic evidence, or when the criteria for organicity are drawn so loosely as to meaningless. In such evaluations one frequently comes across comments such as, "This boy seems poorly coordinated," or, "His fine motor coordination seems to be below par." A lack of specificity and the absence of valid developmental comparisons abound in this approach. On the other hand, viewing such behavior as an expression of anxiety per se involves an implicit assumption that a primary neurotic problem exists. When large numbers of school-age children become enmeshed in these rote approaches, some are bound to be caught up in treatment processes which are irrelevant and detrimental. The adverse social consequences of being labelled brain damaged involve other problems.

Characteristics in the therapist which lead to difficulties in treatment have been noted, but presenting the positive characteristics which lead to successful therapeutic work with adolescents is more difficult. The usual and well-known clichés about good intelligence, compassion, empathy, having a sense of responsibility, good training, having had exposure to different types of diagnostic problems in patients of different ages, utilization of different treatment techniques as indicated, good supervision, and perhaps personal therapy, are obvious. Such lists are widely acknowledged but rarely fulfilled to any extent in the training of most therapists. Elaborations of such traits and backgrounds will not be expanded upon but there should be a knowledge of them. Without such acknowledgement, the descriptions of types of therapy often have a sense of abstractness and unreality. There is also an implication that some type of uniform application by therapists takes place and that this is available for anyone presenting with difficulties. In reality, such a well-systematized scientific application of therapeutic techniques rarely occurs. What makes methodologically sound evaluation for the effectiveness of psychotherapy complicated are the subtleties in individual styles and techniques in a therapist during the actual course of treatment. These have far greater significance than any particular theory of personality or technique to which a therapist may adhere. The results of nearly 400 controlled evaluations of psychotherapy did find that the typical therapy patient is better off than 75 percent of untreated individuals. However, no significant difference was found between different types of psychotherapies.[12]

TYPES OF THERAPEUTIC APPROACHES

Relationship Therapies. Within the group of individually directed treatment efforts, relationship therapies are one of the most frequently utilized. The term is a misnomer since a relationship is essential to any therapeutic contract. Emphasizing the relationship does not deny the significance of the past history of someone, but is rather a therapeutic maneuver to bypass it and focus on contemporary reactive patterns. Acceptance of the adolescent, with his individual needs and grievances, without fearing condemnation or retaliation, is considered the crucial experiential component. It is believed that this approach has overtones of Rankian influence, with its emphasis on the patient's use of the relationship. A similar emphasis developed within some schools of social work.[13] Accordingly, there is a heavy emphasis in these approaches on respect for the individual and his autonomy, an emphasis important in treating adolescents.

Psychological treatments should not be foisted on a patient. An opportunity to form a new relationship with a person which will have merits in its own right can be offered. The implication is that the patient, adolescent or adult, has a right to refuse entering into such a relationship, as well as to make requests of his own for what the therapy is going to entail. Again, therapy is not merely something imposed by a therapist, clinic, or institution. Such a therapeutic posture presumes a degree of cognitive and emotional intactness in an adolescent. The age and level of development of the patient, the degree of repression, and the level of conflict must be considered.

Relationship approaches are similar to Rogerian client-centered therapy and to existential schools of thought. These stress the significance of the here and now. This is in contrast to an emphasis on the painful past or the possibly hopeless future. Dangers of philosophical pessimism or optimism can occur. The restriction that only the present has meaning, if it can be utilized for progressive development of certain capacities and potentials in the future, can omit significant contributions made to personality from earlier childhood. Allen once wrote that therapy commences when the therapist is "brought into a relationship as a supporting and clarifying influence around the patient's need and desire to gain or regain a sense of his own worth."[14] The adolescent is expected to take an active part in directing efforts to his future, in contrast to working through past conflicts and therapy. There is a major point of theoretical disagreement with those therapists who feel that the past cannot be so lightly dismissed. Critics of relationship approaches, when they are used alone, stress that growth cannot progress unless past conflicts are resolved or experiences which have been lacking in the past are given some type of compensation.

Directive Therapies. If an overall survey of approaches used in dealing with adolescents with emotional conflicts were available, some type of directiveness would probably be the most frequently cited method. This would especially be so if types of counseling were included, along with the variety of volunteer programs set up to intervene in the lives of adolescents and their families. This includes not only parental efforts to direct their children's actions, but all of the forms of guidance and rational attempts to influence behavior. Much of an adolescent's life is subjected to such direction, without it being so labeled. These techniques are historically the oldest therapeutic interventions to direct and influence children's behavior.

Directive guidance operates when parents are given advice to carry out certain routines, or to take actions to allay their anxieties about their offspring. For example, parents may be advised to send their son (who has antisocial tendencies) to a camp as a form of treatment. An honest but authoritarian approach is used when a therapist suggests or orders decisions to be made for a child or within a family. The success of the orders is correlated with the wish to please or the need to conform to a particular individual in the adolescent. This may be aided by the transference of omnipotence to the therapist, who gives the suggestion or order, and who permits a change in behavior to occur. Such approaches are seen when adolescent males are put into situations with older male athletes or "big brothers," and try to emulate their ways. It is seen in adolescent girls when they are exposed to the modeling influence of older girls with whom they identify. This is one of the sources of religious influences in changing behavior patterns through identification figures or allowing value shifts which permit shifts in the ego ideal content. The limitation is the instability of these identifications when exposed to pre-existing conflicts or environmental stresses.

Many directive efforts are employed with youths without any attempt to resolve internalized conflicts or alter their character structures. At times direct guidance might utilize threats or coercive efforts ("If you do not obey your parents, we will place you in a residential treatment center"), as well as attempts to persuade a youth rationally to mend his ways. No attempt is made to deal with developmental sources of behavior, but rather the end sought is some kind of change. Some believe it desirable to ignore whatever may have produced the disturbance, so that they see historical material as a set of interesting but unnecessary data.

Many of these practices of guidance are extensions of *educational practices* which educators and parents utilize. Thus, reassurance is given to a young adolescent that he need not feel guilty over certain sexual thoughts or practices, or a therapist reassures an adolescent that a homosexual experience does not make him a homosexual. When anxiety or obsessional symptoms are present, the direct approach might rely on the admonitions of status figures to stop worrying, and in an undetermined number of cases the symptoms become more transient or effect a type of alternative defense. It is with transient or situational reactions that direct techniques seem most efficacious. When a particular symptom or defensive pattern is serving the function of neutralizing painful affect or alleviating conflict, it is much less likely to disappear by fiat. This is similar with longstanding behavior disturbances whose pleasures are quite entrenched and ego-syntonic, as in personality disorders. A variation is to instruct a youth in techniques of self-persuasion, such as exhortations or forms of self-hypnosis. This comes close to the techniques used in sales management courses to enhance the selling capacity by pet talks and exhortations. It may lead to the zealous advocacy by a reformed adolescent to get others to mend their ways.

Hypnosis, as a form of directive therapy, has been advocated for use with younger people. Varieties of hypnotherapy are employed:

1. Direct suggestions under hypnosis to accomplish symptom-removal.

2. Suggestions for attitudes toward something to be altered, such as attitudes about a person or subject in which the goal is to permit more adequate functioning.

3. Cathartic abreaction along the same early lines of psychotherapy as used with adults in the 1890s. When this is used with minors, the justification is that traumatic experiences have been harmful, and a cleansing operation is seen as a desirable therapeutic end result.

4. The use of hypnosis as an adjunctive technique with behavior modification or desensitization procedures is employed where a hierarchical series of low-to high-eliciting anxiety situations are evident.

5. A modified form of hypno-analysis involves therapy sessions carried out in part, or totally, under hypnotic influence. When hypnosis is used with adolescents, in particular, the hypnotist comes to be viewed as an omnipotent, miracle-producing figure. The ease of hypnotizing children is so great that some wonder whether the resistant group is cerebrally injured.[15]

Yet from our knowledge of the strong attachments to adults which children have—being more readily intimidated, and having ego strength to tolerate anxiety-laden material—we should not be surprised at their hypnotic readiness. The above-listed goals for employing hypnosis are rarely seen to be as attainable with adults. In practice, the type of catharsis which some adults seem capable of, is rarely attained with minors. Hypnosis would similarly have little efficacy as the main vehicle for therapeutic communication. This is not only from the old problem of how to use material obtained in an altered state of consciousness, but the generally restricted verbal content produced in most hypnotized adolescents.

If hypnosis has any use with adolescents, it is an adjunctive technique rather than a technique in and of itself.[16] In this context, hypnosis has been used as an accompaniment to individual or family therapy. When a relationship, classification, and interpretation have been carried out, but symptoms remain, hypnosis has been used as an additional vehicle to encourage experimentation with new behaviors, or to give up others. It is then used to bolster ego strength in the hope of permitting a realignment of some intrapsychic structural components. It may thus be used for help in school phobias, or when encopretic symptoms have been present for several years and have not disappeared. It may have use with ego-alien symptoms which persist on a self-perpetuating basis, such as stealing, enuresis, tics, or stuttering. Hypnosis has also found a use in emergency situations, such as vomiting, or symptomatic expressions which are partly conditioned by respondent conditioning via the autonomic nervous system, such as bronchial asthma. In all of these situations, hypnosis is not seen as a substitute for dealing with pathogenic conflicts in the child and his family, but as an accessory. In practice, it often tends to become the primary treatment without further inquiry.

Several decades ago David Levy described what he referred to as "attitude therapy" for use with parents whose attitudes were adversely affecting their children.[17] It was a way of dealing with the capacity and means for attitudinal change in the parents. Alternative ideas or approaches to shift the balance in the relationship between parent and offspring were offered. The approach has similarities with recent suggestions which stress the ascendancy of intellectual processes over upsetting emotions which cause difficulties. An example is the "rational emotive psychotherapy" of Albert Ellis in which self-condemnatory or self-defeating behavior is ascribed to the illogical or inconsistent attitudes of individuals in a person's life. Especially is the finger pointed at authority figures such as parents, teachers, and the prejudices fostered by a culture.[18] These sources of self-defeat are exposed and pointed out by the therapist, who then helps an adolescent re-think such intellectual dead-ends. In effect, this amounts to imposing a different set of values once the illogicality in the old ones has been exposed.

A given, such as a person feeling he needs to be loved at any cost, even at the risk of self-compromise, is an obvious area to be challenged among adolescents. Obtaining dependency gratification above all else or believing their own interests should come last are other naturals. Feelings that sexual curiosity or gratification are not only taboo but bad, are dealt with in this system by rational re-education. Previously unquestioned beliefs and practices are challenged and alternative views offered. The adolescent must be sufficiently enlightened intellectually to understand that it is irrational to expect to be loved by everyone, or by any one person all of the time. Guilt and shame over expressing self-interest as primary are interpreted as rationalization, induced in children by parents and society to control them so parents and other adults are more comfortable.

The result of these rational approaches is to provide a new set of ethical norms which can be internalized. They offer alternative ways of behaving, with comfort for the child being placed first. It should be apparent that in many cases such re-thinking will be resisted strenuously by the families that have used them for generations, because a new philosophy of orientation would be needed for the entire family unit. The inherent conflicts within a culture, and a family unit, were obvious in the mother with obsessional problems when presented with a seventeen-year-old son who found himself tortured if he disobeyed her edicts and if he enjoyed himself too much. Treatment was requested because she became increasingly aware that many of the same tendencies and conflicts which she struggled with had developed in her son. Vacillation and indecisiveness, as well as the use of undoing mechanisms, such as having to take three steps forward and two backward to prevent his mother from dying, were becoming increasingly prominent in the boy. Preciptation into therapy resulted from the mother being unable to answer questions from her son such as why one should, or should not, always have to do his best. Having done this all her life with little pleasure, but rather constant self-criticism, it appeared something she wished to be rid of at age forty-five. Balancing the wishes for autonomy in the adolescent with his rationalizations to oppose others just for the sake of opposition becomes one of the crucial issues.

Reality therapy stresses the discrepancies between what people say and do.[19] If an adolescent who steals cars maintains he really respects and likes people, his disrespect by taking their cars is pointed out as is his personal irresponsibility. Stress is placed on the patient admitting his irresponsible behavior, so that behaviors illustrating responsibility can be promoted. The job of the therapist is to point out and promote alternative behaviors. This may involve direct suggestion and persuasion, but it avoids explanations of intrapsychic mechanisms or constructs, such as unconscious motivations. These are viewed as part of an excuse-giving process by attributing a lack of responsibility to unconscious motivation. This particular distinction seems to fail to distinguish between an understanding of behavior and explaining it from efforts at exculpation. Similarly, labelling an adolescent mentally ill is believed by reality therapists to foster irresponsibility by allowing the label of illness to rationalize their behavior. This comes close to the position of Thomas Szasz in seeing the mental illness category as a myth used to exculpate criminal responsibility.[20]

There are several therapeutic implications in reality approaches, such as ignoring the past history, which is believed unchangeable anyhow. Hence transference problems are ignored and the involvement with the therapist as another human being advocated. The therapist functions not only as a teacher in inculcating different behaviors in an adolescent, and suggesting ways he should behave, but overtly as a pronouncer of moral judgements in firmly labelling behavior as right or wrong. The emphasis on teaching moral responsibility is tantamount to what a competent moral philosopher might do with the young children within his charge, and is reminiscent of the way moral virtures were taught to the young in Greece during the time of Socrates. Conflicts within the family or culture which lead to moral deviations are also relatively ignored, with the assumption that feeling worthwhile will result from following the moral dictates given.

This last point contrasts with the emphasis in rational therapy on the individual accepting responsibility by developing his own value system above and beyond impositions from his family or culture. In reality therapy the emphasis is rather on reinforcing the moral dictates of the community via the authoritative influence of the therapist. A father who becomes aware of car thefts his son has committed would be viewed as making a moral judgement in reporting his son, and losing his own self-respect as well as that of his son if he did not report him. No inquiry into family conflicts being acted out by conscious and unconscious motivations is permitted, such as the possible involvement of the father and others in the behavior for overt or covert reasons.

Abreactive Approaches. Prior to their grouping as a form of psychotherapy, abreactive approaches, which stress the element of catharsis, had a long history. Many societies and organizations have utilized abreaction in the form of confessions and ventilation techniques as part of the requirements or advantages of belonging to a group. Chum relationships for adolescents serve a similar function. There is a history of such approaches in the development of early psychoanalytic efforts to deal with hysterical symptoms. Much therapeutic work was associated with efforts to unravel the mystery of symptom development as well as the effect of undischarged emotions in mental functioning. This early work stressed the original "trauma" which lived on as reminiscences. The theory led to the therapeutic approach of seeking to discharge emotion in the belief that conflicts would then resolve themselves. This theory of trauma, based on a major or rare experience, is still adhered to far too frequently. Work with children has revealed this focusing to be a distortion in contrast to the cumulative events which are experienced in the course of development and which lead to characterological differences and defenses.

With adults, the cathartic goal might be sought by ventilation if the events are primarily conscious. At times, this is aided by drugs to induce relaxation and catharsis, such as pentothal or amytal interviews. Hypnosis could also be used to induce dreamy recall which might lead to an outpouring of affect. This material would later be used in a conscious state for integration. Variations have been used for abreactive purposes, such as inducing dreams on certain themes in a hypnotic state, or when an individual goes to sleep in a customary way. The techniques are employed to overcome periods of resistance or to induce regressions to arrested levels.

How valuable can discharge be per se, without integration into social life and personal history? Some traumatic episodes may be capable of being defused in this reliving manner, so that discharge might be valuable with those who have experienced a catastrophe or with those whose egos are in an overloaded state which they have not been able to assimilate. Even here, the usual technique of permitting a catharsis in a repetitive manner suffices eventually to master the anxiety. An adolescent may ventilate his feelings about many legitimate and alleged injustices. One study noted a group of street corner delinquent boys willingly participated when given a chance to talk into tape recorders about their grievances. However, they actually viewed this as an opportunity to make easy money since they were paid to talk.[21] Despite this, the report stressed the amount of affect and involvement which the boys exhibited. The use of such material beyond its cathartic function is often neglected.

An extension of abreactive approaches has occurred in varieties of adolescent group activities. These take place with or without adult participants and with various degrees of formality, and are often referred to as efforts to expand awareness. They may take place in conjunction with therapists, such as in encounter or sensitivity groups, which employ devices such as role-playing games. Mind expanding drugs may be employed in these ventures (again, sometimes formally, as in an experimental setting, and at other times by adolescents trying out drugs for a variety of motives). The goal may be not simply relief from past transgressions and worries; it may also involve efforts to achieve closeness not available by other means (physical hugging or becoming familiar by bodily contact to lower the inhibitions adolescents have). If such activities are thought of in terms of lowering inhibitions in constricted individuals, they may promote this goal in some and the opposite in others.

The potential for individuals to act out via this medium is quite obvious. The types of activities encompassed under what are called sensitivity groups are too numerous to be counted. They have varied from mixed adolescent discussion groups for purposes of acquaintance or catharsis about social grievances to various degrees of acting out under the label of therapy.

Confusion appears rampant in the ascetic efforts of some of these groups to engage in intellectual discussions about sexual inhibitions. Again, it is very difficult to evaluate these techniques as a form of therapy since many of the participants object to the process being so described, as do those who lead the sessions. Further confusion has resulted from those who lead sessions with no standardized qualifications. The composition of the groups varies from schizoid adolescents to those who see the group as a chance to achieve dominance over peers. Little attention is paid to concepts such as diagnosis or the extent of disturbance present in different youths. Some appear to be extremely disturbed when they are seen later for evaluation for continuing difficulties, while others appear to have a distribution of the usual problems seen in adolescents.

Notice has been given to these approaches since it appears that many youths participate in such meetings. Whether they should be called therapy, any more than any of the other experiences of everyday life, is questionable.

An early form of abreactive therapy applied to children was called "release therapy".[22] It was based on the child acting out his conflicts and powerful affects through the medium of play. In release therapy no attempt is made to interpret feelings, to tie them into a transference relationship, or to advocate new behavior. The goal is rather abreaction on the level of the lowest common denominator to master via repetition and active mastery. Thus, a boy who developed a fear of dogs subsequent to being chased by a barking dog on the way home from school was permitted and encouraged to play out variations on this theme until little anxiety persisted. In treatment there was a restructuring of the play situation to master and control the dog and related arousal. No interpretation was used, and no connections were made between this fear and others, or its possible symbolic connection. Limited use of the technique was proposed from the following criteria:

1. If possible, there should be a definite symptom precipated by a specific event, such as a fright, birth of a sibling, separation, or hospital precedure
2. The fear should not have been present too long
3. Rarely is this technique useful over ten years of age or the preadolescent range

4. The problem should ideally be a past occurrence rather than a chronic state of conflict
5. There should be a family structure which is relatively intact and competent

Unfortunately, in many cases these criteria are ignored and release therapy is used indiscriminately. The result is a heightening of anxiety and the development of additional symptoms, since a little discharge becomes a dangerous thing. These dangers are present in many abreactive approaches when used with the wrong person, at the wrong time, and under the wrong circumstances.

Adjuncts to the expression of emotion are often an integral part of many therapies. The adjuncts may be simple, such as urging and helping an adolescent to participate in athletic or social events or to pursue artistic endeavors. An adolescent with acting out difficulties may be encouraged to participate in aggressive contact sports in the hope this will divert off his acting out potential. This same approach is present when the seventeen-year-old delinquent youth is urged to join the military. An awkward youth may be enrolled in activities to help him improve his coordination or master activities. Types of crafts may be encouraged such as clay, paints, drawing, modeling, games, finger painting—alone or in conjunction with any other type of therapy—where goals vary from emotional discharge to group participation. In other situations some of these activities are used as a medium of communication for interpretive efforts in individual or group therapy.

Music is another expressive means which permits a physiological and psychological impact as a form of therapy. It may stimulate from an otherwise lethargic and withdrawn states, as witnessed in the enormous appeal styles of music have always had among adolescents. Dancing or movement games facilitate discharge and reveal attitudes and conflicts interpersonally and with respect to how an adolescent handles and feels about his body. Dramatics serve similar goals. A variation is the use of puppet shows with latency-age children, where various identity figures are used to portray problems typical of children. Bender and Woltmann once devised such a show with a hero, Casper, who was a curious and uninhibited fellow, immune to harm, who eventually was able to solve his problems.[23] Monkeys, alligators, witches, cannibals, giants, and kind parents are the characters A child audience participates actively. At times the children shout and give advice, or they may be asked to improvise themselves. It is held that children experience a genuine affect and mastery from such an experience.

An example is the child who encourages the puppets to do various things, such as throwing the baby into a garbage can or dropping him down a toilet. Such an experience can be used with other types of therapy, as well as noting the individual distortions a child introduces.

All of these abreactive approaches continue to raise perplexing questions about the nature and limits of psychotherapy in general and with adolescents in particular. All life can be viewed as a therapy in terms of every personal encounter and every dream having the potential for effecting change. Many experiences are not only stimulating but lead to self-reflection or increased peer contact. Many individuals function in the role of influencing adolescents, such as teachers or neighbors, as well as the whole panoply of crises inherent in development before adulthood. These are the substance of child development in coalescence with the biological unfolding of puberty. To call all of these approaches therapy seems a misnomer; to say they may be therapeutic is unquestionable, but that is no more than saying that almost anything in life can be therapeutic at a particular moment.

THE ROLE OF PLAY

While play as an activity, and play therapy as a treatment, are usually thought of as associated with younger children, the nature of play and its relationship to fantasies is desirable knowledge for those who treat adolescents. Forms of dramatic play, as well as techniques stressing catharsis, all utilize play. Role playing activities rely on this as well. Play is a vehicle for communication as well as having specific uses in certain forms of treatment. Academic psychologies, such as Oestalt and field theory, view play as a method of exploring and learning about the world.[24]

In physical activities play is used to test coordination, as well as to promote the use of symbols and fantasy. Sanctioning play in a culture allows confirmation of the reality and meaningfulness of what a child does. Relatively free and non-structured play has a good potential for catharsis or re-enactment of significant themes for children as guided by their own needs at the time. A setting of diversified toys gives a child an opportunity to bring forth certain material. Hence, if model dolls are provided, one would expect different play responses than if toy cars were provided. Similarly, dolls with artificially constructed male and female genitalia give different responses than do typical toy-store dolls.

Theories on the nature of play have included the following:

1. The child has a need to discharge excessive energy
2. Play is a form of practice for activities they will later require as adults
3. Play is a form of relaxation or an escape from emotional fatigue
4. Play is a recapitulation of past stages the human species has lived through
5. Play is a means of discharging affect
6. Play is seeking an outlet for childhood desires since ways accessible to adults are often prohibited

It is apparent that theories of play and their therapeutic uses vary from the elementary to the profound. Play is advocated by some simply because, "It's a lot of fun," which should be justification enough. But in treatment it is used for insights into unconscious material analogous to free association techniques with adults. The role of the therapist is that of a permissive participant to allow play to take place in an atmosphere of friendliness and acceptance.

Hug Hellmuth, the first woman member of the Vienna Psychoanalytic Society, introduced the technique of participating in the play activity of children, as an aid to the diagnosis and treatment of disturbed children.[25] She applied the technique in psychoanalytic work with children and extended it to many other forms of therapy. In turn Melanie Klein used play therapy to attempt psychoanalysis of children.[26] She assumed the free play of children as seen in therapy symbolized wishes, fears, preoccupations, and conflicts. By application of psychoanalytic theory, interpretations were made by observing the context and the sequence of play. Klein objected to misinterpretations which assigned a specific symbolic meaning to various acts which originated in the context of the play situation. Originally using miniature toys which could represent projected family members, interpretations about play were gauged by the manner in which the child responded, similar to an adult responding to verbal interpretations.

Anna Freud differed in not viewing child therapy as capable of utilizing literally the principles taken from adult therapy. Further, not all play was viewed as symbolizing conflict, since this needed determination by way of other crucial factors operating within children and their current situation. While some attach no meaning to play beyond that of permitting expression, this type of reduction seems an oversimplification. Like other means of communication, play also functions at different levels of meaning whether it is primarily verbal or not.

In the tradition of relationship therapy, eight basic principles in the use of play therapy have been given.[27] They are applicable to the relationship with an adolescent where the use of play in a literal sense has become minimal.

1. The therapist must develop a warm, friendly relationship in which good rapport is established as soon as possible
2. The child is accepted as he is
3. The therapist establishes a feeling of permissiveness in the relationship so that the child feels as free as possible to express his feelings
4. The therapist is alert to recognize the *feelings* that are being expressed and reflects them back in such a manner that insight is gained
5. The therapist maintains respect for the ability of the child to solve his own problems if given an opportunity to do so—the responsibility to make choices and to institute change is the patient's and not the therapist's
6. The therapist does not attempt to direct the actions or conversations—the patient leads the way and the therapist follows
7. There is no attempt to hurry therapy since treatment is seen as a gradual process
8. The therapist establishes the limitations necessary to anchor the therapy to the world of reality and make the patient aware of his responsibility in the relationship

These principles have a guideline validity for the commencement of any therapy. Their function beyond the beginning phase does not permit the therapist to progress beyond a relationship. However, play as a relationship treatment is not seen by some as a modality needing anything beyond this level. While a tolerant acceptance of play can be therapeutic in its own right, for many problems it is not sufficient. The assumption that children progress according to their own potential for growth does not recognize the tenacity of defenses and how difficult to modify they are. To the clinician dealing with conflict, such buoyant optimism does not seem realistic. It provides a setting in which a sympathetic and well-intentioned individual may participate in certain play activities, or begin to relate to an adolescent, but it provides no means to go beyond this.

The more profound meaning of play in addition to the above functions has been elaborated by clinicians who do intensive therapy. Therapy which utilizes play is cathartic at times, and the objects and fantasies which a particular child creates are taken as having a special meaning. Play is a vehicle for aggressive activity in which the therapist needs to be aware of the background and be capable of setting limits, without blocking the opportunity to talk about many associated feelings. In this usage play is analogous to the use of dreams, fantasies, or free associations as utilized with adolescents or adults.

Sigmund Freud originally described a play situation of an eighteen-month-old boy when he was considering the *repetition compulsion* principle where painful occurrences of the past continue to be re-enacted by thoughts, acts, or dreams and take precedence over experiencing pleasure.[28] Play was viewed not only as a repetition of experiences but involved motivations to grow up and act out in the manner of adults. Mechanisms for handling aggression are present in play; a child may recreate a punishment, or reconstruct some painful experience such as a hospitalization. Suffering may be imposed on another child willing to submit. A child may seek revenge for what he views as an abandonment by making his mother go away with the safety factor that he can always bring her back in the context of a play situation. Freud's case is interesting in this regard.

> This good little boy, however, had an occasional disturbing habit of taking any small objects he could get hold of and throwing them away from him into a corner, under the bed, and so on, so that hunting for his toys and picking them up was often quite a business. As he did this he gave vent to a loud, long-drawn-out 'O-O-O-O,' accompanied by an expression of interest and satisfaction. His mother and the writer of the present account were agreed in thinking that this was not a mere interjection but represented the German word 'fort' ('gone'). I eventually realized that it was a game and that the only use he made of any of his toys was to play 'gone' with them. One day I made an observation which confirmed my view. The child had a wooden reel with a piece of string tied round it. It never occurred to him to pull it along the floor behind him, for instance, and play at its being a carriage. What he did was to hold the reel by the string and very skillfully throw it over the edge of his curtained cot, so that it disappeared into it, at the same time uttering his expressive 'O-O-O-O.' He then pulled the reel out of the cot again by the string and hailed its reappearance with a joyful 'da' ('there'). This, then was the complete game—disappearance and return. As a rule, one only witnessed its first act, which was repeated untiringly as a game itself, though there is no doubt that the greater pleasure was attached to the second act.

A further observation subsequently confirmed this interpretation fully. One day the child's mother had been away for several hours and on her return was met with the words, 'Baby O-O-O-O!' which was at first incomprehensible. It soon turned out, however, that during this long period of solitude the child had found a method of making *himself* disappear. He had discovered his reflection in a full-length mirror which did not quite reach to the ground, so that by crouching down he could make his mirror-image 'gone.'

The "doctor game" is a fantasy which can be acted out in therapy.[29] The fantasy refers to play material concerning the Oedipus conflict which can persist. It arises developmentally during that period and persists. It reveals conceptions of the sexual act by use of a host of phallic equivalents such as syringes, enemas, knives, and stethoscopes, with the pregnant mother as the sick patient. The doctor is played as a privileged person who denudes and inspects bodies without shame. He concerns himself with urine and feces without being punished, indulges in aggressive acts without guilt, and possesses intimate details about the mysteries of sex and the mother's body. By way of the doctor game, internal conflicts are acted out to an extreme, without running too great a risk of danger.

Play can also be conceptualized developmentally as progressing from autoerotic activities connected with the infant's or mother's body to a transitional object in the intermediate area between an external object and a narcissistic representation of the self. Soft toys make their entry by way of the special object reserved for bedtime or periods of stress, such as separations or hospitalizations.

Various play materials make a chronological entrance based on the following approximate sequence:[30] (1) toys offering opportunities for ego activities are used which are displaced from bodily functions; examples are those which open and shut, or those into which things can be placed or soiled; (2) movable toys representing motility are introduced; (3) building materials permit constructive and destructive play; (4) toys which permit expression of masculine and feminine trends are first used alone and then for phallic exhibitionistic activity, and to act out various triangular relationships within a family. These activities gradually give rise to producing a finished product or achievement.

In time, a transition to a capacity for work is reached. Impulses come under sufficient control and there is an ascendancy of reality testing over pleasure-seeking. Ordinarily, this takes place during latency if a sense of industriousness develops. Games have special meaning for the latency-age child and unfortunately material from games children play is often ignored. The less the degree of concrete acting out of wishes via play in games, the more reliance the child has on wish-fulfilling fantasies and their derivatives. Many areas of personality functioning in the child, as well as in adults, are expressed in games played with the therapist or as reported and observed with peers. Trends of aggression, competition, handling of one's body, and reality testing are examples. Formal games have a quality of strict rule-following and reveal a specific area in which conflicts and striving are played out for a solution or decision. Exaggerated needs to win at all costs are present in some children, while others cannot stand to win. Spontaneous play activity, has more free-floating qualities of free association where primary process thinking is conspicuous.

Although play therapy is frequently used as a cathartic, or for creating a relationship, it reflects levels of development as well as areas of psychopathology. Play activity, when utilized in therapy, raises philosophical issues. To what degree play is work or not, or something beyond simply work, can be settled in part by definition but more promisingly by observation and clinical participation. Even in Freud's example stressing repetition, the correlative aspect of play was the groping for mastery by repeating an experience which the child had been subjected to involuntarily. Play, or acting by play, functioned to gain control over something. This means that play is conceptualized in terms of the need of the ego for mastery: over the self, the body, and social roles. This is not then simply a blind repetition. Play may dramatize what is available in a particular culture at a certain time, but again this is not sufficient without considering the corrective level of development.

Erikson has summed this up:[31] "What has a *common meaning* to all the children in a community (i.e., the idea of having a reel and string represent a living thing on a leash), may have a *special meaning* to some (i.e., all those who have just learned to manipulate reel and string and may thus be ready to enter a new sphere of participation and communal symbolization). Yet all of this may have, in addition, a *unique meaning* to individual children who have lost a person or an animal and therefore endow the game with a particular significance. What these children 'have by the string' is not just any animal—it is the personification of a particular, a significant, and a lost animal—or person. To evaluate play the observer must, of course, have an idea of what all the children of a given age in a given community are apt to play. Only thus can he decide whether or not the unique meaning transcends the common meaning. To understand the unique meaning itself requires careful observation, not only of the play's content and form, but also of accompanying words and visible affects, especially those which lead to what we shall describe as. . .disruption."

Developmentally, play progresses from the autocosmic to the miscrosphere and mascrosphere. *Autocosmic* play centers on the child's own body and originates with repetition of such things as sensual perceptions, kinesthetic sensations, and vocalizations which extend to external objects. The world of *microspheric* play involves toys which a child uses to handle his anxieties and needs for mastery. This may be interfered with in two ways: from the toys not cooperating (they break, get lost, are taken by others), or an immature control system permits an excessive quantity of anxiety-laden material to emerge which leads to a sudden disruption of play or a progressive inability to indulge in play. A failure of mastery is accompanied by regressive phenomena and we then witness autoerotic activities, withdrawal, or self-injurious components. Conversely, a mastery experience either in solitary play or in therapy produces pleasure and raises self-esteem by overcoming fright. The *macrosphere* of play refers to situations involving an interpersonal element with peers. A hierarchy of permissiveness is learned, such as what should be kept in one's private world of fantasy and dreams, what types of autocosmic play are safe, which activities can be permitted expression, and, finally, what can be shared with others.

Each of these levels is uilized at different times. They are called upon as needed in a progressive sequence when things have been depleting or frightening. In summary, play is the equivalent of dealing with experiences by creating model situations which permit mastery of reality by a type of experimentation and planning. "Modern play therapy is based on the observation that a child made insecure by a secret hate against the fear of the natural protectors of his play and family and neighborhood seems able to use the protective sanction of an understanding adult to regain some play peace."[32] The content of play is centered on whatever aspect has been most disconcerting to the ego. From this insight trust in the diagnostic and therapeutic significance of play at all ages has evolved.

LEARNING THEORY: RELEVANCE TO TREATMENT

Conditioning Therapies. Conditioning therapies involve varieties of techniques and assumptions about personality functioning and development. The polemical and evangelistic aspects of some of these approaches will not be focused upon; their merits rather rest upon the contributions they can make to helping conflicted adolescents. Conditioning therapies share a fundamental tenet: psychopathological conditions represent maladaptive habit patterns which have been learned, and by using the same principles, bad habits may be unlearned. Unconscious conflict and motivation are not considered. Insight into conflicts or reconstructions based on the historical aspects of the lifespan of a child and his family are not believed necessary. Psychopathology is viewed as maladaptive behavior in response to external stimulus variables, and a cure lies in manipulating these external variables.

Classical (respondent) learning is used to diminish or eliminate patterns while *instrumental* (operant) learning is employed to reinforce new behaviors. Relief from systematic behavior which is disturbing to a person or his environment, such as in a family setting or antisocial behavior in a community, is conceptualized as a target behavior to modify. An early demonstration often cited is Mary Cover Jones's study in which the fear responses in a child to a rabbit were extinguished by associating the feared object with a pleasant emotion, such as feeding the child when hungry, accompanied by gradual reductions in distances to the source of the fear.[33]

It was early theorized that anxiety itself serves as a drive. Hence, a pattern of behavior that decreased anxiety, such as the development of a symptom, established a reinforcement which becomes entrenched.[34] On that basis a form of treatment for enuretic children was devised consisting of placing an apparatus in a bed which closed a circuit when the bed was wet and led to a bell ringing which woke the child. The goal was an anticipatory warning to urinate before the punishment, or lack of a conditioned response.[35] In more recent years learning techniques have verged closer to those employed in rational therapy or reality therapy.

Mowrer held neurotic symptoms develop because of real guilt associated with thoughts or acts which the superego does not sufficiently inhibit.[36] Neurotic difficulties are viewed as examples of a person acting irresponsibly. This leads to objective guilt and to others condemning the behavior. Becoming healthy means acting more responsibly. This is equated with moral virtues such as honesty, generosity, and reliability. Treatment for the emotionally disturbed is based on developing a greater degree of superego inhibition and stressing a need for more guilt for transgressions of the moral code. Confessional techniques to parents and peers, perhaps with acts of expiation, are viewed as useful and practical aids.

This theoretical explanation for neuroses is diametrically opposed to most views regarding personality conflicts. It seems most applicable to those who have not been exposed to adequate socialization or educational influences or with character deficits. It is in direct conflict with treatment recommendations, made not only by many with a psychodynamic orientation, but also by those who use alternative learning theory formulations. For example, Dollard and Miller feel that the gist of therapy is the permission a person has to talk about taboo topics and transgressions without the fear of condemnation which leads to an extinction of symptoms.[37] The problem is intimately bound to various reinforcements from the environment in a covert and clandestine manner. These are not easily deconditioned, even if the individual submits to attempts at inducing guilt. Nor do characterological problems seem to resolve themselves by a confessional technique more than temporarily, since so many of these youths are oblivious to the things they need to confess.

Conditioning approaches are based on a rather simple paradigm: to weaken or eliminate a symptom, withdraw reinforcement, reinforce a different behavior in order to strengthen it. (This is contingent upon knowing which reinforcer will have the greatest effect on strengthening a response.) For children, food, candy, and toys are used with different reinforcers provided to avoid monotony. A variation is the use of tokens at the end of a session which can be used in exchange for some desired object or privilege. This is a technique tried in correctional or residential treatment settings with adolescents who have impulse control problems. The goal is to reinforce delay of gratification. Reinforcers such as granting a weekend pass might be used. Initial work may begin with a broad base of behavioral shaping in which any type of response within the broad domain that is desired is reinforced, or it may be no more than exposures to appropriate stimuli at first from which schedules of reinforcement are decided upon, such as ration of fixed interval schedule.

The Role of Punishment. The question of punishment merits consideration even without a discussion of the voluminous experimental literature on the subject. Many punitive measures continue to be used by parents, teachers, and therapists inside and outside legal settings. Measures such as deprivation of rewards, confiscation of privileges, isolation techniques, verbal nagging, and cajolery, all involve aversive stimuli to some degree short of the physical infliction of pain.[38] In fact, the most frequent punishment used is the withdrawal of socialization agents, such as parents, as well as techniques of shaming or humiliation. The issue is then not solely an ethical matter, but one which involves conflicting evidence about the efficacy of punishment. In 1913 Thorndike held that reward and punishment had clearly predictable effects. "When a modifiable connection between a situation and a response is made and is accompanied or followed by a satisfying state of affairs, that connection's strength is increased. When the opposite state of affairs prevails, the strength is decreased."[39] By 1932 Thorndike noted many instances in which punishment did not weaken a response strength, which led to altering his viewpoint. "Rewarding a connection always strengthened it substantially; punishing it weakened it little or not at all."[40] Four decades later the same conflicting evidence remains. Some experimental evidence indicates punishment decreases the probability of occurrence of a response or increases its latency; some note a temporary suppressing effect on a response or none at all; and in other experiments a paradoxical effect of punishment is noted, in that a response is strengthened.

It has been noted that if an aversive stimulus is confined to a given response, a greater suppression is achieved, but if it is not, the aversive stimulus results in facilitating the response.[41] Within an operant framework, punishment may actually be defined as a "reduction in the future probability of a specific response as a result of the immediate effect of a stimulus for that response."[42] A stimulus is viewed as punitive if it reduces the projected probability of a future response. Although severe enough punishment may suppress undesirable responses, there is the dilemma that attempts to escape such punishments may be reinforcing. In the therapeutic setting, further treatments may become difficult, while in the less structured general environment there may be greater efforts to escape. This is seen in punitive and shaming approaches to acting out and delinquency in which the effect is to make the offender more devious and dedicated to avoid detection. Unless the substitution of desired responses through positive reinforcement is present, there is great danger of therapeutic backlash.

The appeal of conditioning therapies lies in the simplicity of the theoretical model as well as in the uncomplicated treatment techniques employed. There is also a greater ease of environmental control if the patients are in settings where they are controlled.

Behavior Modification. The most prominent of the current conditioning therapies is represented by behavior modification. These are contemporary therapeutic representations of either classical conditioning or Skinnerian operant psychology. There is an explicit standard that symptomatic relief is sufficient for any treatment measure. Futher, the types of problems most responsive to behavior therapies are behaviors such as enuresis, phobic symptoms, or temper tantrums.[43]

It is interesting that none of the major behavior modification therapies are particularly new, nor are they mutually exclusive. Desensitization procedures are elaborations of Jones' work of over four decades ago, which was viewed as a positive counterconditioning experience. Varieties have been tried over the decades, such as the attempt of Thorne to dissipate fears by training the patient to anticipate the fear and replace it as an inappropriate response.[44] Salter's "conditioned reflex therapy" similarly directs a child or adolescent to assert himself if neurotic anxieties are manifest, or conversely the patient is ordered to abandon aggressive behavior patterns and practice new habits.[45]

"Reciprocal inhibition," as advocated by Wolpe, holds "If a response inhibitory of anxiety can be made to occur in the presence of anxiety-evoking stimuli, it will weaken the bond between these two stimuli and the anxiety."[46] This is a target substitution technique of relaxing responses in contrast to anxiety-evoking ones. It should be noted that auxiliary aids such as hypnosis, autosuggestion, and drugs have been employed in this approach. Varieties of symptomatic pictures are reported to have been alleviated, such as stuttering, tics, phobias, and anxiety states, which represent some of the most prevalent symptom pictures. Anxiety hierarchies are constructed in terms of the most-to-least fear-provoking situation, and the patient is helped to tolerate progressively more threatening situations by uninterrupted relaxation. One of the evaluation difficulties in this approach is the high periodic incidence of multiple phobic behaviors, which occur not only within the course of an established neurosis, but within the course of developmental

Negative reinforcement, a form of punishment, is another variant of conditioning therapies. It utilizes an aversive stimulus for undesirable neurotic responses. Psychopharmacologic agents may induce aversive reactions analogous to the use of Antabuse with alcoholics. Faradic electrical current is more typically used in aversive conditionings. Behavior modification recommends its use for obsessional symptoms, homosexual behavior, adolescents showing transvestite or fetishistic behavior. The therapeutic full circle is striking, since prior to the advent of psychodynamic personality theories, perversions such as fetishism and transvestism were ascribed to accidental childhood experiences which established such behavior by a conditioned reflex. Electrical treatments were used even then as standard treatment, but what was lacking was an explanation based on learning theory to justify the treatments.

Extinction procedures attempt to remove old responses by a lack of reinforcement, or to replace the unconditioned stimuli associated with the eliciting stimuli. An example would be to ignore—and thereby stop—an adolescent exhibiting provocative behavior. Some advocate an exaggerated fear of the symptom as the best way to extinguish it, such as a child with a tic being urged and forced to repeat its performance over and over again. An adolescent with symptoms of a school phobia would be encouraged gradually to approach the school building, subsequently the school room, and then spend gradually increasing durations of time inside the building.[47] For the latter there may be a mixture of operant techniques which are also responded to by rewarding the desired behavior, such as with money or a gift.

A plethora of approaches has been used experimentally with psychotic children as well as with cerebral dysfunction, learning disorders, verbal impairment, and mental deficiency. Most of these are contingent upon the programming of environmental rewards to reinforce the desired responses. There are attempts to modify behavior by manipulating the social consequences of certain behaviors. This may lead to approaches contrary to those customarily employed by therapists. Instead of encouraging withdrawn children to participate in activities, they might be ignored on the theory of not reinforcing detached behavior.[48] A child with violent temper tantrums was reported refractory to treatments of physical restraint coupled with drugs, but he was reported to have been handled successfully merely by placing him in another room until his tantrums ceased.[49]

This is similar to the isolation techniques long employed in inpatient psychiatric units where a quiet room is employed for children whose behavior is disturbing to others, or they are acting in self injurious ways. In other cases they are provided with self-operated shock boxes, analogous to cardiac patients with pacemakers regulated by a box they carry, to impose self-induced shocks when certain thoughts or wishes occur. A wider utilization employing the social millieu is being urged, based on social learning approaches of imitation, modeling, and vicarious reinforcement.

Many of these approaches are advocated for antisocial or socially disruptive behavior. These have extended from temper tantrums in the young to those later classified as negativistic or troublemakers.

The school-age child who is physically or verbally aggressive is treated by instructing teachers to ignore the aggressive acts and respond only to cooperative behavior.[50] Nor have aggressive displays been omitted from the therapeutic armamentarium, since they are seen as responding to positive reinforcement in classroom settings.

Among the studies available is one in which the hyperactivity of nine- and ten-year-old boys, diagnosed as brain-damaged, was controlled by noting the acclaim the boys received for their activities. By reinforcing the entire class for desirable responses in the hyperactives, an increase in their attending behavior was noted. A variation is to program teachers' behavior so that social reinforcers are contingent upon the occurrence of socially acceptable behavior. Assuming that the diagnoses of neurological impairment were valid, this illustrates an old principle: biological causation for a given condition in itself need not imply the necessity of resorting to biological treatments for effectiveness.

Adolescents and delinquents have been exposed to a variety of techniques based on punishment or reinforcement techniques. Being on probation, or institutionalized, is punitive in its own right, apart from the social labelling effect which may actually function as a reinforcer within the delinquent subculture. Conditioning techniques are used with delinquents in an attempt to eliminate specific symptoms, such as lying or stealing, but there have also been treatment measures directed at behavioral traits such as fighting. Rather than merely utilizing the traditional isolation techniques of placing an adolescent in an institution and further isolating him in separate quarters, techniques have been introduced to reinforce adaptive behaviors. Adaptive is a term used by most workers to mean a conformity to institutional rules. Of course, the hope is that conformity will generalize to the outside world upon discharge. All of the criteria used to evaluate the effectiveness of any therapeutic intervention apply here, such as adequacy of data, the variety of apprehension policies in effect, and changes over time with age and developmental status. The most typical positive reinforcement approach, as we have noted, is the giving of tokens to purchase privileges. A treatment plan gives so many tokens for so many hours remaining out of trouble.[51] Similar approaches have outright rewards for appropriate behavior, such as keeping appointments, performing well in academic subjects, behaving according to the rules of the institution, or staying out of trouble.

What type of appraisal is possible for these diverse conditioning therapies in terms of therapeutic methodology and effectiveness?

There are several tenets adhered to by the more zealous of behavior therapists that promote defensive responses, even in those who believe there are contributions to be made from such treatments. Fantastic cure rates are often cited—in the neighborhood of 80 percent—which should give anyone pause.

It is apparent on reviewing the literature that semantic confusion prevails in therapy reports as to the meaning of "cure." When cure is confined by defintion to concrete symptom removal, that cannot be challenged as a goal toward which any therapist and patient may choose to work. Provided that criteria for a given treatment procedure are met, and that a symptomatic individual can be made more comfortable within a few short interviews by particular techniques, this is not something that should be ignored. Nor can the stress on learning principles be anything but praised since the more we learn about maladaptive learning in people, the more we will know about the psychotherapeutic process.[52] All therapies in some form provide rewards or reassurances for behavior deemed desirable. No clinician would deny the effects of repetition on behavior, be this due to psychological factors and conflicts, or the effects of autonomic conditioning. That schedules of reinforcement and habits play a role in behavior, along with the impact of drives and affects which lead to avoidance behaviors, is a position most psychodynamic theorists accept, even though a strict Skinnerian would find surplus in even this brief formulation.

Any form of therapy is subject to the effect of multiple variables. Transference and countertransference are two such variables. With adolescents there is an additional set of factors complicating the assessment of change over time due to developmental changes. This makes the attribution of even a mono-symptom change, due to a specific behavior modifier technique, challengable. It is not an unusual situation to find that symptoms enter states of remission or exacerbation, due to alterations in environmental, physical, or emotional factors. Symptoms also reflect developmental crises. Symptom fluctuation is actually the norm when dealing with conflicted people, and the problem of therapeutic cure is thus far more complicated than an affirmative-or-not answer as to whether a symptom exists at a particular time. Further, it is a rare case where a mono-symptomatic disturbance exists when a thorough history of an adolescent and the family constellation is obtained. Certainly, a position that such a history is not even necessary is subject to criticism.

Nor should the question be confined to nothing but an appraisal of whether a symptom substitution occurs or not. For example, we would rarely expect a phobia to become a compulsion. An entire array of therapeutic maneuvers is involved in addition to specific techniques, such as the quantity and quality of the relationship with the therapist and the multiple personality attributes which a patient and his family members have. A therapist may make suggestions which are explicit or implicit, and the knowledge the participants have about behavior therapy may lead the child to produce responses which the therapist wants and which are thus subtley reinforced along with other direct reinforcements.

It is presumed that all therapists have an emotional investment in the particular brand of therapy which they utilize. That is one more factor which makes appraisal so difficult. It is not that this factor is restricted to one type of therapy, but rather that it is inherent in all types. Although some type of relationship is always present between a clinician and patient, it is not always dealt with. In fact, attempts are made to deny its significance by stressing the impersonality of the relationship is analogous to a surgeon performing an operative procedure.[53] Even here the analogy does not hold, since few surgeons in this day and age view their cutting and stitching skill as the essence of surgery.

Seeking impersonality is a quest for a scientific ideal much like when hypnotism once sought a similar status, and the hypnotizer referred to himself as someone who merely performed a procedure by giving instructions and bringing the patient out of anesthesia. The need to include explanatory parameters of the relationship between an adolescent and his therapist is not only desirable but essential. The entire interpersonal situation requires investigation, as do communication patterns. There is a need for thorough investigation of positions as to whether manipulation of reinforcements, such as giving rewards, does alter overt behaviors over extended periods of time when matched groups and variables are employed. This requires evaluation apart from the other goals of therapy, such as permitting development to progress or developing latent potentials.

Clinicians who use an intrapsychic model, in addition to environmental alterations, believe that intrapsychic conflicts must be dealt with when they have become so entrenched that social rewards are no longer effective. Pathological behavior would continue since previous reinforcements have permitted an internalization process to operate relatively autonomously from the environment. An oppositional character structure would be an example; there an ongoing need exists to continue opposing or challenging authority figures, accompanied by a sense of chronic self-failure.

Interpersonal problems and learning disturbances also intervene. Such behavior may go back to generalizations based on early experiences which continue to influence the developing child and for which insight and dealing with affects are necessary.

Symptom removal may seem irrelevant since one wonders what the "symptom" is, and in fact some would say that such a child has no problems, or that the problems are of a social nature which should be dealt with by changing the culture. This may be particularly so when the problems are of an antisocial nature for which social remedies are proposed in contrast to therapy. A non-behavioristic approach believes treatment has to operate on an entirely different level in dealing with impulses, feelings, and internalized mechanisms regulating self-reward and self-punishment.

Gelfand and Hartmann reviewed the literature on behavior therapy with children, finding it subject to many of the same methodological criticisms present in other therapies.[54] They believe the following criteria need to be employed, and that such standards can be met:

1. Adequate baseline measures for the occurrence of problem behaviors are needed, as well as pro-social responses when applicable. This data could could be collected over a sufficient period of time to provide reliable rate information. It should be collected in a planned manner and not obtained by introspection. A stricture may be entered in terms of how feasible and valid these observations would be. Even if a patient is placed in a maximum observable situation for twenty-four hours a day, such as in a ward where constant observation can take place through one-way mirrors, this would be an artificial situation and isolated from the social experiences otherwise present.

2. A systematic variation of reinforcement contingencies, or other procedures demonstrating control over behavior, is needed. This would permit the re-establishment of problem behavior or the extinguishing of pro-social responses, and their subsequent alteration again. The goal is to demonstrate that target behavior is unmistakably under the control of the therapist rather than due to adventitious factors. This permits conclusions to be drawn from modifier techniques when there are only a few subjects. Where contingency reversal is not feasible, the experimental design of a control group would be treated identically to the experimental subjects, with the exception of

the lack of the systematic application of the contingency. Breaking down the responses into subunits could also be employed.

3. Unbiased behavioral observations are needed in behavior modification approaches as in any therapy evaluation. Less difficulty exists in doing this with discrete behaviors. Procedures such as the automatic recording or filming of target behaviors might be utilized. Observers who are naive about treatment procedures and the use of such evaluation techniques as the establishment of a high inter-observer reliability before the inception of a study, need to consider using such procedures.

4. A final desirable criterion is the longitudinal follow-up of the stability of any changes which have occurred. Again, strict procedures for follow-up evaluation are needed, and not just periodic phone calls or mail out questionnaires.

EGO-ORIENTED THERAPIES

Sector Therapy. Some approaches stress the relationship as a vehicle by which an adolescent can begin to take stock of areas of his life. Sector therapy, when applied to adolescents, selects a particular problem or area where there are difficulties.[55] The reality situation is dealt with, as are the unconscious factors which are contributing to a particular sector. Whatever sector is selected to work on is based on peer relations, learning problems, or acting out problems. The therapeutic technique stressed is that of *sympathetic rejoinder.* Key words and phrases which the adolescent uses pertaining to his symptoms and conflicts are associated with the sector emphasized.

The aim is to lead to associative connections involving deeper conflicts so an alteration in the reactions to others can occur. This approach is also considered a way of strengthening the ego by altering the defenses handicapping the youth. Related to this is the stress on the therapeutic alliance as providing a corrective experience in its own right.[56] There is an active attempt by the therapist to provide a new experience for the patient which is in direct contrast to what he anticipates, based on past experiences with family and older adults. Expectations of rejection, manipulation, or being placed in double-binds are the types of situations anticipated, to which the therapist is alert. Therapy centers on altering these anticipations as well as the need to test and provoke self-destructive repetitions with others. This is done through a positive therapeutic relationship and interpretation of behavior and defenses, but the process does not deal with the transference neurosis or transference reactions per se. Extending therapeutic gains outside of the therapy hour is believed a crucial step as a confirmatory experience.

Adaptational Therapies. Adaptional therapy is closely related to sector therapies. This is based on a view of the organism as maneuvering to stay in a homeostatic balance between physiological and social needs. Although most therapy employing adaptational psychodynamics has been with adults, the implication for treating adolescents is significant since throughout there is an emphasis on ego functions and faulty responses as being at the crux of neurotic conflicts.

Another prominent factor is a stress on feeling and the disordered reactions consequent to attempts at handling these feelings. Beyond a level of hedonistic self-regulation by pleasure, emergency emotions (fear, rage, retroflexed rage, shame, guilt fear, and guilty rage) and welfare emotions (affection, love, pleasurable desire, joy, self-respect, and pride) are regulators. Cognition encompasses emotion and emotional thoughts—the latter using reason and higher intellectual processes. Throughout there is stress on the impact of emergency reactions on the organism in the context of the levels on which they operate.

Conscience is a semi-automatic mechanism of control in which the child learns to anticipate parental demands. Parental reward gives automatized self-rewards, known as self-respect, and moral pride; parental punishment gives automatized self-punishment as a means of expiating one's presumed wrong-doings and reinstating one's self in the loving care of the authority with whom reconciliation is wanted. Conscience achieves security through obedience, but its problem is the control of defiant rage.[57] Early survival becomes associated with the subordination of inner strivings to parental demands. In the course of therapy an emphasis is placed upon the recognition and techniques of dealing with emergency emotions as well as with the accompanying systems which have evolved. The framework of treatment (since the possibilities which contribute to conflict, exemplified in efforts to appease, coerce, expiate, or aggressively cope with anticipated rejection), is limitless. Dependency problems are associated with magical techniques to obtain control over others and the self. With children dependency needs to foster modification of behavior and more realistic and less magical techniques. Encouraging a patient to reproduce many affects toward those who elicited them in the past is considered necessary before an integrated level of adaptation can take place.

Reparative psychotherapy is an application of these viewpoints to personality functioning. Externally disturbing aspects of reality are first handled, such as parental neglect, failure to attend school, or physical problems.[58] Then the emotional factors and defenses are considered, which involves dealing with the accumulated rage associated with these experiences. This may permit development to continue or progress. A thorough reconstructive exploration is not attempted, however, if therapy is confined to these interventions.

Crisis Interventions   Crisis interventions are not independent of other therapeutic approaches since the need for them may arise during the course of any type of therapy. This has many preventive implications for adolescents in or out of treatment. It is mentioned here as an approach which is geared toward therapeutic intervention whenever a *situational* (accidental) crisis is precipitated or a *developmental* crisis unfolds. The former includes events such as the birth of a sibling, loss of a loved one (by death, separation, or divorce), moving away from a familiar setting, or emotional disturbance in a family member. For an adolescent, being hospitalized or becoming a patient of any type, or reacting to an illness in the family members are a few common situational examples.

Developmental crises refer to inevitable crises such as the onset of puberty, expansion of peer social interaction, transferring schools, entering senior high school, dating, and the commencement of sexual activity. There are also the psychological stresses associated with the changed internal and social demands attendant upon different psycho-sexual stages of development. Without recapitulating a general social and preventive psychiatric theory, crises of any type should have a therapeutic handling in their own right. For many adolescents the crises are superimposed on pre-existing emotional problems. The crises place an additional stress from the "flooding" effect. This means that routine handling by existing defenses and coping patterns may not be enough. Ignoring such crises can have two outcomes: it can precipitate or contribute to the consolidation of existing problems, or in some cases it leads to a strengthening of the personality functioning if mastery is achieved.

Intervening appropriately is important as a therapeutic procedure apart from the preventive aspects per se. Whatever the difficulties which have precipitated a crisis, if not handled, they may lead to progressive difficulties. Opportunities arise in dealing with resistances within an adolescent and his family to gain new insights that are useful in therapy. Motivation to deal with painful material is never as prominent as it is during crises. If many environmental contributors are operating, there is a tendency for many people to become involved in the name of helping (teachers, counselors, friends, probation officers, and welfare workers, to name a few). Unfortunately, too many people in the helping role tend to confuse things. They frequently do not share material and even when they try, there is not a common therapeutic framework. The result is an adolescent who drifts and has iatrogenic problems forced on him by this confusion beyond those originally present.

Dealing with crisis situations should not be viewed as more elementary than the sophistication required for doing competent therapy. A knowledge of developmental and psychodynamic models of personality are what give a cogency to intervention and provide a rationale. That knowledge gives power which allows proper steps to be taken is true for every contemporary theory involving child development—from psychoanalysis to "positive disintegration" as elaborated by the Polish child psychiatrist Dabrowski. Crises are viewed by Dabrowski as the acme of a necessary disintegration of personality functioning. After a crisis takes place, a maximum growth can be promoted through secondary integrative mechanisms.

> The positive effect of some forms of disintegration is shown by the fact that children (who have greater plasticity than adults) present many more symptoms of disintegration: animism, magical thinking, difficulty in concentrating attention, overexcitability, and capricious moods.
>
> During periods of developmental crisis (such as the age of opposition and especially puberty), there are more symptoms of disintegration than at other times. The close correlation between personality development and the process of positive disintegration is clear.
>
> Symptoms of positive disintegration are also found in people undergoing severe external stress. They may show signs of disquietude, increased reflections and mediation, self discontentment, anxiety, and sometimes a weakening of the instinct of self-preservation. There are indications both of distress and of growth. Crises are periods of increased insight into oneself, creativity, and personality development.[59]

Transactional Therapies. Transaction or interactional therapy is stimulating, yet perplexing, in its approach to disturbed individuals and their families. It is a therapeutic approach which has borrowed from work in the social sciences, such as communication theory, game theory, and role theory.[60] Symptoms of developmental disturbances in an adolescent are viewed as maneuvers which utilize strategies to obtain what is wanted from other people, institutions, or particular situations. Growing up in a family is viewed as primarily a matter of teaching the members how to play games successfully. Different cultures and social classes favor styles of games, and various tribes and families favor variations of these.[61]

There have been attempts to tie in the basis for a transactional approach with a sociological system of people behaving in ways which are expected because of their roles in a particular social system. When an adolescent is assigned a subservient role and then complies, a state of role complementarity has been selected and chosen. Deviations from this role lead to a reverberating series of personal anxieties and group dislocations. The dubiousness of the theory hinges on the assumption of someone choosing a role, rather than roles being a response to a complex set of factors. Forces are set in motion to restore equilibrium. Role conflicts occur in many situations: with parents, teachers, or peers, as well as in existing cultural conflicts.

The repetition of conflicted behavior is attributed to habit patterns, while others stress the inability of a person in such a situation to handle demands because of the requirement for contradictory roles which contribute to psychopathology. Attributing behaviors and conflicts to unconscious motivations is used by some transactional therapists. However, the implicit assumptions about personality development give an emphasis to interpersonal demands. Various selves evolve which reflect interactional processes with other people, or objects, as well as with the individual's body. Cognitive and perceptual structures are evolved from the cognitive and perceptual fields within which an adolescent participates. These are conceptualized as contributing to the development of systems of self-approval or disapproval.

Attention is called to the enormous debt these theories have to the theory of personality developed by Harry Stack Sullivan. His stress on the "self-system" of the parents is central. When conforming to non-verbalized roles, the "good me" is present; nonconformity to the roles elicits feelings of a "bad me" or even a non-existent self. Events which disturb established patterns of dealing with others lead to anxiety and efforts to obtain relief. This tension and the activities required for relief—security operations because they are addressed to maintaining a feeling of safety in the esteem reflected from other persons."[62] Conflicts arise between strivings which are labelled "bad," although pleasurable, as well as more esoteric aspects of "badness." When such an adolescent is seen in therapy, he has usually accepted his "badness" or self as unappealing and unacceptable. This defective self-image remains perpetually vulnerable to reflected appraisals of others for maintenance of some degree of self-esteem.

The greater the degree of constriction in personality the less capable the person is to relearn and modify his self-esteem system as well as alter his interpersonal relations. Therapy is viewed as an opportunity for the therapist to participate with the adolescent in a joint effort at resolution of presuppositions, perceptual distortions, and parataxic distortions which handicap them. In the process of dealing with thoughts, feelings, and behavior, the distortions are recognized and dealt with. Under no conditions does the therapist accept the distorted reality to which the adolescent has repeatedly been exposed and had reinforced as supposedly representing an objective reality.

Goals of altered self-awareness and self-appraisal are pursued. Sensitivity to affects is crucial so that painful areas can be explored together. The affect may be verbalized to the adolescent initially in terms of the security operations which he has to continue his existence without a catastrophe. Past patterns are utilized when interpreting the distortions. This permits the patient the freedom to initiate and experiment with different patterns interpersonally as well as with respect to self-esteem maneuvers. Such changes in an adolescent inevitably lead to family discomfort, contrary to the requests at the beginning of therapy. What the parents have in mind is something quite different from what is required. This is a therapeutic position which advocates that conflicted areas in an adolescent take precedence over the needs of adults who are dedicated to maintaining the status quo or reverting to patterns which they have long considered normal. This often leads to the necessity for collaborative, or conjoint, efforts to treat other members of the family. These demands on a family may lead to therapist shopping in an effort to find a therapist with a different orientation to the situation or one who will pursue more superficial practices which do not threaten the existing structure.

In particular, the interpersonal approach is useful with the acting out individual who is responding to superego lacunae in a parent. Such parents are burdened with their own unconscious and unresolved acting out wishes. These are conveyed to offspring who

are thus unwittingly duped.[63] Parental influences affect the ego
development of the child in terms of internalizing and adapting to
these unexpressed, yet powerfully effective, sanctions to carry out
forbidden behaviors or not to carry out certain desired behaviors.
Without parental involvement the behavior is likely to lose its
driving force. A contrary situation is where parental impulses
continue to exert their influence and become more overt in
adolescence despite various warnings and exhortations.

> One adolescent boy continued to fight in school, despite repeated warnings and
> expulsion. He was perceived as someone with a 'greater degree of aggression in
> his inherited make-up' than he could handle. At conferences, his father yelled
> at the boy and cursed him out, conveying an excitement in the recapitulation of
> the events. In fact, his behavior toward the boy mirrored the way his son related
> to others—by attempts to intimidate them one way or another.

Contemporary consequences of this approach have resulted in the
therapeutic process being viewed as an empirical operation between
the therapist and adolescent as a microsocial system. This may lead
to a position not to refer to other psychological events or constructs,
such as transference or countertransference. This is a translation of
operational positivism, prevalent in the physical sciences in the
1920s, to the field of human psychotherapy. Although the physical
sciences have long realized the limitations of such a restriction, it
appears to have been transposed anew to areas of psychotherapy.

Explicit and inferred roles occupy much of the substance of
therapy sessions when this model is used, and connections with past
origins are relatively or totally ignored. The therapist directly
communicates many of his reactions to the adolescent as they occur
during therapeutic interviews, as well as deliberately refusing to go
along with many of the demands the patient places on him. This
permits the therapist to deal with the feelings and defenses that
become mobilized in the course of treatment. Direct challenges are
made to some of the behavior going on, such as acting out or
attempts to control others, coupled with support when needed.

Haley emphasized the ploys of patients via symptoms while the
therapist strives to win the contest by pointing out contradictions.[64]
Thus, an adolescent presenting with problems toward authority, as
well as an intense reaction to competitive situations, is described as
attacking others as being selfish and over-aggressive. Therapeutic
maneuvers would attempt to counter this with examples of his own

aggressiveness in therapy as well as in his general life situation. Therapy is viewed as a replay of all the stratagems used for manipulating and contolling others with a successful therapeutic outcome dependent on the patient losing the game so that such attempts are subsequently abandoned.

A plethora of innovations multiply under the aegis of interactional appoaches. Some promote the open expression of sexual or aggressive fantasies as well as direct physical contact. This is reminiscent of Ferenczi's modifications with patients whom he believed had been severely traumatized during development and with whom he introduced a "nursery environment" that permitted indulgent body contact between the therapist and patient.[65] This may be done in groups, such as a group of parents, or fathers and sons, with a therapist present who openly evokes interpersonal feelings through a beginning discussion of suitable topics. The closeness to acting out in some of these treatment activities is the most disturbing element, particularly in a period such as our own, when an increasing demand for doing something about everything is matched by endless groups becoming the treaters. Experimentation with a variety of techniques blurs distinctions between treatment, social activities, acting out, and whatever happens to be passing for treatment at the moment.

WORKING-THROUGH THERAPIES

Differences from Psychotherapy and Indications. Working through therapies seek to go beyond efforts at symptom removal or environmental clarification. They seek clarification of conscious conflicts and resolution of unconscious processes which have been operating antithetically to development. Merely pointing these out to an adolescent, or any patient, has little effect. It is the psychological work through the transference and countertransference which permits change in the multitude of ways a person has been reacting and feeling. In a theoretical sense, the goal is to achieve structural change so that different adaptive techniques can be used in interaction with the environment. For the adolescent in particular, this reorganization seeks to alter developmental distortions and arrests so that ego and superego development may progress. Reconstructive work with a personality presupposes sufficient ego strength to tolerate such inquiry. It does not presuppose that the same degree of reconstruction will be effected with all patients. Rarely will significant change be possible from abreactive sessions per se, or playing through the same theme of support repetitiously in response to crises.

A long-term goal is to place the ego in a position where it can cope with accumulated conflicts or traumatic episodes. By establishing associative links, the pathogenic or repressed part of experiences or ego states is made available for alteration. If little pathogenic potential remains attached, there is a gradual wearing away effect. By putting these feelings into words and interpreting , the therapist lessens the degree of repression which allows the patient to see similarities in his behavior in different situations.

The entire nature of the transference relationship needs consideration. In any interpretive therapy there are adverse influences operating in reality which may work counter to the interpretations offered. For a young person, the therapist has an influence as a real object, in addition to the transference manifestations. Modeling and suggestive influences from the self of the therapist cannot all be subsumed as transference. Hence, the potential for a beneficial therapeutic experience when the therapist can function as an auxiliary superego, for example, when needed, or for accentuating destructive trends in an adolescent from a therapist who misinterprets or presents a destructive self model.[66]

Many of the same elements present in psychoanalyzing an adult are present in reconstructive therapy with adolescents. These are: "To analyze ego resistance before id content and to allow the work of interpretation to move freely between id and ego, following the emergence of material; to proceed from the surface to the depth; to offer the position of the analyst as a transference object for the revival and interpretation of unconscious fantasies and attitudes; to analyze impulses so far as possible in the state of frustration and to avoid their being acted out and gratified; to expect relief of tension, not from catharsis but from the material being lifted from the level of primary process functioning to secondary thought processes; in short, to turn id into ego content."[67] Manipulations are kept to a minimum since they are not regarded as conducive to resolving internalized conflict. Exceptions are made when overtly traumatic or seductive situations are present. Handling resistances, transference, and interpretation of unconscious material, are the substantive tools of therapy.

As far as possible, the aims of analytic therapy in dealing with an adolescent approximate those in any analysis:

1. To obtain as much free and spontaneous material from the patient as possible in an atmosphere conducive to this
2. To shift the balance or relationship between the id, ego, and superego
3. To promote greater tolerance in the superego, as well as for the activities of each of the mental agencies
4. To alter pathological defenses by systematically identifying and altering them
5. To produce intrapsychic modifications
6. To deal with transference reactions, resistance, and manifestations of transference neurosis
7. To use working through to integrate processes and carry out reconstruction.

A necessary question pertains to the indications for such intensive therapy with an adolescent. Since analysis originally was devised with adult transference neuroses in mind, how applicable is it even in the absence of such practical problems as time, expenses, and qualified therapists? These questions become more important when talking about developmental problems, or character disturbances. Extension of adult analysis to types of character problems and psychotic conditions led to considerations of such therapies with some delinquents—those with character deformations, and some borderline conditions.[68] Whether these therapies actually amount to psychoanalysis, or are rather a new application is debatable. A preliminary period of preparatory psychotherapy is usually needed before the adolescent and family are ready to undertake more intensive types of treatment, and the therapist should use such time to assess whether reconstructive therapy should be attempted.

As for the specific indications for analytic types of therapy, the classical neuroses such as the hysterical neuroses, anxiety neuroses, phobias, obsessional neuroses, and depressive disorders are usually listed as prime indicators.[69] Those with inhibitions in ego functions, or with marked ego restrictions, are another group whose symptomatology varies widely. These include the following:

1. Adolescents who spend a great deal of time alone, accompanied by spells of sadness.

2. Those who can perform well only in structured situations, and who react with anxiety attacks or rage if unpredictable demands are made on them (this may also be seen in those with severe nightmares accompanied by other sleep disturbances, such as sleepwalking, which are not reactive to specific eliciting situations).

3. When interest patterns become overwhelmingly centered on one activity, such as an artistic skill or a single athletic activity, to the exclusion of other interests and interpersonal experiences.

4. Cases where regressions in psycho-sexual functioning have commenced and have not merely been transient.

5. Manifest conflicts in gender identity in which persistent and conscious wishes to be of the opposite sex are expressed (questions have been raised about whether latency is already too late to accomplish more than tapering effects due to the pregenital nature of these deep-seated conflicts which can give rise to a host of perverse potentials).

6. Acting-out problems in which the behavior appears related to a strong sense of conscious or unconscious guilt, or is in the service of a need for punishment directly or by provocative inducement. Cases of kleptomania or other types of masochistic phenomena which are being handled by antisocial activity are examples.

7. When traumatic or crisis situations, such as serious medical procedures, parental death, or marital disharmony in parents evoke persistent symptomatology or ego restrictions in an adolescent. An example is a boy whose father was killed in a car accident and who feels unable to ride in cars.

Comparing some of the techniques of psychoanalytically-oriented therapies with psychoanalysis illustrates the differences between them. If the two approaches are not distinguished, the mixture that results may confuse and actually impede the treatment attempted.[70] Goals in psychotherapy usually refer to providing some relief from conflicts with others and the environment. Simply becoming aware of unconscious conflicts furthers such goals, even in the absence of a primary goal of providing insight and awareness of how unconscious conflicts operate. Techniques vary not only by way of which psychotherapeutic approach is chosen, but also in contrast to those used in the psychoanalysis of adults. Alterations in the form of the working alliance, as present with adult patients, always need consideration. Since there is no strict fulfillment of the basic rule, verbalization and behavior tend to blur with acting out. Differences in the transference situation have been noted. Nor is it solely a matter of the number of visits per week, although the frequency and type of content does vary in association with this parameter. The main differences are rather in the way the material is obtained, the type of material deemed important, and how it is used toward different goals.

Even the type of office equipment illustrates differences between general psychotherapeutic techniques versus reconstructive efforts. Consider differences in a young child which highlight the contrasting therapies. With a young child the setting may have enticing toys to stimulate a child into activity and participation. Such things as dolls, a doll house with furnishings, puppets, soldiers, animals, guns, toy dishes, clay, crayons, finger paints, drawing materials, toy cars, airplanes, and a variety of games are the usual paraphernalia. In contrast, when attempting to do analytic work a stimulating office of toys is viewed as a diversion from the child's fantasy life. Activity permits a child an opportunity to use action as a defense and to gain reassurance. If therapy takes the form of an activity project with the therapist, or game-playing, an opportunity is provided for accomplishment and self-reward from efforts and praise from others.

In contrast, in analytic work the goal is to maintain a sufficient degree of working anxiety to deal with powerful motivations and forbidden strivings. To foster such a process requires minimal interferers. Those which are present should be selected for their usefulness in promoting fantasy elaboration. Clinical judgement is needed depending on the individual patient and their age as to when a more strict confinement to verbalization to get at the inner world of play and its derivatives is desirable. Along with this transition there is a minimum of active injection from the therapist, since the goal is not to elucidate the therapist's fantasies or responsive participation to new situations as therapy progresses, but to create the maximum opportunity for the patient to expand about his life and fantasies so that these may be explored.

Permitting an adolescent to expand his derivative fantasies reveals the quality of the therapist as nothing else. The goal is the revelation of the manifestations of the inner life for clinical interpretation and modification instead of giving rewards for activity itself. Nor is it desirable immediately to allay anxiety. It is better to become aware of the thoughts and feelings that are disturbing the patient in their conscious and unconscious aspects. Environmental manipulation or persuasive exhortations are contradictory to these ends. To tolerate not only the patient's anxiety, but the anxiety from those in the environment who are demanding an endless series of "do somethings," demands a high degree of professional and personal security in the clinician. It reflects the competence and emotional security of the therapist who must tolerate the intense emotionality generated without needing to step in and act to alleviate the situation by acts or reassurances.

Such abstinence is believed necessary for the work of reconstructing parts of a personality. Reconstruction is in preference to maintenance of the status quo or seeking alleviation by externalization efforts of ascribing difficulties to the environment if they have become relatively immutable to change.

Sexual material is another area to contrast psychotherapy with reconstructive work. There is a noticeable difference in patients of all ages in the amount and type of sexual material that emerges if therapy is conducted weekly versus several sessions per week. Transference phenomena are part of the difference which promotes the need to express impulses in some direct, disguised, or symbolic manner. In non-reconstructive therapies sexual wishes and fantasies are at best dealt with on a phenomenological level, or at worst by an emphasis on the purely physical aspects of sexual techniques. By adolescence derivatives and associated fantasies are part of therapeutic material which can be used for interpretation when overt sexual themes emerge. Defenses and feelings are dealt with before direct interpretation of impulses.

The Remainder of The Family. Other family members must be involved to some extent, no matter what the type of treatment. Only in a quite theoretical manner can treatment of a juvenile— adolescent or child—proceed without some adult participation, at least to initiate treatment and allow it to continue even if they are not to receive treatment in their own right. There are many ways of dealing with parents and the remainder of the family when one minor member of a family is being seen for individual psychotherapy. Many of these are techniques relevant to treating more than one family member, such as in collaborative or conjoint approaches. If the same therapist is to see the parents separately as well as treat their child, it is often a difficult job to deal with crossed transferences and countertransferences.

Other family members may need treatment as much or more than the primary patient. Elements of competition for time can occur in subtle ways between the different members. If mixed family interviews are added, there is the problem of how to keep the material from individual sessions confidential. If it is not to be kept confidential, what is the advantage of maintaining individual sessions without the advantage of dealing with certain kinds of material which this permits? There is a pervasive feeling in excluded family members that others are being discussed in the absence of an intense relationship that would permit doubts and suspicions to be resolved. This may lead to frequent seeking of reassurances by the adolescent about the confidential relationship with the therapist.

There is also the situation of family members and others who live in the family unit wanting advice on how to handle the adolescent. This has innumerable meanings. Some requests are simply from the uninformed parent who has been accustomed to direct advice-giving by authority figures. Directive therapy encourages this. Thus, an adolescent with school phobia problems may be approached by one or more of the following manipulative techniques: changing teachers, having the parent be available near the school building, providing a homebound teacher, giving tranquilizer medication to lower the anxiety, using aversive conditioning procedures to staying home, and appealing to his desire to learn. In contrast, a reconstructive approach basically views the problem as one that has to be dealt with in terms of the personality structure of the adolescent and family members. Although at certain points in the course of treatment some use adjuncts as supplements to treatment, others (of a purist type) are against even this.

Parental involvement in reconstructive therapy has a different function than being given advice. The parent is relied on to function as part of the reality testing part of the child's ego. In particular, this is needed to help the child appraise the seriousness of certain behaviors. Making decisions which are required during the course of intensive treatment cannot always be left solely to an adolescent. To the extent that a parent is incapable of doing this, they may need some type of therapeutic intervention to help resolve their own ambivalence and conflicts. Apart from such conflicts, parents may be seen periodically. The goal of meetings is to assuage the guilt or competitiveness that is aroused in parents when one of their children becomes deeply involved with a therapist.

There is value in securing a parent who can be a helpful assistant in permitting, if not promoting, therapeutic work. Strict confidentiality is maintained, which itself is viewed as beneficial, since the adolescent becomes aware that feelings and impulses which he has regarded as most dastardly can be tolerated, while the relationship with his parents and the therapist is still maintained. In addition, the therapist becomes a general assistant to the ego development of the patient by permitting blocked or constricted areas to resume functioning. The goal is to aid the patient in resolving problems which impair the capacity to experience pleasure, to choose subject to reality testing and social functioning, and to be able to exercise greater self-control rather than feeling like helpless and ineffectual.

Basic to this achievement is the alleviation of conflicts which lead to suffering on a conscious and unconscious basis, and which are expressed via somatic, interpersonal, or personal constrictions which can all be viewed as destructive.

There is an occasional, but rare, situation when a parent needs to be informed about some material. This is customarily handled by discussing it with the patient and securing his permission. It is made clear to the adolescent that part of therapy consists of the therapist obtaining material from the mother or father which can be brought into therapy, but the confidence of the minor is respected. Again, in contrast to psychotherapy, the criterion for success is not just whether the parents, or some other source, such as a probation officer or a nurse or teacher, says that the person is behaving better. In contrast, equal or more weight is given to psychological criteria utilized within the therapeutic encounter itself. Such criteria refer to the type of material that is being produced, the undoing of repression and other defenses, emerging curiosity about their own problems and those of their family, less stereotyped responses and avoidance behavior and destructive behavior. There are also such indices as the freedom of the patient to produce fantasy-content, his or her reaction to interpretations, and the shifting nature of transference material. Therapeutic work progresses by alternations of dealing with and interpretation of defenses mixed with interpretation of the content as it reflects feelings and impulses. Additional elements used to evaluate progress of intensive therapy are the expansion of conscious content, increasing dominance of ego functioning, progressive clarity of preconscious functioning, and the capacity to form an identification with the therapist.

Very rarely is parental advice-giving considered a primary part of the contract for reconstructive work with adolescnets. There are several reasons for this. First, it is accepted that parents with neurotic offspring have many primary and secondary conflicts of their own. Telling them to get rid of their problems by doing certain things, which is the message of advice-giving, is either naive, redundant, or conducive to accentuating feelings of guilt and hopelessness. It is presumed that if the parents could have changed, they would have, from one of the many advice-giving sources they have almost always consulted beforehand. If deliberate, conscious attempts to produce conflicts in an adolescent are being acted upon by a parent, we are really dealing with a family constellation with major characterological problems. They are rarely interested in therapy beyond some manipulative reason, such as complying with a court order, or making a facsimile attempt at treatment. However, even when problems are largely in the characterological realm, they are not viewed as due to conscious efforts to harm the child, but rather due to a combination of interpersonal, historical, and unconscious mechanisms for handling conflict.

There is a further reason to avoid advice-giving: double-bind situations which result. Not only may the therapist's advice be quoted and misquoted in vain by several family members, but later when the problems are still present, the question of why the problems are still present when everyone has been following the therapist's literal prescription will be raised. All of these maneuvers and resistances must then be dealt with. So, rather than prolong therapy and avoid the pre-existing conflicts, telling the primary patient or family members what to do is usually avoided. "Surely the basic aims of psychoanalysis as a therapeutic measure, child or adult, include goals of broad change in the patient's character structure with particular emphasis upon extension of the sovereignty of the ego and the ultimate heightening of the individual's psychic integration. Clearly, the basic role of the analyst is that of objectivity and his most important activity that of interpretation, not censoring, gratifying, supporting, or educating."[71]

TERMINATION OF TREATMENT

A good deal has been written about the beginning and end of therapy. The customary things mentioned in texts, such as giving adequate notice of termination, working through transference, and separation phenomena, are well-known. There are a few pointers appropriate to terminating with adolescent patients. Two extremes are often encountered: Either therapy ends after a brief period, or it goes on endlessly in some type of protracted dependency relationship. In these closing comments only a few issues are raised about the special difficulties in handling termination. How to deal with the narcissism and separation anxieties of these patients presents the greatest of difficulties. On one hand, there are ambivalent strivings for emancipation from childhood ties; hence, termination of therapy resurrects this element. However, it is not only a recapitulation but part of reality since therapy is ending. Second, the need to come to terms with limits on grandiosity is an experience in itself. This shows up in many ways indicating lack of resolution at termination.

If therapeutic work has taken place, we are aware of the dynamic balance present between the therapist and adolescent patient. What is said and done can be interpreted and reacted to in many ways. Fantasies and cognitive distortions continue to operate. The needs for continuing the relationship, and retaining idealized parts of it, are best appreciated when adult patients are seen years after they were in treatment as adolescents. Manifestations of unresolved transference phenomena are reflected in grossly unrealistic statements made about their therapists from that earlier time. Quotes (or misquotes) from that therapy have been kept alive in their thoughts, and have influenced their choices on important matters such as marital partners and careers. How they have interpreted their therapist's comments or behavior contributed to their choices.

In some cases outcomes have had a painful and tragic overtone. It brings home the point that therapy is not necessarily a harmless tool which either improves a patient or retains status quo. In some cases the old idealizations have given way in adulthood, and the patient is then struggling with feelings of having been betrayed and that he has ruined his life because of decisions made on some false preimse. Bad life experiences make the need greater in adulthood. Not only mistrust and devaluation need to be dealt with before termination, but the anger for being in the predicament where separation must take place. Sadness about separation exists alongside feelings of wanting to continue the therapeutic relationship without parting and without sharing. In turn, greedy possessiveness gives rise to anxiety. To a great extent the work done in these areas over loss will determine whether the feeling of well-being from treatment and its realistic accomplishments will be carried over into the remainder of adolescence and adulthood.

In particular, adolescents with character problems who resort to acting out defenses reflect their narcissistic conflicts. The therapist has been incorporated as part of the narcissistic core, which means that the therapist is perceived as serving needs for greatness, power, ambition, and domination. During the course of treatment grandiose strivings for perfection and power should have been worked on. Failures in being perfect according to the individual ego-ideal system are often manifested in ongoing patterns of delinquent behavior reflecting disillusionment. Mixed with this is the use and manipulation of others based on grandiose needs. Observers describe this in terms of the self-centeredness of adolescents and how they tend to use people.

While these themes should have come up long before the time for termination arrives, the fact of termination raises them anew. It is a situation which an adolescent cannot control, and hence it is in direct conflict with grandiose needs to control the time and place of separating. The termination may be experienced as another traumatic situation imposed on a helpless victim, which is a situation they wish to avoid at all costs. A regression into acting out behaviors, provocative mood instabilities, or episodic psychotic states, can result. These are partial responses to the loss of the therapist as a narcissistic object.

In many ways the psychology of termination can be conceptualized as a variety of the psychology of disappointment. By adolescence, as part of normal development, several stages of losses have been experienced sequentially, as well as whatever individualized losses have transpired. In a perfect world, these preceding losses would have occurred: (1) at the time best for mastery; (2) with the right degree of intensity, and (3) with the proper distancing (not too much or too little) allowed so as to promote growth without undue pain.

However, in adolescents with characterological disturbances, it is in these exact areas that conflicts remain. If treatment has been reasonably successful, the anxiety and pain associated with going one's own way can be tolerated without promoting severe regressions into acting out behavior. Out of this comes the realization that one is not going to be destroyed by the cessation of an attachment, and that one actually may even grow with a greater sense of adequacy. When that happens, we have signs for a successful termination.

In contrast, prominent needs to control and manipulate others indicate that the degree of unbridled narcissism is still quite high. Repetitious patterns of needing to hurt and provoke the self and others will continue if therapy ends prematurely. A parallel assessment takes place on the level of being able to assess assets and liabilities realistically, and then to act on that basis. A boy who applies to a university with one of the most difficult entrance requirements, whose grades are only average, and who, on failing admission, decides not to go to college, has not yet done this; a girl who fails to make the cheerleading team in her high school and then deteriorates into a life of drugs and truancy has not yet mastered her narcissistic conflicts. A boy who has accepted the limitations of his size in terms of not making a school football team, but who then becomes a good performer on the track team has accepted reality without regressing into a pattern of self-defeat. A girl, at the top of her high school class and lauded by most of her teachers, became depressed from her anonymity and average grade performance in a

competitive college situation. In the course of her therapy, she
learned to achieve what was possible for her and also to enjoy other
things in life for the first time. If such a goal is not attainable, what
is therapy and life all about?

REFERENCES

1. *Psychopathological Disorders in Childhood: Theoretical Considerations and a
   Proposed Classification,* Group for the Advancement of Psychiatry, vol. 6, no. 62,
   June 1966.
2. A. Freud, *Normality and Pathology in Childhood,* pp. 58-61 (New York:
   International Universities Press, 1965).
3. M. S. Mahler, On the current status of the infantile neurosis, *Journal of the
   American Psychoanalytic Association* 23(1975): 327-333.
4. A. Aichhorn, *Wayward Youth* (New York: The Viking Press, 1935).
5. K. B. Eissler, Ego-psychological implications of the psychoanalytic treatment of
   delinquents, *The Psychoanalytic Study of the Child* 5(1950):97-121.
6. A. Alpert, Reversibility of pathological fixations associated with maternal
   deprivation in infancy, *The Psychoanalytic Study of the Child* 14(1959):169-185.
7. R. M. Rosenberg and B. C. Mueller, Preschool antisocial children: psychodynamic
   considerations and implications for treatment, *Journal of the American
   Academy of Child Psychiatry* 7(1968):421-441.
8. E. J. Anthony, Developments in child psychotherapy, 6th International Congress
   of Psychotherapy, *Psychotherapy and Psychosomatics* 13(1965):15-28.
9. S. Freud, The interpretation of dreams, *Standard Edition,* p. 485.
10. E. J. Anthony, ed., *The Child in His Family: Children at Psychiatric Risk* (New
    York: John Wiley and Sons, 1974).
11. P. Shaffer, *Equus and Shrivings* (New York: Atheneum, 1975).
12. M.L. Smith and G.V. Glass, Meta-Analysis of Psychotherapy Outcome Studies,
    American Psychologist 32(1977):752-761.
13. J. Taft, *The Dynamics of Therapy in a Controlled Relationship* (New York:
    Macmillan Co., 1933).
14. F. H. Allen, *Psychotherapy with Children,* p. 47 (New York: W. W. Norton and
    Co., 1942).
15. T. Jacobs and J. Jacobs, Hypnotizability of children as related to hemispheric
    references and neurological organization, *American Journal of Clinical Hypno-
    sis* 8(1966):269-274.
16. M. Kaffman, Hypnosis as an adjunct to psychotherapy in child psychiatry,
    Archives of General Psychiatry 18(1968):725-728.
17. D. Levy, Attitude therapy, *American Journal of Orthopsychiatry* 7(1937):103-113.
18. A. Ellis, *Reason and Emotion in Psychotherapy* (New York: Lyle Stuart, 1962).
19. W. Glasser, *Reality Therapy: A New Approach to Psychiatry* (New York: Harper,
    1965).

20. T. Szasz, Psychiatry, ethics, and the criminal law, *Columbia Law Review* 58(1958):183.

21. R. Schwitzgebel, *Streetcorner Research* (Cambridge: Harvard University Press, 1964).

22. D. Levy, Release therapy, *American Journal of Orthopsychiatry* 9(1939):713-736.

23. L. Bender and A. G. Woltmann, The use of puppet shows as a psychotherapeutic method for behavior problems in children, *American Journal of Orthopsychiatry* 6(1936):341-354.

24. S. Millar, *The Psychology of Play* (Baltimore: Penguin Books, 1968).

25. H. Hug-Hellmuth, *Aus dem Seelenleben des Kindes* (Leipzig: Deutriche, 1913).

26. M. Klein, The psychoanalytic play-technique, *American Journal of Orthopsychiatry* 25(1955):223-237.

27. V. M. Axline, *Play Therapy*, p. 75 (Boston: Houghton Mifflin, 1947).

28. S. Freud, Beyond the pleasure principle, *Standard Edition*, pp. 14-15.

29. E. Simmel, The doctor game, *International Journal of Psychoanalysis* 7(1926):470-483.

30. A. Freud, op. cit., p. 80.

31. E. H. Erikson, *Childhood and Society*, 2nd ed., p. 219 (New York: W. W. Norton, 1963).

32. Ibid., pp. 221-222.

33. M. C. Jones, The elimination of children's fears, *Journal of Experimental Psychology* 7(1924):382-930.

34. O. H. Mowrer, A stimulus-response analysis of anxiety and its role as a reinforcing agent, *Psychological Review* 46(1939):553-565.

35. O. H. Mowrer and W. M. Mowrer, Enuresis—a method for its study and treatment, *American Journal of Orthopsychiatry* 8(1938):436-457.

36. O. H. Mowrer, Payment or repayment, *American Psychologist* 18(1963);557-580.

37. T. Dollard and N. Miller, *Personality and Psychotherapy* (New York: McGraw-Hill, 1950).

38. S. Rachman and J. Teasdale, *Aversion Therapy and Behaviur Disorders* (Coral Gables: University of Miami Press, 1969).

39. E. L. Thorndike, *Educational Psychology*, vol. 2, *The Psychology of Learning* (New York: Columbia University Press, 1913).

40. S. T. Thorndike, Reward and punishment in animal learning, *Comparative Psychology Monographs,* vol. 8, no. 39, 1932.

41. R. M. Church, The varied effects of punishment on behavior, *Psychological Review* 70(1963):369-402.

42. N. H. Azrin and W. C. Holz, *Punishment in Operant Behavior: Areas of Research and Application*, ed. by W. K. Honig (New York: Appleton-Century-Crofts, 1906).

43. J. M. Grossberg, Behavior therapy: a review, *Psychological Bulletin* 62(1964):73-88.

44. F. E. Thorne, Directive psychotherapy: VII, Imparting psychological information, *Journal of Clinical Psychology* 2(1946):179-190.

45. A. Salter, *Conditioned Reflex Therapy* (New York: Creative Age Press, 1949).

46. J. Wolpe, *Psychotherapy by Reciprocal Inhibition* (Stanford: Stanford University Press, 1958).

47. A. A. Lazurus, G. C. Davison and D. A. Polefka, Classical and operant factors in the treatment of a school phobia, *Journal of Abnormal Psychology* 70(1965):225-230.

48. D. M. Baer, F. R. Hoines, and M. M. Wolf, Control of nursery school children's behavior by programming social reinforcement from their teachers, (presented at the American Psychological Association, August, 1963).

49. M. Wolf, T. Risley and H. Mees, Application of operant conditioning procedures to the behavior problems of an autistic child, *Behaviour Research Therapy* 1(1964):305-312

50. G. R. Patterson, An application of conditioning techniques to the control of a hyperactive child, *Case Studies in Behavior Modification*, ed. L. P. Ullman and L. Krasner, pp. 370-375 (New York: Holt, Rinehart and Winston, 1965).

51. J. D. Burchard and V. O. Tyler, The modification of delinquent behavior through operant conditioning, *Behaviour Research and Therapy* 2(1965):245-250.

52. E. Wolf, Learning theory and psychoanalysis, *International Journal of Psychiatry* 7(1969):525-535.

53. J. Wolpe and A. A. Lazurus, *Behavior Therapy Techniques* (Oxford: Pergamon Press, 1966).

54. B. S. Brown, L. A. Wienckowski and S. B. Stolz, *Behavior Modification: Perspective on a Current Issue* (Washington, D.C.: Department of Health, Education and Welfare, 1975).

55. F. Deutsch, The associative anamnesis, *Psychoanalytic Quarterly* 8(1939):354-381.

56. F. Alexander, Psychoanalytic contributions to short-term psychotherapy, *Short-Term Psychotherapy*, ed. L. R. Wolberg, (New York: Grune and Stratton, 1965), pp. 84-126.

57. S. Rado, Adaptational psychodynamics: a basic science, *Psychoanalysis of Behavior—Collected Papers*, (New York: Grune and Stratton, 1956), pp. 332-346.

58. G. Goldman, Reparative psychotherapy, *Changing Concepts of Psychoanalytic Medicine*, (New York: Grune and Stratton, 1956),pp. 101-113.

59. K. Dabrowski, The theory of positive disintegration, *International Journal of Psychiatry* 2(1966):237.

60. R. Grinker, A transactional model for psychotherapy, *Contemporary Psychotheories*, ed. M. Stein, (New York: The Free Press, 1960), pp. 190-213.

61. E. Berne, *Games People Play*, (New York: Grove Press, 1964), p. 171.

62. H. S. Sullivan, *The Interpersonal Theory of Psychiatry*, (New York: W. W. Norton, 1953), p. 373.

63. A. M. Johnson and S. A. Szurek, The genesis of antisocial acting out in children and adults, *Psychoanalytic Quarterly* 21(1952):323-343.

64. J. Haley, *Strategies of Psychotherapy* (New York: Grune and Stratton, 1963).

65. S. Ferenczi, Child analysis in the analysis of adults, *International Journal of Psychoanalysis* 12 (1931):468-475.

66. J. Strachey, The nature of the therapeutic action of psycho-analysis, *International Journal of Psychoanalysis* 15(1934):127-159.

67. A. Freud, op. cit., p. 26.

68. O. Kernberg, *Borderline Conditions and Pathological Narcissm* (New York: Jason Aronson, 1975).

69. G. H. J. Pearson, ed., *A Handbook of Child Psychoanalysis* (New York: Basic Books, 1968).

70. H. Arthur, A comparison of the techniques employed in psychotherapy and psychoanalysis of children, *American Journal of Orthopsychiatry* 22(1952)484-498.

71. S. M. Finch and A. C. Cain, Psychoanalysis of children: problems of etiology and treatment, *Modern Psychoanalysis—New Directions and Perspectives*, ed. J. Marmor (New York: Basic Books, 1968).

Index